FROM DATA TO ACTION

CDC's Public Health Surveillance for Women, Infants, and Children

Editors:

Lynne S. Wilcox   James S. Marks

Contributing editors:

José E. Becerra   John L. Kiely

José F. Cordero   Donna F. Stroup

Technical editor: Valerie R. Johnson

Production editor: R. Elliott Churchill

Copy editor: Mescal J. Knighton

Editorial assistant: Patricia S. Huckaby

1994

U.S. DEPARTMENT OF HEALTH & HUMAN SERVICES
Public Health Service
Centers for Disease Control and Prevention

This monograph is the first comprehensive description of the Centers for Disease Control's (CDC) many surveillance and data system activities related to the health of women and children. It illustrates a number of critical public health concerns, spanning the life cycle from infancy to reproductive-age women:

Public health professionals need information on the complexity of health issues among women and children and the interactions of those concerns. A woman at risk for unintended pregnancy is likely to also be at risk for sexually transmitted diseases, including HIV infection. A pregnant woman who begins prenatal care late is at greater risk for pregnancy morbidity and mortality, preterm birth, and early death of her infant. Her child is at risk for inadequate vaccination coverage, poor nutrition, and higher injury rates. When examining data on specific health issues, we must remember the many aspects of the big picture for this population.

Accurate and timely data are important, even essential, for health planning. CDC's current systems can be useful in such planning, but as the commentaries from our colleagues outside CDC note, current reporting systems may be incomplete. A greater investment in data collection and analysis is needed to permit rapid application to public health programs.

A clear potential exists for preventing and reducing many of the most serious health problems of this population. Early and effective access to family planning, prenatal care, and nutrition services are an important part of the solution to unintended pregnancy, sexually transmitted diseases, pregnancy morbidity, and early infant deaths. Effective education and motivation toward healthful behavior can affect intrauterine growth retardation, fetal alcohol syndrome, vaccine-preventable diseases, and injuries among children and adolescents. Assessing the effectiveness of such prevention activities will also require skilled collection and use of data.

This monograph also highlights the interactions and collaboration though-out the public health system to address women and children's health. Many programs across CDC offer useful information for this population. CDC professionals, state and local health officials, and representatives from non-governmental agencies, such as the March of Dimes Foundation, need to communicate regularly with one another to understand the useful collection and application of these and other data.

We are all committed to improving the health of women and children, and we must continue to be vigilant in health surveillance. We hope this book will be useful to our partners in the field of women and children's health.

David Satcher, M.D., Ph.D.
Director, Centers for Disease Control and Prevention

A hundred years ago in the United States, one child in four died before reaching 5 years of age, and the average family lost at least one child, usually to fatal infectious disease. Bearing children was a dangerous enterprise for women as well; maternal mortality was one of the most common causes of death among women aged 15–44 years.

However, since the beginning of the 20th century, our ability to protect the health of reproductive-age women and their children has vastly improved. Maternal deaths are rare events, and most parents can expect every child born to live to adulthood. Yet there are still special health risks for women, children, and adolescents in the United States:

> 22% of pregnant women are hospitalized for complications of pregnancy before delivery, requiring over 2 million hospital days per year
>
> 62,400 women per year are rehospitalized during the postpartum period
>
> 300 to 500 women per year die of pregnancy-related conditions
>
> Over one third of all live births are from unintended pregnancies; among teenagers, over 85% of live births are from unintended pregnancies
>
> Over 500,000 live births occur each year to teen mothers 15–19 years of age
>
> Over 38,000 infants die each year; 25,000 of these infants die in the first 28 days of life
>
> 11% of infants per year are born preterm, and 7% are born with low birth weight
>
> At least 25% of 2-year-old children are not fully vaccinated against childhood diseases
>
> Among children under 2 years of age from low-income families, approximately one child in five has iron deficiency anemia
>
> Over 4,000 children under 10 years of age die each year from unintentional injuries—the leading cause of death in this age-group
>
> Among children and adolescents aged 10–19 years, over 9,000 deaths from unintentional injury and 5,000 deaths from violence occur each year

These risks may be doubled or tripled among disadvantaged populations, such as poor and minority women and children.

Public health practitioners see these numbers as a call for more action to improve the health of women and children. Additional numbers suggest which actions may be most effective. These numbers describe opportunities for health-related prevention programs:

> 35% of women did not use a contraceptive method with their first sexual intercourse, and 7% of women at risk of unintended pregnancy do not use contraception

> 24% of live births are to women who did not receive early prenatal care

> Approximately 20% of live births are to women who smoked during pregnancy; this percentage is more than doubled for live births to women with <12 years of education

> Among high school students, 13% are frequent smokers, 28% are occasional smokers, 31% report episodic heavy alcohol consumption, and 18% of sexually active students do not use contraception

Now, more than ever before in our history, knowledge is power—the power to reach disadvantaged populations, to educate the general public, to legislate effective health laws, and to provide quality health services. As we look into the 21st century, we see rapidly improving technology for collecting, examining, and acting upon data. The "information highway" can serve the public's health as well as its commercial interests. Health-care reform, regardless of its design, will succeed in improving the lives of women and children only with careful attention by the public health community to trends in the application of effective interventions and concomitant improvement in health outcomes. These data will be critical to determining whether available resources are being effectively applied.

This monograph provides an overview of public health surveillance and data programs at the Centers for Disease Control and Prevention that provide information on women and children's health. It offers health practitioners and planners at the local, state, and national levels a better appreciation of the uses and limitations of such data and enables us to think more clearly about future concerns for monitoring health. As a mother notes later in this book, in a few years today's babies will be directing affairs. Let us hope that they will be able to say that we made the most of what we knew.

M. Joycelyn Elders, M.D.
Surgeon General

Table of Contents

**From Data to Action: CDC's Public Health Surveillance
for Women, Infants, and Children**

CDC Maternal and Child Health Monograph

Acknowledgments

This monograph is the product of the collaborative efforts of many persons at the Centers for Disease Control and Prevention. In addition, review and commentary from constituents and colleagues outside CDC enhanced the quality of this report.

Senior editors	Lynne S. Wilcox, M.D., M.P.H., Division of Reproductive Health, National Center for Chronic Disease Prevention and Health Promotion, CDC
	James S. Marks, M.D., M.P.H., Division of Reproductive Health, National Center for Chronic Disease Prevention and Health Promotion, CDC
Contributing editors	José E. Becerra, M.D., M.P.H., Division of Reproductive Health, National Center for Chronic Disease Prevention and Health Promotion, CDC
	José F. Cordero, M.D., M.P.H., Division of Birth Defects and Developmental Disabilities, National Center for Environmental Health, CDC
	John L. Kiely, Ph.D., Division of Health and Utilization Analysis, National Center for Health Statistics, CDC
	Donna F. Stroup, Ph.D., M.Sc., Division of Surveillance and Epidemiology, Epidemiology Program Office, CDC
Technical editor	Valerie R. Johnson, A.B.J., Office of the Director, National Center for Chronic Disease Prevention and Health Promotion, CDC
Production editor	R. Elliott Churchill, M.A., Office of the Director, Epidemiology Program Office, CDC
Copy editor	Mescal J. Knighton, Office of the Director, National Center for Chronic Disease Prevention and Health Promotion, CDC
Editorial assistant	Patricia S. Huckaby, A.A., Division of Reproductive Health, National Center for Chronic Disease Prevention and Health Promotion, CDC
Graphics conversion and standardization	William E. Pamplin, III, B.S., M.A., Corporate Graphics and Publishing

Contributing authors

Melissa M. Adams, M.P.H., Ph.D., Division of Reproductive Health, National Center for Chronic Disease Prevention and Health Promotion, CDC

Hani K. Atrash, M.D., M.P.H., Division of Reproductive Health, National Center for Chronic Disease Prevention and Health Promotion, CDC

Cheryl A. Blackmore, Ph.D., M.P.H., M.S.N., Division of Reproductive Health, National Center for Chronic Disease Prevention and Health Promotion, CDC

Coleen A. Boyle, Ph.D., Division of Birth Defects and Developmental Disabilities, National Center for Environmental Health, CDC

Christine M. Branche-Dorsey, Ph.D., M.S.P.H., Division of Unintentional Injury Prevention, National Center for Injury Prevention and Control, CDC

Kate M. Brett, Ph.D., Division of Epidemiology, National Center for Health Statistics, CDC

Carol Bruce, B.S.N., M.P.H., Division of Reproductive Health, National Center for Chronic Disease Prevention and Health Promotion, CDC

Anjani Chandra, Ph.D., Division of Vital Statistics, National Center for Health Statistics, CDC

Linda D. Clark, M.P.H., R.D., Division of Nutrition, National Center for Chronic Disease Prevention and Health Promotion, CDC

Janet L. Collins, Ph.D., Division of Adolescent and School Health, National Center for Chronic Disease Prevention and Health Promotion, CDC

Margarett K. Davis, M.D., M.P.H., Division of Birth Defects and Developmental Disabilities, National Center for Environmental Health, CDC

Michelle S. Davis, M.S.P.H., Division of Vital Statistics, National Center for Health Statistics, CDC

Pierre Decouflé, Sc.D., Division of Birth Defects and Developmental Disabilities, National Center for Environmental Health, CDC

Nancy S. Doernberg, B.A., Division of Birth Defects and Developmental Disabilities, National Center for Environmental Health, CDC

Larry D. Edmonds, M.S.P.H., Division of Birth Defects and Developmental Disabilities, National Center for Environmental Health, CDC

Tedd V. Ellerbrock, M.D., Division of HIV/AIDS, National Center for Infectious Diseases, CDC

J. David Erickson, D.D.S., Ph.D., Division of Birth Defects and Developmental Disabilities, National Center for Environmental Health, CDC

Patricia L. Fleming, Ph.D., M.S., Division of HIV/AIDS, National Center for Infectious Diseases, CDC

R. Louise Floyd, R.N., D.S.N., Division of Birth Defects and Developmental Disabilities, National Center for Environmental Health, CDC

Robert G. Froehlke, M.D., Department of Pediatrics, Michigan State University

Paula G. Gardner, M.P.H., Division of Vital Statistics, National Center for Health Statistics, CDC

James A. Gaudino, Jr., M.D., M.S., M.P.H., Division of Reproductive Health, National Center for Chronic Disease Prevention and Health Promotion, CDC

Julie A. Gazmararian, Ph.D., M.P.H., Division of Reproductive Health, National Center for Chronic Disease Prevention and Health Promotion, CDC

Mary M. Goodwin, M.A., M.P.A., Division of Reproductive Health, National Center for Chronic Disease Prevention and Health Promotion, CDC

Rachel J. Gorwitz, M.P.H., Division of Sexually Transmitted Diseases and HIV Prevention, National Center for Prevention Services, CDC

Philip L. Graitcer, D.M.D., M.P.H., Office of the Director, National Center for Injury Prevention and Control, CDC

Arlene I. Greenspan, P.T., M.P.H., Dr.P.H., Division of Acute Care, Rehabilitation Research, and Disability Prevention, National Center for Injury Prevention and Control, CDC

Joel R. Greenspan, M.D., M.P.H., Division of Sexually Transmitted Diseases and HIV Prevention, National Center for Prevention Services, CDC

Eileen P. Gunter, R.N., M.P.H., Division of Reproductive Health, National Center for Chronic Disease Prevention and Health Promotion, CDC

Marta Gwinn, M.D., M.P.H., Division of HIV/AIDS, National Center for Infectious Diseases, CDC

Donna L. Hoyert, Ph.D., Division of Vital Statistics, National Center for Health Statistics, CDC

Daniel Hungerford, Dr.P.H., Division of Birth Defects and Developmental Disabilities, National Center for Environmental Health, CDC

Karen J. Hymbaugh, M.P.A., Division of Birth Defects and Developmental Disabilities, National Center for Environmental Health, CDC

Solomon Iyasu, M.B.B.S., M.P.H., Division of Reproductive Health, National Center for Chronic Disease Prevention and Health Promotion, CDC

Levy M. James, M.S., Division of Birth Defects and Developmental Disabilities, National Center for Environmental Health, CDC

Christopher Johnson, M.S.P.H., Division of Reproductive Health, National Center for Chronic Disease Prevention and Health Promotion, CDC

Laura Kann, Ph.D., Division of Adolescent and School Health, National Center for Chronic Disease Prevention and Health Promotion, CDC

John L. Kiely, Ph.D., Division of Health and Utilization Analysis, National Center for Health Statistics, CDC

Michael D. Kogan, Ph.D., M.A., Division of Vital Statistics, National Center for Health Statistics, CDC

Lloyd J. Kolbe, Ph.D., Division of Adolescent and School Health, National Center for Chronic Disease Prevention and Health Promotion, CDC

Lisa M. Koonin, M.N., M.P.H., Division of Reproductive Health, National Center for Chronic Disease Prevention and Health Promotion, CDC

Herschel W. Lawson, M.D., Division of Cancer Prevention and Control, National Center for Chronic Disease Prevention and Health Promotion, CDC

Jennifer J. Luallen, M.D., Division of Unintentional Injury Prevention, National Center for Injury Prevention and Control, CDC

Michele C. Lynberg, Ph.D., M.P.H., Division of Birth Defects and Developmental Disabilities, National Center for Environmental Health, CDC

Marian F. MacDorman, Ph.D., Division of Vital Statistics, National Center for Health Statistics, CDC

James S. Marks, M.D., M.P.H., Division of Reproductive Health, National Center for Chronic Disease Prevention and Health Promotion, CDC

M. Louise Martin, D.V.M., Division of Birth Defects and Developmental Disabilities, National Center for Environmental Health, CDC

Philip W. McClain, M.S., Division of Acute Care, Rehabilitation Research, and Disability Prevention, National Center for Injury Prevention and Control, CDC

Anne B. McClearn, B.A., Division of Birth Defects and Developmental Disabilities, National Center for Environmental Health, CDC

William D. Mosher, Ph.D., Division of Vital Statistics, National Center for Health Statistics, CDC

Allyn K. Nakashima, M.D., Division of Sexually Transmitted Diseases and HIV Prevention, National Center for Prevention Services, CDC

Ibrahim Parvanta, M.S., Division of Nutrition, National Center for Chronic Disease Prevention and Health Promotion, CDC

Geraldine S. Perry, Dr.P.H., R.D., Division of Nutrition, National Center for Chronic Disease Prevention and Health Promotion, CDC

Carol A. Pertowski, M.D., Division of Environmental Hazards and Health Effects, National Center for Environmental Health, CDC

Linda J. Piccinino, M.P.S., Division of Vital Statistics, National Center for Health Statistics, CDC

Jacquelyn A. Polder, B.S.N., M.P.H., Hospital Infections Program, National Center for Infectious Diseases, CDC

Juan G. Rodriguez, M.D., M.P.H. (deceased), formerly with the Division of Unintentional Injury Prevention, National Center for Injury Prevention and Control, CDC

Diane L. Rowley, M.D., M.P.H., Division of Reproductive Health, National Center for Chronic Disease Prevention and Health Promotion, CDC

Julie C. Russell, Ph.D., Division of Unintentional Injury Prevention, National Center for Injury Prevention and Control, CDC

Audrey F. Saftlas, Ph.D., M.P.H., formerly with the Division of Reproductive Health, National Center for Chronic Disease Prevention and Health Promotion, CDC, now with Yale University

Anne Schuchat, M.D., Division of Bacterial and Mycotic Diseases, National Center for Infectious Diseases, CDC

Bettylou Sherry, Ph.D., R.D., Division of Nutrition, National Center for Chronic Disease Prevention and Health Promotion, CDC

Jack C. Smith, M.S., Division of Reproductive Health, National Center for Chronic Disease Prevention and Health Promotion, CDC

Suzanne M. Smith, M.D., M.P.H., Division of Unintentional Injury Prevention, National Center for Injury Prevention and Control, CDC

Joseph E. Sniezek, M.D., M.P.H., Division of Acute Care, Rehabilitation Research, and Disability Prevention, National Center for Injury Prevention and Control, CDC

Alison M. Spitz, M.S., M.P.H., Division of Reproductive Health, National Center for Chronic Disease Prevention and Health Promotion, CDC

Paul A. Stehr-Green, Dr.P.H., M.P.H., National Immunization Program, CDC

Peter M. Strebel, M.B.Ch.B., M.P.H., National Immunization Program, CDC

David Thurman, M.D., M.P.H., Division of Acute Care, Rehabilitation Research, and Disability Prevention, National Center for Injury Prevention and Control, CDC

Stephanie J. Ventura, A.M., Division of Vital Statistics, National Center for Health Statistics, CDC

Charles W. Warren, Ph.D., Division of Adolescent and School Health, National Center for Chronic Disease Prevention and Health Promotion, CDC

Melinda Wharton, M.D., M.P.H., National Immunization Program, CDC

Linda A. Webster, Ph.D., Division of Sexually Transmitted Diseases and HIV Prevention, National Center for Prevention Services, CDC

Lynne S. Wilcox, M.D., M.P.H., Division of Reproductive Health, National Center for Chronic Disease Prevention and Health Promotion, CDC

Jacqueline B. Wilson, M.P.H., Division of Vital Statistics, National Center for Health Statistics, CDC

Marshalyn Yeargin-Allsopp, M.D., Division of Birth Defects and Developmental Disabilities, National Center for Environmental Health, CDC

Ray Yip, M.D., M.P.H., Division of Nutrition, National Center for Chronic Disease Prevention and Health Promotion, CDC

Stella Yu, Sc.D., M.P.H., R.D., Division of Vital Statistics, National Center for Health Statistics, CDC

S. Christine Zahniser, B.S.N., M.P.H., Division of Cancer Prevention and Control, National Center for Chronic Disease Prevention and Health Promotion, CDC

Colette L. Zyrkowski, M.P.H., R.D., Division of Nutrition, National Center for Chronic Disease Prevention and Health Promotion, CDC

Commentary authors from outside CDC

Sara Reed DePersio, M.D., M.P.H.,Deputy Commissioner, Personal Health Services, Oklahoma State Department of Health, Oklahoma City, Oklahoma

William H. Hollinshead, M.D., M.P.H., Medical Director, Division of Family Health, Rhode Island Department of Health, Providence, Rhode Island

Kay A. Johnson, M.P.H., M.Ed., Director, Policy and Government Affairs, March of Dimes Birth Defects Foundation, Washington, D.C.

Samuel S. Kessel, M.D., M.P.H., Director, Division of Systems, Education, and Science, Maternal and Child Health Bureau, Health Resources and Services Administration, Rockville, Maryland

Audrey H. Nora, M.D., M.P.H., Director, Maternal and Child Health Bureau, Health Resources and Services Administration, Rockville, Maryland

Magda G. Peck, Sc.D., Executive Director, CityMatCH, Chief, Section on Child Health Policy, Assistant Professor, Pediatrics, University of Nebraska Medical Center, Omaha, Nebraska

Deborah Klein Walker, Ed.D., Assistant Commissioner, Bureau of Family and Community Health, Massachusetts Department of Public Health, Boston, Massachusetts

Reviewers from outside CDC who evaluated draft versions of the monograph

Sara Reed DePersio, M.D., M.P.H., Deputy Commissioner, Personal Health Services, Oklahoma State Department of Health, Oklahoma City, Oklahoma

Edward P. Ehlinger, M.D., M.S.P.H., Director, Personal Health Services, Public Health Center, Department of Health and Family Support, Minneapolis, Minnesota

William H. Hollinshead, M.D., M.P.H., Medical Director, Division of Family Health, Rhode Island Department of Health, Providence, Rhode Island

Kay A. Johnson, M.P.H., M.Ed., Director, Policy and Government Affairs, March of Dimes Birth Defects Foundation, Washington, D.C.

Samuel S. Kessel, M.D., M.P.H., Director, Division of Systems, Education, and Science, Maternal and Child Health Bureau, Health Resources and Services Administration, Rockville, Maryland

Patricia K. Nicol, M.D., M.P.H., Director, Division of Maternal and Child Health, Department for Health Services, Cabinet for Human Resources, Commonwealth of Kentucky, Frankfort, Kentucky

Audrey H. Nora, M.D., M.P.H., Director, Maternal and Child Health Bureau, Health Resources and Services Administration, Rockville, Maryland

Magda G. Peck, Sc.D., Executive Director, CityMatCH, Chief, Section on Child Health Policy, Assistant Professor, Pediatrics, University of Nebraska Medical Center, Omaha, Nebraska

Donna J. Petersen, M.H.S., Sc.D., Director, Maternal and Child Health Division, Minnesota Department of Health, Minneapolis, Minnesota

Roger Taillefer, M.Ed., Assistant Director, Office of Family and Community Health, Division of Public Health Services, Department of Health and Human Services, State of New Hampshire, Concord, New Hampshire

Deborah Klein Walker, Ed.D., Assistant Commissioner, Bureau of Family and Community Health, Massachusetts Department of Public Health, Boston, Massachusetts

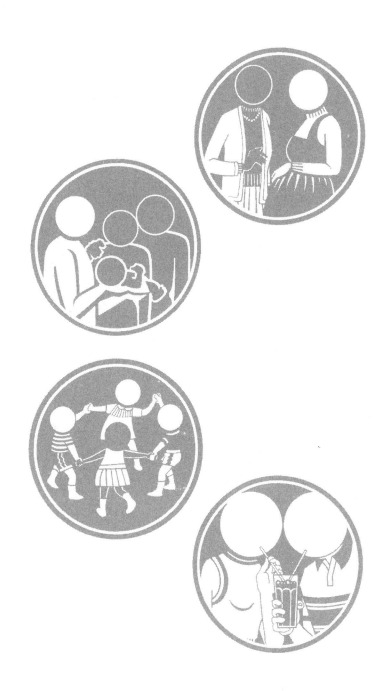

COMMENTARY

on CDC's Public Health Surveillance for Women, Infants, and Children from the Health Resources and Services Administration

The quantitative and qualitative collection, analysis, and use of public health data are critical ingredients for effective problem solving and are fundamental to the development of an infrastructure to solve women and children's health problems at the state and local levels. Data analysis should be a central component of efforts to identify maternal and child health needs, to design appropriate program interventions, to manage and evaluate those interventions, and to monitor our progress toward achieving the *Healthy Children 2000* objectives *(1)*.

The collection and analysis of data to improve decision making is increasingly the focus of policy and program formulation at the national, state, and local levels. Recently, for example, amendments to Title V of the Social Security Act (Maternal and Child Health Services Block Grant) emphasize public and private partnerships to secure the necessary infrastructure for a comprehensive, family-centered system of health services for all women, infants, children (including those with special needs), and adolescents in our nation. This legislation requires the collection of maternal and child health data to establish accountability in identifying services provided and their respective cost-effectiveness in improving health care. This information is to be incorporated into state-level decisions on planning and resource allocation in order to effect quantitative problem solving. The goal is for states to make informed decisions and to realize their maximum potential in improving the health of children and families, despite limited health-care dollars.

Decisions surrounding the allocation of dollars, particularly under health-care reform, must be focused on outcomes and system performance measures and be driven by the best information available, not anecdotes. This requires quality data. CDC and the Maternal and Child Health Bureau of the Health Resources and Services Administration are focusing on the development, analysis, and use of maternal and child health data in response to the need to better establish accountability, effectiveness, and efficiency.

In this regard, *From Data to Action: CDC's Public Health Surveillance for Women, Infants, and Children* is an important reference for state and local health officers. Not only does this monograph provide a useful inventory of CDC surveillance data sources, but it also provides an important background to help health officers better understand the uses of these data. As states become more adept at using and understanding their data, the information in this monograph will become increasingly useful.

Audrey H. Nora, M.D., M.P.H.
Director
Maternal and Child Health Bureau
Health Resources and Services Administration
Rockville, Maryland

Samuel S. Kessel, M.D., M.P.H.
Director
Division of Systems, Education, and Science
Maternal and Child Health Bureau
Health Resources and Services Administration
Rockville, Maryland

REFERENCE

1.   Public Health Service. Healthy children 2000: national health promotion and disease prevention objectives selected for mothers, infants, children, adolescents, and youth. Adapted
from: Public Health Service. Healthy people 2000: national health promotion and disease
prevention objectives—full report, with commentary. Washington, DC: US Department of
Health and Human Services, Public Health Service, 1991; DHHS publication no.
(PHS)91-50212.

COMMENTARY

on CDC's Public Health Surveillance
for Women, Infants, and Children
from the March of Dimes Birth Defects Foundation

Improving the health of women, infants, and children has been a goal of public health efforts since the turn of the last century. Surveillance data have been critical to these efforts. In the early 1900s, Julia Lathrop, first chief of the Children's Bureau, summarized the importance of data when she said that "if the government can investigate and report, the conscience and power of local communities can be depended upon for local action." Lathrop saw the federal role as "securing actual data of current value [to stimulate] general interest in better legislation and enforcement" (1).

This monograph explores topics of longstanding importance to the health of women, infants, and children. Maternal mortality and morbidity as well as fetal and infant deaths are of continuing concern, along with associated conditions such as infectious diseases, preterm births, and birth defects. In addition, newer issues, such as human immunodeficiency virus infection, injuries, and developmental disabilities, indicate the increasing view of public health defined more broadly than in the earlier decades of this century. Recognition and measurement of the behaviors and conditions that contribute to unintended pregnancy and to adolescent and pregnancy health risks enhance public health professionals' ability to address these critical issues. The study of these indicators can provide fundamental clues to improving the health of women and children.

Several themes illustrate the challenges of the surveillance of women and children's outcomes. First, surveillance data and epidemiologic studies rarely differentiate among etiologic pathways. Without more detailed information and investigation of causes, the data cannot yield the knowledge needed to design preventive interventions.

Second, no indicator has widespread meaning until standard definitions are used, reporting is consistent, and attention is given to data quality. Some key examples include the need for more standardization in fetal death reporting, better reporting of data regarding the last menstrual period to determine gestational age, and improved diagnosis of birth defects. Although CDC can provide definitions and guidance, standardization is needed at the state, local, and clinical levels to improve data quality.

The need for more usable information on behavioral risk factors is a third theme echoed throughout this monograph. Basic surveillance is conducted through vital statistics systems, population-based surveys, hospital-discharge data systems, disease-reporting and case-finding systems, and convenience and sentinel sampling. However, efforts to link this information to behavioral risk factor data and to improve the quality of such data are only beginning. The Youth Risk Behavior Surveillance System and the Pregnancy Risk Assessment Monitoring System are useful examples of approaches to collecting this important information. States must participate in and facilitate such efforts if they are to succeed in surveillance.

A final theme is related to the role of technology in future surveillance efforts. Computer and communications technology have enabled us to transmit information instantaneously as well as to manage large amounts of data. Nearly every author in this monograph has predicted that the future may bring dramatic changes to surveillance. The message is clear—we have a tremendous technological potential to apply as we reach the year 2000.

An example of how this monograph can be applied is detailed in the recent report, *Toward Improving the Outcome of Pregnancy: The 90s and Beyond,* which sets out recommendations that were developed by a committee of 30 experts and approved by more than 20 national organizations *(2).* These recommendations reinforce the need for state perinatal data systems to conduct surveillance of outcomes as well as behavioral and other risks. In addition, community-level perinatal mortality review programs and local-area perinatal boards to coordinate data and other activities are recommended. This monograph provides technical details that can be used to carry out these recommendations, particularly by states establishing perinatal data systems and by communities creating local systems.

In the process of health-care reform, we must pay attention to public health surveillance efforts. This is particularly true because the use of outcome data has been proposed as a strategy to measure the quality and effectiveness of public health and medical interventions. If health-care reform policies aim to use surveillance data to assess outcomes, the challenge to public health agencies will be to assure that these questions are answered satisfactorily. This monograph defines key questions that must be answered to meet this challenge. For example, what is the meaning of the selected indicator? Are the data timely and accurate? Do the data permit valid comparisons to be made among providers, populations, or geographic areas?

The potential for improving public health today far exceeds the imagination of the professionals who established the nation's first major public health efforts at the turn of the last century. Never before have we had a greater understanding of the data's importance and how we can use such data to take action on recognized problems affecting the health of women, infants, and children.

Kay A. Johnson, M.P.H., M.Ed.
Director
Policy and Government Affairs
March of Dimes Birth Defects Foundation
Washington, D.C.

REFERENCES

1. Skocpol T. Protecting soldiers and mothers: the political origins of social policy in the United States. Cambridge, Massachusetts: Harvard University Press, 1992:488.

2. Committee on Perinatal Health. Toward improving the outcome of pregnancy: the 90s and beyond. White Plains, New York: March of Dimes Birth Defects Foundation, 1993.

Using this Monograph

The chapters in this monograph are organized according to a reproductive health view of the life cycle. The first section describes the experience of reproductive-aged women: conception and contraception, infertility, sexually transmitted diseases, health behaviors, and pregnancy. The second section addresses birth outcomes and infant health and includes topics related to birth weight, fetal and infant survival, and birth defects. The third section discusses the health of the growing child, including immunization, infectious diseases, nutrition, injuries, lead poisoning, fetal alcohol syndrome, and developmental disabilities. The fourth section closes the cycle, as adolescents move from the health risks of childhood to the exposures of young adulthood and reproductive maturity. This organization should make it easier to identify the topics most relevant to readers.

Each chapter describes surveillance for a public health topic in terms of 1) public health importance, 2) a brief history of the program, 3) CDC surveillance systems, 4) general surveillance findings, 5) methodologic and interpretive issues, 6) examples of uses of the surveillance data, and 7) future issues regarding the measured health event or surveillance system. To help you identify the most useful information on each topic and surveillance activity, several appendixes are included. To learn more about specific surveillance activities, you may consult with the contact people listed in Appendix A. Appendix B permits you to quickly identify which surveillance activities include the topics of interest; these surveillance activities can then be identified in the text by using the index page references. We have provided an abbreviated listing in Appendix C indicating the organizational location of CDC authors and contact persons included in this monograph to guide readers through the sometimes confusing lists of titles, divisions, and centers within a large government agency. Appendix D is a glossary of abbreviations found in this monograph and some of the most important epidemiologic definitions.

This monograph is not intended to provide step-by-step instructions on the analysis of surveillance data. It does discuss how to evaluate the usefulness of data published from these data-collection systems, and it provides examples, references, and contact persons for public health professionals who would like to know more about analytic approaches. In addition, this monograph does not exhaust the list of surveillance programs at CDC that include reproductive and child health data. It does not, for example, describe CDC's surveillance activities related to reproductive tract cancers in women or sexually transmitted diseases in men, although these are important reproductive health concerns. A number of national surveys at CDC provide information related to women and children's health, but here we have focused particularly on information from the National Survey of Family Growth, the National Hospital Discharge Survey, and the National Maternal and Infant Health Survey, with briefer references to other national surveys. As with any monograph, there are topics omitted that could have been included, and topics included that could have received more attention. Nevertheless, we believe these chapters will be useful in addressing many surveillance issues in the field of women and children's health.

Overview

Lynne S. Wilcox, M.D., M.P.H.,[1] and James S. Marks, M.D., M.P.H.[1]

INTRODUCTION

Public health professionals have always been concerned with measuring the events of the life cycle—birth, infancy, childhood, adolescence, sexual maturity, and childbearing. Good health policy requires accurate, timely public health data, and public health planners need to know the data that are available and how to use that information. In turn, public health data systems need to respond to the needs of program managers and health planners by providing and interpreting numbers that can be translated into appropriate action. The demand for such information is rapidly increasing in the public health community and will become even more critical as the United States moves into the twenty-first century.

This monograph is a step toward making the surveillance systems of the Centers for Disease Control and Prevention (CDC) more accessible to persons concerned with the health of women, infants, and children. It describes the state of the art for surveillance at CDC and discusses applications of public health data. We hope that this monograph will aid health professionals in collecting, examining, and applying data to improve the health of women and children.

Early Health Data on Women and Children

In the latter half of the nineteenth century, scientists and clinicians interested in public health issues began to recognize the importance of collecting adequate data to address the health of American women and children. Infant death rates were considered a critical measure of the population's health in the general sanitation reform movements that occurred in the United States and Europe during this period (1). One of the best known early U.S. reports on public health data was *Shattuck's Report of the Sanitary Commission of Massachusetts, 1850*, which described the health of the citizens of Massachusetts (2). This extensive report described infant and maternal mortality and recommended that public health programs conduct sanitary surveillance, immunization activities, and well-baby programs. The extremely high death rates among children of poor, urban immigrants also were of special concern, as described in the 1857 American Medical Association *Report on Infant Mortality in Large Cities, the Sources of Its Increase and the Means of Its Diminution* (3).

By the late 1870s, many city and state health departments were calculating the infantile death rate, a measure of the ratio of deaths to children <5 years of age to all deaths in the community (1). Health officials also were beginning to recognize the importance of distinguishing deaths among children <1 year of age from deaths among older children and of examining the seasonal changes in causes of death. These more precise data led to the identification of annual epidemics of summer diarrheal deaths among the youngest infants in urban environments. Reports of these epidemics, published each summer in city newspapers, drew public attention to the influence of environment and nutrition on infant health. By the 1890s, these concerns had led to the operation of hygienic milk stations by private philanthropists and city

[1] Division of Reproductive Health
National Center for Chronic Disease Prevention
and Health Promotion
Centers for Disease Control and Prevention
Atlanta, Georgia

health departments to provide safe milk for urban infants (1,4).

At the turn of the century, the U.S. Bureau of the Census began publishing national census data that included infant mortality rates and covered 41% of the national population (5). Fifteen cities reported infant mortality rates of >200 deaths per 1,000 live births. In 1906, a summary of causes of infant deaths from 1900–1904 reported that the most common causes were "digestive and diarrheal diseases," "congenital problems," and "respiratory disease" (6). These rates were based on estimates of the numbers of live births (although births were registered in a number of cities, a national birth-registration area was not established until 1915). In 1908, the New York City Health Department established a Division of Child Hygiene, one of the first city bureaus of child health in the country. The division's early programs used the city birth register to identify every newborn in a Lower East Side health district and then send a public health nurse to teach new mothers appropriate infant care (4). Four years later, the federal Children's Bureau was created in the Department of Labor with the primary responsibility of studying and reducing infant mortality (7).

During the second decade of the twentieth century, health professionals became increasingly aware that protecting the health of pregnant women might significantly improve infant health, and prenatal care became a more popular concept. The importance of prenatal care was emphasized in 1913 with the publication of the first national reports of neonatal deaths. This information from the 1910 census described infant deaths occurring within 1 day, 1 week, 1 month, and 1 year of birth (8). "Premature birth," "congenital debility," and "malformations" were reported as the top causes of death in the neonatal period, whereas "diarrhea and enteritis," "respiratory disease," and "premature birth" were the overall most common causes of death in the first year of life. These reports illustrated that neither clean milk nor maternal classes on infant care would address a large portion of the causes of infant mortality, and that clinicians needed to pay greater attention to the health of the mother before the infant's birth.

That same year, the Children's Bureau published the first edition of its pamphlet, Prenatal Care (9).

The Children's Bureau encouraged birth registration and also conducted a series of community evaluations, beginning in 1913, to examine the determinants of infant mortality. These evaluations included the recording of all infant births and deaths, household surveys to interview the families of these infants, and the collection of standardized data on community sanitation, civic organization of the community, and economics. These survey data confirmed the distribution of causes of infant death that were being reported by the census bureau and provided quantitative evidence of the effect of long-suspected risk factors—such as age, parity, and family income—on the survival of infants (1,7).

During World War I, interest in children's health increased with the recognition that disturbingly high numbers of American draftees were not healthy enough for military service. The Children's Bureau identified 1918 as "Children's Year" and used the special event as an opportunity to convince state legislatures to improve birth registration, create divisions of child health, and expand well-baby and prenatal care in urban and rural settings. Maternal mortality also gained greater public attention. In 1917, the Children's Bureau submitted a report to Congress on Maternal Mortality from All Conditions Connected with Childbirth in the United States and Certain Other Countries, stating that in 1913, maternal mortality was the second most common cause of death (after tuberculosis) among females aged 15–44 years (10). By 1920, the health of pregnant women and the health of their infants were considered linked in public health programs for maternal and infant welfare.

Women and children's health was further bolstered after the Great Depression's effects on the welfare of families led to the passage of the Social Security Act of 1935. This act provided for state maternal and child health services, or Title V programs. Over the succeeding decades, this act served as a source of federal support for state health programs, and, at times, for research into women and children's health *(1)*. More recently, the Omnibus Budget Reconciliation Act of 1989 linked the use of Title V funds to state assessment and reporting requirements, increasing states' focus on the use of women and children's health data.

Shortly after World War II, the concept of public health surveillance became embodied in the Communicable Disease Center, the precursor agency of the Centers for Disease Control and Prevention (CDC) *(11)*. Over the past 40 years, CDC's surveillance activities—initially oriented to a few infectious diseases—have expanded to encompass both emerging infectious diseases and numerous noninfectious causes of morbidity and mortality among women and children. The Cutter vaccine incident of 1955—when vaccine contaminated with live polio virus caused polio among newly vaccinated children—was an early indication of the importance of surveillance for a childhood illness and led directly to the formation of the poliomyelitis surveillance program at CDC. In 1957, the Public Health Service's Venereal Disease Division, with its emphasis on aggressive use of field data to control reproductive tract infection, was transferred to CDC.

CDC became responsible for the national polio immunization program in 1961, and the Vaccine Assistance Act of 1962 eventually provided funds for a major pediatric immunization and surveillance program covering polio, diphtheria, pertussis, tetanus, and measles. CDC programs in family planning and birth defects surveillance were also begun during the 1960s. The Public Health Service Ten-State Nutrition Survey of the late 1960s, which demonstrated that millions of U.S. children and young women were malnourished, signaled the beginning of CDC's pregnancy and pediatric nutrition surveillance activities in the 1970s.

In the 1980s, new CDC programs related to women and children's health have included the development of injury and violence surveillance systems, the emergence of acquired immunodeficiency syndrome as a major health concern, and the expansion of CDC to include the National Center for Health Statistics, with its

vital statistics and survey data. More recent CDC surveillance activities are described throughout this monograph, illustrating the continuing interaction among health trends, data collection resources, and public policy.

Modern Concerns About Women and Children's Health Data

The 10-fold to 100-fold decreases in infant and maternal mortality since 1900 are the results of twentieth century interventions to improve the health of women and children *(12)*. Changes in the primary causes of infant deaths—from digestive and diarrheal diseases in 1900 to birth defects, sudden infant death syndrome, and preterm delivery in 1988 *(12)*—reflect innovative developments in medical therapy and public health practice. Nevertheless, the United States continues to have many of the serious discrepancies first identified in the 1850s— health differences between rich and poor, minority and white, and urban and rural populations. Infant and child mortality remains a core measure of our society's strengths and priorities. Similarly, for maternal mortality and morbidity in the United States and in the developing world, education and poverty remain important predictors of risk. High levels of unintended pregnancy, sexually transmitted diseases, and abortion in the United States illustrate the continuing need for society to address the health concerns of women throughout their reproductive years.

How does public health surveillance address these issues? In its 1988 report, *The Future of Public Health*, the Institute of Medicine recommends that "every public health agency regularly and systematically collect, assemble, analyze, and make available information on the health of the community, including statistics on health status, community health needs, and epidemiologic and other health problems." This report emphasizes the need for data collection and analysis at local, state, and national levels *(13)*. Most importantly, the theme of that report and this monograph is that community health data be used systematically to evaluate and improve health programs and policies.

Local and state health departments routinely examine information on the primary causes of mortality and morbidity and the populations at highest risk for these outcomes. They also provide health services and, increasingly, must evaluate these services—determining who needs health care, who is receiving services, and how effective are the services. To answer these questions, health departments must regularly collect, analyze, and interpret public health data. With Medicaid costs rising, state revenues decreasing, and health-care reform developing, the need to identify the most efficient and effective public health response in each community is more critical than ever.

For decades, the CDC has worked with state health departments in the surveillance and analysis of health data. Traditionally, this partnership has focused on examining infectious disease concerns. More recently, CDC has also assisted states in examining the epidemiology of noninfectious chronic diseases, injuries, and environmental health problems. Women and children's health focuses on a specific population rather than a specific disease or a bundle of diagnoses; it addresses major socioeconomic, cultural, and health system concerns. CDC programs approach this population from many directions—such as immunization, injury control, the monitoring and prevention of birth defects and developmental disabilities, family planning and prevention of adolescent pregnancy, and behavioral risk factor surveillance—reflecting the broad distribution of health problems and risk factors that affect women and children.

The use of epidemiology, data surveillance and analysis, and program evaluation has become an essential aspect of strong maternal and child health programs. The goal of this monograph is to describe the various surveillance activities and data collection systems at CDC that are relevant to the health of women and children. This information will be useful to state and local public health professionals, university maternal and child health educators, and others concerned with women and children's health. In addition to describing CDC's surveillance programs, we also discuss data interpretation issues and provide examples of how the data have been used effectively in public health practice.

SURVEILLANCE OF WOMEN AND CHILDREN'S HEALTH

What is Public Health Surveillance?

According to CDC's formal definition *(14)*—

> Public health surveillance is the ongoing systematic collection, analysis, and interpretation of health data essential to the planning, implementation, and evaluation of public health practice, closely integrated with the timely dissemination of these data to those who need to know. The final link in the surveillance chain is the application of these data to prevention and control. A surveillance system includes a functional capacity for data collection, analysis, and dissemination linked to public health programs.

In broad terms, public health surveillance is the monitoring of diseases, injuries and conditions for their frequency, risk factors, consequences, and health service requirements *(15)*. This monitoring carries with it a responsibility for examining and interpreting the reported data, recommending and implementing public health action, and evaluating that action through continued surveillance. Ideally, all portions of the health system contribute to this cycle. The principles of public health surveillance are described elsewhere *(16)*.

What events should have a high priority for surveillance? The numbers of affected individuals, the severity of the condition, the costs of the condition to society, the availability of preventive or curative treatments, and the importance of the event as a sentinel indication are all considerations in determining surveillance need *(15)*. Health policy or public interest may emphasize the surveillance of events in special groups, such as minority or adolescent populations. These general surveillance concerns also apply to the surveillance of women and children's health. Many health events of special interest to maternal and child health programs are described in the Public Health Service's *Healthy People 2000 (17)*.

In establishing and maintaining surveillance systems at the local, state, or federal level, we must consider several general feasibility issues, such as the quality of data, timeliness of reporting, confidentiality, and costs:

- The quality of data affects the conclusions that can be drawn, and frequently a trade-off must be made between the amount and accuracy of gathered data. To ensure good data quality, we must appropriately refine surveillance definitions, design data collection instruments, train data collectors, and supervise data entry activities.

- Timely availability of information is particularly important for public program planning. Provisional infant mortality rates, with a limited number of variables, are reported 3–4 months after the month of occurrence of the deaths. However, to analyze infant mortality patterns using extensive data from vital records, we must wait until the subsequent calendar year is completed and all children born in the first year have had time to reach 1 year of age. Thus, >2 years must pass from the birth of the first infant in the cohort year before a linked infant birth-death file can be prepared for analysis. In a recent feasibility study of the national linkage of infant birth-death files to Medicaid service files, Mamer estimated that with all systems operating at present efficiency, the earliest such a file could be available would be 5 years after the birth of the first infant in the study year (18).

- Data must be collected at the individual level to permit the linkage of information from one data set to another. Individual identifying information such as name, date of birth, and address are needed for successful linkage; however, the collection of these data increases concerns over confidentiality.

- The costs of the data collection system must be weighed against the program improvements that may result from more accurate and timely data (19). With limited resources, many public health programs have difficulty supporting data gathering and analysis activities while service needs

remain unmet. Nevertheless, this service obligation must be balanced with the recognition of the importance of quality, timely information for effective management of limited resources and for supporting budget justifications. Failure to establish coherent, consistent data systems retards a health department's ability to target programs effectively and to identify those activities that are not cost-effective.

Measurement Issues

Although feasibility issues exist for any women and children's health surveillance system, measurement issues are more specific to the defined purpose of each surveillance activity. These purposes may include questions related to level of use, risk exposures, health outcomes, health services use, and data linkages. Many of the measurement issues described here in general terms are discussed in relation to specific surveillance programs in other chapters in this monograph.

LEVEL OF USE

Health officials at the local, state, and national levels have certain common data needs, but they also may need to collect different types of information for health issues unique to their location. The importance of states' constitutional role in public health means that they need answers to questions regarding their local conditions. National data or data from other regions of the country may be limited in their relevance to local concerns. For example, national surveys frequently use the term "Hispanic" in describing ethnicity, without further delineation. Yet differences in neonatal and postneonatal mortality risks have been identified among Puerto Rican, Cuban American, and Mexican American populations (20). Nevertheless, national data are useful for comparisons with local data and can serve as a first step in assessment if local data are not available. The surveillance systems described in this monograph include discussions of whether data are available at the state level and how they have been used by health departments and other agencies.

RISK EXPOSURES AND HEALTH OUTCOMES

In establishing data surveillance and analysis systems, health officials must decide what exposures and outcomes need evaluation. *Healthy Communities 2000: Model Standards (21)* notes the importance of establishing community health status (outcome) objectives. This document suggests surveillance and data system goals that include the ability "to detect and monitor conditions contributing to morbidity and mortality in the community," a concept that includes the measurement of risk exposures as well as health outcomes.

Exposures include preexisting conditions, such as diabetes, and risk factors, such as smoking, which can lead to a health condition. They also include factors, such as early prenatal care, which can protect against an adverse health outcome. Some important questions must be asked regarding the measurement of exposures: Will the system be able to identify the medical, demographic, and socioeconomic characteristics that put a community, family, or individual at a high risk for poor health outcomes? How accurate are measures of prenatal care, child day-care use, drug and alcohol use, immunization status, economic conditions, and other risk factors?

The examination of race and ethnicity as a health exposure requires special attention. The designation of race and ethnicity is often problematic, and definitions may vary from one data collection activity to another. Race is frequently a marker for a variety of cultural, economic, and medical factors, and these factors must be taken into account when assessing the effects of race on health outcomes. Following a 1993 CDC workshop on the use of race and ethnicity in public health surveillance *(22)*, attendees recommended that all CDC surveillance reports that included analyses by race should indicate the reasons for measuring race and interpret the meaning of this variable. In keeping with this recommendation, many of the chapters in this monograph discuss the use of race as a variable in the various surveillance activities.

Outcomes may also be a variety of health events, such as deaths due to sudden infant death syndrome, or hospitalizations due to preeclampsia. When measuring outcomes, health planners must also consider a number of questions: Can hospitalizations be counted? Are complications of labor and delivery recorded? Are all outpatient visits reflected in the data? Ideally, definitions of each exposure and outcome should be formally described and should be consistent throughout the surveillance period. The 1989 revision of the U.S. Standard Certificate of Live Birth is an example of recent attempts to increase states' collection of information on exposures and outcomes *(23)*. The revised certificate gathers new information on exposures, such as medical and behavioral risk factors, and on outcomes such as abnormal conditions of the infant.

HEALTH SERVICES USE

The purpose of tracking health services usually is to address questions regarding the numbers of clients, the unmet need for services, and the effectiveness of the services provided. Frequently, measures of service use are not population-based but are drawn from clinics or health programs selected for administrative purposes. To determine the extent of need for services, and to compare services provided in the program with services delivered outside the program, health policy analysts may link program data to population information. Service-based data sets need to be evaluated to determine what population-based data are necessary to answer health policy questions regarding unmet service needs and the effectiveness of program services that are provided.

DATA LINKAGES

Linkages between health-risk or service data and population outcome data are useful for estimating unmet service needs and comparing health-care use and outcomes between health program recipients and other population groups. In establishing data linkages, the analyst must address concerns such as unique identifying information that permits person-specific linkage and delineation of family units so that maternal and child care service data can be linked. Data linkage has only recently become technically feasible with the availability of less expensive but powerful computer hardware and software. Health data can now be entered into personal computers at local health departments and be transmitted electronically to mainframes at the state level for analysis. Linkages once handled manually can now be performed through automated linking protocols, so that linked data are produced faster and with less cost.

A number of reports have come from the linkage of population and program data sets. Yip, for example, linked Special Supplemental Food Program for Women, Infants, and Children (WIC) data from the Pediatric Nutrition Surveillance System (program services) and Tennessee birth certificates (vital records) to identify whether children at a high risk of nutritional deficiency were enrolled in WIC programs (24).

As was evident at the Maternal, Infant, and Child Health Programs Data Analysis and Tracking Approaches Conference in 1992, states are particularly eager to link data sets (Atrash HK, unpublished data, 1992). In fact, the need for linkage of records was mentioned by virtually every state. Emphasis was placed on linkages among WIC, vital statistics, Medicaid, and other data sources including the Community Health Services Information System, Integrated Services Information System, hospital discharge data, Pregnancy Risk Assessment Monitoring System, Pregnancy Nutrition Surveillance System, and census data. States also expressed interest in cross-agency linkages among health, education, hospital, criminal justice, motor vehicle, and social services agencies, as well as in linked birth and death records.

CDC DATA COLLECTION SYSTEMS

Public health data collection systems used at CDC include not only traditional public health casefinding, disease-reporting, and sentinel surveillance activities but also such important data sources as vital records, population surveys, and hospital discharge data (25) (the surveillance activities described in this monograph are presented by category in Table 1). Not all of these systems meet CDC's formal definition of surveillance, and not all of them were originally designed for public health surveillance. However, these systems can provide health planners with useful,

regularly updated information that will improve their ability to prevent and control health problems among women and children.

Vital Statistics Systems

Vital statistics systems are a type of population-based system. The current U.S. vital records system has many of the advantages of an ideal data system. It gathers individual-level data; permits aggregation from the individual to the community, state, and national levels; has consistent definitions across jurisdictions; provides enough identifying information to avoid duplication of records and permit linkage to other data systems. This system measures critical outcomes (such as births, deaths, fetal deaths, and abortions) and, for births and fetal deaths, provides enough exposure information to help identify people at high risk because of geographic, temporal, and personal characteristics. These substantial advantages, as well as this system's historical role, make vital records a strong base on which to build a coherent, responsive data system. Topics in this monograph drawn from vital records data include low birth weight and preterm delivery, maternal and infant mortality, and fetal deaths.

Despite these considerable strengths, the vital records system has disadvantages as well. Often the risk exposure information is not sufficiently detailed to assure specificity or program relevance. Vital statistics systems rarely provide adequate service use measures for the major service programs (e.g., WIC, Medicaid) or for private sources of health care. Beyond the birth period, these systems provide no measure of morbidity outcomes. Furthermore, vital records contain no information on costs of outcomes or services.

Vital records data and programs have several limitations. Serious concerns have been raised regarding data quality, especially for risk factor information, because the information is often gathered by persons untrained in systematic data collection. Timeliness may also be a concern because many months may lapse before all vital records are available on a birth cohort. Moreover, vital statistics programs require substantial resource investments in every state.

TABLE 1. Systems of collecting data for women and children's health — CDC, 1994

Vital statistics	Population surveys	Hospital discharge data systems	Disease-reporting and case-finding surveillance	Convenience and sentinel surveillance
Birth registration	National Survey of Family Growth	National Hospital Discharge Survey	Sexually transmitted diseases surveillance	Pregnancy Nutrition Surveillance System
Death registration				Pediatric Nutrition Surveillance System
Fetal death reporting	Pregnancy Risk Assessment Monitoring System	Birth Defects Monitoring Program	Abortion surveillance	
Linked birth/infant death database	HIV Seroprevalence Survey in Childbearing Women	Ectopic pregnancy and maternal morbidity surveillance	AIDS case reporting	HIV infection reporting
Current Mortality Sample (provisional)	Youth Risk Behavior Surveillance System		Pregnancy mortality surveillance	Gonococcal Isolate Surveillance Project
	National Maternal and Infant Health Survey		Metropolitan Atlanta Congenital Defects Program	
	National Health Interview Survey		National childhood lead poisoning surveillance	
	National Health and Nutrition Examination Surveys		Metropolitan Atlanta Developmental Disabilities Surveillance Program	
			National Bacterial Meningitis Reporting System	
			National Notifiable Diseases Surveillance System	

Population Surveys

Population surveys permit the assessment of key factors from all members of the population or from a representative sample. A sampling design is developed so that all members of the population have a known probability of being in the sample. Data may be collected through mailed questionnaires, telephone interviews, in-person interviews, or other approaches that permit data gathering on an individual level. Because the probability of being included in the sample is known for each individual, population surveys can be used to estimate the health experience of the entire population.

Among the important advantages of such surveys is that they provide information on the important risks and services affecting the entire population, including persons who use no health services or who obtain services in the private sector. These surveys also can directly provide data on overall population exposures, outcomes, and service needs. A variety of states have conducted population surveys to gather information needed for tracking and planning purposes. A national example of a population survey is the periodic National Maternal and Infant Health Surveys (formerly the National Natality Surveys), conducted most recently in 1988 by the National Center for Health Statistics.

16

Population surveys have several disadvantages related to linkage and feasibility. Frequently, direct linkage of data from surveys to individual data in other systems is not possible, because surveys are only a sample of the population and are often anonymous. Feasibility issues include the high costs of conducting such surveys. Although the data collected on interviewed individuals is often more complete and accurate than vital records data, conclusions may be inappropriate if many people refuse to participate in the survey (response bias). Such surveys also may miss rare events and may not provide sufficient data on population subgroups or small geographic areas. The timeliness of data collection and analysis may also be a problem.

Hospital Discharge Data Systems

Hospital discharge data systems provide estimates of the causes of major morbidity and mortality in the population. The National Hospital Discharge Survey, for example, provides population-based estimates of the numbers of Americans hospitalized each year as well as their medical diagnoses at discharge. The degree to which hospital admissions reflect the prevalence of a health event depends on the severity and emergency nature of the outcomes. For example, most fetal deaths in utero will require hospitalization of the mother, whereas early spontaneous abortions are less likely to result in hospitalization.

The advantages of these systems depend in part on how representative they are of all hospitalizations in a population. The National Hospital Discharge Survey is a population-based sample, and state-specific hospital discharge systems generally include most hospitals in the state. These systems can be used to estimate hospitalization rates of the entire population.

The disadvantages of hospital discharge data systems include the limited information provided for each patient—age, race, insurance, hospital length of stay, and diagnostic or procedural codes. Risk factor information important for public health purposes, such as the patient's smoking habits, are not included in these data. Because of confidentiality concerns, linking multiple records for the same patient across different hospital admissions often is impossible. For example, a discharge data system may be used to report how many hospital admissions for infant injuries occurred in a year but not how many individual children were hospitalized for injury during that period.

Disease-Reporting and Case-Finding Surveillance Systems

Disease or injury reporting and case-finding systems are probably closest to the traditional image of public health surveillance programs. These systems are generally established, defined, and supported by a public health program and aim to capture all identifications of the health events of interest within specified geographic areas or reporting groups.

These reporting systems have sometimes been classified as passive or active, depending on whether public health personnel simply record voluntary reports of cases or actively search for cases through telephone calls to health providers or through other approaches. Data in these systems are collected in many ways and from a variety of sources, such as hospital records, laboratory reports, and school health documents.

One of the advantages of these systems is timeliness, because most of these surveillance systems are oriented toward early and regular reporting of health events. In addition, the quality of data may be very good if the system includes a major investment of resources in case-finding activities. Such systems usually have formal definitions for the health outcomes of interest, so the health events that are reported are accurately identified.

Many surveillance systems acknowledge that underreporting is a common problem. Another disadvantage may include cost, depending on the investment of public health resources in case-finding. In addition, confidentiality concerns may reduce the willingness of local health providers to identify cases for the surveillance—they may be concerned that their patients will be embarrassed or annoyed by contacts from the health department staff. Finally, information on

17

exposures may be limited, depending on the surveillance system's design. For example, race and ethnicity data are often not available in laboratory reporting systems.

Convenience Sample and Sentinel Surveillance

Convenience sample surveillance refers to examining a population that is readily accessible but not necessarily representative of the population of interest. Sentinel surveillance uses a similar approach; it is not based on a known probability system of sampling but on past experience that surveillance reports from a certain sample have provided a quick indication of health events in the general population. Some overlaps exist between these types of surveillance and the disease-reporting surveillance systems already described.

The Pediatric Nutrition Surveillance System and the Pregnancy Nutrition Surveillance System are examples of convenience samples that include pregnant women and children from public health programs that address the needs of low-income populations. Although accurate population rates of nutritional disorders cannot be obtained from these systems, they provide health policy makers with useful information on a large portion of low-income families in the United States.

The anonymous human immunodeficiency virus (HIV) seroprevalence surveillance of certain population groups, such as childbearing women, is an example of a sentinel surveillance system. When using these systems to make health policy decisions, we must assume that the data are a qualitative, if not a quantitative, representation of a broader population's health experience. For example, if the system detects increases in the frequency of a health event among the monitored population, we may assume that the same trend is occurring in populations that are not directly monitored, although the rate of the event in other populations is not known precisely. Sentinel surveillance activities traditionally serve as early warning systems—changes in health trends in these systems may indicate the need for short-term investment in more population-based (and more expensive) surveillance to address public health crises.

Advantages of these systems are low cost and timeliness, because they are specifically intended to be less expensive than a population-based approach and to provide data rapidly. The greatest disadvantages are usually the limited quality of the collected data and the fact that the information is not population-based. However, for certain sentinel events, such as childhood meningitis, even a few cases call for public health action, regardless of whether a population rate can be determined. Other drawbacks may include a paucity of exposure information and an inability to link this information to other data sets, although some convenience sample systems do provide detailed data.

CONCLUSION

One of the Children's Bureau's first steps in translating data into public health action was to prepare public information pamphlets on prenatal and infant care. From 1914–1921, almost 1.5 million copies of *Infant Care* were distributed to American women *(26)*. In turn, women across the country sent the bureau honest, poignant letters describing their expectations and experiences with labor and delivery, child rearing and child loss, infertility, birth control, and a host of other reproductive and family health concerns. In 1921, a pregnant woman wrote for information to prepare her for her fourth delivery if the physician did not arrive in time, as had happened with two of her first three deliveries. Despite inadequate medical care, Mrs. M.A. of Minnesota was relatively lucky, as she notes of her third delivery *(26)*:

> Had no Dr. at all, but being a more experienced Mother and having my mother and a neighbor Lady with me, we got along fine. I have 3 boys. . . . Naturally, I am much interested in the things being done for children. I consider them the Nations most important asset. . . . In the course of a few years the Babies of today will be directing affairs. . . . I wish to say that I appreciate your work very much, tho I am only one of the many common-place "Ma's."

It is for the nation's most important asset, the mothers of today and their babies, that this monograph is written.

REFERENCES

1. Meckel RA. Save the babies: American public health reform and the prevention of infant mortality, 1850–1929. Baltimore, Maryland: The Johns Hopkins University Press, 1990.

2. Shattuck L. Report of the Sanitary Commission of Massachusetts, 1850. Facsimile ed. Cambridge, Massachusetts: Harvard University Press, 1948. Cited in: Meckel RA. Save the babies: American public health reform and the prevention of infant mortality, 1850–1929. Baltimore, Maryland: The Johns Hopkins University Press, 1990.

3. Reese DM. Report on infant mortality in large cities, the sources of its increase and the means of its diminution. Transactions of the American Medical Association 1857;10:102. Cited in: Meckel RA. Save the babies: American public health reform and the prevention of infant mortality, 1850–1929. Baltimore, Maryland: The Johns Hopkins University Press, 1990.

4. Rosen G. A history of public health. New York: MD Publications, 1958.

5. National Office of Vital Statistics. Vital Statistics of the United States, 1950, 2 vols. Washington, DC: US Department of Health, Education, and Welfare, National Office of Vital Statistics, 1954. Cited in: Meckel RA. Save the babies: American public health reform and the prevention of infant mortality, 1850–1929. Baltimore, Maryland: The Johns Hopkins University Press, 1990.

6. US Census Bureau. Mortality statistics, 1900–1904. Washington, DC: US Census Bureau, 1906. Cited in: Meckel RA. Save the babies: American public health reform and the prevention of infant mortality, 1850–1929. Baltimore, Maryland: The Johns Hopkins University Press, 1990.

7. Parker JK, Carpenter EM. Julia Lathrop and the Children's Bureau: the emergence of an institution. Soc Sci Rev 1981;55:60–77.

8. US Department of Commerce, Bureau of the Census. Mortality statistics, 1910. Washington, DC:US Department of Commerce, Bureau of the Census, 1913. Cited in: Meckel RA. Save the babies: American public health reform and the prevention of infant mortality, 1850–1929. Baltimore, Maryland: The Johns Hopkins University Press, 1990.

9. West MB Mrs. Prenatal care. In: Children's Bureau. Baby-saving campaigns. Washington, DC: US Department of Labor, Children's Bureau, 1913. Cited in: Meckel RA. Save the babies: American public health reform and the prevention of infant mortality, 1850–1929. Baltimore, Maryland: The Johns Hopkins University Press, 1990.

10. Meigs GL. Maternal mortality from all conditions connected with childbirth in the United States and certain other countries. Washington DC: US Department of Labor, Children's Bureau, 1917. Cited in: Meckel RA. Save the babies: American public health reform and the prevention of infant mortality, 1850–1929. Baltimore, Maryland: The Johns Hopkins University Press, 1990.

11. Etheridge EW. Sentinel for health: a history of the Centers for Disease Control. Berkeley, California: University of California Press, 1992.

12. NCHS, US Department of Health and Human Services. Vital statistics of the United States 1988. Vol II—mortality, part A. Hyattsville, Maryland: Public Health Service, CDC, 1991; DHHS publication no. (PHS)91-1101.

13. Institute of Medicine. The future of public health. Washington, DC: National Academy Press, 1988.

14. Thacker SB, Berkelman RL. Public health surveillance in the United States. Epidemiol Rev 1988;10:164–190.

15. Teutsch SM. Planning a surveillance System In: Teutsch SM, Churchill RE, eds. Principles and practice of public health surveillance. New York: Oxford University Press, 1993.

16. Teutsch SM, Churchill RE, eds. Principles and practice of public health surveillance. New York: Oxford University Press, 1993.

17. Public Health Service. Healthy people 2000: national health promotion and disease prevention objectives—full report, with commentary. Washington, DC: US Department of Health and Human Services, 1991; DHHS publication no. (PHS) 91-50212.

18. Mamer J. Measuring prenatal care effectiveness: linking birth, infant death, and Medicaid files. Princeton, New Jersey: Mathematica Policy Research, 1992.

19. Thacker SB, Berkelman RL, Stroup DF. The science of public health surveillance. J Public Health Policy 1989;10:187–203.

20. Becerra JE, Hogue CJR, Atrash HK, Pérez N. Infant mortality among Hispanics: a portrait of heterogeneity. JAMA 1991;265:217–21.

21. American Public Health Association. Healthy communities 2000: model standards. Guidelines for community attainment of the year 2000 national health objectives. 3rd ed. Washington, DC: US Government Printing Office, 1991.

22. CDC. Use of race and ethnicity in public health surveillance. Summary of the CDC/ATSDR Workshop. MMWR 1993;42(No.RR–10):1–16.

23. Ventura SJ. Advance report of new data from the 1989 birth certificate. Hyattsville, Maryland: US Department of Health and Human Services, Public Health Service, CDC, NCHS, 1992. (Monthly vital statistics report: vol. 40, no. 12, suppl.)

24. Yip R, Fleshood L, Spillman TC, Binkin NJ, Wong FL, Trowbridge FL. Using linked program and birth records to evaluate coverage and targeting in Tennessee's WIC program. Public Health Rep 1991: 106;176–81.

25. Stroup NE, Zack MM, Wharton M. Sources of routinely collected data for surveillance. In: Teutsch SM, Churchill RE, eds. Principles and practice of public health surveillance. New York: Oxford University Press, 1993.

26. Ladd-Taylor M. Raising a baby the government way: mothers' letters to the Children's Bureau, 1915–1932. New Brunswick, New Jersey: Rutgers University Press, 1986.

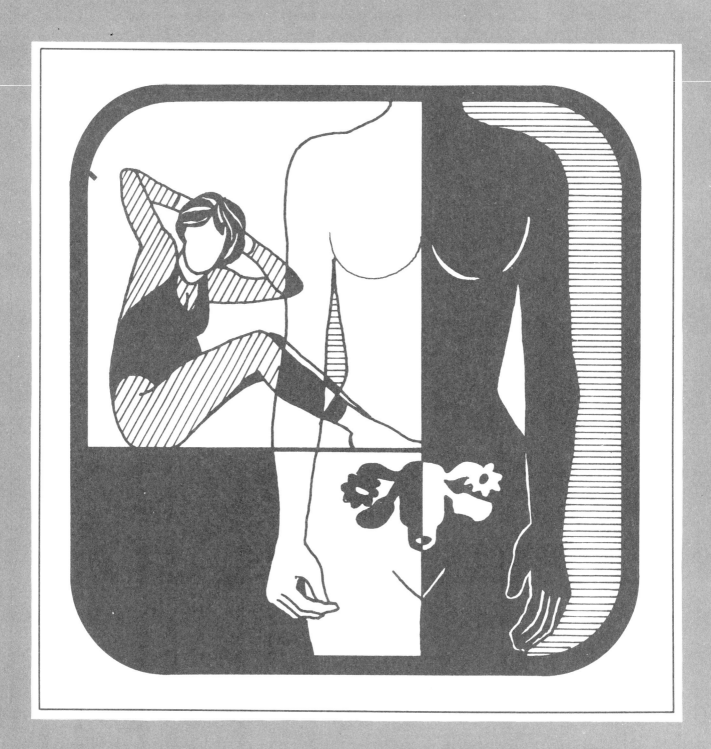

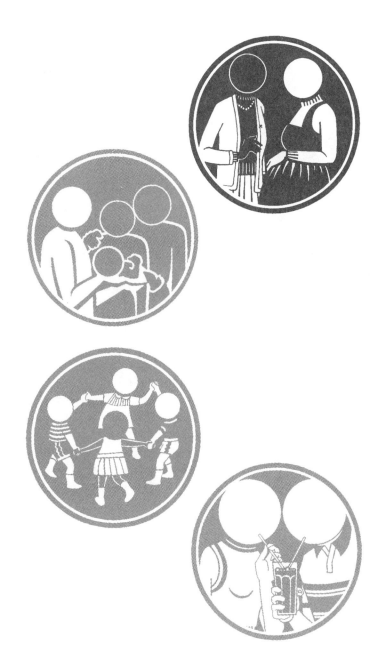

COMMENTARY

on Reproductive Health of Women
from the Oklahoma State Department of Health

With health system reform on the horizon, public health practitioners must move swiftly and carefully to establish surveillance systems that capture and disseminate the information needed to study the reproductive health status and outcomes of women, both within and outside of health-care systems. The decision to allocate scarce resources to developing surveillance systems when women and children are going without acute care services—let alone primary and preventive health care—is difficult. The executive and legislative branches of government as well as other government and private funders tend to reward direct care services and frequently discount the need to collect the information required to determine if those direct care services are appropriate or effective.

For decades, public health practice related to reproductive health has emphasized the collection of data from vital statistics (prenatal care and maternal mortality) or special disease reporting systems (infectious diseases and their sequelae). Few states have ongoing systems of collecting, analyzing, and interpreting health data necessary for planning, conducting, and evaluating public health practice as it relates to pregnancy, contraception, and periconception risk reduction. In addition, states have deemphasized maternal mortality studies, yet new and deadly infectious diseases may have profound implications for women of childbearing age. This monograph assists states in taking a closer look at a variety of methods for collecting and examining data that can be used in planning public health programs.

Public agencies also struggle to meet the ever-growing demands for prenatal, child health, nutrition, social, and special health services to families who are caught up in a cycle of poverty, unintended childbearing, unsafe living conditions, and behavioral practices that promote poor health. Even more discouraging than crowded waiting rooms in clinics and long waiting lists is the knowledge that an unknown number of potential users of health care need to be encouraged to use clinical preventive care and primary care services. States must develop and use effective health surveillance programs if they are to identify these potential users.

Unintended pregnancy has long been recognized as an important issue for women, families, and the future of children. An expert panel on health policy identified unintended pregnancy as one of four most important precursors of unnecessary illness (1). In recognition of society's interest in well-spaced and wanted children, the federal government began funding family planning programs in the late 1960s. In the early years, these federally funded family planning programs sought to measure the effectiveness of services by studying health service data for the population served by a particular provider or grantee. Sampling techniques were used to select medical records for audit to determine whether a person wanting to postpone pregnancy or to seek permanent sterilization achieved that goal. Clinical effectiveness indicators selected for nationwide collection, however, emphasized specific health-care services and education received by users rather than reproductive outcomes related to individual decisions about the number and spacing of children. Family planning programs were able to measure certain aspects of the health of the populations that they served and the preconception care and counseling given to participants who desired pregnancy in the future. However, these programs were generally not expected to measure the effectiveness of their services in reducing unintended pregnancy in the total population. Until recently, states have not had systems to collect population-based information, comparable from state to state, about the prevalence of unintended pregnancy. With the establishment of the Pregnancy Risk Assessment Monitoring System (PRAMS), participating states have now begun to acquire and use unintended pregnancy data that were never before available. State population-based data indicating that nearly half of all live births and nearly 9 out of 10 births among minority teenagers were unintended at the time of conception is a shocking revelation and commentary on the health status of women. All states need to consider how establishing a PRAMS program could help them acquire needed population-based reproductive health information on unintended pregnancy and contraceptive knowledge and use.

In the late 1980s, **infant mortality** became a household word in describing and measuring the status of health and social services at the national, state, and local levels. Much attention was focused on strategies to reduce infant deaths. Gradually, as the relationships between healthy mothers and healthy babies have been studied and more clearly articulated, the link between women's health and infants' health has become more apparent. Over the past decade, we can see how this important public health issue has evolved:

- In 1985, the Institute of Medicine's report *Preventing Low Birthweight* emphasized the notion of prepregnancy consultation and care to identify and reduce risks associated with poor pregnancy outcomes and the contribution of family planning to reducing the incidence of low birth weight *(2)*.

- In 1989, in a report of the Public Health Service Expert Panel on the Content of Prenatal Care, *Caring for our Future: The Content of Prenatal Care*, panel members emphasized preconception care for all women, with the assertion that "the preconception visit may be the single most important health care visit when viewed in the context of its effect on pregnancy" *(3)*.

- In 1993, the March of Dimes released *Toward Improving the Outcome of Pregnancy: The 90s and Beyond*, recommending a perinatal care system that provides a framework for ensuring optimal health for every woman and baby. Other key recommendations include the provision of age-appropriate reproductive health information for every schoolchild in grades K–12; new strategies to provide reproductive health information to each woman of childbearing age, routine family planning counseling and services, annual preconception or interconception visits, and a prepregnancy visit as a standard component of care *(4)*.

Armed with these recommendations, the current challenges for reproductive health care advocates relate to the anticipated changes in the way health-care services are provided and financed. We must ensure that the new health-care system addresses population-based preventive health care currently provided by public health agencies or recommended by panels of experts who have examined these issues.

Healthy People 2000, which outlines the national health promotion and disease prevention objectives, challenges the health-care system by establishing goals for the nation and each locality to achieve by the turn of the century—goals relating to reproductive health, the health of women, and the surveillance and data needs to evaluate these goals (5). States and localities that can best describe the comprehensive reproductive health status of their populations will have a clear advantage in meeting the goals of *Healthy People 2000*.

Sara Reed DePersio, M.D., M.P.H.
Deputy Commissioner
Personal Health Services
Oklahoma State Department of Health
Oklahoma City, Oklahoma

REFERENCES

1. Amler RW, Dull HB. Closing the gap: the burden of unnecessary illness. New York: Oxford University Press, 1987.

2. Institute of Medicine. Preventing low birthweight. Washington, DC: National Academy Press, 1985.

3. Public Health Service. Caring for our future: the content of prenatal care. A report of the Public Health Service Expert Panel on the Content of Prenatal Care. Washington, DC: US Department of Health and Human Services, 1989.

4. Committee on Perinatal Health. Toward improving the outcome of pregnancy: the 90s and beyond. White Plains, New York: March of Dimes Birth Defects Foundation, 1993.

5. Public Health Service. Healthy people 2000: national health promotion and disease prevention objectives—full report, with commentary. Washington, DC: US Department of Health and Human Services, Public Health Service, 1991; DHHS publication no. (PHS)91-50212.

Contraception

William D. Mosher, Ph.D.[1]

PUBLIC HEALTH IMPORTANCE

Public health researchers and practitioners need to know about the prevalence, choice, and effectiveness of contraception for a number of compelling reasons. Use of contraception is the most important factor affecting the U.S. birthrate. Oral contraceptives (OCs), the leading method, are among the most studied drugs in the United States. Female sterilization by tubal ligation, the second leading method of contraception, is also the second leading reason for hospitalization among women of reproductive age—second only to childbirth. In a recent review of the literature, investigators argued that in general, use of contraception slightly reduces health risks, except for OC users at risk of heart disease and intrauterine device (IUD) users at risk of sexually transmitted diseases (STDs) *(1)*. The use of condoms reduces the risk of transmitting STDs including human immunodeficiency virus (HIV), the virus that causes acquired immunodeficiency syndrome (AIDS). Moreover, when women make medical visits to obtain birth control services, they often receive important health screening and primary medical care *(2, 3)*. For additional information about related topics and surveillance activities, see the Infertility, Unintended Pregnancy and Childbearing, and Pregnancy in Adolescents chapters.

HISTORY OF DATA COLLECTION

National data on the use of contraception were first gathered in the Growth of American Families (GAF) study in 1955. The GAF study was intended to help explain trends and differences in birthrates in the United States by collecting data on contraception, infertility, and births expected in the future. The GAF survey, which was sponsored by the Rockefeller Foundation and conducted by the Scripps Foundation and the University of Michigan, was repeated in 1960. Renamed the National Fertility Survey, the survey was conducted in 1965 and 1970 by the Office of Population Research at Princeton University, and it was funded by the National Institute of Child Health and Human Development, part of the National Institutes of Health. These surveys documented the ineffective contraceptive practices of the 1950s; increased use of the pill, IUD, and sterilization by married couples; and the role of these methods in reducing unintended childbearing in the United States from 1960 through 1973 *(4)*. This information was used extensively in reports by the Commission on Population Growth and the American Future *(5)*, and it was used to help establish the Title X Population Research and Family Planning Programs in 1970 *(4)*.

These surveys produced so much valuable data on contraception and other factors affecting the birthrate and women's health that they were taken over by the National Center for Health Statistics (NCHS) in the early 1970s. The first National Survey of Family Growth (NSFG) was conducted in 1973, and the second was conducted in 1976. These surveys included all currently and formerly married women; women who had never been married were included only if they had had one or more births. (In other words,

---

[1] Division of Vital Statistics
National Center for Health Statistics
Centers for Disease Control and Prevention
Hyattsville, Maryland

women who had never been married and had never had children were excluded. The rationale for this exclusion was that the women included in the survey presumably were or had been sexually active at some time in their lives.) About 9,800 women were interviewed in 1973, and 8,600 were interviewed in 1976. These findings have been reported in numerous reports and articles (6).

Beginning with the 1982 NSFG, NCHS decided to expand the survey to include women of all marital statuses. So the 1982 and 1988 NSFGs were conducted with national samples of about 8,000 women of all marital statuses and included data on all major factors affecting the birthrate and closely related health topics: heterosexual intercourse, marriage and divorce, contraception, sterilization, infertility, breast-feeding, miscarriage and stillbirth, and the social and health factors that affect them (7). The NSFG is the principal national source of data on the use of contraception, its effectiveness in actual use, and where women obtain contraceptives.

CDC SURVEILLANCE ACTIVITIES

The NSFG is conducted by the Family Growth Survey Branch of NCHS, which recently became part of CDC. The data are collected in face-to-face interviews with national samples of noninstitutionalized U.S. females 15–44 years of age. (Homeless and institutionalized women are not covered.) The interviews are conducted by professional female interviewers specially trained to administer the questionnaire. In 1988, of the 8,450 women interviewed, 2,771 were black, 5,354 were white, and 325 were of other races. Interviews lasted an averaged of 70 minutes and were conducted by using a preprinted standardized questionnaire. The content of the interview included a detailed contraceptive history, including the first contraceptive method ever used, methods used between each pregnancy, and the current method used. For the 4-year period just before the interview, questions were also asked, month by month, to determine whether the woman was using contraception, and if so, which method; and whether she was pregnant, sterile, not having intercourse, or not using a method.

This kind of information allows us to calculate contraceptive failure rates using life-table methods (8).

Some NSFG findings in this and other chapters of this monograph, are shown by race and Hispanic origin. Differences between non-Hispanic white women vs. black and Hispanic women are often associated with the lower income and educational levels of minority women, their limited access to health care and health insurance, the neighborhoods in which they live, and other factors. The causes of these differences merit further research; however, the data shown here should be useful to health providers who wish to target the delivery of medical services such as birth control counseling and STD and cancer screening.

One limitation of the NSFG is that the sample is not large enough to provide data for individual states. CDC has undertaken some state surveys, which are described in the Interpretation Issues section of this chapter.

GENERAL FINDINGS

Contraceptive Use at First Intercourse

Contraceptive use at first intercourse is an important indicator of early use of contraception in general. One recent study found that adolescents who do not use contraception at first intercourse are four times as likely to have a premarital pregnancy as those who do use a method, and that one fifth of all premarital first pregnancies to teenagers occur in the first month after they begin intercourse. Use at first intercourse is also important as a measure of protection from STDs, including HIV—particularly because the most common method used at first intercourse is the condom. Other common methods used at first intercourse are the pill, and—among whites only—withdrawal (9).

TRENDS

The percentage of females (or their partners) who used a contraceptive at first intercourse increased in the 1980s, from 53% in 1980–1982 to 65% in 1983–1988. This increase occurred primarily among white females (55% in 1980–1982 to 70% in 1983–1988), mainly because of a sharp increase in condom use by their partners (27% in 1980–1982 to 42% in 1983–1988) (Table 1). No significant change in use at first intercourse was observed among black females in the 1980s.

GROUP DIFFERENCES

Hispanic females were the least likely to use a method at their first intercourse of any group identified (32%); white Jewish females were most likely to do so (68%). Females who had intercourse before the age of 15 years, who grew up in single-parent families, who were fundamentalist Protestants, and whose mothers did not graduate from high school were the least likely to use a method at first intercourse. These differences emphasize the crucial role of social and economic opportunity as well as family, neighborhood, and cultural factors in contraceptive use *(9)*.

Contraceptive Use at the Time of Interview

Most women reported that they had used contraception by the date of interview. In 1982 and 1988, about 7% of females aged 15–44 years were at risk of unintended pregnancy and were not using a contraceptive method. (Women are not at risk of unintended pregnancy if they are sterile, pregnant, trying to become pregnant, or not having intercourse.) Many unintended pregnancies result from this relatively small group of nonusers of contraception. The remaining unintended pregnancies are the result of inconsistent or incorrect contraceptive use (see the Efficacy section of this chapter).

TRENDS

The sweeping and very dramatic changes in contraceptive use in the past half century have been documented in the eight national fertility surveys

TABLE 1. Percentage of females* who used a method of contraception at first premarital intercourse, by method, race, and year of first intercourse — United States, 1965–1988

Race and year of first intercourse	Any method	Pill	Condom	Withdrawal	Other
All races[†]					
1965–1969	45.8	8.6[§]	24.0	9.5	3.7
1970–1974	44.4	12.1	21.0	7.3	4.0
1975–1979	46.5[¶]	12.8	22.0	7.5	4.2
1980–1982	53.1[¶]	14.2	26.7[¶]	8.4	3.8
1983–1988	65.4	12.1	41.8	8.9	2.8
Non-Hispanic white					
1965–1969	49.6	9.5	24.6	11.3	4.2
1970–1974	47.1	12.8	22.8	8.1	3.9
1975–1979	50.2[§]	13.6	23.7[§]	8.0	4.8
1980–1982	55.0[¶]	14.5	27.7[¶]	8.7	4.1
1983–1988	69.8	11.2	45.4	10.0	3.2
Non-Hispanic black					
1965–1969	35.8	7.1	24.7[§]	2.1	1.6
1970–1974	34.9[§]	10.9	17.0[§]	4.0	3.0
1975–1979	45.3[§]	14.6	24.3	2.5	3.8
1980–1982	54.2	18.9	29.2	3.4	2.6
1983–1988	58.0	22.8	32.4	2.9	0.9

* Includes females aged 15–44 years who have had premarital intercourse; percentages for the four methods may not total the percentage for *any method* because of rounding.
† *All races* includes respondents of *other* races as well as females of Hispanic origin.
§ Significance refers to the difference between the marked category and the category below it; p<0.05.
¶ p<0.001.

Source: National Survey of Family Growth.

discussed in this chapter. In the 1950s, the leading methods were the condom, the diaphragm, and the rhythm method, and nonuse was quite common (10); the result was the highest birthrate since the turn of the century. By 1973, more effective contraception drove the birthrate down to fewer than two children per woman. The pill was by far the leading method, but male sterilization, female sterilization, and the use of IUD had become more common (11). By 1982, use of the pill had dropped sharply, and female sterilization had increased. By 1988, use of the IUD virtually disappeared because the two major American makers of IUDs withdrew them from the U.S. market; use of the pill increased among college-educated white women, and female sterilization increased among minorities and less educated women. Condom use increased among young women in the 1980s as diaphragm use decreased (12).

Why has sterilization—especially female sterilization—become so popular? Female sterilization alone is the second leading method, just behind the pill, and when male and female sterilization are combined, they lead all other methods of contraception. For example, the percentage of married couples with a sterilization operation of some kind—tubal ligation, hysterectomy, or vasectomy—soared from 16% in 1965 to 42% in 1988. About 65% of couples with wives aged 35–44 years (nearly two out of three) opted for surgical sterilization in 1988 (13). The reason for this increase lies partly in the high failure rates for other methods. But another important reason is that the period of childbearing has been compressed to a very small number of years, usually while the woman is in her 20s. By age 30, three fourths of women who have ever been married have had all the births they want. The typical woman being sterilized is married, is about 30 years of age, and has two or three children. This leaves many married couples with about 15 years in which they are fertile but do not want any more babies. They want a method that is safe and very effective in preventing pregnancy. Moreover, sterilization is often performed as an outpatient procedure, which is frequently covered by health insurance, so its cost to the patient is modest. For many married couples and for other women who are sure that they want no

more children, sterilization may be a reasonable choice (7, p. 210) (see also the Unintended Pregnancy and Childbearing chapter).

GROUP DIFFERENCES

In 1988, low-income and minority groups relied heavily on tubal ligation. Of all women using contraception, 52% of women with less than a high school education opted for female sterilization, compared with only 21% of college-educated women (Table 2); and about 38% of black women opted for female sterilization, compared with 26% of white women. These patterns strongly suggest that the temporary contraceptive methods available then were not meeting women's needs.

Efficacy

The efficacy of contraceptive methods has been measured by every NSFG since the 1970s. In the most recent study, the failure rates—the average probability of having an unintended pregnancy in a year of using a particular method—were as follows: the pill, 7%; the condom, 16%; the diaphragm, 22%; periodic abstinence (calendar and temperature rhythm methods as well as natural family planning), 31%; and spermicides, 30%. Thus, the average annual failure rate varied from 1 in 14 for the pill to 1 in 5 for the diaphragm and 1 in 3 for periodic abstinence methods. The average failure rate for all methods except sterilization was 14%; the failure rates for black (18%), Hispanic (17%), low-income (21%), and teenage females (26%) were higher than they were for other groups (8). For example, low-income women's heavy reliance on sterilization may be explained in part by the fact that their contraceptive failure rate is 21%, compared with 10% for women with higher incomes (see Table 4 in reference 8).

Use of Family Planning Services

The NSFG also has the only patient-based national data on use of family planning and birth control services in the United States. About 20 million females aged 15–44 years (35%) had one visit or more for family planning services in 1988, about the same number as in 1982 (14). Women aged 20–24 years were the most likely to have

TABLE 2. Percentage of contraceptive users aged 15–44 years who rely on various methods, by selected characteristics — United States, 1982 and 1988

Characteristics	Female sterilization		Male sterilization		Pill		IUD		Condom	
	1982	1988	1982	1988	1982	1988	1982	1988	1982	1988
Total	23	28*	11	12	28	31	7	2*	12	15*
Age (years)										
15–19	0	2	0	0	64	59	1	0	21	33*
20–24	5	5	4	2	55	68†	4	0*	11	15
25–29	14	17	6	6	35	45*	10	1†	11	16*
30–34	31	33	15	14	16	22*	9	3†	12	12
35–39	42	45	18	20	6	5	8	3*	12	12
40–44	45	51	23	22	1	3	6	4	11	11
Marital status										
Never married	4	6	2	2	53	59	5	1†	12	20†
Currently married	27	31*	16	17	19	21	7	2†	14	14
Formerly married	39	51*	3	4	28	25	12	4*	2	6*
Education (years)§										
0–11	40	52*	8	7	22	23	12	4*	9	6
12	27	34†	14	15	28	29	6	2†	9	11
≥13	19	21	11	13	24	29*	8	2†	14	16
Income (% of poverty level)										
0–149	26	37†	6	4	36	36	8	3*	9	13*
150–299	25	32*	10	12	26	29	7	2†	12	14
≥300	21	22	14	14	26	30	7	2†	14	16
Fertility intentions										
More children	0	0	0	0	51	59*	6	1†	15	22†
No more children	40	46*	19	19	13	13	7	3†	10	10
Race/ethnicity										
Hispanic	23	32	5	4	30	33	19	5†	7	14*
Non-Hispanic white	22	26*	13	14	26	30	6	2†	13	15
Non-Hispanic black	30	38†	2	1	38	38	9	3†	6	10*

* Change from 1982 to 1988 is significant (p<0.05).
† Change from 1982 to 1988 is significant (p<0.01).
§ Education data are for women aged 20–44 years only.

Source: National Survey of Family Growth.

had a family planning visit (59%), typically to obtain OCs, which require regular visits. The percentage of women who had a family planning visit declined to 53% for those aged 25–29 years, 35% for those aged 30–34 years, 17% for those aged 35–39 years, and 6% for those aged 40–44 years.

SOURCE OF SERVICE

Women in varying income groups were about equally likely to obtain family planning services in 1982 and 1988, but they differed strongly in where they obtained these services. The family planning programs, established by Title X of the Public Health Service Act in 1970, were created to serve minorities, low-income women, and teenagers—groups that rely most heavily on sub-sidized public clinics for their family planning services. Of the 20 million women who used family planning services in 1988, about 64% obtained those services from a private physician, group practice, or health maintenance organization; 36% used a clinic. About 53% of black women and only 32% of white women used a clinic at their most recent visit; 60% of low-income women and 27% of higher-income women used a clinic. About 62% of teenagers obtained their family planning services from clinics. These differences probably are related to the fact that minority and low-income women are less likely to have health insurance or adequate income to pay the fees of a private physician, and they are less likely to have a regular source of medical care. Other factors, such as the location of private physicians' offices and clinics and the availability of trans-portation, may also help to explain the greater use of clinics by low-income women and minorities (14).

OTHER MEDICAL SERVICES

NSFG data show that women who obtain family planning services often obtain related medical services that they might otherwise not obtain at all. For example, 54% of women who obtained family planning services at a clinic had received a test for an STD in the last 12 months, compared with 34% of those who obtained family planning services from a private physician, and only 16% of those who obtained no family planning ser-vices in the past year (2). Family planning visits

are also important occasions for other health screenings: >90% of women who received family planning services in the last 12 months received a Papanicolaou (Pap) smear or pelvic examination, a breast physical examination, or a blood pressure test, regardless of who provided the service or who paid for the visit. Only about half of women who received no family planning services had had these tests in the last 12 months (3). These findings suggest that many women are getting some or all of their primary medical care during family planning visits.

INTERPRETATION ISSUES

The NSFG data on contraceptive use, choice, efficacy, and family planning services have sev-eral strengths. First, they are based on large national samples of 8,000 women or more. Second, the large sample of black women per-mits reliable estimates for subgroups of black women. Third, the large overall sample size allows national estimates that have small sampling errors and small confidence intervals, and it allows esti-mates for many subgroups. Fourth, the ability to identify women who used Title X clinics (in 1988 only) has permitted detailed profiles of the demographic and health characteristics of that population. Fifth, we can identify the region, met-ropolitan status, and income level of women in the sample, which allows us to estimate the num-ber of women at risk of unintended pregnancy and the number of women in need of family planning services for regions and other subgroups (15). Sixth, the NSFG estimates of contraceptive efficacy are based on actual national averages—not small self-selected, highly motivated groups—so they give an accurate picture of the chances of an average patient's having an unin-tended pregnancy with a particular method of contraception. Seventh, in sharp contrast to some surveillance systems, the NSFG data have a rich supply of independent variables—characteristics to help explain contraceptive behavior.

The data do, however, have some limitations. First, although the data cover more independent variables—more characteristics to explain contra-ceptive use—than most surveillance data systems do, even more detail would be helpful. More detail is to be collected in the 1994 NSFG.

Second, the data collected before the 1994 survey have not been available at frequent enough intervals. Therefore, the 1994 survey is to be followed by telephone follow-up interviews 20 and 40 months after initial interview. Third, not all abortions have been reported in these surveys until now, and this has led to questions about the accuracy of the data on contraceptive effectiveness. Efforts have been made, however, to correct the contraceptive failure rates, and they appear to yield good results (8). Furthermore, in the 1994 NSFG, surveyors are attempting to increase the reporting of abortions by using self-administered questionnaires, rewording questions, and employing other means. Fourth, the NSFG has large enough samples of white and black women to make separate, detailed estimates for these groups but not enough cases to make estimates for specific subgroups of Asians or American Indians. Past NSFG surveys have not included enough Hispanic women to make estimates for subgroups, but the 1994 NSFG does.

Fifth, although the sample sizes are large, they are not large enough to permit estimates for individual states or local areas. If estimates for a state are needed, we recommend using estimates from the latest NSFG. If your state's composition by race, age, or other characteristics differs substantially from national averages, the NSFG public use tape can be used to make estimates for the metropolitan and nonmetropolitan regions of each of the four census regions, specific for race or age. If your state's population has a large Hispanic population (Texas, Arizona, New Mexico, Florida, and New York), a large Asian population (Hawaii and California), or large numbers of a particular religious group (i.e., Mormons, Utah and Idaho), and if you know that those groups have different patterns of contraceptive use than white or black women of the same age and education level, then state-specific data may be needed. For most states, however, estimates from the NSFG should be very useful.

Data for states or Public Health Service regions may be available from the NSFG in the future. In the meantime, CDC can assist states with particular needs in two ways: first, by conducting workshops to train people to use NSFG data to make estimates of family planning needs and contraceptive use at the state level; and second, by helping states to conduct state-level surveys that collect data necessary to measure contraceptive use at the date of interview.

These state-level surveys are conducted by telephone and are based on questionnaires similar to the NSFG but shortened and simplified. One such survey, covering females aged 15–44 years, was conducted in New York State (excluding New York City) in 1988 (16); another was conducted in Idaho in 1985 (17). Others have been conducted in Hawaii and Arizona. CDC also provided assistance for a survey based on face-to-face interviews with 3,175 women aged 15–49 years in Puerto Rico in 1982 (18). The results of this survey have been used to develop family planning policy in Puerto Rico.

Data on contraceptive use for high school students in grades 9–12 are available from CDC's Youth Risk Behavior Surveillance System, conducted by CDC in collaboration with state departments of education. State-level surveys were conducted in 23 states and 10 cities in 1991; a national Youth Risk Behavior Survey was also conducted (19). These surveys are limited to high school students, most of whom are aged 14–17 years. The major advantages of Youth Risk Behavior Survey data are that they are available for many specific states and are released quickly. The major limitation is that very few demographic characteristics are available to examine subgroup differences in contraceptive use or to study the determinants of use or method choice.

Another source of national contraception data that illustrates some of the relative strengths of NSFG data is an annual survey, conducted by the Ortho Corporation and based on a self-administered questionnaire that respondents receive and return by mail (20). The overall response rate (74%) was somewhat lower than the NSFG response rate (79%). Even more serious is the fact that the response rate was much lower for youths aged 15–17 years (51%), unmarried women (60%), and women of races other than white (about 50%). Furthermore, the figures could not be adjusted by race and parity, something that can be and is done with NSFG data (21). Comparisons of NSFG data on live births, for example, with data from the birth registration system suggest that the quality of NSFG data is generally very high.

EXAMPLES OF USING DATA

The Office of Population Affairs uses NSFG data for its Annual Report to the Congress on Family Planning Services and Population Research (22); for profiling people who use Title X family planning clinics; and for assessing the rates of sexual activity, contraceptive use, and pregnancy among teenaged youths. The contraception information and other data are used by the National Institute of Child Health and Human Development and the Office of Population Affairs for answering data requests on a wide variety of topics, including contraception, and for grant and contract research. NSFG data are also used for research and information purposes by other federal agencies, including CDC and the Administration for Children and Families.

The data were used for monitoring our progress in meeting the 1990 health objectives for the nation and are now being used to monitor our progress in meeting the year 2000 objectives outlined in *Healthy People 2000 (23)*. NSFG data are used for seven of the objectives on family planning (5.1 through 5.7), two on HIV risk reduction (18.3 and 18.4), and two on STD risk reduction (19.9 and 19.10). The NSFG also has data that could be used to track a number of the other objectives.

FUTURE ISSUES

The introduction of new contraceptive methods, including the female condom or pouch, Norplant® System, and Depo-Provera®, may affect trends in contraceptive use. Another potentially important factor is the continued danger of HIV infection, which may further increase condom use.

In 1994, the NSFG was to include a national sample of 10,500 females aged 15–44 years, including about 3,000 black women, 1,800 Hispanic women, and 5,700 white and other women. The interviews, scheduled for September ber 1994 to February 1995, are being done with laptop computers, which are expected to make the interviews easier to conduct and to produce higher quality data on contraceptive effectiveness and other topics. Data from the 1994 survey should be available in early 1996.

Better measures of multiple method use (such as use of the pill to prevent pregnancy and use of the condom to prevent STDs) and better measures of the consistency of contraceptive use will be obtained. Because the 1994 survey is to be followed by telephone follow-up interviews in 1996 and 1997, the range and usefulness of the data will increase to meet the changing needs of the 1990s.

ADDITIONAL RESOURCES

- Public use computer tapes of the NSFG data are produced and are available from the National Technical Information Service of the U.S. Department of Commerce, Springfield, VA 22161.

- A list of reports from the most recent NSFG and application forms for the public use data tapes are available from the Family Growth Survey Branch, National Center for Health Statistics, 6525 Belcrest Road, Room 840, Hyattsville, MD 20782.

- For further information about state-level surveys and workshops, contact the Behavioral Epidemiology and Demographic Research Branch, Division of Reproductive Health, National Center for Chronic Disease Prevention and Health Promotion, Centers for Disease Control and Prevention, Mail Stop K–35, 4770 Buford Highway, NE, Atlanta, GA 30341-3724.

REFERENCES

1. Harlap S, Kost K, Forrest JD. Preventing pregnancy, protecting health: a new look at birth control choices in the United States. New York: Alan Guttmacher Institute, 1991.

2. Mosher WD, Aral SO. Testing for sexually transmitted diseases among women of reproductive age: United States, 1988. Fam Plann Perspect 1991;23:216–21.

3. Wilcox LS, Mosher WD. Factors associated with obtaining health screening among women of reproductive age. Public Health Rep 1993;108:76–86.

4. Westoff CF. The yield of the imperfect: the National Fertility Study. Demography 1975;12:573–80.

5. The Commission on Population Growth and the American Future. Population and the American future. New York: The New American Library Inc., 1972.

6. Mosher WD. Fertility and family planning in the 1970s: the National Survey of Family Growth. Fam Plann Perspect 1982;14:314–20.

7. Mosher WD. Fertility and family planning in the United States: insights from the National Survey of Family Growth. Fam Plann Perspect 1988;20:207–17.

8. Jones EF, Forrest JD. Contraceptive failure rates based on the 1988 NSFG. Fam Plann Perspect 1992;24: 12–9.

9. Mosher WD, McNally JW. Contraceptive use at first premarital intercourse: United States, 1965–1988. Fam Plann Perspect 1991;23:108–16.

10. Goldscheider C, Mosher WD. Religious affiliation and contraceptive usage: changing American patterns, 1955–82. Stud Fam Plann 1988;19:48–57.

11. Mosher WD, Westoff CF. Trends in contraceptive practice: United States, 1965–76. Hyattsville, Maryland: US Department of Health and Human Services, Public Health Service, NCHS, 1982. (Vital and health statistics; series 23, no. 10.)

12. Mosher WD. Contraceptive practice in the United States, 1982–1988. Fam Plann Perspect 1990;22: 198–205.

13. Mosher WD, Pratt WF. Fecundity and infertility in the United States, 1965–88. Hyattsville, Maryland: US Department of Health and Human Services, Public Health Service, CDC, NCHS, 1990. (Advance data from vital and health statistics; no. 192.)

14. Mosher WD. Use of family planning services in the United States, 1982 and 1988. Hyattsville, Maryland: US Department of Health and Human Services, Public Health Service, CDC, NCHS, 1990. (Advance data from vital and health statistics; no. 184.)

15. Henshaw SK, Forrest JD. Women at risk of unintended pregnancy, 1990 estimates: the need for family planning services, each state and county. New York: Alan Guttmacher Institute, 1993.

16. Walsh RW, Woelfel ML, Shuttleworth A, Spitz A, Goldberg HI, Morris L. New York Reproductive Health Survey, 1989. Atlanta: CDC, 1989.

17. Scofield N, Koppanyi Z, Spitz AM, Goldberg HI, Morris L. Idaho Female Health Survey, 1985: final report. Atlanta: CDC, 1987.

18. Herold JM, Warren CW, Smith JC, Rochat RW, Martinez R, Vera M. Contraceptive use and the need for family planning in Puerto Rico. Fam Plann Perspect 1986;18:185–92.

19. CDC. Selected behaviors that increase risk for HIV infection, other sexually transmitted diseases, and unintended pregnancy among high school students— United States, 1991. MMWR 1992;41:945–50.

20. Forrest JD, Fordyce RR. U.S. women's contraceptive attitudes and practice: how have they changed in the 1980s? Fam Plann Perspect 1988;20:112–8.

21. Judkins DR, Mosher WD, Botman S. National Survey of Family Growth: design, estimation, and inference. Hyattsville, Maryland: US Department of Health and Human Services, Public Health Service, CDC, NCHS, 1991. (Vital and health statistics; series 2, no. 109.)

22. Secretary of Health and Human Services. Family planning and five year plan: report for fiscal year 1990. Washington, DC: US Department of Health and Human Services, 1992.

23. Public Health Service. Healthy people 2000: national health promotion and disease prevention objectives— full report, with commentary. Washington, DC: US Department of Health and Human Services, Public Health Service, 1991; DHHS publication no. (PHS) 91-50212.

Sexually Transmitted Diseases

Rachel J. Gorwitz, M.P.H.,[1] Linda A. Webster, Ph.D.,[1]
Allyn K. Nakashima, M.D.,[1] and Joel R. Greenspan, M.D., M.P.H.[1]

PUBLIC HEALTH IMPORTANCE

Sexually transmitted diseases (STDs) continue to be among the most important public health problems in the United States. An estimated 12 million persons acquire sexually transmitted infections each year in the United States. Two thirds of STD cases occur in persons <25 years of age, and 3 million teenagers are infected with STDs annually (1). In addition to contributing to increased morbidity, mortality, and health-care costs among sexually active adolescents and adults, sexually transmitted infections and their potential long-term outcomes or sequelae have a significant effect on maternal and child health. In women, untreated or inadequately treated sexually transmitted infections can result in upper genital tract infection or pelvic inflammatory disease (PID), which can in turn lead to infertility, ectopic pregnancy, and chronic pelvic pain syndromes. In up to two thirds of acutely infected pregnant women, STDs are preventable causes of adverse outcomes of pregnancy such as fetal loss (including stillbirth and spontaneous abortion), low birth weight or prematurity, and congenital infection (2).

Cases of primary and secondary (P&S) syphilis increased annually in the United States between 1986 and 1990. In 1990, health officials reported more than 50,000 cases of P&S syphilis—the most cases reported in any year for the past 40 years (3). Between 1986 and 1990, increases in the P&S syphilis rate were much more dramatic for women than for men. Specifically, the rate of P&S syphilis increased 46% among men but 140% among women during this period. Although reports of P&S syphilis cases declined between 1991 and 1990, this apparent reduction in incidence did not occur uniformly among men and women or in different regions of the country.

For pregnant women with untreated syphilis, the risk of fetal death is 40% (1). Infants born to women with untreated syphilis may suffer brain damage, blindness, or bone deformities. In 1991, more than 4,300 cases of congenital syphilis were reported among infants <1 year of age, but even this high number is probably a substantial underestimate (1). Congenital syphilis is almost entirely preventable if pregnant women receive appropriate diagnosis and treatment. Congenital syphilis is therefore an important sentinel health event that reflects inadequacies in prenatal care and STD control services in the community.

Gonorrhea is the most frequently reported communicable disease in the United States (1). Overall, reported gonorrhea cases have declined in recent years, but an increasing proportion of gonococcal infections are caused by strains of gonorrhea that are resistant to clinical doses of one or several antibiotics. Effective therapy is available for all strains of gonorrhea that have been isolated in the United States, but new therapies to treat resistant strains can be as much as 10 times as expensive as penicillin. Approximately 10%–20% of women who acquire gonorrhea develop acute PID (1). Gonococcal eye infections (conjunctivitis) may occur as a result of mother-to-infant transmission during birth. Gonorrhea is also associated with septic abortions, prematurity, and other complications that may affect the fetus during pregnancy (1).

[1] Division of Sexually Transmitted Diseases and HIV Prevention
National Center for Prevention Services
Centers for Disease Control and Prevention
Atlanta, Georgia

An estimated 4 million cases of genital chlamydial infections occur annually, making *Chlamydia trachomatis* the most common sexually transmitted bacterial pathogen in the United States *(4)*. Numerous studies have reported a high prevalence of chlamydial infection among sexually active persons of all socioeconomic strata *(1)*. Chlamydial infection is curable. However, chlamydial infections in women are frequently not detected until after damage has occurred to the upper genital tract. Up to 75% of women with uncomplicated chlamydial infection experience no symptoms, and only recently have accurate, relatively inexpensive screening and diagnostic tests for chlamydia become widely available. Chlamydial infections account for one fourth to one half of the 1 million recognized cases of PID in the United States each year *(5)*. These infections—in addition to *C. trachomatis* infections of the fallopian tube not clinically recognized as PID—contribute significantly to the increasing number of women who experience ectopic pregnancy or involuntary infertility. Infants with infected mothers can acquire a chlamydial infection at birth from contact with infected cervicovaginal secretions. Perinatal chlamydial infections are the most common cause of neonatal conjunctivitis and are a frequent cause of infant pneumonia, which may predispose a child to respiratory problems later in life *(1)*.

All of these infections are curable, provided they are clinically recognized and treated before permanent damage to the upper genital tract or transmission to the fetus has occurred. However, all are associated with and may facilitate the transmission or acquisition of human immunodeficiency virus (HIV) infection, which is not curable and which may also be transmitted perinatally from infected mother to infant. Both ulcerative STDs (including syphilis) and nonulcerative STDs (including gonorrhea and chlamydial infection) can increase the risk of HIV transmission approximately threefold to fivefold, according to the results of multiple studies based on clinical or laboratory evidence of STDs adjusted for sexual behavior *(6–8)*.

Abstinence or limiting sexual intercourse to one mutually monogamous uninfected partner are the only totally effective strategies to prevent STDs, including HIV infection. However, properly using condoms and reducing the number of sex partners can decrease a person's risk of infection. During the 1980s, an increasing proportion of adolescent women reported that they had had premarital sex *(9)*. Furthermore, first sexual experiences occurred at younger ages during this period. Early initiation of sexual intercourse is associated with an increased number of sex partners. In addition, recent studies have revealed that condom use increased among sexually active adolescents during the 1980s but that fewer than half of the adolescents who used condoms did so all the time *(10)*. These behavior patterns have placed many female adolescents at increased risk of acquiring sexually transmitted infections, having unintended pregnancies, and transmitting infections to their offspring (for additional information about related topics and surveillance activities, see the Human Immunodeficiency Virus, Infertility, Pregnancy-Related Morbidity, Youth Risk Behavior, and Pregnancy in Adolescents chapters).

HISTORY OF DATA COLLECTION

In the late 1930s, a number of states began to require premarital blood tests, antenatal screening for syphilis, and reporting of syphilis and gonorrhea cases. Since 1941, state health departments have reported cases of syphilis (including congenital syphilis) and gonorrhea annually to CDC. In 1972, a national gonorrhea control program was initiated. Federal funds were appropriated to state and local areas to establish screening programs to identify asymptomatic women with gonococcal infection. Within 1 year, more than 8 million women who were receiving pelvic examinations for other reasons were also screened for gonorrhea.

CDC SURVEILLANCE ACTIVITIES

National surveillance of sexually transmitted infections other than HIV infection is the responsibility of CDC's National Center for Prevention Services. Cases of STDs are reported to CDC by health departments in the 50 states, the District of Columbia, selected cities,

U.S. dependencies and possessions, and independent nations in free association with the United States. Health departments use standardized forms to submit data electronically or on hard copy.

Most areas generally adhere to the STD case definitions found in *Case Definitions for Public Health Surveillance (11)*, although some areas have different case definitions, data collection policies, and systems for collecting surveillance data.

CDC receives data monthly, quarterly, and annually from state health departments in the form of summary statistics. Monthly reports include summary data for syphilis, by county and state. Quarterly reports include summary data for syphilis, gonorrhea, and other STDs, by sex and source of report (public, private, or military) for the 50 states, 64 large cities (most with a population of >200,000), and outlying areas of the United States. Annual reports include summary data for syphilis and gonorrhea, by age, race, and sex for the 50 states and six large cities. In addition, data on antimicrobial susceptibility in *Neisseria gonorrhoeae* are collected through the Gonococcal Isolate Surveillance Project, a sentinel system of 26 STD clinics and five laboratories located throughout the United States. Each week, states also provide CDC with provisional data on syphilis and gonorrhea for inclusion in the *Morbidity and Mortality Weekly Report*.

In 1983, CDC began collecting detailed demographic and clinical data on cases of congenital syphilis for national public health surveillance. State and local health departments send CDC case reports that include the reporting state as well as the infant's date of birth, vital status, birth weight, gestational age, signs of congenital syphilis, and case classification. These reports also include the mother's age and race/ethnicity, whether she sought prenatal care, the date of her first prenatal care visit, the date she was treated for syphilis, and the treatment she received.

In 1989, a new surveillance case definition for congenital syphilis was introduced, and by January 1, 1992, all reporting areas had started using this new definition. The new case definition has greater sensitivity than the former definition. In addition, many areas greatly enhanced their active case finding for congenital syphilis during this time. These factors contributed to a dramatic increase in reported cases of congenital syphilis during 1989–1991.

STD incidence (per 100,000 population) are calculated annually by using Bureau of the Census population estimates or published intercensus estimates based on Bureau of the Census population estimates, which include information on area (county, state), age (5-year age-groups), race (white, black, Asian/Pacific Islander, American Indian/Alaska Native), and, beginning in 1990, ethnicity (Hispanic). Many cities do not have a separate health jurisdiction that collects and reports data on cases of STDs. For these cities, case numbers and incidences are considered to be equal to those of the county or counties in which the city is located. For the remaining cities, incidences are calculated by using population estimates based on Bureau of the Census estimates and the results of a 1989 marketing survey conducted by Market Statistics, Inc., of New York.

The accessibility of line-listed (individual case) or aggregate STD surveillance data at the state or local level varies from area to area. In some areas, lack of equipment or trained personnel precludes the creation of computerized databases containing line-listed data. In some other areas, STD program data are entered onto a central mainframe computer system located at the state health department, which is not set up to allow access to and analyses of data beyond the creation of routine, standardized reports. State and local investigators and program officials who wish to perform additional analyses of local data that are not easily accessible through their programs may contact CDC to obtain copies of the aggregate data that have been submitted to CDC.

CDC's annual surveillance report on STDs consists of five parts: a national profile, which consists primarily of figures that provide an overview of the STD situation in the United States; regional profiles and state profiles, which provide regional maps of P&S syphilis rates, state-specific trends of P&S syphilis and gonorrhea, and county-specific maps of P&S syphilis cases and rates; tables for general reference; and an appendix containing detailed information about the sources and limitations of the data used to prepare the report *(12)*. Data from the Gonococcal Isolate Surveillance Project are also included in the CDC surveillance report and are presented in more detail in a separate annual report *(13)*.

GENERAL FINDINGS

During the second half of the 1980s, the United States witnessed an epidemic of P&S syphilis that resulted in the highest reported rates since the 1940s. In 1991, the number of reported cases of P&S syphilis in the United States declined for the first time since 1985 *(12)*. The decline in the number and rate of reported cases of syphilis in 1991 occurred among both males and females; however, the male-to-female rate ratio decreased steadily from 1984 through 1991, reflecting the larger increase in rates among females during the epidemic period and the smaller decrease in rates among females from 1990 through 1991 *(3)*.

The number and rate of reported syphilis cases declined in every region of the United States except the Midwest, where the total P&S syphilis rate increased 37.3% between 1990 and 1991. Despite the increase in syphilis rates in the Midwest, the highest rates of P&S syphilis continue to be seen in the South. In 1992, nine states, all located in the South, reported P&S syphilis rates for women that were at least twice the year 2000 objective of 10 per 100,000 people (Figure 1). During the epidemic period, the most dramatic increase in P&S syphilis rates among women involved those aged 20–24 years; the rates continue to be highest for this age-group *(1)*. From 1981 through 1991, 10%–12% of the reported morbidity from P&S syphilis in the United States affected youths aged 10–19 years. P&S syphilis rates for adolescent females were much higher in 1991 than in 1981, reflecting the dramatic increase in syphilis among females of all ages in the latter half of the 1980s. Differences in race- and ethnic-specific P&S syphilis rates among females aged 15–19 years increased steadily from 1986 through 1990 (see Figure 6 in Webster et al. [*14*]). Specifically, rates for black females in this age-group increased more than 150% from 1986 through 1990 compared with increases

FIGURE 1. Rates of primary and secondary syphilis for women, by state—United States, 1992*

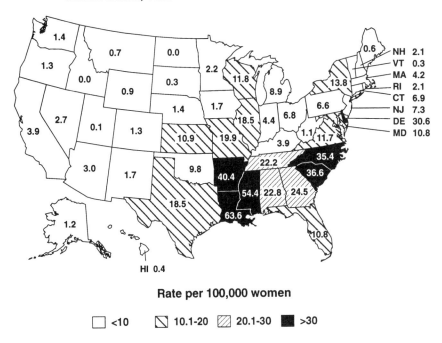

Rate per 100,000 women

☐ <10   ◨ 10.1-20   ▨ 20.1-30   ■ >30

* The U.S. rate of primary and secondary syphilis was 12.5 per 100,000 women. The year 2000 objective is to reduce this rate to 10 per 100,000.

FIGURE 2. Rates of congenital syphilis for infants <1 year of age, by state—United States, 1992*

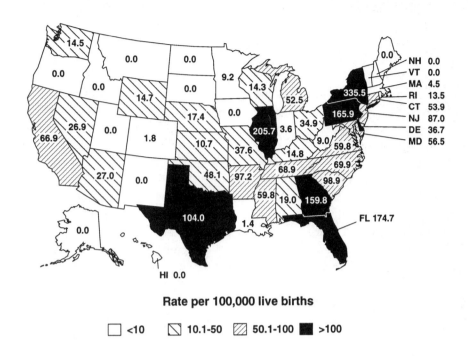

NH   0.0
VT   0.0
MA   4.5
RI   13.5
CT   53.9
NJ   87.0
DE   36.7
MD   56.5

FL 174.7

HI 0.0

Rate per 100,000 live births

☐ <10   �«10.1-50»   ▨ 50.1-100   ■ >100

* The U.S. rate of congenital syphilis was 94.7 per 100,000 live births. The year 2000 objective is to reduce this rate to 50 per 100,000 live births.

of <50% for non-Hispanic white and Hispanic females *(14)*. Such comparisons of racial/ethnic groups may help program planners to target prevention efforts to groups at greatest risk. Differences in risk among racial/ethnic groups may reflect social, economic, behavioral, or other factors, rather than race/ethnicity directly. Further analyses are needed to better understand these associations.

In the 1980s, a rise in reported cases of congenital syphilis paralleled the epidemic of P&S syphilis among women *(1)*. Rates of congenital syphilis for infants <1 year of age have increased steadily from 4.3 cases per 100,000 live births in 1983 to 103.4 in 1991—more than double the year 2000 objective of 50. Some of the large increases in the number of congenital syphilis cases reported since 1988 were related to the changes in the surveillance case definition and the case-finding activity mentioned previously; however, these changes cannot fully account for the overall increasing trend. Geographic differences in congenital syphilis rates reflect both true differences in dis-

ease incidence and the degree to which active case finding is pursued in a given area (Figure 2).

In an analysis of the characteristics of U.S. infants with congenital syphilis and their mothers for 1983–1990, the most common factor contributing to the occurrence of congenital syphilis was a lack of prenatal care (*CDC, unpublished data, 1993*). Among mothers who were tested for syphilis before delivery, the most common contributing factor to the occurrence of congenital syphilis in their offspring was receiving late treatment for syphilis, which was predominantly associated with not being tested for syphilis until the last 30 days of pregnancy. The second most common contributing factor among mothers tested for syphilis before delivery was acquiring syphilis after one or more seronegative test results during pregnancy (late infection). Twelve percent of the pregnant women who came to delivery with untreated syphilis had received prenatal care but were not tested for syphilis before delivery.

Although gonorrhea rates overall have decreased since the mid-1970s, these declines have not been observed in all demographic groups. Gonorrhea rates for adolescents increased or remained unchanged from 1981 through 1991, whereas the rates for older age-groups decreased. From 24% to 30% of the reported morbidity from gonorrhea during that period occurred among adolescents. Gonorrhea rates for adolescent females were consistently higher than rates for adolescent males during this 11-year period. Since 1984, rates of gonorrhea for females have been the highest for those aged 15–19 years (Figure 3). Although still fairly low relative to rates for other age-groups, rates of gonorrhea for females aged 10–14 years actually increased 51.2% between 1981 and 1991 (14). Among adolescent females, different patterns of reported disease morbidity were observed for whites, blacks, and Hispanics. Among females aged 10–14 years, gonorrhea rates increased for both black and Hispanic females from 1987 through 1991, whereas the rates decreased for white females during that same period. In addition, even though the overall rates of gonorrhea for females aged 15–19 years decreased during the decade, race-specific analyses indicated that the decrease occurred only among white and Hispanic females (see Figures 3 and 4 in Webster et al. [14]). Gonorrhea rates for black females aged 15–19 years remained relatively unchanged during the 11-year period. In 1991, approximately 5.2% of black females aged 15–19 years had gonorrhea. The reported gonorrhea rates for black adolescents were high in all regions of the country, ranging from approximately 3.5% in the West to 7.3% in the Northeast (regional analyses exclude adolescents from New York, Kentucky, and Maryland). These comparisons of gonorrhea rates among racial/ethnic groups reveal epidemic levels of gonorrhea for black adolescents that may reflect social, economic, behavioral, or other factors, rather than race/ethnicity directly. Despite the potential limitations of the categories of race and ethnicity, such information can be helpful in targeting prevention efforts to groups at greatest risk.

Surveillance of chlamydial infections is incomplete in many areas of the country. A combination of factors limit our ability to document the incidence and prevalence of genital chlamydial infections: 1) a large percentage of asymptomatic infections that can only be detected through active screening programs; 2) a lack of inexpensive, widely available diagnostic tests for chlamydia; 3) limited resources to support screening activities; 4) a lack of public health laws in many states requiring that health-care providers and laboratories report cases; and 5) a lack of local resources to manage and report information on the large number of chlamydial infections. Therefore, the number of chlamydia cases reported to CDC by most state health departments reflects the degree of local interest in chlamydia as a public health problem and initial attempts to resolve reporting limitations rather than true disease burdens or trends. The absence of a comprehensive nationwide surveillance system for chlamydia has necessitated the use of nongonococcal urethritis as a surrogate in monitoring trends in chlamydial infections and the use of gonorrhea case counts to estimate the number of chlamydial infections each year (15).

A few states have established wide-ranging chlamydia prevention programs that include the surveillance of cases, screening and treatment of asymptomatic women, and treatment of infected partners. In 1991, 28 (78%) of the 36 states that had chlamydia reporting legislation reported chlamydial infection rates that were above the year 2000 objective of 170 cases per 100,000 population (16). Rates of chlamydia were highest in the Midwest and West, where legislators have committed substantial resources for organized screening programs. In areas where screening programs are in place, reported rates of chlamydia for women far exceed those for men, reflecting increased detection of asymptomatic infection in women through screening. These low rates for men suggest that many sex partners of women with chlamydia have undiagnosed, untreated, or unreported cases of chlamydial infection.

The prevalence of genital chlamydial infection among women ranges from 8% to 40% (17). From 8% to 12% of pregnant females may have chlamydial infections (1). Those at highest risk are unwed teenagers living in urban areas, where the prevalence is often 20% to 30%. However, in large screening projects, analyses of the prevalence of chlamydial infec-

FIGURE 3. Age-specific rates of gonorrhea for females 15–44 years of age — United States, 1981–1991

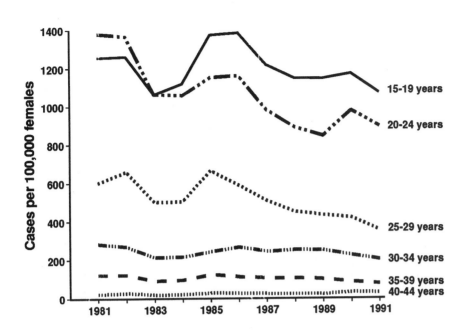

tion among women demonstrate much less variation by age, race, and geographic location than analyses of the prevalence of gonorrhea and syphilis, indicating the need for a large and comprehensive chlamydia-control program (1).

INTERPRETATION ISSUES

When interpreting data collected through these systems, we must consider several limitations of STD surveillance systems:

- Areas differ in their ability to resolve differences in total cases derived from monthly, quarterly, and annual reports. Therefore, depending on the database used, discrepancies may exist in total cases reported for a given period. In most instances, these discrepancies represent <5% of total reported cases and have a minimal effect on national totals for cases and rates. However, for a specific area, the discrepancies may be larger.

- The percentage of STD cases for which race, ethnicity, and age were unknown or

unspecified differs considerably, depending on the year and area. In 1983 and 1984, up to 25% of total U.S. cases were in this category (12).

- Although most areas use the same standardized case definitions for STDs, some areas have significantly different case definitions, data collection policies, and systems for collecting surveillance data. Therefore, we should use caution when interpreting comparisons of case numbers and rates between areas. Because case definitions and surveillance activities within a given area remain relatively stable, however, trends should be minimally affected.

- In many areas, reporting from publicly supported institutions (e.g , STD clinics) was more complete than from other sources (e.g., private practitioners). Therefore, data may not be representative of the entire population under consideration (national, state, or local).

- Because of the new, more sensitive case definition for congenital syphilis and the introduction of greatly enhanced active case finding for congenital syphilis in many areas, the number of reported cases of congenital syphilis increased dramatically during 1989–1991. As is true of any change, a period of transition during which trends cannot be clearly interpreted has resulted. Because all reporting areas had started using the new case definition for reporting cases of congenital syphilis by January 1, 1992, the reliability of trends should be stable for data reported after this date.

- Many areas do not have laws or policies for the uniform reporting of chlamydia cases, and the numbers of reported cases are much lower than expected or are zero. In addition, trends in some areas may be more representative of increases in reporting rather than actual trends in disease. As areas develop chlamydia prevention and control programs, including improved surveillance to monitor trends, the data should improve and become more representative of true trends in disease.

EXAMPLES OF USING DATA

STD surveillance systems are an integral part of program management at all levels of STD prevention in the United States. The role of these surveillance systems is to provide program managers with the morbidity information necessary for problem definition, priority setting, resource allocation, and program evaluation.

In 1991, the New York City Health Department began operating a new active surveillance system for congenital syphilis. All mothers are tested for syphilis at delivery, and the infants of women who come to delivery with untreated or inadequately treated syphilis are classified as confirmed, compatible, or stillbirth cases of congenital syphilis, according to the new congenital syphilis surveillance case definition

introduced in 1989. Full-time disease intervention specialists have been assigned to each of the hospitals where the largest numbers of congenital syphilis cases are diagnosed. These individuals are responsible for monitoring the laboratory reports of all women admitted to the hospital for delivery each day and, for those women with reactive syphilis serologies, reviewing public health departments' syphilis reactor files to determine whether these mothers have recently been treated for syphilis. This information is used to help determine the status of the infant for surveillance purposes and to aid the clinician in selecting a treatment plan. In addition to providing greater assurance that all infants who may have been congenitally infected with syphilis are receiving appropriate treatment, New York's surveillance program has helped public health officials to determine the extent of the congenital syphilis problem and to identify high-risk populations and geographic areas. This information is useful in guiding resource allocation and developing appropriate intervention programs for persons at risk.

In Wisconsin, family planning providers throughout the state played a leading role in developing and implementing a statewide *C. trachomatis*-control program that was established in 1985 *(18)*. This program selectively screens women visiting family planning clinics throughout the state, provides treatment and counseling for infected male partners of family planning clinic clients, and provides universal screening of patients at the state's largest STD clinic. The program also offers low-cost, high-volume testing in centralized laboratories, mandates the reporting of *C. trachomatis* infections, and maintains a computerized chlamydia case registry.

Data from the Wisconsin case registry and from targeted studies have been used to guide the development of the chlamydia-control program and to evaluate its effectiveness. Epidemiologic studies were conducted to assess risk factors for chlamydial infection among women visiting urban and rural family planning clinics in Wisconsin. The results of these studies were used to develop selective screening criteria that has enabled clinic personnel to identify a high proportion of the chlamydial infections among their clients, using a limited amount of resources. An analysis of data from the chlamydia case registry revealed that the number of reported chlamydia cases has declined since 1988 among women visiting family planning clinics but not among persons in other groups. Because the decline occurred in the presence of continued selective screening and a relatively constant volume of testing, it probably was not the result of decreased detection or reporting of infections. Program evaluators have assessed the effect of this program by using the results of these analyses combined with the results of epidemiologic follow-up studies showing that the prevalence of chlamydial infection decreased by 50% between 1985 and 1990 among women visiting a subset of Wisconsin family planning clinics.

An additional analysis of Wisconsin's chlamydia case registry data assessed the risk factors for recurrent chlamydial infections in women; these recurrent infections are believed to be primarily responsible for the associated tubal scarring that causes serious reproductive sequelae (*CDC, unpublished data, 1993*). The results of this analysis—which revealed that the risk for recurrent *C. trachomatis* infection is markedly elevated in adolescent females—can be used by program planners to help them develop targeted intervention strategies and to advocate the appropriation of resources to address STDs among adolescents.

FUTURE ISSUES

The highest priority for STD surveillance is to expand organized approaches to detecting chlamydial infections and treating women with these infections. More accurate measures of the number of chlamydial infections and trends in chlamydial infection rates are needed to justify, develop, and evaluate chlamydia-control programs. As of early 1993, 43 states had enacted laws or regulations requiring the reporting of chlamydia. To encourage the consistent reporting of chlamydial infections by all laboratories and health-care providers, every state should have mandatory reporting laws. Because up to

25% of men and 70% of women with chlamydial infections may be asymptomatic, however, periodic expanded screening efforts must also be initiated to better estimate the prevalence of chlamydial infections in local communities.

Such screening efforts should be carried out in a variety of settings such as prenatal clinics, family planning clinics, STD clinics, adolescent health clinics, correctional facilities, detention centers, hospital emergency rooms, university health centers, health maintenance organizations, and drug treatment centers. The prevalence of chlamydial infections in local communities can then be estimated from the number of persons tested and the number of persons with positive test results. In addition, these expanded screening efforts could serve as a way of identifying asymptomatically infected persons who continue to contribute to the transmission of chlamydial infections in a community.

Ongoing, universal screening for chlamydia should be conducted within a small number of clinic populations (sentinel surveillance sites) in local communities. In addition to laboratory test result data, information on the demographic characteristics and selected risk factors of all screened patients should be collected at these sites. These data will allow STD program personnel to estimate disease frequency, determine secular trends, and focus prevention programs by identifying persons at high risk for the disease. Furthermore, monitoring secular trends in these sentinel sites should help programs to evaluate their chlamydia prevention efforts. For example, decreases in reported episodes of chlamydial infections in these sites could indicate that the majority of preexisting cases had resulted in diagnosis and treatment and that the system was now detecting mainly new infections (i.e., a movement from prevalent to incident disease detection). Alternatively, these decreases could indicate a true decline in the rate of disease transmission resulting from routine screening, appropriate treatment, or partner notification.

Another high-priority issue for the future is the development of better methods of measuring the prevalence and incidence of PID and other long-term outcomes of sexually transmitted infections. A more accurate assessment of the extent and distribution of these conditions is needed to justify, develop, and evaluate prevention programs. Developing and implementing methods of measuring the prevalence and incidence of viral STDs (including herpes and genital warts) and vaginitis is an additional goal for the future. Currently, data on the prevalence and incidence of these infections are limited to estimates of trends in physicians' office practices *(12)*.

Finally, public health officials must work to improve the local infrastructure for collecting and analyzing STD surveillance data. These data must be used proactively to define specific high-risk groups and thus better focus program resources. In addition, STD surveillance data should be combined with meaningful measures of program activity to help determine the most effective strategies for preventing and controlling STDs in different high-risk populations.

REFERENCES

1. CDC. Division of STD/HIV Prevention: Annual report, 1992. Atlanta: US Department of Health and Human Services, Public Health Service, CDC, 1992.

2. Wasserheit JN, Holmes KK. Reproductive tract infections: challenges for international health policy, programs, and research. In: Germain A, Holmes KK, Piot P, Wasserheit JN, eds. Reproductive tract infections: global impact and priorities for women's reproductive health. New York: Plenum Press, 1992: 7–33.

3. Webster LA, Rolfs RT. Surveillance for primary and secondary syphilis—United States, 1991. MMWR 1993;42 (no. SS-3):13–9.

4. Washington AE, Johnson RE, Sanders LL Jr. Chlamydia trachomatis infections in the United States: what are they costing us? JAMA 1987;257:2070–2.

5. CDC. Chlamydia trachomatis infections: policy guidelines for prevention and control. Atlanta: US Department of Health and Human Services, Public Health Service, CDC, 1985.

6. Wasserheit JN. Epidemiological synergy: interrelationships between human immunodeficiency virus infection and other sexually transmitted diseases. Sex Transm Dis 1992;19:61–77.

7. Pepin J, Plummer FA, Brunham RC, Piot P, Cameron DW, Ronald AR. The interaction of HIV infection and other sexually transmitted diseases: an opportunity for intervention. AIDS 1989;3:3–9.

8. Laga M, Manoka AT, Nzila N, et al. Genital chlamydial infection among prostitutes in Kinshasa: prevalence, incidence, risk factors and interaction with HIV. In: Bowie WR, Caldwell HD, Jones RP, et al., eds. Chlamydial infections: proceedings of the Seventh International Symposium on Human Chlamydial Infections. Cambridge, England: Cambridge University Press, 1990:584–7.

9. CDC. Premarital sexual experience among adolescent women—United States, 1970–1988. MMWR 1991;39: 929–32.

10. Cates W Jr. The epidemiology and control of sexually transmitted diseases in adolescents. In: Schydlower M, Shafer MA, eds. AIDS and other sexually transmitted diseases. Philadelphia: Hanley and Belfus, Inc., 1990:409–27.

11. CDC. Case definitions for public health surveillance. MMWR 1990;39(no.RR-13):1–43.

12. CDC. Sexually transmitted disease surveillance, 1991. Atlanta: US Department of Health and Human Services, Public Health Service, 1992.

13. National Center for Prevention Services. Gonococcal Isolate Surveillance Project: 1991 annual report. Atlanta: US Department of Health and Human Services, Public Health Service, CDC, 1991.

14. Webster LA, Berman SM, Greenspan JR. Surveillance for gonorrhea and primary and secondary syphilis among adolescents, United States—1981–1991. MMWR 1993;42(no.SS-3):1–11.

15. Washington AE, Johnson RE, Sanders LL, Barnes RC, Alexander ER. Incidence of Chlamydia trachomatis infections in the United States: using reported Neisseria gonorrhoeae as a surrogate. In: Oriel D, Ridgway G, Schachter J, Taylor-Robinson D, Ward M, eds. Chlamydial infections. Cambridge, England: Cambridge University Press, 1986:487–90.

16. Webster LA, Greenspan JR, Nakashima AK, Johnson RE. An evaluation of surveillance for Chlamydia trachomatis infections in the United States, 1987–1991. MMWR 1993;42(no.SS-3):21–7.

17. Cates W, Wasserheit JN. Genital chlamydial infections: epidemiology and reproductive sequelae. Am J Obstet Gynecol 1991;164:1771–81.

18. Addiss DG, Vaughn ML, Hillis SD, Amsterdam L, Davis JP. History and essential features of the Wisconsin Chlamydia Trachomatis Control Program. Fam Plann Perspect 1993 (in press).

Human Immunodeficiency Virus

Patricia L. Fleming, Ph.D., M.S.,[1] and Marta Gwinn, M.D., M.P.H.[1]

PUBLIC HEALTH IMPORTANCE

From 1981 through 1992, as a result of the human immunodeficiency virus (HIV) epidemic in the United States, 253,448 cases of acquired immunodeficiency syndrome (AIDS) were reported to CDC; 27,485 (11%) involved adult and adolescent females ≥13 years of age, and 4,249 (2%) involved children <13 years of age (1). About 68% of persons reported with AIDS are known to have died. Women account for an increasing proportion of AIDS cases (13% in 1992), and 85% of females with AIDS are in their childbearing years (15–44 years).

CDC projects that the number of women and children with AIDS will increase significantly in the next few years and that persons of minority races and ethnicities will increasingly be disproportionately affected by the epidemic (2-4). The incubation period from HIV infection to severe immunodeficiency characterized as AIDS is long and variable, averaging 10 years or more. In the early years of the epidemic, most infections occurred among men who had sex with men and injection drug-using men and women; these two transmission modes account for the largest proportion of cumulative AIDS cases. A few years later, as a result of heterosexual transmission, more women sex-partners were infected with HIV. From HIV-infected women, children acquired infection perinatally. Once an HIV-infected person has progressed to having AIDS, the prognosis is poor, with most adults dying within 2 years.* In the coming years, we face the prospect of increasing morbidity and mortality from HIV-related disease among women and children.

Since the first cases of AIDS were identified and reported to CDC in 1981, we have recognized that the HIV epidemic is of great social, economic, and public health significance. Several factors contribute to the magnitude of the epidemic's effects:

- The virus is principally transmitted sexually, parenterally, or perinatally (5). Worldwide, most persons who are infected or are at risk of infection are sexually active young men and women. They become ill and die in their prime years of productivity. Thus, HIV incurs an enormous societal cost. A unique aspect is that in the United States and other western countries, most HIV-infected persons are men who had sex with other men, or injection drug-using men and women or their sex-partners. Thus, HIV is concentrated in populations that may be socially or economically disenfranchised. Another unique aspect is that the epidemic among women is reflected in the epidemic among infants and children. Since heat treatment of blood products and effective blood-screening programs were initiated in the mid-1980s, new infections from HIV-contaminated blood have been virtually eliminated, and the number and proportion of infections in children due to receipt of blood or blood products have gradually decreased. Now, most children with AIDS are infected perinatally

---

* Estimates of survival time from AIDS diagnosis to death depend on how AIDS is defined. Under the 1987 surveillance case definition, the median survival time from AIDS diagnosis was <2 years in most published reports. The 1993 expansion of the surveillance definition of AIDS is expected to increase median survival time, because a large proportion of persons with AIDS will meet the case definition at an earlier stage of the disease.

[1] Division of HIV/AIDS
National Center for Infectious Diseases
Centers for Disease Control and Prevention
Atlanta, Georgia

(>90% of 771 U.S. pediatric AIDS cases reported in 1992).

- In most cases, only in the late stages of the disease do infected persons show signs of illness attributed to HIV. As a result, these persons frequently seek medical attention and learn of their diagnosis only after they have become clinically ill and, likely, after a number of years of sexual activity or needle-sharing. Because disease progression is much more rapid in children than adults, women may first recognize their risk of HIV infection when their child becomes ill or is diagnosed with AIDS. Late diagnosis and recognition of infection impedes public health efforts to prevent further transmission. By the time infected persons become aware of their infection, receive counseling and treatment, and modify their high-risk behaviors, the virus may have already been transmitted to others.

- The principal target of HIV is the immune system. By progressively attacking and destroying the T-lymphocytes responsible for mounting the immune response, HIV renders the host vulnerable to secondary infection by a variety of ubiquitous opportunistic infections that ultimately cause illness and death. In general, manifestations of late-stage disease are similar for men and women; approximately 50% of adults are reported as having *Pneumocystis carinii* pneumonia, the most common AIDS-defining opportunistic infection (6). However, the complexity and variety of clinical manifestations of HIV infection challenge health-care providers' ability to recognize the disease and provide treatment.

- In the past decade, through surveillance, epidemiologists have characterized the populations affected by HIV. Substantial advances have been made in understanding the structure of the virus, disease pathogenesis, and natural history, and various treatment regimens have been developed that can prevent the complications of immunodeficiency. Nevertheless, much remains to be learned about the virus itself and about the physiologic response to infection. Most importantly, no curative agents or effective vaccines are yet available, and a recent European study has called into question the effectiveness of zidovudine (the drug most commonly used to treat HIV infection) in delaying disease progression.

Worldwide more than 15 million persons are believed to be infected with HIV in what is now considered a global pandemic (7). Prospects for prevention and control worldwide are complicated by poverty, the lack of adequate medical services, as well as the low cultural status of women. The epidemic is growing rapidly in some parts of the world, such as Africa and Asia, where heterosexual contact appears to be the predominant mode of HIV transmission. The percentage of adults with HIV/AIDS who are women is approaching 50% (for additional information about related topics and surveillance activities, see the Sexually Transmitted Diseases and Youth Risk Behavior chapters).

HISTORY OF DATA COLLECTION

Historically, surveillance for HIV/AIDS has been accomplished largely through three data collection systems: AIDS case reporting, HIV infection reporting, and measurements of HIV seroprevalence in selected populations. AIDS surveillance was initiated in 1981 when the epidemic was first recognized. Persons with severe immunosuppression, opportunistic infections, or malignancies characterizing severe morbidity associated with HIV infection are reported to state and local health departments as meeting the standard case definition for AIDS (8,9). The surveillance of AIDS cases has provided a population-based estimate of the incidence and prevalence of the most severe morbidity associated with HIV infection and has characterized the demographic and HIV-exposure categories of persons so affected.

Following the development of the serologic antibody test for HIV in 1985, several states began reporting confirmed cases of HIV infection as an adjunct to AIDS surveillance programs to enhance public health planning (10). By early 1993, 25 states required the reporting of persons with HIV infection. Although HIV surveillance data provide information on some persons who are more recently infected than persons with AIDS, these data do not completely represent all persons with

HIV infection because not all of these persons seek or are offered HIV testing.

Surveillance of HIV antibody prevalence in selected sentinel populations has also been conducted to more completely characterize the distribution of HIV infection in the United States. In 1987, CDC instituted a national HIV serologic surveillance system known as the Family of Surveys (Table 1) *(11)*. HIV seroprevalence data are collected without personal identifiers through surveys of childbearing women; clients of sexually transmitted disease, tuberculosis, and substance abuse treatment clinics; hospitalized persons in selected facilities in high-AIDS incidence cities and in other settings where persons with HIV infection may be surveyed.

Data from HIV/AIDS surveillance and seroprevalence surveys have been useful in focusing and evaluating prevention programs, planning and implementing services for HIV-infected persons, and allocating resources. Much of what is known about the epidemiology of HIV/AIDS in the United States has come from national AIDS surveillance programs and HIV seroprevalence surveys.

CDC SURVEILLANCE ACTIVITIES

To monitor the HIV epidemic and forecast the public health resources that will be needed for prevention activities and the care of infected persons, CDC's National Center for Infectious Diseases conducts and coordinates HIV/AIDS surveillance activities through cooperative agreements with state and local health departments. Funding to conduct HIV/AIDS surveillance ensures that these departments use standardized methods, data-collection forms, and computer software developed by CDC. State and local health departments collect information, including the patient's and physician's names, the patient's mode of HIV exposure, demographic data (age, race/ethnicity,[†] sex, date of birth, date

of death), clinical data, and laboratory criteria. Information is obtained by active surveillance methods, including on-site medical record reviews by health department personnel and in-person or telephone contacts with infection control nurses, physicians, or other health-care providers. Personnel enter the data into their local databases and each month send CDC encrypted data without personal identifiers; CDC can identify unique cases at the national level by using an alphanumeric code (soundex) based on the patient's surname and a state-assigned patient number. Data are collected under a federal assurance of confidentiality and are maintained in accordance with strict security and confidentiality protections.

CDC regularly releases aggregated AIDS surveillance data for public use. These data are population-based; rates are calculated by using U.S. population estimates developed by the U.S. Bureau of the Census. Numbers of cases and rates of AIDS incidence in the population are published quarterly by CDC *(1)* and can be obtained from the National AIDS Clearinghouse. In addition, a public-use data set available through the National AIDS Clearinghouse is widely used by public health planners and academic researchers (see the Additional Resources section of this chapter).

TABLE 1. Sentinel populations in the family of HIV seroprevalence surveys*

Sentinel population	Data sources
Persons with sexually transmitted diseases (STDs)	Health department, STD clinics
Injection drug users entering treatment	Drug treatment clinics
Women seeking reproductive health services	Women's health clinics
Tuberculosis (TB) patients	Health departments, TB clinics
Hospital patients	Hospitals
Outpatients	Labs, physicians' networks
Childbearing women	Neonatal metabolic screening programs
Blood donors	Blood donation centers
Military recruits	HIV screening program (Department of Defense)
Job Corps entrants	HIV screening program (Department of Labor)

* Adapted from Pappaioanou et al. *(11)*.

† HIV/AIDS surveillance reports collect information on five racial/ethnic categories as designated by the U.S. Office of Management and Budget: white (not Hispanic), black (not Hispanic), Hispanic, American Indian/Alaska Native, and Asian/Pacific Islander. Dissemination of HIV/AIDS surveillance and seroprevalence data for racial/ethnic categories is consistent with U.S. Public Health Service objectives emphasizing the prevention of HIV/AIDS in minority populations.

Surveillance Case Definition for Adults and Adolescents

Our progressive understanding of the clinical spectrum of HIV-related diseases has resulted in several revisions to the surveillance case definition for AIDS in adults and adolescents ≥13 years of age. The original definition relied on diagnosis (by definitive methods such as culture, biopsy, histology) of specific opportunistic infections (e.g., *P. carinii* pneumonia) and malignancies resulting from cell-mediated immune deficiency. In 1985, HIV antibody testing became widely available, and inclusion of serologic evidence of HIV infection was incorporated into the case definition. In 1987, the case definition was substantially expanded to include other HIV-related conditions, such as HIV encephalopathy and wasting syndrome, as well as the presumptive diagnosis of several of the opportunistic infections in the presence of documented HIV infection *(8)*.

In 1993, the case definition was again expanded to include a direct measure of the severe immunosuppression caused by HIV—a depressed CD4+ T-lymphocyte count (<200 cells/μL or <14%), in part, to reflect standards of medical practice (laboratory measurements of immunosuppression direct patient management including antiretroviral therapy and prophylaxis against *P. carinii* pneumonia). In addition, the 1993 case definition added several conditions for which clinical management is complicated by HIV—pulmonary tuberculosis, recurrent pneumonia, and invasive cervical cancer in the presence of documented HIV infection *(9)*. Recurrent pneumonia is a frequent cause of HIV-related mortality. The addition of both pulmonary tuberculosis and invasive cervical cancer highlights conditions of public health importance, and the addition of invasive cervical cancer should improve providers' awareness of the need for gynecologic care among HIV-infected women.

AIDS cases are typically identified in hospital settings because the case definition captures severe morbidity characteristic of end-stage illness, which usually requires inpatient care. In addition to medical record reviews, routine reviews of death certificates are conducted to identify cases. Since the 1993 case definition became effective, some states have required laboratory-initiated reporting of CD4+ T-lymphocyte counts as an adjunct to provider-based surveillance.

Surveillance Case Definition for Children

Developing comprehensive revisions to the current 1987 AIDS surveillance case definition for children *(8)* and the clinical classification system for pediatric HIV disease *(12)* has posed numerous challenges. The spectrum of HIV-related diseases and the natural history of HIV infection are less well described for children than for adults. Diseases seen in immunocompromised children with HIV infection overlap with diseases seen commonly in uninfected children. Moreover, because maternal HIV antibody may not be cleared until 18 months of age, laboratory diagnosis of HIV disease in infancy has been difficult. However, recent improvements in early diagnostic tests (e.g., polymerase chain reaction), are improving clinicians' ability to diagnose HIV disease and provide treatment earlier in infancy. To more completely describe the effects of this epidemic in children and to promote and evaluate early identification and intervention programs, the Council of State and Territorial Epidemiologists has proposed substantially expanding surveillance for HIV infection in children. CDC is currently considering this proposal.

HIV Infection Reporting

Twenty-five states require the reporting, by name, of adults with documented HIV infection, and 26 states have similar requirements for reporting children with HIV infection. However, most of these states have low-to-moderate AIDS incidence annually; together they account for less than one fourth of cumulative AIDS cases. CDC has provided technical assistance to these states since 1989 and has funded active surveillance for HIV infection in these states since 1992. States have implemented HIV reporting for a variety of public health reasons, for example, to better plan for needed resources, monitor emerging trends in selected populations (e.g., adolescents), and facilitate referrals to prevention and treatment programs. In reporting data to CDC, states use a standardized definition of HIV seropositivity *(13)*. Reports may emanate from public HIV testing facilities, private physicians, hospitals, or laboratories. Reporting requirements vary by state, with most states requiring reporting from laboratories and health-care providers. Most states also provide sites where persons may be tested anonymously and reporting is not conducted. HIV reporting data do not completely capture all persons with HIV infection and may be biased by self-selection for HIV testing, overrepresentation of groups targeted by HIV screening programs, and the availability of anonymous testing (14).

Seroprevalence Surveys

Seroprevalence surveys provide a measure of the current prevalence of HIV infection by sampling segments of the population. These surveys assist in identifying populations that need to be targeted for HIV testing programs and prophylactic treatment to slow progression to AIDS as well as at-risk segments of the population that need to be targeted for prevention activities.

CDC's surveys of HIV seroprevalence among women are conducted in selected settings, such as women's reproductive health clinics. The largest of these surveys is a national, population-based survey of childbearing women, initiated in 1988 (15). This ongoing survey is based on systematic testing for HIV antibody of residual newborn dried-blood specimens collected by heel-stick onto filter paper for routine metabolic screening. All personal identifying information is permanently removed from specimens before enzyme immunoassay and Western blot tests are conducted. Data collected include demographics and HIV-1 Western blot antibody banding patterns. Because the survey is blinded, no behavioral risk information is obtained. The targeted population for the survey includes nearly all women who deliver a live-born infant in a hospital; thus, the prevalence of infection among childbearing women can be calculated directly from the survey data.

In general, seroprevalence surveys do not measure incident infection; however, the national survey of childbearing women is an exception. Although this survey is designed to measure the prevalence of infection among women delivering infants in the United States, it also indirectly measures the incidence of infection among infants

who acquire the disease perinatally from their mothers (15). We can use estimates of HIV prevalence among childbearing women to estimate the number of infected children born each year in the United States by applying estimated rates of vertical transmission from mother to child (25%–35%) to the number of women with HIV infection who deliver live-born infants each year.

Through cooperative agreements, CDC conducts these seroprevalence surveys in collaboration with state and local health departments in 39 states, the District of Columbia, Puerto Rico, and the Virgin Islands of the United States; similar surveys in an additional five states have been supported by the National Institute of Child Health and Human Development. Data are released in a summary available from the National AIDS Clearinghouse (16).

GENERAL FINDINGS

AIDS

The number of reported AIDS cases continues to increase each year, but overall, the rate of increase has slowed in the last several years (Figure 1, p. 57). The characteristics of AIDS cases vary among children, adolescents, men, and women (Table 2, p. 55). Though the number and proportion of AIDS cases are substantially lower among women than among men, AIDS incidence has significantly increased among women in the past several years. Minorities, especially blacks and Hispanics, account for the majority of cases among women (75%) and children (78%). Fifty percent of all cases among women are attributed to injection drug use. However, an increasing proportion of these cases is attributed to heterosexual contact. About 60% of cases related to heterosexual transmission are attributed to sexual contact with an injection drug user. Therefore, HIV prevention and treatment efforts must address substance abuse by women and their sex partners. CDC projects that minorities will account for an increasing proportion of cases among men, women, and children in the coming years. In contrast, the number of cases associated with exposure to blood or blood products will most likely continue to decline with time because of the effective HIV screening programs in place since 1985. AIDS case reporting has been shown to be >90% complete in some studies *(17)*, so it can provide a basis for monitoring these trends over time in the population, depending on the resources committed to AIDS case surveillance.

About 85% of the cases reported among adult and adolescent females have involved those aged 15–44 years. Data reported in 1992 show that women accounted for >13% of adult cases (Table 3) but 11% of cumulative cases (Table 2) and that ≥90% of cases among children resulted from perinatal transmission. Among the 25%–35% of infants who will be found to be truly HIV-infected after the clearing of maternal antibody, HIV may have been transmitted intrapartum, peripartum, or postpartum via breast-feeding. Reported perinatal transmission rates have varied in different studies, in part because of differences in the stage of maternal disease *(18)*.

About 46% of 3,665 perinatally acquired cases reported have been associated with maternal injection drug use, and 20% have been associated with maternal sexual contact with an injection drug-using partner. Maternal HIV infection acquired through other heterosexual contact or through unknown or unreported exposure accounts for the remaining 34% of these cases. Although progression to AIDS occurs more rapidly in children than in adults, the ages when AIDS is diagnosed vary. Among children diagnosed with AIDS who acquired HIV perinatally, 44% had AIDS diagnoses at <1 year of age, and 81% had diagnoses before the age of 5 years. Some perinatally infected children, however, have had AIDS diagnoses at ≥10 years of age.

In the past, the epidemic among women and children has been concentrated in large urban areas in the Northeast—particularly in New York and New Jersey, which account for 46% of AIDS cases among women and 37% among children. Recently, however, we have seen evidence of increasing numbers of AIDS cases attributed to heterosexual transmission outside the Northeast, particularly in the southeastern states *(19)*. Though the vast majority of cases (85%) are reported from large metropolitan statistical areas

(MSAs) with populations of ≥500,000, the proportion of cases among residents of smaller MSAs or non-MSAs has increased steadily.

Monitoring trends in reported AIDS indicator disease has provided a useful minimum estimate of morbidity caused by selected conditions and has provided an indirect measure of the effects of the Public Health Service's recommendations regarding *P. carinii* pneumonia prophylaxis. Most case reports include only one AIDS indicator disease, and records rarely reflect the subsequent diagnosis of additional manifestations of AIDS. However, knowing the pattern of reported AIDS indicator diseases may help clinical practitioners to promptly identify and treat women and children with HIV infection. *P. carinii* pneumonia, esophageal candidiasis, and HIV wasting are the most commonly reported AIDS indicator diseases among women *(6)*.

In contrast, although the leading AIDS indicator disease among children is *P. carinii* pneumonia, lymphoid interstitial pneumonitis and recurrent bacterial infections are the other most commonly reported conditions. In addition, among AIDS cases in children, the frequency of AIDS indicator diseases varies with age *(18)*.

HIV Infection

HIV reporting provides a minimum estimate of the number of infected persons who have been tested for HIV, who may require ongoing counseling to prevent further transmission, and who will require ongoing medical care and social services. HIV data have assisted state/local governments and community-based programs in planning needed programs and services. In HIV-reporting states, the mean ratio of newly reported persons with HIV infection to newly reported persons with AIDS is approximately 2:1, with relatively higher proportions of young (aged 13–24 years), female, and black persons among those reported with HIV infection vs. AIDS *(CDC, unpublished data, 1992)*. Though these data do not reflect the prevalence of infection in a community, HIV reporting can facilitate referrals to intervention programs and provide a framework for evaluating access to prevention and treatment services *(14)*.

**TABLE 2. Persons reported with AIDS, by age at diagnosis, race/ethnicity, and exposure categories —
United States, 1981–1992**

Age-group (years)	Adults and adolescents (≥13 years)				Children (<13 years) (N = 4,249)	
	Males (N = 221,714)		Females (N = 27,485)			
	No.	(%)	No.	(%)	No.	(%)
< 5					3,432	(81)
5–12					817	(19)
13–19	671	(1)	275	(1)		
20–29	41,323	(19)	6,972	(25)		
30–39	103,118	(47)	12,800	(47)		
40–49	53,350	(24)	4,637	(17)		
50–64	20,351	(9)	1,987	(7)		
≥ 65	2,901	(1)	814	(3)		
Race/Ethnicity*						
White, not Hispanic	124,827	(52)	6,927	(25)	871	(20
Black, not Hispanic	59,135	(30)	14,551	(53)	2,311	(54)
Hispanic	35,427	(17)	5,745	(21)	1,027	(24)
Asian/Pacific Islander	1,448	(1)	143	(1)	19	(<1)
Native American/Alaska Native	374	(<1)	61	(<1)	13	(<1)
Exposure Category						
Men who have sex with men	142,626	(64)				
Injection drug use	43,786	(20)	13,626	(50)		
Men who have sex with men and inject drugs	15,899	(7)				
Hemophilia or coagulation disorder	1,983	(1)	43	(<1)	188	(4)
Heterosexual contact	6,419	(3)	9,835	(39)		
Receipt of blood transfusions	3,036	(1)	1,944	(7)	306	(7)
Other/undetermined	7,965	(4)	2,037	(7)	90	(2)
Mothers with or at risk for HIV infection					3,665	(86)

* Excludes persons whose race/ethnicity is unknown.

Seroprevalence

In the 1992 survey of childbearing women, the highest HIV prevalence rates were among women delivering infants in New York (0.60%), Puerto Rico (0.59%), and Florida (0.55%), with most states having rates of <0.10% (Figure 2, p. 59) (CDC, unpublished data, 1992). The 1992 weighted national estimate of HIV prevalence among child-bearing women (based on data available December 1993) was 0.17%. From this estimate, we have determined that approximately 7,000 births among HIV-seropositive women occurred in 1992. We could expect approximately 1,400–2,100 of infants born in 1992 to be infected with HIV. If no effective therapies are provided to these children early in the course of infection, we can assume that these estimates signal substantial increases in the number of children with AIDS in the coming years.

Additional information on HIV prevalence is available from other unlinked surveys, conducted since 1988 in a variety of clinical settings in

TABLE 3. Persons reported with AIDS, by age at diagnosis, race/ethnicity, and exposure categories — United States, 1992

| | Adults and adolescents (≥13 years) | | | | Children (<13 years) (N = 771) | |
| | Males (N = 40,080) | | Females (N = 6,255) | | | |
Age-group (years)	No.	(%)	No.	(%)	No.	(%)
< 5					625	(81)
5–12					146	(19)
13–19	98	(<1)	61	(1)		
20–29	6,523	(16)	1,460	(23)		
30–39	18,359	(46)	2,854	(46)		
40–49	10,668	(27)	1,303	(21)		
50–64	3,831	(10)	445	(7)		
≥ 65	601	(1)	132	(2)		
Race/Ethnicity*						
White, not Hispanic	20,743	(52)	1,458	(23)	128	(17)
Black, Not Hispanic	12,035	(30)	3,394	(54)	468	(61)
Hispanic	6,782	(17)	1,337	(21)	166	(22)
Asian/Pacific Islander	276	(1)	36	(1)	2	(<1)
Native American/Alaska Native	94	(<1)	16	(<1)	3	(<1)
Exposure Category						
Men who have sex with men	23,936	(60)				
Injection drug use	8,610	(21)	2,815	(45)		
Men who have sex with men and inject drugs	2,429	(6)				
Hemophilia or coagulation disorder	313	(1)	3	(<1)	21	(3)
Heterosexual contact	1,677	(4)	2,437	(39)		
Receipt of blood transfusions	397	(1)	276	(4)	19	(2)
Other/undetermined	2,718	(7)	724	(12)	34	(4)
Mothers with or at risk for HIV infection					697	(90)

* Excludes persons whose race/ethnicity is unknown.

approximately 40 metropolitan areas *(11,16)*. These surveys also are based on HIV antibody testing of discarded blood specimens routinely collected for other purposes, after all personal identifiers have been permanently removed. For example, in 1988–1990, surveys of HIV prevalence among women visiting sexually transmitted disease clinics revealed a median prevalence of 0.7%, with rates of >5% in some clinics. Median HIV prevalences varied for women visiting prenatal (0.8%), family planning (0.2%), or abortion clinics (0.1%) in 1988–1989. The prevalence of HIV infection among 564,000 women applying for military service since routine screen-

ing was introduced in 1985 has remained fairly stable at approximately 0.06%. However, rates have varied by geographic area, with the highest rates observed among female military service applicants from New York City and cities in northern New Jersey (≥0.5%).

INTERPRETATION ISSUES

After a person is infected with HIV, disease progression follows a long and variable course, from mild or no symptoms in the early stages to severe end-stage morbidity and death. Along the clini-

FIGURE 1. AIDS cases reported to CDC, 1981–1992

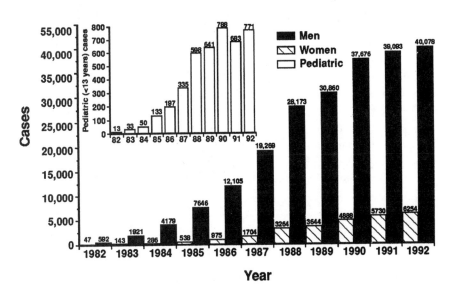

cal spectrum of HIV disease, public health surveillance can take place, with varying degrees of completeness, at discrete points marked by laboratory or clinical indicators of the stages of disease. The information that can be collected on each individual depends on the reporting source and the methods of data collection. Ongoing evaluation programs assess the validity and accuracy of surveillance and seroprevalence data as well as the timeliness and completeness of reporting.

Surveillance for AIDS captures those HIV-infected persons who manifest an AIDS-defining condition and are detected largely through provider reporting, systematic medical record reviews, or death certificate reviews. However, clinical information tends to overrepresent the conditions that are present when the person first meets the AIDS case definition. Subsequent clinical events are not completely or systematically captured.

Because information is obtained largely from medical records, surveillance activities are able to obtain complete demographic, laboratory, clinical, and HIV-exposure information. For example, only 4% of cumulative AIDS cases have an undetermined mode of HIV transmission (1). These cases are prioritized for follow-up investigation by state and local health departments. Recently, CDC has observed an increase in heterosexually acquired AIDS cases (20). A pilot study to validate the risk information on men in

this transmission group suggested that some misclassification in the mode of transmission may have occurred (21). A study to validate HIV risk information collected in surveillance is currently under way.

In validation studies of the completeness of AIDS case reporting, investigators have matched AIDS registries with hospital discharge registries and outpatient clinic databases and established a high degree (>90%) of completeness as a result of federal funding for active case-finding (17). Because of the completeness of case ascertainment and of information on cases, AIDS surveillance data are useful in monitoring trends over time in the epidemic's effects, by sex, age, race/ethnicity, and HIV-exposure group. The completeness and timeliness of reporting under the 1993 expanded AIDS surveillance case definition may vary among different populations. A number of factors may contribute to this variation. Areas with high AIDS incidence may experience increased demands on resources in order to report a large and growing number of cases, resulting in longer reporting lags and incomplete case ascertainment. Moreover, persons who meet the immunologic criteria for AIDS may be clinically well and therefore not recognize their risk or undergo HIV and CD4+ T-lymphocyte testing. These persons will likely develop an AIDS-defining opportunistic infection eventually, and they may be reported at a later stage of disease progression. The 1993 AIDS case definition is expected to capture an increasing proportion of outpatient cases because the newly included clinical and immunologic conditions occur among some persons who are not so severely ill as to require hospitalization. Thus, reporting of these patients, who may be seen in private care settings, is likely to be less complete. In the future, the data may have inherent biases, which will also reflect increased access to and use of HIV and CD4+ T-lymphocyte testing as well as follow-up care. Similar limitations apply to HIV infection reporting data. Evaluation of the completeness and representativeness of HIV and AIDS surveillance data will remain an important ongoing priority (22).

Another limitation to consider is the lag that occurs between the date AIDS is diagnosed and the date the case is reported to CDC. Approximately 85% of cases are reported to CDC within 1 year of diagnosis. Similarly, lags occur in the reporting of AIDS-related mortality. Therefore, to accurately monitor trends and forecast the future effects of this epidemic, surveillance data are analyzed by using statistical adjustments to account for delays in the reporting of newly diagnosed AIDS cases (23).

Health departments' confidence in the usefulness of HIV/AIDS surveillance data depends largely on the completeness and accuracy of the reporting systems. To promote providers' compliance with case-reporting requirements, we must ensure the confidentiality of reported information. HIV/AIDS surveillance data are protected with a federal assurance of confidentiality. To protect the physical security and confidentiality of HIV/AIDS surveillance data, CDC and state and local health departments have instituted policies and procedures including restricted access to case reports, alarm systems, and legal statutes with penalties for the unauthorized disclosure of patient information (9).

In general, HIV seroprevalence surveys are conducted in selected geographic areas to measure prevalent HIV infection in targeted populations at sites such as sentinel hospitals, sexually transmitted disease clinics, and substance abuse treatment clinics. To protect confidentiality and reduce selection bias, these surveys usually are conducted in an anonymous, unlinked fashion, with-

out personal identifiers. Thus, the information that is collected usually is limited to selected demographic characteristics. Detailed information on clinical status and mode of HIV transmission is usually not available. Monitoring trends over time by risk group or clinical characteristics is not feasible for most surveys. The completeness of reporting demographic data varies markedly among states participating in CDC's national survey of childbearing women. Few states can provide the details needed to estimate HIV prevalence among childbearing women (or the incidence among children), by age, race, or other demographic group. Nevertheless, this survey provides complete, relatively unbiased estimates of HIV seroprevalence, measured in time and place, among women delivering live-born infants (15). Therefore, this national survey provides an invaluable adjunct to the surveillance of AIDS among women and children by providing information on the current effects of the epidemic on these populations, only a small proportion of which have developed AIDS.

EXAMPLES OF USING DATA

Data from HIV/AIDS surveillance systems are collected for the purposes of disease prevention and control. Public health planning requires timely dissemination of complete, accurate data that reflect the effects of the disease in the population. National, state, and local legislators, public health professionals, and health-care practitioners use surveillance data extensively to document the need for resources and to target prevention and treatment services to populations at risk of HIV infection. For effective public health promotion and early intervention to prevent the further spread of HIV, surveillance data must adequately characterize affected populations. The examples that follow illustrate how HIV/AIDS surveillance and seroprevalence data have been used to develop policies and programs that have directly affected the course of this epidemic (14,24).

At the national level, CDC has used both HIV/AIDS surveillance data and information on seroprevalence in selected populations to plan, target, and implement counseling and testing services (24). The completeness of coverage of these testing/prevention programs can be assessed by comparing data from seroprevalence surveys with

FIGURE 2. HIV seroprevalence among childbearing women—
United States, 1991

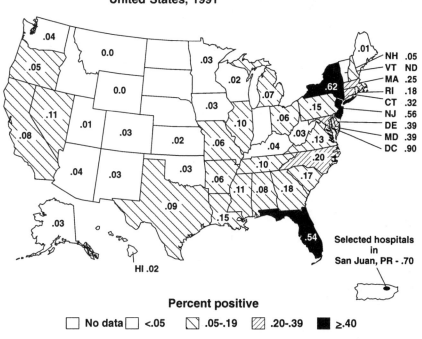

HIV/AIDS surveillance data. For example, the effectiveness of policies to offer HIV testing routinely to pregnant women can be assessed by comparing the number of HIV-infected women from the survey of childbearing women in a given period with the number of women reported with HIV/AIDS who delivered an infant during the same period. Various government public health agencies also use HIV/AIDS surveillance data to mobilize funds and distribute resources and programs to areas and populations most in need. For example, the Health Resources and Services Administration awards funds for HIV/AIDS consortia, which provide direct patient care services, on the basis of the level of AIDS incidence in eligible states and communities. The National Institute on Drug Abuse allocates funding for needle-exchange programs on the basis of AIDS data on injection drug users and seroprevalence rates in drug-treatment clinic surveys. In addition, the Department of Housing and Urban Development uses surveillance data to identify cities needing assistance in providing homes and shelter for AIDS patients. The National Institutes of Health uses the data to prioritize research programs on the manifestations of HIV disease, to target populations for natural history/disease pathogenesis studies, and to identify populations for clinical therapy trials and vaccine research.

At the state and local levels, HIV/AIDS surveillance and seroprevalence data are used to predict the future effects of the epidemic so as to plan for needed medical and social resources. Data are provided to policy makers, the medical community, and the public through routine dissemination of surveillance data and seroprevalence survey findings via newsletters, press reports, professional meetings, and information/education campaigns. For example, some states with high prevalences of HIV used data from the national survey of childbearing women to establish uniform recommendations that obstetricians and gynecologists routinely offer voluntary prenatal HIV testing to women. States also have used data collected through their HIV infection reporting systems and surveys of Job Corps applicants to implement age-specific and culturally sensitive prevention programs targeted to teens. Local community-based organizations often use surveillance and seroprevalence data from hospitals and clinics to apply for funds; plan and develop prevention, treatment, and social support services; and evaluate the acceptability and effects of these services (24).

Another important use of surveillance data is to examine changes in incidence and prevalence over time, and therefore, indirectly evaluate the effects of prevention programs. Persons with newly acquired HIV infection represent the failure of prevention activities. HIV reporting and seroprevalence data help to characterize persons who do not access counseling and testing services or who do not effectively adopt HIV prevention behaviors. The effectiveness of therapies that aim to prevent or delay disease progression can be monitored indirectly through the prevalence of AIDS-defining opportunistic infections. Careful monitoring of temporal trends in these surveillance systems is a very useful means of evaluating the effects of prevention and therapeutic strategies.

FUTURE ISSUES

We must address a broad range of issues to change the course of the HIV epidemic: promoting and adopting prevention strategies; enhancing public awareness of HIV; ensuring the confidentiality of patient information in medical-care settings and public health surveillance systems; and improving access to and availability of services for persons with HIV infection. To reduce the HIV epidemic's effects on women, we must increase women's access to early, ongoing preventive services (including gynecologic care) as well as care and treatment services. By improving prevention efforts targeted to women, we can reduce the incidence and prevalence of HIV among women, which will ultimately reduce the number of infected infants. We also need to increase the proportion of injection drug users who are in substance abuse treatment programs in order to reduce the incidence of HIV infection among drug users and their sex and needle-sharing partners. If current or future therapies can delay or prevent disease progression, we can reduce the incidence of AIDS by ensuring early access to life-prolonging therapies among persons already infected. To monitor the effects of intervention programs, we must focus on specific surveillance and data needs that have been identified through collaborations between state/local health departments and CDC: monitoring HIV infection and related diseases; assessing public knowledge and HIV-related risk behaviors; and monitoring the effectiveness of prevention and treatment services.

Providing preventive and therapeutic services to women and children requires a flexible and responsive medical and social structure to accommodate the multiple burdens of poverty, drug abuse, and inadequate health care in households where the woman, her spouse or partner, and her children may all be infected with HIV (5). HIV afflicts families as a group; mothers of adult children with HIV, wives and partners of men with HIV infection, mothers of infants and young children with HIV infection, all provide both primary care and financial support to families. In 1990, HIV was the sixth leading cause of death among women aged 25–44 years (25). The orphaned children of HIV-infected women who have died represent a growing social concern (26). Most of these children are not infected and will require extensive resources in the future. Further, CDC projects that women, children, and minorities—especially blacks and Hispanics—will be disproportionately affected by the epidemic in the foreseeable future (3,4).

HIV/AIDS surveillance programs and seroprevalence surveys, at national and state/local levels, must continue to effectively monitor the epidemic so that we can characterize HIV-infected persons in need of interventions and services and assess the effects of interventions on the epidemic's spread. Data collected through HIV/AIDS surveillance and seroprevalence surveys are important tools that improve the ability of communities to plan for and meet the needs of affected populations.

ADDITIONAL RESOURCES

For additional information on AIDS surveillance data, contact the CDC National AIDS Clearinghouse, P.O. Box 6003, Rockville, MD 20849-6003; (800) 458-5231.

REFERENCES

1. CDC. HIV/AIDS surveillance report. Atlanta: US Department of Health and Human Services, Public Health Service, CDC, February 1993:1–23.

2. CDC. Estimates of HIV prevalence and projected AIDS cases: summary of a workshop, October 31– November 1, 1989. MMWR 1990;39:110–2,117–9.

3. CDC. HIV prevalence estimates and AIDS case projections for the United States: report based upon a workshop. MMWR 1990;39(No. RR-16):1–31.

4. CDC. Projections of the number of persons diagnosed with AIDS and the number of immunosuppressed HIV-infected persons, United States, 1992–1994. MMWR 1992;41 (No. RR-18):1–29.

5. Fleming PL, Gwinn M, Oxtoby MJ. Epidemiology of HIV infection. In: Yogev R, Connor E, eds. Management of HIV infection in infants and children. St. Louis, Missouri: Mosby Year Book, 1992:7–22.

6. Fleming PL, Ciesielski CA, Byers RH, Castro KG, Berkelman RL. Gender differences in reported AIDS-indicative diagnoses. J Infect Dis 1993;168:61–7.

7. Mann JM, Makadon HJ, Silin J. What can we expect from the 1993 International Conference on AIDS? JAMA 1993;269:2895–6.

8. Council of State and Territorial Epidemiologists, CDC. Revision of the CDC surveillance case definition for acquired immunodeficiency syndrome. MMWR 1987; 36:1–15S.

9. CDC. 1993 revised classification system for HIV infection and expanded surveillance case definition for AIDS among adolescents and adults. MMWR 1992;41(No. RR-17):1–19.

10. CDC. Update: public health surveillance for HIV-infection—United States, 1989 and 1990. MMWR 1990;39:853,859–61.

11. Pappaioanou M, Dondero TJ, Petersen LR, Onorato IM, Sanchez CD, Curren JW. The family of HIV sero-prevalence surveys: objectives, methods, and uses of sentinel surveillance for HIV in the United States. Public Health Rep 1990;105:113–9.

12. CDC. Classification system for human immunodeficiency virus (HIV) infection in children under 13 years of age. MMWR 1987;36:225–230, 235.

13. CDC. Interpretation and use of the Western blot assay for serodiagnosis of human immunodeficiency virus type 1 infections. MMWR 1989;38(no. S-7):1–7.

14. CDC. Public health uses of HIV-infection reports—South Carolina, 1986–1991. MMWR 1992;41:245–9.

15. Gwinn M, Pappaioanou M, George JR, et al. Prevalence of HIV infection in childbearing women in the United States. JAMA 1991;265:1704–8.

16. CDC. National HIV serosurveillance summary. Results though 1990. Atlanta: US Department of Health and Human Services, Public Health Service, CDC, 1991.

17. Rosenblum L, Buehler JW, Morgan MW, et al. The completeness of AIDS case reporting, 1988: a multisite collaborative surveillance project. Am J Public Health 1992;82:1495–9.

18. Oxtoby MJ. Perinatally acquired HIV infection. In: Pizzo PA, Wilfert CM, eds. Pediatric AIDS: the challenge of HIV infection in infants, children, and adolescents. Baltimore: Williams and Wilkins, 1991.

19. CDC. Update: acquired immunodeficiency syndrome—United States, 1991. MMWR 1992;41:463–8.

20. CDC. Update: acquired immunodeficiency syndrome—United States, 1992. MMWR 1993;42:547–57.

21. Nwanyanwu OC, Conti LA, Ciesielski CA, et al. Increasing frequency of heterosexually transmitted AIDS in southern Florida: artifact or reality? Am J Public Health 1993;83:571–3.

22. CDC. Impact of the expanded AIDS surveillance case definition on AIDS case reporting—United States, first quarter, 1993. MMWR 1993;42:308–10.

23. Karon JM, Devine OJ, Morgan WM. Predicting AIDS incidence by extrapolating from recent trends. In: Castillo-Chavez C, Levin S, eds. Mathematical and statistical approaches to AIDS epidemiology: lecture notes in biomathematics. Vol 83. Berlin: Springer-Verlag, 1989.

24. Onorato IM, Gwinn M, Dondero TJ. From HIV serosurveillance to prevention: lessons from the CDC's family of surveys. Public Health Rep 1994 (in press).

25. Selik RM, Chu SY, Buehler JW. HIV infection as leading cause of death among young adults in US cities and states. JAMA 1993;269:2991–4.

26. Caldwell MB, Fleming PL, Oxtoby MJ. Estimated number of AIDS orphans in the United States. Pediatrics 1992;90:482.

Infertility

Anjani Chandra, Ph.D.[1]

PUBLIC HEALTH IMPORTANCE

Physicians in the United States typically classify couples as infertile if they have been unable to conceive a pregnancy after 12 months or more without contraception. In 1988, this definition could be applied to about 2.3 million U.S. couples with wives aged 15–44 years, or one in 12 married women (1). Another useful measure of infertility is impaired fecundity, which includes unmarried as well as married women and encompasses problems with pregnancy loss as well with becoming pregnant. In 1988, 4.9 million women—or one in 12 females aged 15–44 years—had impaired fecundity. Among married women, 3.1 million, or one in 10, had impaired fecundity.

The rates of infertility in less industrialized nations are markedly higher, and infectious diseases are responsible for a greater proportion of infertility than in the United States and other industrialized nations (2–5). Despite the low and relatively constant levels of infertility over the past three decades, a number of demographic and social factors have contributed to the misperception of an **infertility epidemic** in the United States (1–6).

- Delayed childbearing and the aging of baby boomers have increased the absolute numbers of couples trying to have their first children at ages when it is considerably more difficult. Because older couples have fewer years in which to achieve their desired family size, they may seek help more quickly, thereby inflating the demand for infertility services.

- Dramatic increases in physician visits for infertility have drawn immense media interest. In 1968, 600,000 office visits were for infertility services compared with 1.7 million in 1991. Between 1982 and 1988, the number of women reporting a visit for infertility services in the previous year grew by 25%.

- The number of physicians trained to provide specialized infertility services has soared over the past 20 years.

- New infertility drugs and treatment procedures have been developed in the last two decades. With each new treatment option, tremendous publicity has been generated about infertility and the resulting medical, legal, and ethical issues of infertility services. As more hope for overcoming infertility is created, more people may be motivated to seek medical help.

- The decreased number of infants, especially white infants, available for adoption has increased the proportions of couples of all ages who seek medical and legal assistance to have a baby (7).

Although infertility does not represent a serious public health threat in the United States, it carries significant personal, societal, and economic consequences that call for surveillance and action. Diagnosis and treatment are very costly, time-consuming, and invasive, and they can place immense stress on marital and family relations. Clearly, the financial and personal costs pose a significant barrier to many who face the disappointments of infertility. National data sources describing infertile couples may suggest ways to

[1] Division of Vital Statistics
National Center for Health Statistics
Centers for Disease Control and Prevention
Hyattsville, Maryland

prevent infertility and improve access to infertility services.

One of the Public Health Service's year 2000 national health objectives is to reduce the prevalence of infertility from 8% to 6.5% (8). Much of this reduction will depend on our success in identifying risk factors for infertility and lowering the rates of risk factors that are preventable—primarily sexually transmitted diseases (STDs) and pelvic inflammatory disease (PID). Because of the relatively high prevalence and young age distribution of STDs in the United States, their impact on PID, ectopic pregnancy, and infertility may not be seen for many years (9). Only by regularly monitoring these trends can we accurately estimate the total need for infertility services in the coming decades.

The wide social and economic disparities in infertility services sought by American women represent yet another reason for monitoring infertility in the United States. Women who seek infertility services are not representative of all women who are infertile (10,11). Continued surveillance is critical for shedding light on these inequities and identifying the barriers that women face in meeting their childbearing goals. For both men and women, infertility frustrates one of the most basic of human desires (6).

Moreover, as greater numbers of couples seek medical help with infertility, the need to ensure the quality and cost-effectiveness of the services received becomes more urgent. Medical care for persons with infertility poses unique challenges to professionals striving to ensure standardization and quality control, largely because the potential to help infertile couples varies widely. Many demographic, behavioral, and clinical factors determine the prognosis for each infertile couple. In addition to identifying predictors of success, infertility services research has addressed other questions such as these (12):

- What constitutes a standard infertility workup?

- What are the most accurate and cost-effective diagnostic tools for specific classes of infertility?

- How are treatment success rates affected by the diagnostic mix of patients and the different definitions of **success**?

- How much should services cost, and to what extent should insurance cover these costs?

The national surveillance data presented in this chapter cannot answer these questions directly, but they provide the demographic and epidemiologic backdrop needed to evaluate clinic-based studies, which are known to be based on highly selected groups of infertile individuals—namely, those who actually pursue medical help (for additional information about related topics and surveillance activities, see the Contraception and Sexually Transmitted Diseases chapters).

HISTORY OF DATA COLLECTION

In the United States, only one source has provided reliable national data on infertility: the National Survey of Family Growth (NSFG) and its predecessor surveys, the Growth of American Families Study in 1955 and 1960 and the National Fertility Survey in 1965 and 1970 (see the Contraception chapter for background information). Since 1973, CDC's National Center for Health Statistics (NCHS) has periodically conducted the NSFG to ask national samples of women about their pregnancies, reproductive health, infertility, and basic social and economic characteristics. To date, four NSFGs have been conducted—in 1973, 1976, 1982, and 1988. Work is presently underway on the 1994 NSFG, which will contain an enhanced set of infertility questions.

Between 1978 and 1984, the World Health Organization conducted a multinational, multicenter study of infertility in both developed and developing countries, collecting data on 2,500 couples. The chief purpose of this study was to provide a standardized approach for diagnosing infertility. Because the study was clinic-based, investigators were unable to estimate the prevalence of infertility. Nevertheless, these findings represent the largest database of demographic, epidemiologic, and clinical information on couples seeking medical help for infertility *(2)*.

Several data sources provide information on infertility services and service providers. In addition to collecting data on services in the 1982 and 1988 NSFGs, NCHS has conducted the National Ambulatory Medical Care Survey and found that nearly 400,000 new patients are seen for infertility each year—at more than double the rate in 1966. In 1991, 1.7 million physicians' visits were made in which infertility was mentioned as at least one of three top reasons for the visit. In 1985, the Alan Guttmacher Institute surveyed private physicians in four specialties: obstetrics/gynecology, urology, general/family practice, and surgery. These data sources, along with several European studies *(6,13,14)*, have given comparable pictures of the levels and predictors of service-seeking among infertile couples. On average, less than two thirds of infertile couples seek medical help, and the rates of service-seeking are highest among persons who are well educated, older, and of a higher-than-average income status.

CDC SURVEILLANCE ACTIVITIES

Definition of Terms

The NSFG produces data on two measures of infertility: **infertility status** and **impaired fecundity. Infertility status** reflects the standard medical definition of infertility used in the United States—a case in which a married couple is not surgically sterilized, has not used contraception, and has not become pregnant for at least 12 months *(15)*.

In the 1982 and 1988 NSFGs, an **impaired fecundity** measure was formulated to determine if it was difficult, impossible, or dangerous for a woman to become pregnant or carry a pregnancy to term. This broader measure of infertility has potentially greater utility for planning and monitoring services because it 1) includes women regardless of marital status,* and 2) encompasses

problems with pregnancy loss as well as with getting pregnant. The goal of individuals with fertility problems is, after all, to have a healthy baby.

Women who did not report any sterilizing operations (e.g., tubal ligation, hysterectomy) were classified as having impaired fecundity on the basis of their answers to the following series of questions:

- Some women find it physically impossible to have (more) children. As far as you know, is it physically possible or impossible for you to conceive a(nother) baby, that is, to get pregnant (again)?

- What about your husband? Is it physically possible or impossible for him to father a(nother) child?

- Some people are able to have a baby but have difficulty getting pregnant or holding onto the baby. As far as you know, is there any problem or difficulty for you (and your husband) to conceive or deliver a(nother) baby?

- Does your husband have any difficulty fathering a child?

- Has a doctor ever told you **never** to become pregnant (again)?

Women were considered to have impaired fecundity if they gave any of the following responses:

- They said it was impossible or physically difficult to conceive or deliver a baby.

- They said that a doctor had told them never to become pregnant again because the pregnancy would pose a danger to them, the baby, or both.

- They said they or their husbands were infertile (were continuously married, did not use contraception, and did not become pregnant) for 36 months or more.

---

* The impaired fecundity measure was used in the 1976 NSFG, but the 1982 NSFG was the first cycle to include women of all marital statuses. Trends since 1976 can be examined for currently married women only.

Use of Medical Services for Infertility

In the 1982 and 1988 NSFGs, all women, regardless of marital or contraceptive status, were asked the following questions about using infertility services:

- Have you (or your husband) ever been to a doctor or clinic to talk about ways to help you become pregnant?

- (Not counting routine care or advice about a pregnancy), have you (or your husband) ever been to a doctor or clinic to talk about ways to help you prevent a miscarriage?

Women who answered "yes" to either of these questions were considered to have sought medical help for infertility. In the 1982 survey, women were asked an open-ended question about specific services they or their husbands received, and in the 1988 survey, women identified specific services from a list (Table 1).

GENERAL FINDINGS

NSFG data indicate that one in 12 currently married American women (8%) was infertile in 1988. This overall rate did not change **significantly** between 1965 and 1988, nor did infertility rates change within specific age-groups (Figure 1).

In the 1988 NSFG, about 4.9 million married and unmarried females aged 15–44 years (one in 12) were found to have impaired fecundity. Among women who were married at the time of the survey, about 3.1 million women (roughly one in 10) had impaired fecundity compared with 2.3 million women (one in 12) who were infertile. These rates had changed little since 1982.

The precise role of factors such as age on infertility is challenging to identify because risk

TABLE 1. Use of infertility services among females aged 15–44 years — United States, 1988

Type of service	Number of women (in thousands)	Percentage of women who ever used services	Percentage of all females aged 15–44 years (N = 57.9 million)
Any infertility services	6,756	100.0	12
Advice on becoming pregnant (e.g., timing of intercourse)	3,537	52	6
Tests on male partner	2,224	33	4
Tests on female partner	2,105	31	4
Ovulation drugs	1,901	28	3
Bed rest	1,560	23	3
Treatment of blocked tubes	1,018	15	2
Advice on starting or stopping contraception	946	14	2
Artificial insemination	369	6	1
In vitro fertilization	145	2	0.3
Other	1,070	16	2

FIGURE 1. Prevalence of infertility among married females* aged 15–44 years — United States, 1965–1988

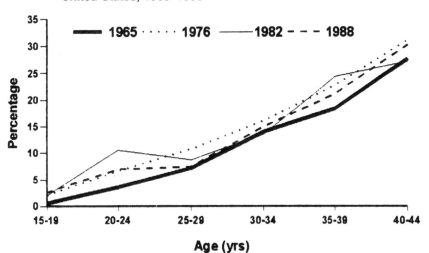

* Excluding surgically sterilized females.

factors and demographic characteristics are often highly intercorrelated. The NSFG, as a primarily demographic fertility survey, gives us data on factors such as age, parity, race, and the use of infertility services, whereas epidemiologic studies provide information pertaining to important medical and behavioral factors related to infertility.

Because the definition of impaired fecundity includes unmarried women and women having difficulties carrying to term, we focus on this broader measure of infertility when presenting NSFG data. For the most part, the 12-month infertility status measure shows similar trends, levels, and correlates, and we discuss these issues when appropriate.

Age and Parity

Population- and clinic-based research studies have demonstrated that fertility declines as women get older; the debate generally centers on the critical age, with most studies showing substantial declines after age 35 or 40 years (16,17). Age and parity (the number of live births) are discussed together here because their role in fertility problems is closely linked.

Impaired fecundity increases with age, particularly after age 35, and the rates are higher among women with no previous births (parity 0) (Table

2). These nulliparous women are referred to as having **primary** impaired fecundity, whereas women experiencing difficulty having a second or higher-order birth are referred to as having **secondary** impaired fecundity. Among women who have had one or more births, impaired fecundity does not increase significantly with age, largely because surgical sterilization occurs more frequently among older women, and fewer older women are **at risk** of impaired fecundity.

Using the 12-month definition among currently married women and excluding surgically sterilized women, CDC researchers found that age-specific infertility rates (all parities taken together) have remained fairly constant in the United States since 1965 (within the sampling error of each survey), but they observed a distinct rise in infertility with increasing age (Figure 1). With regard to parity, between 1965 and 1988, the proportion of infertile couples trying to have a first birth (i.e., primary infertility) increased dramatically, from one in six to one in two married infertile couples. These figures reflect the trends of delayed marriage and delayed childbearing in marriage throughout the past 30 years.

Education and Occupation

Education level and occupational status are frequently used as proxy measures for socioeco-

TABLE 2. Number of females aged 15–44 years and percentage distribution* of those who are fecund, by fecundity status, parity, and age — United States, 1982 and 1988

Parity, by age	All women (no. in thousands)		Surgically sterile (%)		Impaired fecundity (%)		Fecund (%)	
	1988	1982	1988	1982	1988	1982	1988	1982
All parity								
15–44 years	57,900	54,099	28.0	25.2	8.4	8.4	63.6	66.3
15–24 years	18,592	20,150	2.2	2.3	4.8	4.3	93.0	93.4
25–34 years	21,726	19,644	25.6	25.9	9.6	10.0	64.7	64.2
35–44 years	17,582	14,305	58.3	57.0	10.6	12.1	31.0	31.0
0 parity								
15–44 years	25,129	22,941	4.3	3.1	8.8	8.4	86.9	88.5
15–24 years	14,978	15,547	0.2	0.1	4.1	4.1	95.7	95.8
25–34 years	7,252	5,628	4.7	5.1	13.4	14.7	82.0	80.2
35–44 years	2,899	1,766	25.0	23.0	21.4	25.7	53.6	51.3
≥1 parity								
15–44 years	32,771	31,158	46.1	41.7	8.1	8.5	45.8	49.9
15–24 years	3,164	4,603	10.5	9.6	7.7	5.2	81.8	85.2
25–34 years	14,474	14,016	36.1	34.2	7.8	8.1	56.1	57.8
35–44 years	14,683	12,539	64.8	61.7	8.5	10.1	26.7	28.1

* Because of rounding, percentages may not total 100%.

nomic status, but they have some limitations. NSFG data from 1982 suggest that infertile women (using the 12-month definition and including only married women) were less likely to have an education level beyond high school, and they were more likely to work in lower-status jobs (10,18). When all women are included, regardless of marital status, however, education and occupation are unrelated to impaired fecundity (11). These factors are closely linked to the use of medical care for infertility, which contributes to the impression that infertility is more frequent among women with higher education or higher-status jobs.

Race and Ethnicity

Analyses of 1982 NSFG data had suggested that infertile couples are more likely to be black than white and that this race gap is widest for couples with secondary infertility (18). The apparent link between race and infertility, particularly infertility due to tubal or pelvic problems, is confounded by socioeconomic differences in factors associated with infertility as well as in patterns of seeking services for infertility. For example, rates of STDs and PID have been found to be higher among blacks than among whites (9,10).

Infertile black women are less likely to seek medical help than infertile white women (10,11,18). This is probably related to the fact that black women, on average, have lower levels of education and income than white women.

CDC investigators found that neither race nor Hispanic origin is related to impaired fecundity after controlling for a history of PID treatment (Wilcox LS, Mosher WD, unpublished data, 1994).

Behavioral Factors

The National Fertility Survey and NSFG data do not include sufficient details for assessing behavioral factors; however, numerous epidemiologic and clinical studies have well characterized the behavioral risk factors for specific classes of infertility. Cigarette smoking has been tied to longer time to conception, ovulatory and tubal disorders, and fetal and early infant death. In addition, women whose mothers smoked during pregnancy were found to take longer to become pregnant themselves (19). The precise effects of caffeine consumption, alcohol use, and other drug use are still under investigation and pose many difficulties in defining and measuring exposure.

The role of certain birth control methods, such as intrauterine device (IUDs) and oral contraceptives, also continue to be investigated. Only specific types of IUDs (e.g., the Dalkon Shield) and high-estrogen-dose birth control pills appear to place women at risk of developing fertility problems (20,21). The complex mechanisms whereby sexually transmitted infections can lead to PID, ectopic pregnancy, and infertility have been described elsewhere (9).

Use of Services

The 1982 and 1988 NSFG found that the most common service sought was advice on becoming pregnant; more than half of the women who received any services reported getting instructions on timing intercourse during the fertile period of the menstrual cycle or measuring basal body temperature to predict the time of ovulation. Nearly one third of service-seekers reported infertility testing for themselves or their husbands. Ovulation drug treatment was the most common specialized treatment—sought by 28% of service-seekers and 3% of all females aged 15–44 years (Table 1).

Between the 1982 and 1988 NSFG surveys, the number of women who reported using infertility services in the previous 12 months increased 25%—from 1.08 to 1.35 million women (1). Service-seekers in both surveys were more likely to be white, college-educated, married, and of a higher-income status than infertile women who never sought medical help for infertility (10,11,18).

In 1988, users of infertility services were more likely than nonusers to be non-Hispanic white, college-educated, of a higher income status, >30 years of age, nulliparous, or ever married (Table 3). For example, infertile women >30 years of age who had never been pregnant were 1.5 times as likely to seek medical help than were their counterparts <30 years of age (58% vs. 39%). The percentage of women who received infertility services rose steadily with income, ranging from 24% to 52%. College-educated women were 50% more likely to have received services than were high school graduates (60% vs. about 40%).

Thus, women who use infertility services represent a highly selected subgroup of the population of infertile females. Studies in other industrialized nations have reached similar conclusions—that the need for infertility services is unmet among persons with low incomes and less education (2,4,13,14).

INTERPRETATION ISSUES

Numerous studies have shown that the way that infertility is defined can affect the estimates of

TABLE 3. Percentage of females* aged 15–44 years receiving any infertility services, by selected characteristics — United States, 1988

Characteristic	Any service
Total	43
Race/ethnicity	
Hispanic	31
Non-Hispanic white	47
Non-Hispanic black	30
Education (years)[†]	
0–11	32
12	40
13–15	42
≥16	60
Income[§]	
0–149	24
150–399	43
≥400	52
Age/parity[¶]	
15–29/0	39
15–29/≥1	29
30–44/0	58
30–44/≥1	42
Marital status	
Never married	24
Currently married	48
Previously married	38

* Among 5.3 million females with impaired fecundity or infertility.
[†] Among women aged 20–44 years.
[§] Percentage of poverty level income; among women aged 20–44 years.
[¶] For age/parity groups, 15–29/0 and 15–29/≥1 indicate women aged 15–29 years with 0 or ≥1 parity; 30–44/0 and 30–44/≥1 indicate women aged 30–44 years with 0 or ≥1 parity.

prevalence, the identification of risk factors, and prognosis (2,22–24). For example, the standard medical definition in the United States is 12 months of unprotected intercourse without pregnancy, whereas the World Health Organization and many European countries use a 24-month criterion. The results of demographic studies of conception indicate that the average waiting time to conception is 7.5 months, which means that about 10% of women will not become pregnant after 12 months of trying, and about 5% will not become pregnant after 24 months (25). The NSFG prevalence estimate of 8% of married women is well in line with these figures. Some infertile women, identified in the NSFGs or in clinical studies, may simply represent the **tail** of the normal distribution of waiting times to conception; after additional months, some of them may become pregnant, regardless of whether they receive medical help. Amidst this statistical debate, we should further consider that the usefulness of the 12-month or 24-month criterion depends on many other factors—most importantly, age and medical history. For example, a woman whose fallopian tubes are completely blocked or whose husband produces no sperm (azoospermia) will be infertile after one month as well as after many years of trying to conceive, unless medical help is obtained.

In addition to the time frame used to define infertility, another methodologic issue affecting prevalence and prognosis is the definition of primary and secondary infertility (26). Secondary infertility, in which a prior pregnancy has occurred, generally carries a better prognosis for future fertility than primary infertility, in which no prior pregnancy has occurred. Clinicians recognize that infertility is often a couple-based problem—that is, either partner may be able to get pregnant with someone else, but they have difficulty conceiving with each other. Clinicians have not reached a consensus, however, about how to define prior fertility status. A couple-based definition of primary infertility would require that no prior pregnancy had occurred in the partnership, whereas secondary infertility would mean that one or more pregnancies had occurred. Woman-based definitions are often used in clinical practice. Under these definitions, a woman who has never been pregnant would be classified as having primary infertility, whereas a

woman who has ever been pregnant would be classified as having secondary infertility. When presenting their published results, investigators do not always clarify which definitions of primary and secondary infertility they used, and this omission can lead to confusing estimates of prevalence and prognosis.

EXAMPLES OF USING DATA

Although the NSFG does not provide infertility data for individual states, this survey, along with other surveillance and epidemiologic research on infertility, has been used extensively over the past 15 years to formulate and justify state-level, infertility-related legislation in numerous areas (6):

- Insurance policies.

- Standardization of diagnosis and treatment procedures, and other quality-control measures.

- Registry of in vitro fertilization procedures and other assisted reproductive technologies.

- Targeted prevention programs.

More recently, national surveillance efforts have played a key role in encouraging the enactment of federal statutes for the regulation and quality control of infertility services (e.g, the In Vitro Fertilization Registry conducted by the American Fertility Society) and insurance coverage in a growing number of states.

FUTURE ISSUES

Results on infertility and infertility services from the 1994 NSFG should be available in 1996. This survey design includes periodic follow-up interviews that will allow us to examine factors associated with infertility and the use of services over time.

Although we have limited new information on the population prevalence and other epidemiologic characteristics of infertile couples, several recent studies (12) may help us acquire a more complete picture of who is infertile, who seeks services, and what services are most helpful. These studies have focused on the epidemiologic and psychosocial evaluation of specific aspects of infertility services:

- Evaluations of the prognostic value and cost-effectiveness of some standard diagnostic techniques, such as the postcoital test and the timed endometrial biopsy.

- Establishment of more accurate prognostic guidelines for the use of various treatments, most notably in vitro fertilization and artificial insemination.

- Identification of more accurate and clinically relevant diagnosis groups to minimize fruitless or inappropriate treatment.

- Investigation of adverse effects of infertility treatments on women and their babies as well as the short- and long-term effects of service-seeking on personal and family well-being.

Future studies should address the difficult economic, legal, and ethical questions raised by infertility. For example, surrogate motherhood and donor embryos spark considerable debate over a person's **right** to have children and draw further public attention to infertility. Another challenge for translating data into policy is evident with research on fertility and age. Given that infertility rates generally increase with a woman's age, particularly over age 35 or 40, **and** given that the trends of delayed marriage and childbearing are unlikely to reverse, policies and interventions should focus on better educating women about their fertility prognosis and helping them achieve their desired family size.

Furthermore, because epidemiologic studies have given mixed results on risk factors, including age and STD history, more multidisciplinary research is needed to clarify the effects of these factors on fertility as well as the ramifications of specific prevention goals. This information will be critical for targeting prevention efforts more appropriately and realistically as well as for making services more responsive to the needs of infertile individuals.

REFERENCES

1. Mosher WD, Pratt WF. Fecundity and infertility in the United States, 1965–88. Hyattsville, Maryland: US Department of Health and Human Services, Public Health Service, CDC, 1990. (Advance data from vital and health statistics; no. 192).

2. Cates W, Farley TMM, Rowe PJ. Patterns of infertility in the developed and developing worlds. In: Rowe PJ, Vikhlyaeva EM, eds. Diagnosis and treatment of infertility. Toronto: Hans Huber Publishers (for the World Health Organization), 1988:57–67.

3. De Schryver A, Meheus A. Epidemiology of sexually transmitted diseases: the global picture. Bull World Health Organ 1990;68:639–54.

4. Högberg U, Sandström A, Nilsson NG. Reproductive patterns among Swedish women born 1936–1960. Acta Obstet Gynecol Scand 1992;71:207–14.

5. Thonneau P, Marchand S, Tallec A, et al. Incidence and main causes of infertility in a resident population (1,850,000) of three French regions (1988–1989). Hum Reprod 1991;6:811–6.

6. Office of Technology Assessment, US Congress. Infertility: medical and social choices. Washington: US Government Printing Office, 1988; publication no. OTA-BA-358.

7. Bachrach CA, Stolley KS, London KA. Relinquishment of premarital births: evidence from national survey data. Fam Plann Perspect 1992;24:27–32,48.

8. Public Health Service. Healthy people 2000: national health promotion and disease prevention objectives—full report, with commentary. Washington, DC: US Department of Health and Human Services, Public Health Service, 1991; DHHS publication no. (PHS) 91-50212.

9. Cates W Jr, Rolfs RT Jr, Aral SO. Sexually transmitted diseases, pelvic inflammatory disease, and infertility. Epidemiol Rev 1990;12:199–220.

10. Kalmuss D. The use of infertility services among fertility-impaired couples. Demography 1987;24:575–85.

11. Wilcox LS, Mosher WD. Use of infertility services in the United States. Obstet Gynecol 1993;82:122–7.

12. Chandra A, Gray RH. Epidemiology of infertility. Curr Opin Obstet Gynecol 1991;3:169–75.

13. Templeton A, Fraser C, Thompson B. The epidemiology of infertility in Aberdeen. BMJ 1990;301:148–52.

14. Templeton A, Fraser C, Thompson B. Infertility—epidemiology and referral practice. Hum Reprod 1991;6:1391–4.

15. Mosher WD. Reproductive impairments in the United States, 1965–1982. Demography 1985;22:415–30.

16.	Menken J, Trussell J, Larsen U. Age and infertility. Science 1986;233:1389–93.

17.	Newcomb WW, Rodriguez M, Johnson JWC. Reproduction in the older gravida: a literature review. J Reprod Med 1991;36:839–45.

18.	Hirsch MB, Mosher WD. Characteristics of infertile women in the United States and their use of infertility services. Fertil Steril 1987;47:618–25.

19.	Weinberg CR, Wilcox AJ, Baird DD. Reduced fecundability in women with prenatal exposure to cigarette smoking. Am J Epidemiol 1989;129:1072–8.

20.	Bracken MB, Hellenbrand KG, Holford TR. Conception delay after oral contraceptive use: the effect of estrogen dose. Fertil Steril 1990;53:21–7.

21.	Cramer DW, Goldman MB, Schiff I, et al. The relationship of tubal infertility to barrier method and oral contraceptive use. JAMA 1987;257:2446–50.

22.	Greenhall E, Vessey M. The prevalence of subfertility: a review of the current confusion and a report of two new studies. Fertil Steril 1990;54:978–83.

23.	Marchbanks PA, Peterson HB, Rubin GL, Wingo PA, Cancer and Steroid Hormone Study Group. Research on infertility: definition makes a difference. Am J Epidemiol 1989;130:259–67.

24.	McFalls JA Jr. The risks of reproductive impairment in the later years of childbearing. Ann Rev Sociol 1990;16: 491–519.

25.	Bongaarts J, Potter RG. Fertility, biology, and behavior: an analysis of the proximate determinants. New York: Academic Press, 1983.

26.	Collins JA, Garner JB, Wilson EH, Wrixon W, Casper RF. A proportional hazards analysis of the clinical characteristics of infertile couples. Am J Obstet Gynecol 1984;148:527–32.

Unintended Pregnancy and Childbearing

Linda J. Piccinino, M.P.S.[1]

PUBLIC HEALTH IMPORTANCE

Unintended pregnancies and births* are attracting national attention as public health problems that are once again on the rise. Although we have witnessed almost two decades of decline since 1965 (1), recent data for women who were ever married indicate that the prevalence of unintended births increased during the 1980s. Preliminary data for 1990 reveal that the level has reached a new high of 39% (Figure 1) (2). This increase suggests a reversal of the trend that we saw from 1965 to 1982.

Because unintended births constitute what appears to be an increasing proportion of all recent births from 1982 to 1990, the health and social costs of this increase could grow. A higher prevalence of unintended pregnancies and births implies that women are unnecessarily being exposed to the risk of additional morbidity and mortality.

A further consequence of unintended births is the postponement of prenatal care. Between

1982 and 1988, the receipt of prenatal care services was more likely to be delayed beyond the first trimester if the birth was unintended. Only about half (55%) of babies that were unwanted received early prenatal care, whereas almost three fourths (72%) of babies that were wanted at conception received such care (3).

Other research suggests that unintended births lead to more child abuse and neglect. In a relevant study of single mothers with very low incomes, Zuravin found that unintended births increased the risk of child abuse and neglect, especially in large families (4).

Unintended births largely result from failures in contraceptive use (5). Unintended births that occur because a woman has failed to use a contraceptive method correctly or because the method itself failed have important implications for family planning programs and for contraceptive development. Method failure indicates the need for better efforts to ensure proper and consistent use of modern methods as well as reliable backups for when these methods fail. Even with the array of effective methods currently available, additional methods are needed to satisfy user preferences. No one method is likely to be **perfect** for a woman over her entire reproductive life.

With mistimed births, factors such as changes in marital status, career crises, and gain or loss of employment can substantially affect the preferred timing of a birth even though it may be wanted eventually. A young woman who becomes pregnant in college at age 19, who

---

* The following are definitions of some terms used in this chapter (see glossary for additional definitions).

Unintended pregnancies include all pregnancies that were unintended (mistimed or unwanted) at conception—including those that result in live births, miscarriages, stillbirths, and abortions.

Unintended live births include two types of pregnancy outcomes—**mistimed births**, which occur sooner in a woman's life than she had intended and eventually are wanted, and **unwanted births.**

Wantedness status refers to whether the mother considered the pregnancy to be wanted, mistimed, or unwanted at conception.

Recent births are those births occurring within exactly 5 years before the mother's survey interview date for 1982 and 1988 and within 2 years before her interview for the 1990 reinterview survey.

---

[1] Division of Vital Statistics
National Center for Health Statistics
Centers for Disease Control and Prevention
Hyattsville, Maryland

really wanted to have her first birth at age 23 when she finished college, for example, might experience a need to delay or even terminate her education and career plans.

The problem of unintended pregnancies has become more pronounced in recent years because of the shorter duration of time in which women actually want to become pregnant. Women now spend many of their childbearing years trying to avoid unintended pregnancy because they tend to delay marriage and desire smaller families. The fact that many women experience long periods when they do not wish to become pregnant is an important issue for health-care providers and policymakers alike (for additional information about related topics and surveillance activities, see the Contraception, Legal Induced Abortion, Behavioral Risk Factors Before and During Pregnancy, Infant Mortality, and Pregnancy in Adolescents chapters).

HISTORY OF DATA COLLECTION

Since 1973, CDC's National Center for Health Statistics (NCHS) has conducted the National Survey of Family Growth (NSFG), collecting data on the wantedness status of pregnancies. Since then, data from three subsequent cycles of surveys (and a telephone reinterview survey) have allowed intersurvey comparisons and analysis of trends over time. Interviewing for the Cycle V NSFG began in 1994.

The CDC has also collected data on the wantedness status of pregnancies in other national and state surveys. In 1987, CDC collaborated with several states and the District of Columbia to establish an ongoing system for the surveillance of selected maternal behaviors. This system, known as the Pregnancy Risk Assessment Monitoring System (PRAMS), is designed to collect annual data to supplement vital records and to supply states with data to plan and assess their perinatal health programs (6). In 1988, NCHS conducted the first National Maternal and Infant Health Survey (NMIHS). The NMIHS is based on a sample of births in a particular year and focuses on the health of mothers and their infants. This survey is scheduled to be conducted again in 1996.

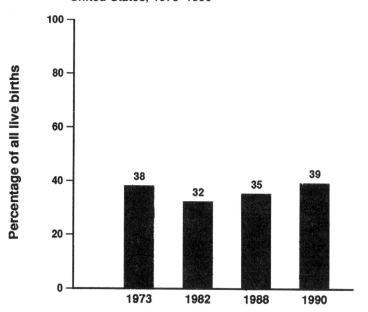

FIGURE 1. Percentage of recent live births* that were unintended pregnancies to ever-married women aged 15–44 years — United States, 1973–1990

* Births within exact 5 years of interview date.

Source: CDC/NCHS. NSFG, 1973 to 1988. Telephone reinterview, 1990 (preliminary data).

Since 1982, data on the wantedness status of all pregnancies have been collected annually for all female respondents participating in the National Longitudinal Survey of Youth (NLSY). This survey is conducted by the Center for Human Resource Research at the Ohio State University under the administration of the U.S. Department of Labor's Bureau of Labor Statistics. Although these data are constrained by the original 1979 NLSY cohort age-range (14–21 years), when weighted, they represent a national sample of women—aged 25–32 years on January 1, 1990 (or aged 14–21 years on January 1, 1979)—who have had at least one pregnancy (7). Most of the pregnancies in the sample are to younger women; the oldest women in the sample who have had pregnancies reached the age of 32 years by the latest survey.

Questions about whether the pregnancy was wanted, mistimed, or unwanted at conception were asked while the pregnancy was ongoing, in most cases; therefore, the data provide prospective measures of the wantedness status of births. A recent study using the NLSY focused on the wantedness status of first births and looked at the

74

factors that might be linked to whether a woman says that she wanted her first birth at the time of her pregnancy. The study findings suggest that marital status and race are important predictors of the wantedness status of first births to these women *(8)*.

CDC SURVEILLANCE ACTIVITIES

National Survey of Family Growth

The NSFG has always been a nationally representative sample of women of childbearing age. All women surveyed are from the noninstitutionalized population of the United States. Cycles I through IV of the NSFG were based on multistage area probability samples. The 1973 and 1976 surveys interviewed only females aged 15–44 years who were ever married; women of all marital statuses were interviewed for the first time in the Cycle III survey in 1982. In the Cycle IV survey, interviews were conducted from January through August 1988 with 8,450 women of all marital statuses. A telephone reinterview survey was conducted in 1990 on a subsample of 5,686 women who had been interviewed in 1988. Wantedness status information for women in the 1990 survey who were pregnant at the time of the 1988 survey was taken from the 1988 NSFG data tape for the tables presented in this chapter.

Sources of NSFG data include 1) the many NCHS Advance Data and Series 23 reports; 2) journal articles by researchers at NCHS and elsewhere; 3) conference presentations and publications; and 4) public use data tapes and tape documentation (information on how to order these resources can be found in the Contraception chapter).

The NSFG classified unintended pregnancies or births as those that were mistimed or unwanted at the time of conception. The following series of questions in the 1988 survey were used to classify pregnancies as intended (wanted), mistimed, or unwanted at conception:

1. At the time you became pregnant with (baby's name/the pregnancy that ended in month/year), did you, yourself, actually want to have a(nother) baby at **some** time?

2. Those who answered "yes" to question 1 were then asked: Did you become pregnant sooner than you wanted, later than you wanted, or at about the right time? Those who answered "no" to question 1 continued with the rest of the questionnaire.

3. In the Cycle IV survey, those who answered "don't know" to question 1 were then asked: It is sometimes difficult to recall these things but, just before the pregnancy began, would you say you probably wanted a(nother) baby at **some** time or probably not?

In the NSFG, pregnancies that were wanted but occurred sooner than the woman would have liked were considered mistimed. A pregnancy was classified as mistimed if the woman wanted a(nother) baby eventually, but not as soon as the pregnancy occurred (for example, she became pregnant at the age of 18 years but actually wanted to have her first child at the age of 21 years).

Pregnancies were labeled unwanted if the woman answered "no" to questions 1 or 3; that is, she reported that she did not or probably did not want a child at any time in the future. If the woman never wanted the pregnancy (for example, she wanted only two children, but became pregnant with her third child), the pregnancy was considered unwanted. Also, a pregnancy was considered unwanted at conception if 1) the woman stopped or did not use contraception for reasons other than trying to get pregnant, or 2) she became pregnant while using contraception and did not want a(nother) baby.

Pregnancy Risk Assessment Monitoring System

Information on various topics is collected from new mothers through a self-administered questionnaire mailed to them 2–6 months after delivery. Topics include the wantedness status of the birth, including the mother's attitudes and feelings about her pregnancy.

National Maternal and Infant Health Survey

The 1988 NMIHS data on unintended births can be analyzed along with a variety of accompanying health and socioeconomic measures. Women were asked to think back to just before they became pregnant and to state whether they wanted to become pregnant at that time. They also were asked about the outcome, any complications of the pregnancy, employment status around delivery, smoking and other health habits, prenatal care, income, and characteristics of the baby's father (9).

GENERAL FINDINGS

Unintended births are again at levels experienced in the early 1970s (Figure 1). According to 1988 NSFG data, more than one third (39%) of recent births to women of childbearing age, regardless of their marital status, were unintended (27% of these births were mistimed and 12% were unwanted) (Table 1). Thus, more than two thirds (68%) of the unintended births to women surveyed in 1988 were mistimed.

Between 1982 and 1988, the proportion of unintended births that were unwanted has been much smaller than the proportion of those that have been mistimed, however this proportion has increased for women overall, and also for black and white women (with the exception of white women aged 35–44 years) (Table 1). The percentage of births that were unintended was 36% for white women, but 59% for black women, partially because of the larger proportion of births among unmarried black women. Nevertheless, since 1982, the proportion of births among white women that were mistimed has increased slightly but declined among black women.

Data in the tables shown by race do not imply that differences are related to racial or genetic characteristics of the women per se. Such differences are more likely related to variations in

TABLE 1. Percentage of intended and unintended live births* among females aged 15–44 years, by race and age of mother — United States, 1982 and 1988

| Race and age (years) | Total† | Intended | | Unintended | | | | | |
| | | | | Mistimed | | Unwanted | | Total Unintended | |
		1982	1988	1982	1988	1982	1988	1982	1988
All races¶	100.0	63.5	60.6	26.6	26.8	9.8	12.3	36.4	39.1
15–19	100.0	20.7	14.8	64.5	63.4	14.9	21.8	79.3	85.2
20–24	100.0	49.6	45.7	42.7	41.1	8.0	13.0	50.4	54.1
25–34	100.0	71.8	66.6	19.4	23.1	8.8	10.1	28.2	33.2
35–44	100.0	71.8	68.3	10.4	13.5	17.7	18.1	28.0	31.6
White	100.0	66.9	63.8	25.5	26.8	7.7	9.2	33.1	36.0
15–19	100.0	20.7	17.0	71.4	65.3	7.9	17.6	79.3	82.9
20–24	100.0	52.4	49.4	42.3	42.6	5.3	7.7	47.6	50.3
25–34	100.0	74.5	68.2	18.5	23.5	7.0	8.1	25.5	31.6
35–44	100.0	74.0	71.6	10.2	14.0	15.8	14.1	26.0	28.1
Black	100.0	45.1	40.4	32.6	30.2	22.1	29.0	54.7	59.2
15–19	100.0	19.1	11.7	50.9	58.1	30.0	30.2	80.9	88.3
20–24	100.0	38.7	33.8	41.3	35.6	20.0	30.7	61.3	66.3
25–34	100.0	53.1	51.3	25.0	24.4	21.6	23.5	46.6	47.9
35–44	100.0	57.9	38.7	15.7	14.8	24.4	46.5	40.1	61.3

* Includes births occurring <5 years from the date of interview.
† Total includes births of unknown wantedness status.
¶ All races includes white, black and other races. Other races are not shown separately.

Source: National Survey of Family Growth, 1982 and 1988.

income and educational levels, with minority women often being associated with lower income and educational levels, limited access to health care and insurance, and other factors. These socioeconomic differences require further investigation if we are to better understand the underlying causes of these differentials.

The prevalence of recent births that were unintended over all age-groups increased between 1982 and 1988 (Table 1). For black women (except those aged 35–44 years) and white women classified by age in 1988, the percentage of births that were unintended declined with age. The probability of contraceptive failure also declines as women get older, which partially accounts for the decrease in mistimed births among older women (5). However, as has been true for the past decade, most unintended births are mistimed births. Unwanted births cluster at the youngest and oldest age-groups (Table 1).

The highest percentage of births that were unintended among all races, and among black and white women separately, is among females aged 15–19 years. As Trussell observed (10), one out of every 10 women in this age-group become pregnant each year. Data for 1988 reveal that of all recent pregnancies among these young women, roughly five out of six (>85%) are unintended. This is an increase of almost 6 percentage points since 1982. Trussell also notes that only a minority of sexually active teens **always** rely on contraception, and that even fewer of them use the most effective methods.

A comparison of births among black teens aged 15–19 years and white teens indicate that although black teens have about the same level of unintended births as white teens (83% for white teens, 88% for black teens), the proportion of unintended births that were unwanted is almost twice as high for black teens as it is for white teens. Although the proportion is lower among white teens, it is rising. The proportion of births that were unwanted seems to have stabilized at about 30% for black teens; however, this is a high level.

If teens were to have more access to contraceptives, and to better education about how to use those methods effectively, some researchers

maintain that there would be a group of teenagers, comprised mostly of poor black and Hispanic women, that still would show little change in the incidence of unintended births. Teens, too, generally are poor at anticipating when intercourse will occur, and thus often are unprepared with respect to birth control. They also are prone to believe that their risk of pregnancy is small (10) (for additional information, see the Pregnancy in Adolescents chapter).

In 1982, about 8% of recent births to women who had ever been married, were unwanted. By 1988, however, this increased to >10% (Table 2). The proportion of births that were mistimed has remained relatively constant since 1973 at about one fourth of all births. In 1988, however, mistimed births were two and one-half times as common (25%) as unwanted births (10%).

Among subgroups of women who had ever been married, the proportion of births that were unwanted increased with age in all three survey years (Table 2). At the same time, the proportion of mistimed births declined with age. Young females who had ever been married (aged 15–24 years), both black and white, had the largest proportion of mistimed births. These unwanted births stayed at a relatively low level, although in 1988, the proportion of births that were unwanted was more than twice as high for blacks as for whites of the same age. Overall, the largest proportion of births that were unwanted occurred among older women aged 35–44 years (18% in 1988). This high figure is an average of all races, inflated by the particularly high proportion of unwanted births among black women aged 35–44 years (44% in 1988).

In a regression analysis of the determinants of unwanted births to ever-married, Williams used NSFG final data from 1973 and 1982 and NSFG preliminary data from 1988 and found that age and income were strong predictors of unwanted childbearing (11). During all survey years, births to women aged ≥30 years were much more likely to have been unwanted than births to younger women. These unwanted births tend to be higher order births (e.g., a third birth to a woman who only wanted and already had two babies). Births that were unwanted at conception occurred most often to women at or below the poverty level.

77

TABLE 2. Percentage of intended and unintended live births* among females aged 15–44 years who have ever been married, by race and age of mothers — United States, 1973, 1982, and 1988

| Race and age (years) | Total[†] | Intended | | | Unintended | | | | | |
| | | | | | Mistimed | | | Unwanted | | |
		1973	1982	1988	1973	1982	1988	1973	1982	1988
All races[¶]										
All ages	100.0	61.6	68.1	64.6	24.0	24.0	24.9	14.3	7.7	10.4
15–24	100.0	52.4	50.5	48.5	39.4	43.8	42.6	8.0	5.7	8.6
25–34	100.0	68.0	74.6	67.7	18.3	18.5	23.1	13.5	6.7	9.0
35–44	100.0	54.7	71.4	69.9	9.5	11.3	12.2	35.6	17.1	17.7
White										
All ages	100.0	64.2	69.6	65.5	23.4	23.6	25.4	12.3	6.7	8.8
15–24	100.0	55.0	51.1	48.9	38.3	44.1	43.4	6.5	4.8	7.4
25–34	100.0	70.3	76.5	68.6	18.0	17.6	23.4	11.6	5.8	7.8
35–44	100.0	57.8	73.2	72.4	9.8	11.2	12.7	32.2	15.6	14.6
Black										
All ages	100.0	40.6	55.6	50.5	28.9	28.1	26.2	30.5	15.9	22.8
15–24	100.0	36.6	45.1	48.1	45.9	40.2	36.3	17.5	14.8	15.6
25–34	100.0	46.4	59.0	53.8	20.1	25.2	26.4	33.4	15.6	19.1
35–44	100.0	31.0	60.9	42.1	5.6	16.6	13.6	63.4	20.4	44.4

* Includes births occurring <5 years from the date of interview.

[†] Total includes births of unknown wantedness status.

[¶] All races includes white, black and other races. Other races are not shown separately.

Source: National Survey of Family Growth, 1973, 1982, and 1988.

Williams *(11)* notes that "although the national family planning program in this country was initially instituted to target women with incomes at or below poverty level . . . these are the women among whom unwanted childbearing has been increasing."

Other observers have speculated about the principal reasons for this shortfall: 1) public expenditures for family planning services, after controlling for inflation, have fallen by one third since 1980 *(12)*; and 2) increasing clinic costs and funding cuts have weakened the ability of family planning clinics to provide clients with services, particularly contraceptive services and sexually transmitted disease screening and treatment to low-income women and teenagers *(13,14)*.

INTERPRETATION ISSUES

Women at Risk

Not all women are at risk of an unintended pregnancy at a given point in time. NSFG data show

that in 1988, about 33% of females aged 15–44 years were not at risk of an unintended pregnancy at the time of the survey. Several reasons for this include 1) the women had never had intercourse (almost 12%); 2) they were not currently having intercourse (7%); 3) they were pregnant, had just delivered, or were trying to become pregnant (9%); or 4) they were sterile for noncontraceptive reasons, such as a hysterectomy (6%). These proportions vary depending on the age of the woman and relect different patterns of reproductive behavior by age-group *(15)*. The remaining 67%—roughly 39 million women—were at risk of a mistimed or unwanted pregnancy.

Abortion Underreporting

Most studies of unintended pregnancy focus on live births, because not all surveyed women report all of the abortions that they have had. Abortion underreporting has been a significant problem in fertility surveys in the United States and worldwide. In the NSFG, for example, only about 35% of the estimated number of abortions that occurred in the United States from 1984 through 1987 were actually reported in the 1988 survey (5).

In reports using the 1988 NSFG data, pregnancies were presented in two ways: 1) the total of live births, miscarriages, and stillbirths only, and 2) the total of live births, miscarriages, stillbirths, and abortions, adjusted for underreporting of abortion (Table 3).

These data indicate that >40% of live births, miscarriages, and stillbirths—some 9 million pregnancies—were unintended. Moreover, 39% of live births occurring within 5 years of the interview were unintended. We know that underreporting of abortion necessarily implies the underreporting of unintended pregnancies, primarily those resulting from failures in the use of contraceptive methods (5). To account for this factor, virtually all reported pregnancies that ended in abortion were assumed to be unintended. The number of abortions was then adjusted to estimate the total proportion of pregnancies that were unintended, as follows:

- The total (reported) number of live births and miscarriages/stillbirths was first calculated.

- Recent data were used to estimate the number of abortions that were unreported, by taking the number of total abortions for 1984 through 1988 (16) and subtracting the number of abortions that were reported in the 1988 survey.

- Of all the pregnancies ending in abortion that were reported, 100% were assumed to be unintended, or 2,885,000 pregnancies ending in abortion (the actual reported percentage was not 100, although it was close because 1) some women did not understand the question properly, 2) they had **wanted pregnancies** that ended in therapeutic abortion because of fetal defects, or 3) they had **wanted pregnancies** that ended in abortion because their relationships with their partners dissolved).

- Of all the pregnancies ending in abortion that were unreported (4,927,000), all were assumed to be unintended. The estimated totals for reported and unreported abortions were then added, producing a total of 7,812,000 unintended pregnancies ending in abortion.

TABLE 3. Number of recent pregnancies* among females aged 15–44 years, by wantedness status of pregnancies at conception and pregnancy outcomes — United States, 1988

	Total[†]	Unintended	
	N (in thousands)	Percentage	N (in thousands)
Total[§]	22,791	40.5	9,226
Live births	18,910	39.2	7,406
Miscarriages and stillbirths	3,881	46.9	1,820
Total[¶]	30,603	55.9	17,038
Live births	18,910	39.2	7,406
Miscarriages and stillbirths	3,881	46.9	1,820
Abortions**	7,812	100.0	7,812

* Pregnancies completed <5 years from the date of interview.
† Total includes intended and unintended pregnancies and pregnancies of unknown wantedness status. Totals may not add exactly due to rounding.
§ Total excludes abortions and current pregnancies.
¶ Total excludes current pregnancies.
** Estimated, adjusted for underreporting. Assumes 100% of abortions are unintended pregnancies.

Source: National Survey of Family Growth, 1988 (16).

- When the adjusted number of unintended pregnancies ending in abortions was added to the total of live births, miscarriages, and stillbirths, an estimated 55.9% of all pregnancies were found to be unintended—approximately 17 million recent pregnancies between 1984 and 1988.

In sum, more than half of all recent pregnancies to women of childbearing age were unintended, compared with 39% of live births.

Retrospective vs. Prospective Data

The NSFG is a cross-sectional survey and therefore must rely on women to report retrospectively what they felt about the wantedness status of a pregnancy at conception. The NLSY is now attempting to measure intentions very close to the actual time of conception and to prospectively track the pregnancy through to its outcome, instead of collecting the wantedness status retrospectively (17). In future telephone reinterviews, the NSFG will attempt to make such measurements for a national sample of females covering the entire range of reproductive ages (15–44 years).

EXAMPLES OF USING DATA

A special feature of the population-based PRAMS is that it provides state-specific data on unintended births. With these data, states can plan and assess programs for subgroups of women at risk of having unwanted or mistimed births. PRAMS also enables states to compare data from their home state with data from other PRAMS states.

At least one state has used PRAMS data to assess the characteristics and outcomes of teen mothers. Data for Oklahoma show that more than two thirds (68%) of teen births are unintended at the time of conception (18).

Data from the Oklahoma PRAMS have also been used to assess the characteristics of women with unintended pregnancy, including behaviors conducive to poor pregnancy outcomes (19). After finding that 44% of live births are unintended at conception, the Oklahoma

family planning program adjusted its priorities to meet the increasing demands in clinics and, ultimately, to achieve the year 2000 objective of reducing unintended pregnancies to no more than 30% of all pregnancies.

The principal limitations of PRAMS are that 1) not all states are included (only about 13 states and the District of Columbia at present), and 2) the data are not available for public use because they belong to the individual states.

FUTURE ISSUES

National objectives for the year 2000 include targeting women at risk of unintended pregnancies and curbing the level of teenage pregnancy. The goals are to improve family planning by 1) reducing the number of teenage pregnancies by 30%, to a maximum of 50 per 1,000 girls aged <17 years) (objective 5.1); and 2) reducing the proportion of all pregnancies that are unintended to 30% (objective 5.2). Currently, an estimated 56% of all recent pregnancies are unintended (Table 3) (20).

Cycle V of the NSFG, which began field interviews this year, is one of the major surveys that will provide future data on unintended pregnancy. The interest that funding agencies have taken in unintended childbearing has meant valuable support for continued survey research in this area. Another round of surveys that will provide data on the intention status of pregnancies is the series of Fertility and Family Surveys, which have been under way in several countries in Europe. These surveys are being coordinated, with assistance from NCHS, by the United Nations Economic Commission for Europe (ECE) in ECE member countries. Many of these countries' surveys will include questions on the wantedness status of pregnancies and on contraceptive use.

CDC currently is undertaking a reproductive health telephone survey of about 3,000 women aged 18–44 years in Arizona; Mexican-American women will be oversampled. All women who have ever been pregnant are being asked a standard set of questions on the wantedness status of pregnancy as well as a new test question designed to allow them to hear all of the wantedness status options in one question. CDC also plans to continue supporting PRAMS, which includes questions regarding the intendedness of pregnancy.

In the future, efforts should focus on improving the reliability of birth control method use. Although modern contraceptive use was at a high level, the percentage of births that were unintended increased. Many of these unintended pregnancies could have been prevented with proper and consistent use of reliable contraception. At present, although highly effective, reversible contraceptive methods exist, we have no guarantee that they will be used correctly during every act of sexual intercourse. Reversible methods for which data are available have contraceptive failure rates ranging from 8% (the pill) to about 25% (periodic abstinence or spermicides) in the first year of use (5).

One of the greatest challenges for health-care providers will be to help women cope with prolonged exposure to the risk of unintended pregnancy and to help them successfully plan their pregnancies. Because more women want fewer children and are delaying childbearing, the average length of time they plan to be pregnant is significantly diminished. A great number of women in the United States, therefore, spend several years trying to avoid unintended pregnancies and births, and many are not succeeding.

REFERENCES

1. Pratt WF, Mosher WD, Bachrach CA, Horn MC. Understanding U.S. Fertility: findings from the national survey of family growth, cycle III. Popul Bull 1984;39:1–43.

2. Piccinino LJ. Unintended pregnancy and childbearing in the United States: 1973–1990. Hyattsville, Maryland: US Department of Health and Human Services, Public Health Service, CDC, NCHS, 1994 (in press). (Advance data from vital and health statistics.)

3. Chandra A. Health aspects of pregnancy and childbirth. United States, 1982–1988. Data from the National Survey of Family Growth Series 23, Hyattsville, Maryland: US Department of Health and Human Services, Public Health Service, CDC, NCHS, 1994 (in press).

4. Zuravin SJ. Unplanned childbearing and family size: their relationship to child neglect and abuse. Fam Plann Perspect 23:155–61.

5. Jones EF, Forrest JD. Contraceptive failure rates based on the 1988 NSFG. Fam Plann Perspect 1992;24:12–9.

6. Adams MM, Shulman HB, Bruce C, Hogue C, Brogan D. The Pregnancy Risk Assessment Monitoring System: design, questionnaire, data collection and response rates. Paediat Perinat Epidemiol 1991;5:333–45.

7. Center for Human Resource Research. NLS Handbook 1992, The National Longitudinal Surveys. Columbus, Ohio: Ohio State University, 1992.

8. Abma JC, Mott FL. Determinants of pregnancy wantedness: profiling the population from an interventionist perspective. Presented at the International Symposium on Public Policies Toward Unwanted Pregnancies, Pittsburgh, Pennsylvania, November 1990.

9. Teitelbaum M. Intended and unintended pregnancies: women's prenatal care coverage and pregnancy experience. Presented at the American Public Health Association annual meeting, Atlanta, Georgia, November 10–14, 1991.

10. Trussell J. Teenage pregnancy in the United States. Fam Plann Perspect 1988;20:262–72.

11. Williams LB. Determinants of unintended childbearing among ever-married women in the United States: 1973–1988. Fam Plann Perspect 1991;23:212–21.

12. Gold RB, Daley D. Public funding of contraceptive, sterilization and abortion services, Fiscal Year 1990. Family Planning Perspectives 1991;23:204–11.

13. Donovan P. Family planning clinics: facing higher costs and sicker patients. Fam Plann Perspect 1991;23:198–203.

14. Cates W Jr, Stone KM. Family planning, sexually transmitted diseases and contraceptive choice: a literature update part II. Fam Plann Perspect 1992;24:122–8.

15. Forrest JD, Singh S. The sexual and reproductive behavior of American women, 1982–1988. Fam Plann Perspect 1990;22:206–14.

16. Ventura SJ, Taffel SM, Mosher WD, Henshaw S. Trends in pregnancies and pregnancy rates, United States, 1980–1988. Hyattsville, Maryland: US Department of Health and Human Services, Public Health Service, CDC, NCHS, 1992. (Monthly vital statistics report; vol. 41, no. 6, suppl.)

17. Baydar N, Grady W. Predictors of birth planning status and its consequences for children. Presented at the Population Association of America annual meeting, Cincinnati, Ohio, April 1–3, 1993.

18. Oklahoma State Department of Health. Maternal characteristics and outcomes of teenage women in Oklahoma. PRAMS-GRAM 1992; 2:1–4.

19.   DePersio SR, Chen W, Blose D, Lorenz R, Thomas W, Zenker PN. Unintended childbearing: Pregnancy Risk Assessment Monitoring System—Oklahoma. MMWR 1992;41: 933–6.

20.   Public Health Service. Healthy people 2000: National health promotion and disease prevention objectives—full report, with commentary. Washington, DC: US Department of Health and Human Services. Public Health Service, 1991; DHHS publication no.(PHS)91-50212.

Legal Induced Abortion

Lisa M. Koonin, M.N., M.P.H.,[1] and Jack C. Smith, M.S.[1]

PUBLIC HEALTH IMPORTANCE

Legal induced abortion is one of the most frequently performed surgical procedures in the United States. Each year since 1980, the number of abortions in this country has remained relatively stable at approximately 1.3–1.4 million abortions per year (1). Recent reports show that in 1991, 339 abortions were provided for every 1,000 live births and that about 24 of every 1,000 females of reproductive age (15–44 years old) had an abortion (1).

Induced abortions usually are linked to unintended pregnancies, which often occur despite the use of contraception (2–4). In the mid-1980s, about 1.2 million of the live births that occurred each year were unintended (either mistimed or unwanted at conception) (5). Improving contraceptive practices as well as access to and education about safe, effective, and low-cost contraception and family planning services may help minimize the need for abortion in this country (6).

Fewer than one woman in 100 develops a major complication from induced abortion, and fewer than one in 100,000 dies (7,8). The risk of morbidity and mortality from legal abortion is directly related to gestational age at the time of abortion—the earlier the gestation, the safer the procedure (9,10).

The surveillance of legal induced abortion is important for numerous reasons. Surveillance is used to identify characteristics of those who have abortions, in particular, women at high risk of

unintended pregnancy. Ongoing surveillance is essential to monitor trends in the number, ratio, and rate of abortions in this country.* We need statistics on the number of pregnancies ending in abortion to add to birth and fetal death statistics so that we can accurately estimate pregnancy rates and calculate other outcome rates, such as the rate of ectopic pregnancies per 1,000 pregnancies. In turn, abortion and pregnancy rates can be used to evaluate the effectiveness of family planning and unintended pregnancy prevention programs. This is especially important for teenage pregnancy programs, because a large proportion of teenage pregnancies are terminated by abortion (1). Ongoing surveillance also gives us an opportunity to assess changes in clinical practice patterns related to abortion, such as changes in types of procedure over time. Finally, abortion data are used as denominators to calculate abortion morbidity rates and mortality rates.

Legal abortion rates vary widely among countries—ranging from a high of >100 abortions per 1,000 women of reproductive age in the former Soviet Union to a low of 5 per 1,000 in the Netherlands. The induced abortion rate in the United States (24 per 1,000) is higher than rates reported by Australia, Canada, and most Western European countries; the U.S. rate is lower than rates reported by the former Soviet Union, China, Cuba, and Eastern European countries (11). Abortion rates for teenagers are much higher in the United States than in most Western European countries and in some Eastern European countries (11) (for additional information about related topics and surveillance

---

* The **ratio** is the number of abortions per 1,000 live births. The **rate** is the number of abortions per 1,000 females 15–44 years old.

[1] Division of Reproductive Health
National Center for Chronic Disease Prevention
   and Health Promotion
Centers for Disease Control and Prevention
Atlanta, Georgia

83

activities, see the Unintended Pregnancy and Childbearing and the Pregnancy in Adolescents chapters).

HISTORY OF DATA COLLECTION

During the late 1960s and early 1970s, a new reproductive health event, legal induced abortion, was emerging as a result of judicial and legislative changes occurring in this country. At that time, the incidence of induced abortion in the United States was unknown. In 1969, recognizing both the importance of abortion as a public health issue and the need for national abortion statistics, CDC began the continuous epidemiologic surveillance of abortion in the United States.

That same year, CDC published the first report of legal induced abortions. The term **legal** was used to contrast those abortions with illegal procedures or self-induced procedures that still occurred. Since then, reports of annual data for 1969–1990 have been published regularly.

To assess morbidity associated with legal induced abortion from 1971 through 1978, CDC sponsored a multicenter, observational study of complications following legal induced abortion (12). This study, known as the Joint Program for the Study of Abortion (JPSA), continued the initial investigation (JPSA I) sponsored by the Population Council of New York. On the basis of data from about 80,000 abortions performed in 32 institutions between 1971 and 1975 (JPSA II) and 84,000 abortions performed in 13 institutions between 1975 and 1978 (JPSA III), CDC offered the medical community recommendations, which have significantly reduced the number and severity of abortion complications and the number of related deaths in this country.

Today, abortion statistics are compiled by CDC's National Center for Chronic Disease Prevention and Health Promotion (NCCDPHP) and National Center for Health Statistics (NCHS) as well as the Alan Guttmacher Institute, an independent, nonprofit research organization. Abortion data compiled by NCHS are collected from participating states and registration areas. Information on each induced abortion are provided to NCHS on magnetic tape as a part of the Vital Statistics

Cooperative Program. In 1988, the last year for which statistics were reported, NCHS reports included data from 14 states[†] and New York City (13). The Alan Guttmacher Institute conducts periodic direct surveys of abortion providers in the United States (14); however, the institute does not conduct continuous annual surveys or collect information on the characteristics of women obtaining abortions.

CDC SURVEILLANCE ACTIVITIES

NCCDPHP is responsible for national surveillance to document the number and characteristics of women obtaining abortions, and NCHS is responsible for compiling abortion data in selected states. On occasion, NCCDPHP and NCHS collaborate in producing abortion surveillance reports.

A legal induced abortion is defined as a procedure performed by a licensed physician or someone acting under the supervision of a licensed physician, with the intent to "terminate a suspected or known intrauterine pregnancy and to produce a nonviable fetus at any gestational age" (9). Data on the reasons for the legal induced abortion are not collected by many states and are not provided to NCCDPHP.

Until the late 1970s, state health departments had independently developed their own abortion reporting forms or had used fetal death reporting forms, which were problematic for reporting induced abortions. In 1977, with the assistance of state health departments, NCHS developed a model abortion reporting form to collect demographic information and data on gestational age and the type of procedure performed; the form does not include personal identifiers of the woman. This reporting form has been modified periodically and serves as the primary tool for collecting abortion statistics in most states.

NCCDPHP compiles tabular data, aggregated at the state and area levels, received from 52 reporting areas: 50 states, New York City, and the District of Columbia. The total number of legal

---

† States include Colorado, Indiana, Kansas, Maine, Missouri, Montana, New York, Oregon, Rhode Island, South Carolina, Tennessee, Utah, Vermont, and Virginia.

induced abortions are available from all reporting areas, most of which provide information on the characteristics of women obtaining abortions. Each year, in about 45 reporting areas, data are provided from the central health agencies.§ In the remaining reporting areas, data are provided from hospitals and other medical facilities. No patient or physician identifiers are provided to CDC. Data are reported by the state in which the abortion occurred. CDC checks the data for numerical accuracy and for consistency with published state reports and resolves discrepancies by communicating with health department personnel. Data are stored in secured files.

CDC computes abortion-to-live-birth ratios by using the number of abortions in a given category (e.g., by state, age, or race) as the numerator and the number of live births (reported by state and area health departments) in the same category as denominators. Abortion rates are computed by using the number of abortions as numerators and Current Population Survey data for females aged 15–44 years as denominators.

Preliminary annual data on legal induced abortions are published in the *Morbidity and Mortality Weekly Report (MMWR)*, and a final and more comprehensive report is published later in the *MMWR's CDC Surveillance Summaries*. National numbers, ratios, and rates of abortions are presented in each report. State-specific characteristics of women obtaining abortions are presented in the *Surveillance Summaries* only.

GENERAL FINDINGS

From 1970 to 1982, the reported number of legal abortions in the United States increased every year; the largest percentage increase occurred during 1970–1972 (Figure 1). From 1976 to 1982, the annual rate of increase slowed continuously, reaching a low of 0.2% for 1981–1982. Since 1980, the number of abortions has remained relatively stable, with only small (<5%) year-to-year fluctuations. The abortion ratio increased each year from 1970 to 1980, remained relatively stable until 1988,

and since then has decreased somewhat each year (Figure 1).

Women who have abortions in this country tend to be young, white, unmarried, and having the procedure for the first time. Specifically, women 20–24 years of age have approximately one third of all abortions, whereas women younger <15 years of age have about 1%. Abortion ratios are highest for women at the age extremes—<19 years (particularly <15 years) and ≥40 years of age (Figure 2). Women aged 30–34 years have the lowest ratios. Among teenagers, the abortion ratio is highest for those <15 years old and lowest for those 19 years old.

Most reported legal abortions are performed before 8 weeks of gestation, and more than three fourths are done before 13 weeks. Approximately 4% of abortions are performed at 16–20 weeks of gestation, and 1% at ≥21 weeks. Approximately 99% of legal abortions are performed by curettage (which is consistent with the fact that 94% of abortions are performed in the first trimester or early second trimester of pregnancy), and <1% are performed by intrauterine saline or prostaglandin instillation. Hysterectomy and hysterotomy are rarely used to perform abortions.

Abortion ratios vary by race and ethnicity, although these variations are probably related to socioeconomic differences rather than to race per se. Almost two thirds of women obtaining abortions are white; however, the abortion ratio for blacks is about two times higher than that for white women, and the ratio for women of other races (Asian-Pacific Islander, Native American, Alaska Native, or race listed as other) is 1.3 times higher than that for white women. In 1990, the abortion ratios for Hispanics were similar to those for whites. When the proportion of women undergoing legal abortion is analyzed by race and age-group, few differences are found between whites and blacks except among girls <15 years old; the percentage of girls who had an abortion was over twice that of white girls in this age-group (Table 1).

Over three fourths of women who have legal induced abortion are unmarried. The abortion ratio is 11 times higher for unmarried women than for married women.

---

§ Agencies include state health departments and the health departments of New York City and the District of Columbia.

FIGURE 1. Legal abortions — United States, 1970–1990*

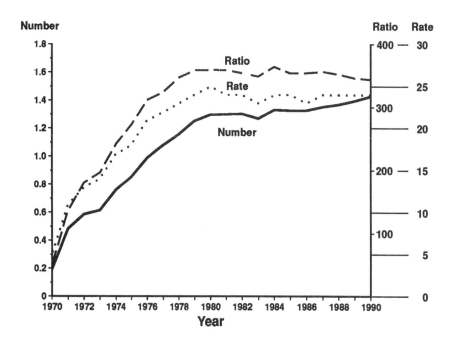

* Number of abortions are in millions of women, ratio is number of abortions per 1,000 live births, and rate is number of abortions per 1,000 women aged 15–44 years.

Source: CDC abortion surveillance.

FIGURE 2. Abortion ratio, by age-group — United States, 1990

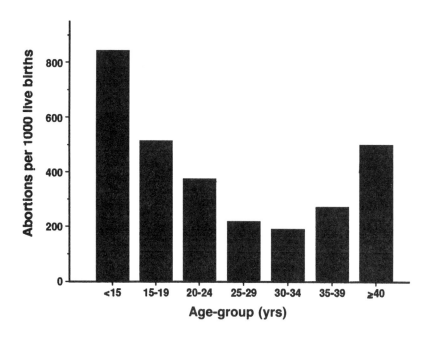

Source: CDC abortion surveillance.

**TABLE 1. Number and percentage of reported legal abortions, by race and age-group —
United States, 1990**

| Age-group* (years) | Race | | | | | |
| | White† | | Black and other races | | Total | |
	No.	%	No.	%	No.	%
< 15	2,215	0.6	2,597	1.3	4,812	0.8
15–19	88,731	22.3	41,597	20.1	130,328	21.5
20–24	132,427	33.2	68,922	33.3	201,349	33.2
25–29	87,044	21.8	49,242	23.8	136,286	22.5
30–34	52,741	13.2	28,171	13.6	80,912	13.4
35–39	27,571	6.9	12,919	6.3	40,490	6.7
≥ 40	8,022	2.0	3,229	1.6	11,251	1.9
Total§	398,751	100.0	206,677	100.0	605,428	100.0

* Excludes persons of unknown ages.
† Includes Hispanics.
§ Reported by 30 states and New York City.

Source: CDC, National Abortion Surveillance *(17)*.

The abortion ratio is highest for women who had no live births and lowest for women who had one live birth. Approximately half of women obtaining abortions are having the procedure for the first time, whereas approximately 15% have had at least two previous abortions.

Overall, most women obtain abortions during the first 12 weeks of pregnancy. However, girls <15 years of age are more likely to obtain abortions later in pregnancy than older women. The proportion of women obtaining an early abortion (<8 weeks) increases with age, and the proportion obtaining a late abortion (≥16 weeks) decreases with age. Black women of all ages tend to obtain abortions later in pregnancy than white women.

About 99% of abortions at <12 weeks of gestation are performed by curettage (primarily suction procedures). Beyond 12 weeks of gestation, the most common procedure again is curettage, which is usually reported as dilatation and evacuation. Most intrauterine instillations involve the use of saline and are usually performed at ≥16 weeks of gestation.

For all racial groups, educational level strongly influences when an abortion is performed *(15)*.

For example, in 1988, among white women who obtained an abortion, 60% of those with college educations (≥16 years of school completed) had an early abortion (<8 weeks), compared with 46% of those who completed high school only. Among minority women who obtained an abortion, about 53% of those with college educations had an early abortion compared with 42% of those who completed high school only.

Also in 1988, about 88% of women who obtained abortions lived in metropolitan areas *(15)*. For these women, the abortion ratio was about 2.2 times greater than the ratio for women who lived in nonmetropolitan areas (373 vs. 168 abortions per 1,000 live births). This difference varied by race. For example, the abortion ratio for minority women living in metropolitan areas was 2.8 times the ratio for those living in nonmetropolitan areas (599 vs. 210 abortions per 1,000 live births). In contrast, the abortion ratio for white women living in metropolitan areas was 1.9 times that of white women living in nonmetropolitan areas (302 vs. 162 abortions per 1,000 live births).

Areas with the highest incidence of legal induced abortion include California, New York City, Texas, and Illinois; the lowest incidence occurs in Wyoming, South Dakota, Alaska, and Idaho

(Table 2) *(1,16)*. Data on women whose state of residence is known indicate that approximately 92% have the abortion performed within that state.

INTERPRETATION ISSUES

Since the 1970s, legal induced abortion has spurred much public controversy, which has affected national and state surveillance activities. In recent years, the abortion issue has influenced a significant number of public policy decisions, including issues related to the public funding of abortions, fetal tissue research, international family planning program development and support, and the possible availability of certain abortion-inducing medications, such as RU 486.

Despite NCCDPHP's ability to monitor national abortion trends, these data have several significant limitations. In 1990, approximately 28% of the abortions were reported from states that do not have centralized reporting; these areas could provide no information on the characteristics of women obtaining abortions. Representativeness is limited when data from all states are not available. In addition, because the number of states that report such information varies from year to year, we must use caution when making temporal comparisons. Nevertheless, the data available from CDC's abortion surveillance system are particularly useful because national characteristic data of women who obtain abortions are not collected by any other system. Also, because this is a continuous surveillance activity, data for each year since 1969 have been compiled, tabulated, and reported.

Differences in the data reported to NCCDPHP and NCHS also must be considered. For example, legal induced abortion data reported to NCHS contain demographic data—including information on educational level and area of residence (metropolitan or nonmetropolitan)—not available from states that provide data to NCCDPHP. The NCHS data system also enables detailed cross-tabulation of these and other characteristics. Because NCHS data are from a limited number of states, they cannot be used to represent national statistics. In 1988, NCCDPHP received the same number of reported abortions

as did NCHS for the selected states in their system—these NCHS abortion data represented approximately 22% of all abortions reported to NCCDPHP in that year.

The Alan Guttmacher Institute reports higher numbers of abortions in a given year than does NCCDPHP. However, the institute does not conduct abortion surveillance annually; in the 1980s, data were not collected for 1983, 1986, and 1989. The number of abortions reported to CDC has consistently been about 19% lower than the number ascertained by the Alan Guttmacher Institute *(17)*. Methodologic differences account for this discrepancy. The institute uses an active survey technique to contact all identifiable abortion providers, whereas NCCDPHP primarily compiles data collected by state health departments. The smaller number of abortions reported to NCCDPHP from health departments is likely the result of inconsistencies among states in abortion reporting requirements and methods. Specifically, the completeness of state health department data varies widely because 1) some states require reporting from all licensed facilities whereas others have a voluntary abortion reporting system, 2) the types of providers that must report vary among states, and 3) the completeness of reporting varies among states. These factors probably contribute to underreporting in some states, which can lead to an underestimation of the national abortion rate and ratio.

Because legal induced abortions are usually performed in licensed medical facilities and most states use a standard abortion reporting form for data collection, we suspect that overreporting of abortions (false positives) is rare. However, the data collection forms filled out by providers may contain incomplete data, which in turn would be submitted to NCCDPHP for inclusion in national statistics.

NCCDPHP's definition of legal induced abortion is very similar to the definitions used by NCHS and the Alan Guttmacher Institute. NCHS uses the term **induced termination of pregnancy** in its reports and defines it as the "purposeful interruption of an intrauterine pregnancy with the intention other than to produce a live-born infant, and which does not result in a live birth . . . and excludes management of prolonged retention of

TABLE 2. Reported number, ratio, and rate of legal abortions and percentage of abortions obtained by out-of-state residents, by state of occurrence — United States, 1990

State	Number of abortions*	Ratio†	Rate§	Abortions obtained by out-of-state residents (%)¶
Alabama	15,012**	237	16	NR
Alaska	1,489**	125	11	NR
Arizona	15,783	229	19	2.5
Arkansas	5,953	163	11	3.2
California	357,579††	585	50	NR
Colorado	12,679	237	16	8.2
Connecticut	18,776	375§§	24	NR
Delaware	5,557	500	34	NR
District of Columbia	19,969	NR¶¶	NR	52.9
Florida	66,071	332	24	NR
Georgia	39,245	349	24	8.3
Hawaii	4,748	232	18	0.8
Idaho	1,390	85	6	9.0
Illinois	67,350	345	25	NR
Indiana	14,351	167	11	3.6
Iowa	7,166**	182	12	NR
Kansas	7,516†††	193§§	14	46.5
Kentucky	10,921	202	13	29.3
Louisiana	13,020	181	13	NR
Maine	4,607	266	16	12.6
Maryland	22,425	279§§	19	6.8
Massachusetts	39,739	430	27	3.9
Michigan	36,183	236	16	4.2
Minnesota	17,156	252	17	10.7
Mississippi	6,842	157	11	22.7
Missouri	16,366	207	14	10.8
Montana	3,365	290	19	23.6
Nebraska	6,346	260	18	20.2
Nevada	7,226	331	26	11.2
New Hampshire	4,259**	243	16	NR
New Jersey	41,358	337	23	3.0
New Mexico	5,288	194	15	3.9
New York	159,098	545	37	3.4
City	102,202§§§	787	NR	2.9
State	56,896	351	NR	4.2
North Carolina	36,494	349	23	8.3
North Dakota	1,723	186	12	38.2
Ohio	32,165	193	13	9.6
Oklahoma	10,708**	225§§	15	NR
Oregon	13,658	319	21	9.7
Pennsylvania	52,143	305	19	5.9
Rhode Island	7,782	512§§	33	21.7
South Carolina	13,285	227	16	6.1
South Dakota	946	86	6	19.4

TABLE 2. Reported number, ratio, and rate of legal abortions and percentage of abortions obtained by out-of-state residents, by state of occurrence — United States, 1990 — continued

State	Number of abortions*	Ratio†	Rate§	Abortions obtained by out-of-state residents (%)¶
Tennessee	21,144	282	18	17.4
Texas	92,580	293	23	3.9
Utah	4,786	132	12	15.2
Vermont	3,184	384	23	29.8
Virginia	32,992	334	21	6.0
Washington	31,443	397	27	4.9
West Virginia	2,500	111	6	11.7
Wisconsin	16,848	232	15	6.1
Wyoming	363	52	4	12.4
Total	1,429,577	345¶¶¶	24	8.2

* Abortion data from central health agency unless otherwise noted.
† Abortions per 1,000 live births (live-birth data from central health agency unless otherwise specified).
§ Abortions per 1,000 women aged 15–44 years (from Bureau of the Census, Current Population Survey, March 1990).
¶ Based on number of abortions for which residence status of women was known.
** Reported from hospitals and/or other medical facilities in state.
†† CDC estimate.
§§ Live births reported by NCHS (16).
¶¶ >1,000 abortions per 1,000 live births.
*** >1,000 abortions per 1,000 women aged 15–44 years.
††† Excludes 330 Kansas residents obtaining abortions in other states.
§§§ Reported from New York City Health Department.
¶¶¶ Differs from the preliminary ratio (344) published in MMWR (1).
NR: Not reported.

products of conception following fetal death" (18).

Because of multiple levels of reporting—from the facility or doctor to the state health department and then to NCCDPHP—reporting complexity is part of this surveillance system. This complexity is exacerbated by the political sensitivities and legal issues surrounding abortion in every state. This creates a surveillance situation that is dynamic and not completely in the control of the state health agency collecting data.

The timeliness of surveillance data can be described as having two components: 1) the interval between the performance of the abortion and the reporting of the event to the state health department and subsequently NCCDPHP, and 2) the interval between the receipt of such data by NCCDPHP and dissemination of the results of the analysis. Since 1991, the interval between the abortion and publication of a report has been about 3 years.

EXAMPLES OF USING DATA

CDC's need for abortion data at the national level is used by states to justify state legislation requiring abortion reporting. In turn, states compare their data with national data to make and assess policy and program decisions related to abortion. States also use abortion data to monitor teen pregnancy prevention programs and to plan for providing family planning and STD treatment and prevention services to groups at high risk for unintended pregnancies.

FUTURE ISSUES

Although no year 2000 objectives specifically call for reducing the number of legal induced abortions provided in this country, several objectives indirectly address this issue:

- Objective 5.1: Reducing teen pregnancies.

- Objective 5.2: Reducing the proportion of pregnancies that are unintended.

- Objective 5.7: Increasing the effectiveness with which family planning methods are used.

Achieving these objectives will affect the need for abortion services *(19)* and will require all states to collect abortion data needed to fully assess our progress in reducing abortions.

Not all states have recognized the need for state-based abortion surveillance, and some states have recognized the need but have been unable to gather information because of the sensitivities that abortion generates. Data on the number and characteristics of women having abortions in all states are needed to have an accurate picture of legal induced abortion in this country. Moreover, a larger emphasis must be placed on preventing unintended pregnancy, particularly among teenagers. States that do not have age- and race/ethnicity-specific data on abortions will be in a weak position for assessing their needs, addressing teen pregnancy and unintended pregnancy in high-risk groups, and evaluating the effectiveness of their programs.

Ultimately, recent judicial rulings, executive orders, and legislative changes related to parental consent for abortions for minors, restrictions on the availability of services, the possible availability of RU 486, and the funding of abortion services may affect the number of abortions performed, the characteristics of women having abortions, and the methods used for abortion surveillance. Therefore, ongoing abortion surveillance continues to be a dynamic process that can contribute valuable information about an important public health issue.

REFERENCES

1. Koonin LM, Smith JC, Ramick M. Abortion surveillance—United States, 1990. MMWR 1993;42:(No. SS-6).

2. Jones EF, Forrest JD. Contraceptive failure rates based on the 1988 NSFG. Fam Plann Perspect 1992;24: 12–9.

3. Henshaw SK, Silverman J. The characteristics and prior contraceptive use of U.S. abortion patients. 1988;20:158–68.

4. Torres A, Forrest JD. Why do women have abortions? Fam Plann Perspect 1988;20:169–76.

5. Williams L, Pratt WF. Wanted and unwanted childbearing in the United States 1973–88. Hyattsville, Maryland: US Department of Health and Human Services, Public Health Service, CDC, NCHS, 1990. (Advance data from vital and health statistics; no. 189.)

6. Westoff CF. Contraceptive paths towards the reduction of unintended pregnancy and abortion. Fam Plann Perspect 1988;20:4–13.

7. Koonin LM, Smith JC, Ramick M, Lawson H. Abortion surveillance—United States, 1989. MMWR 1992;41 (No. SS-5):1–34.

8. Grimes DA, Cates W Jr. Complications from legally induced abortions: a review. Obstet Gynecol Surv 1979;34:177–91.

9. CDC. Abortion surveillance, 1981. 1985:1–51.

10. Berger GS, Tietze C, Pakter J, Katz SH. Maternal mortality associated with legal abortions in New York State: July 1 1970–June 30, 1972. Obstet Gynecol 1974;43:315–26.

11. Henshaw SK. Induced abortions: a world review, 1990. Fam Plann Perspect 1990;22:76–89.

12. CDC. Abortion surveillance: United States, 1974. Atlanta: CDC, 1976:1–49.

13. Kochanek KD. Induced terminations of pregnancy: reporting states, 1988. Hyattsville, Maryland: US Department of Health and Human Services, Public Health Service, CDC, NCHS, 1991; DHHS publication no. (PHS)91-1120. (Monthly vital statistics report; vol. 39, no. 12, suppl.)

14. Henshaw SK, Forrest JD, Van Vort J. Abortion services in the United States, 1987 and 1988. Fam Plann Perspect 1990;22:102–8.

15. Koonin LM, Kochanek KD, Smith JC, Ramick M. Abortion surveillance, United States, 1988. MMWR 1991;40(No. SS-1):15–42.

16. NCHS. Advance report of final natality statistics, 1990. Hyattsville, Maryland: US Department of Health and Human Services, Public Health Service, CDC, 1993. (Monthly vital statistics report; vol. 41, no. 9, suppl.)

17. Atrash HK, Lawson HW, Smith JC. Legal abortions in the US: trends and mortality. Contemp Obstet Gynecol 1990;58–69.

18. National Center for Health Statistics. Model state vital statistics act and regulations. 1992 revision. Hyattsville, Maryland: US Department of Health and Human Services, Public Health Service, CDC, 1994 (in press).

19. Public Health Service. Healthy people 2000—full report, with commentary. Washington, DC: US Department of Health and Human Services, Public Health service, 1991; DHHS publication no. (PHS)91-50212.

Behavioral Risk Factors Before and During Pregnancy

Mary M. Goodwin, M.A., M.P.A.,[1] Carol Bruce, B.S.N., M.P.H.,[1]
S. Christine Zahniser, B.S.N., M.P.H.,[2]
Michael D. Kogan, Ph.D., M.A.,[3] Eileen P. Gunter, R.N., M.P.H.,[1]
and Christopher Johnson, M.S.P.H.[1]

PUBLIC HEALTH IMPORTANCE

Infant mortality and low birth weight continue to pose important public health problems in the United States. Although U.S. infant mortality has decreased steadily in recent decades, the rate of decrease slowed from an annual average of 5% in the 1970s to an annual average of 3% in the 1980s. Between 1989 and 1990, U.S. infant mortality decreased by 6%, from 9.8 to 9.2 infant deaths per 1,000 live births. Despite this encouraging statistic, infant mortality remains higher in the United States than in many other developed countries (1). Low birth weight, which contributes heavily to U.S. infant mortality and morbidity, has declined very little in the last two decades. In 1970, 7.9% of all U.S. live births were classified as low birth weight, whereas in 1989 the percentage remained at 7.1% (2).

Studies have suggested that women's behaviors during the periconceptional and prenatal periods are related to infant mortality and low birth weight. Types of behavior just before and during pregnancy that have been determined to be associated with infant mortality and morbidity include delayed or no prenatal care and use of cigarettes, alcohol, and illicit drugs. In addition, researchers are interested in other behavior thought to be related to pregnancy outcome, such as weight gain, planning status of pregnancy, physical activity before and during pregnancy, and psychosocial stress. Of all known behavioral risk factors, smoking and alcohol use before and during pregnancy have received the most attention because

of the availability of data and their recognized associations with pregnancy outcome (3,4) (for additional information about related topics and surveillance activities, see the Contraception, Prenatal Care, Pregnancy-Related Nutrition, Infant Mortality, and Fetal Alcohol Syndrome chapters).

HISTORY OF DATA COLLECTION

The effects of women's behavior on pregnancy outcome and infant health have stimulated researchers' interest in obtaining data to examine this complex relationship. Three principal sources of data have been used for this purpose: vital records, periodic cross-sectional surveys, and ongoing surveillance systems (Table 1). Vital records have been the primary tool for surveillance of maternal status during pregnancy and the condition of infants at birth. Additions of items

[1] Division of Reproductive Health
    National Center for Chronic Disease Prevention
        and Health Promotion
    Centers for Disease Control and Prevention
    Atlanta, Georgia

[2] Division of Cancer Prevention and Control
    National Center for Chronic Disease Prevention
        and Health Promotion
    Centers for Disease Control and Prevention
    Atlanta, Georgia

[3] Division of Vital Statistics
    National Center for Health Statistics
    Centers for Disease Control and Prevention
    Hyattsville, Maryland

TABLE 1. Data sources on maternal risk behavior during the periconceptional and prenatal periods

Data source	Population	Survey years	Behavioral risk factors	
			Just before pregnancy	During pregnancy
Birth certificates	All U.S. live births	Annual	NA	Smoking and alcohol use; weight gain
National Natality Surveys (NNS)	Stratified sample of U.S. live births to married women only	1963, 1964–1966, 1967–1969, 1972, 1980	Smoking and alcohol use, by amount; intendedness of pregnancy (1980 NNS)	Smoking and alcohol use, by amount; weight gain (1980 NNS)
National Maternal and Infant Health Survey (NMIHS)	Stratified sample of U.S. live births, infant deaths, and fetal deaths	1988–1991	Smoking, alcohol and illicit drug use, by amount; physical activity; intendedness of pregnancy	Smoking, alcohol and illicit drug use, by amount; physical acitivity; weight gain; use of prenatal care
Pregnancy Risk Assessment Monitoring System* (PRAMS)	Stratified sample of live births in state	Ongoing; cycles beginning in 1987 and 1990	Smoking, alcohol use, by amount; intendedness of pregnancy	Smoking, alcohol use, by amount; stressful events; weight gain; use of prenatal care

* Participants include Alabama, Alaska, California, District of Columbia, Florida, Georgia, Indiana, Maine, Michigan, New York, Oklahoma, South Carolina, Washington, and West Virginia.

to the birth certificate and format changes introduced in 1989 have increased the information that birth certificates provide. Nevertheless, they provide limited data on maternal behavior during pregnancy and no information on women's behavior before conception.

Cross-sectional surveys conducted by CDC's National Center for Health Statistics (NCHS), such as the National Survey of Family Growth (NSFG) and the National Maternal and Infant Health Survey (NMIHS), have obtained nationally representative information regarding the health aspects of pregnancy and childbirth. In addition, the NMIHS has been designed to complement data available from vital records with more detailed information regarding women's behavior before and during pregnancy. The NSFG and the NMIHS provide unique sources of nationally representative data; however, they

are conducted intermittently and both are of limited use for analysis at state and local levels.

To provide a state-specific supplement to vital records, CDC's National Center for Chronic Disease Prevention and Health Promotion initiated a cooperative agreement in 1987 with the District of Columbia and five states to design and establish the Pregnancy Risk Assessment Monitoring System (PRAMS). Since then, eight additional states have started participating in PRAMS. PRAMS participants include Alabama, Alaska, California, District of Columbia, Florida, Georgia, Indiana, Maine, Michigan, New York (excluding New York City), Oklahoma, South Carolina, Washington, and West Virginia. CDC provides these states with financial and technical support for developing, conducting, and maintaining their PRAMS projects.

PRAMS is an ongoing, population-based surveillance system that obtains self-reported behavioral information from new mothers. This information is linked to birth certificate data for analysis. PRAMS is designed to generate state-specific data and it allows comparisons between states through the use of standardized data collection methods. PRAMS data have been used to estimate the prevalence of behavioral risk factors, to assess the effects of behavioral risk factors on infant mortality and birth weight, and to target intervention programs. Currently, PRAMS surveillance covers about one third of U.S. births.

In addition to the population-based surveillance systems and surveys covered in this chapter, a variety of other data collection mechanisms obtain behavioral risk information from subgroups of women. For example, CDC's Pregnancy Nutrition Surveillance System (PNSS) has monitored behavioral and nutritional risk factors among low-income women in selected states since 1979. PNSS collects prospective data on alcohol use, smoking, and weight gain during pregnancy from women who receive prenatal care in a public health setting (see the Pregnancy-Related Nutrition chapter).

CDC SURVEILLANCE ACTIVITIES

Vital records constitute the only perinatal database for the U.S. population. Revisions in the U.S. Standard Birth Certificate in 1989 were designed to improve surveillance of pregnancy outcome and related factors (5). The 1989 revisions added several new items and replaced open-ended questions with a check-box format designed to make data collection more uniform and complete. Before 1989, behavioral risk information was recorded or birth certificates in open-ended comment boxes captioned **complications of pregnancy** and **concurrent illnesses or conditions affecting the pregnancy**. The responses to these questions were not included on NCHS's computerized national natality files. These items have now been replaced by check-boxes that collect categorical information on cigarette smoking, use of alcohol, and weight gain during pregnancy. These data are now available on national natality files.

Although the revised birth certificate is a useful surveillance tool to determine trends in pregnancy outcome, the scope of prenatal behavioral information it collects is limited. Smoking and alcohol use questions are restricted to use at any time during pregnancy, and average amount consumed per week over the entire pregnancy. The data therefore fail to account for changing patterns of the use of these substances during pregnancy. Changing use patterns are particularly important in regards to alcohol use, which poses the greatest risk for anatomic anomalies when consumed heavily during the periconceptional period. Because of the lack of specificity in question design and the lack of uniformity in the way birth certificate information is collected, birth certificates may underestimate the prevalence of some risk behaviors during pregnancy (6).

Despite these limitations, the birth certificate is a useful source of clinically reported birth outcome information, and it furnishes an excellent sampling frame for surveys such as the NMIHS and surveillance systems such as PRAMS. Additionally, vital records include variables that can be used to identify groups of special interest for which oversampling might be indicated.

To obtain additional data that could be linked to birth outcome information in vital records, NCHS has conducted the NMIHS and related earlier surveys such as the National Natality Surveys (NNS). These surveys are based on national samples drawn from vital records of live births, infant deaths, and late fetal deaths (7).

The NMIHS is primarily a mail survey; only nonrespondents are contacted for a personal or telephone interview. Collected data are linked to data in birth certificates and health-care provider records. NMIHS data are collected from mothers 6–30 months after the birth of the child to assess their behavior before and during pregnancy, their health, the pregnancy outcome, and the infant's health. Known and potential risk factors covered on the NMIHS questionnaire include weight gain during pregnancy, physical activity, and the use of cigarettes, alcohol, and illicit drugs just before and during pregnancy. The 1988 NMIHS was the first in the series to collect information from all women regardless of their marital status; previous NNS cycles collected data only from married women. The survey design oversamples high-risk groups in the natality component, including low- and very-low-birth-weight infants, African-American infants, and in Texas only, Hispanic infants.

The NNS and NMIHS contributed the first nationally representative estimates of the prevalence of behavioral risk factors before and during pregnancy among women who recently gave birth. These surveys continue to provide important supplements to vital records data. In addition, the NMIHS follow-up surveys, in which respondents are recontacted after 2–3 years, are an important source of longitudinal data that allow us to examine maternal risk behavior from the periconceptional period through early childhood.

Like the NMIHS, PRAMS also samples from birth certificates. The sampling frame consists of all live births occurring during a specified period in a given state. The system's primary data collection method consists of statewide mail surveillance with telephone follow-up for nonrespondents *(8)*. Every month, each PRAMS state draws a stratified systematic sample of 100–200 births from recently processed birth certificates. Unlike the NMIHS, which must wait for the states to send their records to NCHS before sampling, PRAMS's monthly samples for mail surveillance require only that the birth certificate has been logged into the state vital statistics registry system. This allows PRAMS projects to contact a new mother within 2–6 months after the delivery.

Although stratification variables differ among PRAMS states, all states oversample births in subpopulations with an increased risk of poor birth outcomes (Table 2). PRAMS data are entered at the state health agency. CDC then weights the data on the basis of sample design, nonresponse, and omissions from the sampling frame.

The PRAMS questionnaire is structured into two parts: a core portion that is identical for all states, and a state-specific portion. Core questions related to maternal behavior and birth outcomes include focus on the use of cigarettes and alcohol before and during pregnancy, intendedness of pregnancy, and stressful events during pregnancy.

State-specific questions related to maternal behavior before and during pregnancy address such topics as mental health and social support, occupation and physical activity, drug use, and physical abuse.

Data collection by mail with telephone follow-up for nonrespondents has worked well in most PRAMS states. However, in states with large urban populations in which response rates by mail tend to be low, mail surveillance is supplemented with hospital-based surveillance in defined geographical areas with telephone follow-up for nonrespondents. Births in subpopulations with traditionally low-response rates by mail are sampled from the delivery logs of targeted hospitals. Reaching new mothers while they are still in the hospital after delivery has provided a feasible and effective method for collecting data from women who are less likely to respond by mail.

GENERAL FINDINGS

Birth Certificates

Analyses of national data from the revised 1989 birth certificate regarding behavioral risks during pregnancy have focused on smoking, use of alcohol, and weight gain during pregnancy *(9,10)*. Here are some selected findings on these topics:

- Nineteen percent of women who gave birth in 1989 reported smoking during pregnancy. Smoking varied according to the mother's level of education and adequacy of prenatal care. Mothers with 9–11 years of education were about eight times as likely to smoke (42%) as were college graduates (5%). Mothers whose care was inadequate were twice as likely to have smoked during pregnancy (32%) as were those with adequate care (16%).

- Controlling for race, adequacy of prenatal care, and mother's educational level, babies born to mothers who smoked during pregnancy were at a greater risk of having a low birth weight. Whereas 6% of babies born to nonsmoking mothers had a low birth weight, 11.4% babies born to mothers who reported

TABLE 2. Stratification variables and stratum-specific response rates for the Pregnancy Risk Assessment Monitoring System, by state, 1990–1991*

State	Stratification variables	Stratum		No.†	Response rate
Alaska	Maternal race, adequacy of prenatal care	Inadequate prenatal care	Native Alaskan	503	68.4
		Adequate prenatal care	Native Alaskan	540	74.9
		Inadequate prenatal care	non-Native Alaskan	541	72.0
		Adequate prenatal care	non-Native Alaskan	727	82.9
Maine	Birth weight	<2,500 g		259	75.0
		≥2,500 g		381	73.7
Michigan	Maternal race, birth weight	Black (mail)	<2,500 g	348	49.7
		Black (hospital)	<2,500 g	186	78.5
		Other races	<2,500 g	367	73.8
		Black (mail)	≥2,500 g	354	58.5
		Black (hospital)	≥2,500 g	233	83.3
		Other races	≥2,500 g	414	84.3
Oklahoma	Birth weight	<1,500 g		228	65.9
		1,500–2,499 g		195	59.3
		2,500–3,999 g		260	70.3
		≥4,000 g		293	79.6
West Virginia	Adequacy of prenatal care, birth weight	Inadequate prenatal care	<2,500 g	201	62.2
		Adequate prenatal care	<2,500 g	250	74.4
		Inadequate prenatal care	≥2,500 g	218	75.4
		Adequate prenatal care	≥2,500 g	204	82.6

* Includes only states with 1 year or more of weighted PRAMS data. States initiating PRAMS in 1990 began data collection in spring 1993 and therefore are not included.
† No. = number of women; all data were collected during 1990–1991, but the number of months' worth of data vary.

smoking during pregnancy had a low birth weight.

- Four percent of women who gave birth in 1989 reported using alcohol during pregnancy. Among women who reported drinking during pregnancy, 61% reported consuming one drink or less per week, and 21% said they consumed three or more drinks per week.

- Among women who reported having three or more drinks per week, 15–20% of their babies had a low birth weight compared with 7% of mothers who did not drink.

- Approximately 17% of white mothers and 27% of African-American mothers with gestations of >40 weeks gained <20 lbs. during pregnancy. This is below the 1990 National Institute of Medicine's recommended weight gain of 25–35 lbs. for an average-sized woman. Women most at risk for insufficient weight gain included those with less than a high school education, unmarried women, and women whose attendant at birth was not a physician or midwife. Differences found by racial group may be attributable to economic, social, or other factors.

States have used birth certificates to look at such topics as the relationship between smoking during pregnancy and conditions such as low birth weight, sudden infant death syndrome (SIDS), and other complications of pregnancy (11–14). States have also used birth certificates to describe patterns of smoking during pregnancy among subgroups of women (15).

National Maternal and Infant Health Survey and National Natality Survey

Numerous analyses of NMIHS and NNS data have addressed behavioral risk factors such as tobacco, alcohol, and drug use before and during pregnancy; weight gain during pregnancy; physical activity and stress during pregnancy; and unintended or unwanted pregnancy:

- Results from the 1988 NMIHS indicate that age, race, marital status, and depression (but not occupation) were significantly related to

alcohol consumption just before and during pregnancy (16).

- Among mothers with live births included in the 1988 NMIHS, women who drank more during pregnancy also smoked more, were younger and less educated, and gave birth to babies whose gestational age was less than the gestational age of babies born to women who drank at lower levels or not at all (17).

- 1988 NMIHS data revealed that both intrauterine and passive exposure to cigarette smoke were associated with an increased risk of SIDS (18).

- An analysis of live births from the 1988 NMIHS indicated that African-American women were significantly less likely to receive prenatal advice on smoking and alcohol cessation than were white women (19).

- A study of data from the 1967 and 1980 NNS revealed that among married mothers, level of education was strongly associated with the decrease in prevalence of smoking during pregnancy. Between 1967 and 1980, whereas prevalence of smoking during pregnancy decreased from 48% to 43% among mothers with <12 years of education, it decreased from 34% to 11% among mothers with >12 years of education (20).

- Results from the 1980 NNS revealed an association between whether the pregnancy was wanted and the likelihood that a smoker would stop smoking after her pregnancy is confirmed. Wanting the birth to have occurred earlier or at that time was associated with a 23% decrease in the probability that the woman would quit smoking (21).

Pregnancy Risk Assessment Monitoring System

CDC's major areas of PRAMS analysis— conducted with combined data sets for four participating states—have addressed smoking and alcohol use during pregnancy:

- The prevalence of smoking before, during, and after pregnancy among women receiving publicly funded prenatal care was 2.3 to 3.4 times the comparable prevalence among women who received care from private providers.

- Although many smokers reduced or quit smoking while they were pregnant, most resumed or increased their smoking to nearly prepregnancy levels within 3–6 months after delivery (Table 3) (3).

- The prevalence of drinking during the last 3 months of pregnancy is relatively low: 11.7% of mothers reported light drinking (one to six drinks per week), 0.2% reported moderate drinking (seven to 13 drinks per week), and 0.03% reported heavy drinking (14 drinks or more per week) (Table 4) (4).

- The prevalence of drinking during the 3 months before conception was much higher, with 31.9%–53.8% of mothers reporting light drinking; 1.6%–3.0% reporting moderate drinking; and 0.6%–1.3% reporting heavy drinking (4).

- Between 66% and 75% of PRAMS respondents received prenatal counseling about alcohol's effects. Heavy drinkers were more likely than light drinkers to receive such counseling (4).

- A comparison of PRAMS data with information from birth certificates indicates that the reporting of alcohol use during pregnancy is significantly higher on the self-reported PRAMS questionnaire than on the birth certificate (4).

State-Specific Findings from PRAMS

OKLAHOMA

Oklahoma publishes PRAMS findings in a quarterly newsletter, the *Oklahoma PRAMS-GRAM*, which is distributed to public and private health care providers; university faculty in medicine, nursing, and public health; legislators; state maternal and child health directors; and professional organizations (22). Oklahoma has also published its PRAMS findings in *Morbidity and Mortality Weekly Report* (23). These data focus on topics such as the prevalence of alcohol and cigarette consumption during pregnancy as well as unintended pregnancy:

- One in 10 Oklahoma mothers reported consuming alcohol during the last 3 months of pregnancy, with <1% consuming seven drinks or more per week during the last trimester.

- One in seven mothers (14.6%) reported that they were not asked by their prenatal care provider if they drank alcohol.

- Mothers who smoked during pregnancy were found to be 2.3 times more likely to deliver a low-birth-weight infant than were mothers who did not smoke.

TABLE 3. Percentage distribution of cigarette consumption (in relation to prepregnancy amount) during the last 3 months of pregnancy and 3–6 months postpartum among 2,473 women who smoked before pregnancy — Maine, Michigan, Oklahoma, and West Virginia, 1988–1989

Timing	Cigarette consumption					
	Quit		Reduced		Smoked same or more	
	%	(SE)*	%	(SE)*	%	(SE)*
Last 3 months of pregnancy	29.4	(2.1)	39.1	(2.3)	31.5	(2.2)
3–6 months postpartum	13.4	(1.5)	18.4	(1.7)	8.2	(2.1)

*SE, standard error.

Source: Adams MM, Brogan DJ, Kendrick JS, et al. (3).

TABLE 4. Percentage distribution of alcohol consumption 3 months before and during the last 3 months of pregnancy among 6,319 women — Maine, Michigan, Oklahoma, and West Virginia, 1988–1989

	Alcohol consumption									
	None		Light <7 drinks/week		Moderate 7–13 drinks/week		Heavy ≥14 drinks/week		Unknown	
Timing	%	(SE)*	%	(SE)*	%	(SE)*	%	(SE)*	%	(SE)*
3 months before pregnancy	47.4	(1.4)	44.2	(1.4)	2.4	(0.05)	1.0	(0.3)	4.9	(0.5)
Last 3 months of pregnancy	85.3	(1.0)	11.7	(0.9)	0.2	(0.1)	0.03	(0.02)	2.8	(0.4)

* SE, standard error.

Source: Bruce FC, Adams MM, Shulman HB, et al. *(4)*.

- One in five mothers reported that they smoked cigarettes during the last 3 months of pregnancy.

- About 44% of respondents reported that their most recent pregnancy was unintended.

- More than two thirds (69.4%) of respondents <20 years of age reported that their most recent pregnancy was unintended, and 14% of infants were delivered to females <20 years of age.

MAINE

Maine has published a report describing its PRAMS research methodology and providing general findings from the first four years of surveillance to state government agencies, public and private health agencies, and professional associations *(24)*. These findings relate to the use of alcohol and cigarettes during pregnancy:

- About 40% of respondents reported consuming alcohol during the last trimester of pregnancy.

- Similar to Oklahoma, Maine found that <1% of women reported consuming seven drinks or more a week during the last 3 months of pregnancy.

- Approximately 25% of respondents who gave birth in 1991 reported smoking during the last trimester of pregnancy.

- One in 10 women reported smoking at least one pack of cigarettes a day during the last trimester of pregnancy.

- About half of WIC recipients reported smoking during their most recent pregnancy.

WEST VIRGINIA

West Virginia's analyses of PRAMS data have focused on smoking because the prevalence of smoking among West Virginia women of reproductive age is comparatively high. Results have been presented at numerous state conferences and have been regularly distributed to state agencies and other organizations:

- About 39% of women who received Medicaid smoked during pregnancy compared with 21% of women not on Medicaid *(25)*.

- After controlling for age, PRAMS officials found that recipients of Medicaid were still 1.8 times more likely to smoke during pregnancy than were women not on Medicaid.

- Medicaid recipients who smoked gave birth to infants who at term weighed, on average, about 306 g (11 oz) less than infants born to nonsmoking, non-Medicaid recipients.

INTERPRETATION ISSUES

Currently we have no national reporting system to provide detailed, prospectively collected information about women's behavior during pregnancy. Despite the 1989 expansions in the scope and specificity of information collected on the birth certificate, vital records do not provide the level of detailed behavioral information necessary to study important aspects of women's behaviors, such as the timing of tobacco and alcohol consumption during pregnancy, and their relationship to birth outcome.

The NMIHS and PRAMS provide estimates of the prevalence of women's pregnancy-related behaviors that may be associated with poor outcome. NMIHS data provide important information regarding national trends in women's risk behavior before and during pregnancy. PRAMS collects data about women's behavior that can be used by state health departments to inform program decision makers. PRAMS also offers states the opportunity to participate in sampling design, data collection, and questionnaire development, thus strengthening their ability to make program decisions based on state-specific scientific information.

Despite their differences, the NMIHS and PRAMS face comparable methodologic considerations because of similarities in data collection. The NMIHS and PRAMS data are both designed to supplement birth certificate information. Both data collection systems use birth certificates as a sampling frame, which has several advantages. Sampling from birth certificates allows the NMIHS to obtain a nationally representative sample. For PRAMS, the sample drawn from each participating state's birth certificates is representative of the state population; therefore, findings can be generalized to the state. Vital records also allow both data collection systems to oversample populations of special interest.

A disadvantage of using birth certificates is that data must be collected retrospectively, increasing the chance of recall bias or inability to contact the selected woman. In addition, the extent to which pregnancy outcome may influence a woman's recall and reporting of behavior is unknown. Retrospective data collection means that sensitivity and predictive value of a positive test are difficult to determine.

For both the NMIHS and PRAMS, a final birth certificate file is necessary to assess sample bias and weight the data. Reliance on vital records means that both the NMIHS and PRAMS are dependent on varying state time frames for recording and finalizing birth certificate files. Delays in vital records processing at the state level hinder the timeliness of data collection and production of weighted data sets.

Because the NMIHS and PRAMS questionnaires are primarily self-administered and collected by mail, they may provide a more accurate report of risky behaviors such as smoking and alcohol use during pregnancy than would be obtained in face-to-face interviews. Some research indicates that respondents are less likely to report high-risk behavior directly to a clinician or interviewer (26–28). Even though confidentiality is stressed during interviews women may be self-conscious about the possible adverse effects of their behavior and therefore not report honestly.

Self-administered questionnaires have the advantage of not introducing bias resulting from the presence of an interviewer. However, they are limited in their ability to obtain complex medical information, which would require lengthier, more difficult questions. Further, because interpretation of a question is left to the respondent, ensuring uniform interpretation is difficult. In contrast, an interviewer-administered questionnaire allows for probing when the respondent fails to understand a question or provide an appropriate response.

The greatest challenge presented by mail questionnaires is low response, particularly among highly mobile or disadvantaged subpopulations. Both the NMIHS and PRAMS send two mailings before contact is attempted by phone or, in the

101

case of the NMIHS, by personal interview. The total response rate to the mail component of the 1988 NMIHS was 30.3%, excluding follow-up attempts for nonresponders. Response to the mail component of PRAMS has been better, ranging from about 33.6% in Washington, D.C., to approximately 77.1% in West Virginia (8). To boost overall response rates, the NMIHS used census interviewers to conduct home visits for face-to-face data collection. PRAMS has developed and established hospital surveillance, which has increased overall response rates. However, the addition of both home interviews and hospital surveillance has increased the labor intensity and cost of conducting the NMIHS and PRAMS.

EXAMPLES OF USING DATA

Dissemination of findings is an essential component of any survey or surveillance system. Birth certificate and national survey data have been used to describe national trends and set national goals for improving the health of women and children. Baseline data used to determine national year 2000 objectives for women and children's health are derived from birth certificate and national survey information (29). These data have also been the basis of a large body of scientific research concerning maternal behavior and its influence on birth outcomes. Many findings from these studies have enhanced our understanding of how behavior and birth outcome are linked and have influenced women and children's health programs.

The addition of behavioral risk information to the birth certificate will provide states with ready estimates of the overall prevalence of smoking and alcohol use during pregnancy. States are already using such information to target public health resources. In Georgia, a study of prenatal smoking information from birth certificates was instrumental in expanding Georgia Medicaid to cover smoking cessation programs for pregnant women (Rochat R, unpublished data, 1993).

States participating in PRAMS have found that PRAMS data can provide the basis for state-specific research. Using PRAMS data, states have documented the need to strengthen women and children's health services; monitored their progress toward meeting public health goals; and

informed health-care providers and the public about the prevalences of certain types of behavior during pregnancy. They have used PRAMS data to measure progress toward meeting year 2000 objectives in the areas of prenatal weight gain, maternal smoking, breast-feeding, births among teenagers, and alcohol consumption. Below are brief descriptions of some ways PRAMS findings have helped shape policies and programs.

Maine's commissioner of health has developed a series of plans calling for expansion of women and children's health services for young mothers. PRAMS data have been incorporated into a working document titled *Teen and Young Adult Health: Annual Action Plan, FY '90–'91*, which documents the need for improved pregnancy management services for teens and young mothers (30). Using data on smoking behavior, Maine is also producing a brochure for health care providers designed to reinforce the importance of counseling pregnant women about the effects of smoking.

The *Oklahoma PRAMS-GRAM* reaches a wide spectrum of public health providers, policy makers, and the general public (22). On the basis of research findings, the *PRAMS-GRAM* makes program recommendations aimed at achieving year 2000 goals for improved women and children's health. PRAMS data regarding alcohol consumption during pregnancy was instrumental in the establishment of a state fetal alcohol syndrome (FAS) prevention center, which will help communities establish FAS prevention projects and work with state community leaders to improve policies aimed at preventing FAS. In addition, the governor and the commissioner of health have used PRAMS data to develop public health policies and strategies regarding women and children's health *(Oklahoma State Department of Health, unpublished data, 1993)*.

FUTURE ISSUES

Meaningful data systems are necessary if the United States is to monitor its progress toward improved public health. National and state public health organizations are under increasing pressure to inform health-care providers, policy makers, and the public about the status of infant health and to translate data into improved health services for women and children. In recognition of this fact, goals for improved public health surveillance systems form an integral part of the national health objectives in *Healthy People 2000* (29).

Meeting these challenges will require the continuation of periodic national surveys. In 1991, a follow-up survey of women interviewed for the 1988 NMIHS was conducted to obtain longitudinal data on the progress of their children. In addition, a new cycle of the NMIHS is being planned for 1996 or 1997, with subsequent follow-up at 2-year intervals. The cohort will be followed at least until the children reach 6 years of age.

State health departments will also be required to enhance their capacity to collect and analyze state-specific data on women and children's health. PRAMS responds to these needs directly by building data collection and analytic capacity within state health departments. PRAMS states are developing analysis projects in collaboration with university faculty, private health promotion organizations, and CDC. Such collaborative relationships will enhance the quality and timeliness of new PRAMS analyses. In addition, PRAMS data will help states monitor their progress toward attaining national public health goals by providing state-specific data addressing 16 of the year 2000 objectives for women and children's health and family planning.

As new research findings modify our understanding of factors that affect infant health, data collection systems must evolve as well. Future evaluation needs include 1) regular assessment of response rates by mode of contact, 2) periodic evaluation of data collection and sampling methodology, and 3) periodic revision of information collected in questionnaires. The revision of information obtained in questionnaires will be particularly important as our knowledge of behavioral risk factors increases. PRAMS is designed to be an ongoing surveillance activity of state health departments in the area of infant health, with PRAMS states functioning more independently over time. Given the availability of resources, CDC hopes to extend PRAMS to every state, thus providing them with access to a unique

source of information about how periconceptional and perinatal behavior are linked to infant health. The participation of all states will also provide us with a new source of national data and strengthen our ability to conduct comparisons between states.

Several changes under way will help to improve the efficiency of longitudinal studies and surveillance systems like the NMIHS and PRAMS. More timely registration of vital records through the Electronic Birth Certificate System will reduce the time between the mother's delivery and her receipt of the survey. Improvements in the birth certificate registry will help NCHS and PRAMS states to quickly release data that are needed by health professionals and agencies to measure their progress and target resources. For new PRAMS states, greater standardization of PRAMS methodology will streamline the start-up process and ease operation of the surveillance system.

The global goal of data collection systems like the NMIHS and PRAMS is to provide a quantitative basis for improved policies and programs that reduce infant mortality and morbidity. In regard to behavioral risk factors during the periconceptional and perinatal periods, the information these data systems collect can improve our understanding of women's behavior and our knowledge of how to reduce the prevalence of behavioral risk factors. In the future, improved data systems and prompt dissemination of findings will continue to strengthen the link between surveillance and improvements in women and children's health policies and services.

REFERENCES

1. CDC. Infant mortality—United States, 1990. MMWR 1993; 42:161–5.

2. NCHS. Health, United States, 1991. Hyattsville, Maryland: US Department of Health and Human Services, Public Health Service, CDC, 1992.

3. Adams MM, Brogan DJ, Kendrick JS, et al. Smoking, pregnancy, and source of prenatal care: results from the Pregnancy Risk Assessment Monitoring System. Obstet Gynecol 1992;80:738–44.

4. Bruce FC, Adams MM, Shulman HB, et al. Alcohol use before and during pregnancy. Am J Prev Med 1993;9:267–73.

5. Luke B, Keith LG. The United States Standard Certificate of Live Birth: a critical commentary. J Reprod Med 1991;36:587–91.

6. Bruce FC, Adams MM, Shulman HB, PRAMS Working Group. How well is alcohol use reported in birth certificates? Presented at the annual meeting of the American Public Health Association, Atlanta, Georgia, November 10–14, 1991.

7. Sanderson M, Placek PJ, Keppel KG. The 1988 National Maternal and Infant Health Survey: design, content, and data availability. BIRTH 1991;18:26–31.

8. Adams MM, Shulman HB, Bruce FC, Hogue C, Brogan D, PRAMS Working Group. The Pregnancy Risk Assessment Monitoring System: design, questionnaire, data collection, and response rates. Pediatr Perinatal Epidemiol 1991;5:333–46.

9. NCHS. Advance report of new data from the 1989 birth certificate. Hyattsville, Maryland: US Department of Health and Human Services, Public Health Service, CDC, 1992. (Monthly vital statistics report; vol. 40, no. 12, suppl.)

10. CDC. Pregnancy risks determined from birth certificate data—United States, 1989. MMWR, 1992; 41:556–63.

11. Georgia Department of Human Resources. Low birthweight among smokers and nonsmokers in Georgia. Georgia Epidemiol Rep 1991;7(3):1–2.

12. Li D-K, Daling JR. Maternal smoking, low birth weight, and ethnicity in relation to sudden infant death syndrome. Am J Epidemiol 1991;134:958–64.

13. Malloy MH, Hoffman HJ, Peterson DR. Sudden infant death syndrome and maternal smoking. Am J Public Health 1992;82:1380–2.

14. Myhra W, Davis M, Mueller BA, Hickok D. Maternal smoking and the risk of polyhydramnios. Am J Public Health 1992;82: 176–9.

15. Davis RL, Helgerson SD, Waller P. Smoking during pregnancy among northwest Native Americans. Public Health Rep 1992;107:66–9.

16. Hanna E, Faden V, Dufour M. Do pregnant women alter their drinking behavior? If not, why not? Presented at the annual meeting of the American Public Health Association, Washington, DC, November 8–12, 1992.

17. Faden V, Graubard B, Dufour M. Drinking by expectant mothers: what does it mean for their babies? Presented at the annual meeting of the American Public Health Association, Washington, DC, November 8–12, 1992.

18. Schoendorf KC, Kiely JL. Relationship of sudden infant death syndrome to maternal smoking during and after pregnancy. Pediatrics 1992;90:905–8.

19. Kogan MD, Kotelchuck M, Alexander GR, Johnson WE. Racial disparities in reported prenatal care advice from health care providers. Am J Public Health, 1993 (in press).

20. Klienman JC, Kopstein A. Smoking during pregnancy, 1967–80. Am J Public Health 1987;77:823–5.

21. Weller R, Eberstein IW, Bailey M. Pregnancy wantedness and maternal behavior during pregnancy. Demography 1987;24:407–12.

22. Oklahoma State Department of Health, Maternal and Child Health Services. Oklahoma PRAMS-GRAM 1991–1992; vols. 1 and 2.

23. CDC. Unintended childbearing: pregnancy risk assessment monitoring system—Oklahoma, 1988–1991. MMWR 1992;41:933–6.

24. Maine Department of Human Services, Office of Data, Research, and Vital Statistics. PRAMS—The first four years. Augusta, Maine: Maine Department of Human Services, 1992.

25. West Virginia Bureau of Public Health. Medicaid-funded pregnancy and birth in West Virginia: 1989. Charleston, West Virginia: West Virginia Bureau of Public Health, 1989.

26. Dillman DA. Mail and telephone surveys: the total design method. New York: John Wiley & Sons, 1978.

27. Weissfeld JL, Holloway JJ, Kirscht JP. Effects of deceptive self-reports of quitting on the results of treatment trials for smoking: a quantitative assessment. J Clin Epidemiol 1989;42:231–43.

28. Wagenknecht LE, Burke GL, Perkins LL, Haley NJ, Friedman GD. Misclassification of smoking status in the cardia study: a comparison of self-report with serum cotinine levels. Am J Public Health 1992;82:33–6.

29. US Department of Health and Human Services, Public Health Service. Healthy people 2000: national health promotion and disease prevention objectives—full report, with commentary. Washington, DC: US Department of Health and Human Services, Public Health Service, 1991; DHHS publication no. (PHS)91-50212.

30. Maine Department of Human Services. Teen and young adult health: annual action plan, FY '90–'91. Augusta, Maine: Maine Department of Human Services, 1990.

Prenatal Care

John L. Kiely, Ph.D.,[1] and Michael D. Kogan, Ph.D., M.A.[2]

PUBLIC HEALTH IMPORTANCE

Prenatal care has been recognized as the cornerstone of our health-care system for pregnant women since the beginning of the twentieth century. During the first decade of the century, Mrs. William Lowell Putnam initiated a prenatal service at Boston Lying-In Hospital in which pregnant women were visited by a nurse every 10 days and instructed in self-care. Women were urged to report as early in pregnancy as possible. Meanwhile, in New York City, a program of organized prenatal care was begun in 1907 by Dr. Josephine Baker. In 1915, J. Whitbridge Williams found that dystocia, toxemia, and preterm birth could be reduced if prenatal care included instruction for the pregnant woman in personal hygiene, rest, and diet, along with a competent obstetrical examination (1). The approach to prenatal care was based originally on the detection and treatment of preeclampsia, and later, preterm birth. The emphasis in the delivery of prenatal care services has continued to change from focusing on conditions of the mother to conditions of the fetus, as disparities in birth weight and infant mortality have remained or increased.

A number of studies have indicated a relationship between the use of prenatal care services and birth outcomes (2–16). Adequate use of prenatal care has been associated with improved birth weights and the amelioration of the risk of preterm delivery (5,6,15). Inadequate use of prenatal care has been associated with increased risks of low-birth-weight births, premature births, neonatal mortality, infant mortality, and maternal mortality (1–4,9–11,13,14). Several researchers have suggested that the beneficial effects of prenatal care are strongest among socially disadvantaged women (7,8,12,16).

The importance of prenatal care as a public health priority has been reinforced recently by a study in which investigators analyzed results from the 1980 U.S. National Natality Survey (NNS), the 1981 French National Natality Survey, a 1979 sample of Danish births, and a 1979–1980 survey performed in one Belgian province (17). The proportion of women who began prenatal care late (after 15 weeks of gestation) was highest in the United States (21.2%) and lowest in France (4%). Across all maternal ages, parities, and educational levels, late initiation of prenatal care was more frequent in the United States. Fewer financial barriers characterize the care delivery systems in the three European countries (18), which may explain why women of low-socioeconomic status begin prenatal care earlier there than they do in the United States (for additional information about related topics and surveillance activities, see the Contraception, Behavioral Risk Factors Before and During Pregnancy, Pregnancy-Related Morbidity, Pregnancy-Related Mortality, Low Birth Weight and Intrauterine Growth Retardation, Infant Mortality, and Pregnancy in Adolescents chapters).

[1] Division of Health and Utilization Analysis
National Center for Health Statistics
Centers for Disease Control and Prevention
Hyattsville, Maryland

[2] Division of Vital Statistics
National Center for Health Statistics
Centers for Disease Control and Prevention
Hyattsville, Maryland

HISTORY OF DATA COLLECTION

Data from the U.S. Standard Certificate of Live Birth have been used in prenatal care surveillance since 1968, when a question about **the month of pregnancy that prenatal care began** was added to the certificate. Data on the number of prenatal visits have been collected and published since 1972.

Because birth certificate data on the total number of prenatal visits provide no information regarding the timing of visits, and because information on the timing of visits does not reveal whether care has been continuous, the Institute of Medicine in 1973 developed a composite index incorporating both the month of the first prenatal visit and the total number of visits into one summary utilization measure (19). Using guidelines from the American College of Obstetricians and Gynecologists, the Institute of Medicine adjusted timing and quantity of prenatal visits for length of gestation and combined the two measures to yield a measure of the use of prenatal care. Under this classification scheme, the use of prenatal care could be placed in three categories: adequate, intermediate, and inadequate.

This system was modified by Gortmaker in 1979 (4) and is now commonly used in the surveillance of prenatal care. It is called the Adequacy of Care Index or, more commonly, the Kessner Index. In 1987, Alexander and Corneley markedly improved the Kessner Index by categorizing pregnant women into six groups: those receiving no care, inadequate care, intermediate care, adequate care, and intensive care and those for whom such information is missing or unknown (20). The **intensive** group includes women who made a relatively excessive number of visits given the month that prenatal care began and the duration of pregnancy. Intensive, repeated use of prenatal care services is assumed to indicate potential morbidity or complications.

Over the past 15 years, birth certificate data have been used in numerous U.S. surveys of prenatal care. In the 1980 NNS, for example, the National Center for Health Statistics (NCHS) collected data from a representative sample of

9,941 birth certificates for 1980. Survey staff conducted detailed interviews with most of the mothers represented by those births, and they collected additional data from hospital and physician questionnaires.

During the 1982 and 1983 interviews conducted for the National Survey of Family Growth (NSFG), NCHS began collecting data on prenatal care and method of payment at delivery for women who had live births in the period beginning January 1979 (21). Several years later, in the 1988 National Maternal and Infant Health Survey (NMIHS), NCHS began studying risk factors such as inadequate prenatal care, inadequate weight gain during pregnancy, as well as smoking and alcohol and drug use during pregnancy (22). Maternal behaviors during pregnancy also are monitored via the Pregnancy Risk Assessment Monitoring System (PRAMS)—a state-based surveillance system, established by CDC in 1987, that uses mail and telephone questionnaires to solicit information from women. Thirteen states and the District of Columbia are participating in PRAMS (23).

CDC SURVEILLANCE ACTIVITIES

Vital Statistics

Data on prenatal care are collected on birth certificates filed in each of the states through their vital registration systems. Although vital registration is a state activity, NCHS promotes uniformity in the data collected via recommended standard certificates. These standard certificates are developed in cooperation with state vital statistics offices and providers and users of the information. They are revised about every 10 years.

The state data are provided on computer tapes to NCHS, which then compiles them into national data and disseminates them annually. The primary vehicles for dissemination are 1) the *Advance Report of Final Natality Statistics (24)*, which contains summary tabulations; 2) *Vital Statistics of the United States, Volume I, Natality (25)*, which contains detailed tabulations; 3) public-use computer tapes; and 4) periodic analytic reports.

Generally, national natality files are available within 18–24 months of the end of the data year. State-level data are available from all of these files. With only a few exceptions, all characteristics are shown, by state, in the published annual natality volumes, *Vital Statistics of the United States, Volume I, Natality (25)*.*

In surveillance activities that use data from birth certificates, prenatal care utilization is monitored by using one of four measures:

- **Some prenatal care vs. no prenatal care.** This is probably the least useful of the four prenatal care measures because of tremendous variability contained in the **presence of prenatal care category.**

- **Month or trimester of first prenatal care visit.** The month or trimester of the first prenatal visit provides more information about the opportunity to detect problems by virtue of how early in pregnancy the first visit occurs. However, this information alone provides no evidence of what occurs subsequent to the first visit. Heterogeneity exists within any group of women who begin prenatal care in the same gestational month or trimester because the number of visits can range widely. A recent investigation indicated that the timing of prenatal visits differs across racial and ethnic groups *(26)*. Although the timing of the first prenatal visit has often been used as a measure of the adequacy of prenatal care received, it is limited because early care does not always mean continuous care.

- **Total number of prenatal care visits.** The total number of prenatal visits provides more information about the extent of provider content. However, use of this variable by itself provides no information regarding the timing of the visits.

- **A composite measure such as the Kessner Index.** This classification system is better than the other three measures because it combines the month of the first prenatal visit with the total number of visits to establish a measure of the use of prenatal care *(19)*.

Ongoing Surveillance

CDC oversees two ongoing surveillance systems that collect data on prenatal care—the NSFG and PRAMS. The NSFG is a probability household survey of females aged 15–44 years in the civilian noninstitutionalized population. In 1982 and 1983, 7,969 women were interviewed. In addition to garnering data on women's reproductive and family planning histories, the NSFG also collects information on prenatal care and method of payment at delivery.

CDC established PRAMS to collect data on maternal behaviors that influence pregnancy outcomes. Thus far, Alabama, Alaska, California, the District of Columbia, Florida, Georgia, Indiana, Maine, Michigan, New York (excluding New York City), Oklahoma, South Carolina, Washington, and West Virginia have established 5 PRAMS programs *(23)*. Through PRAMS, states conduct population-based surveillance of maternal behaviors during women's pregnancies and during the early infancy of their children. PRAMS data also supplement birth certificate data and provide information that can be used to identify needs and target interventions. To allow multistate comparisons of PRAMS findings, states use standardized data collection methods. In each state, mothers are sampled monthly from a sampling frame of recently processed resident birth certificates. Mothers are then mailed a 14-page questionnaire 3–6 months after delivery. If no response is received, a second questionnaire is mailed; if the woman still does not respond, PRAMS staff attempt to administer the questionnaire by telephone. The questionnaire also asks detailed questions about the mother's use of prenatal care. Collection procedures are described in detail elsewhere *(23)*.

---

* Reports on the use of prenatal care based on natality files include data on mothers of live-born infants only. Thus, most of the findings reported in this chapter refer to live births. Because induced abortions are of little interest in studies of the use of prenatal care, only two minor problems arise with using the number of live births as an index of the number of pregnant women. First, mothers of multiple infants are counted more than once. Second, women whose pregnancies result in fetal deaths are not included at all. However, in the United States in 1991, 2.31% of live births were twins and 0.08% were triplets or higher order multiple births. Of pregnancies that progressed to 20 weeks of gestation, 0.73% resulted in fetal deaths and 99.23% resulted in live births. Thus, for the purpose of reports on the use of prenatal care, very little difference exists between proportions of *live births* and proportions of *women*.

GENERAL FINDINGS

The most detailed review of studies of risk factors for insufficient prenatal care is a report, issued by the Institute of Medicine in 1988, entitled *Prenatal Care: Reaching Mothers, Reaching Infants* *(27,28)*. Much of the following discussion of variables related to the use of prenatal care is based on this report.

Demographic Risk Factors

RACE AND ETHNICITY

Among white women with live births in 1990, 79.2% began care in the first trimester of pregnancy, and 4.9% received late or no care. Black women were far less likely than white women to begin care early (60.6%) and twice as likely to receive late prenatal care (11.3%) or no care (4.9%) *(29)*. Hispanic mothers were substantially less likely than non-Hispanic white mothers to obtain late or no care, but they were more likely than non-Hispanic black mothers to begin care late or not at all. Native American women were more likely than either white or black women to obtain late or no care. These racial differences are not likely related to race per se but instead to socioeconomic factors such as income, educational level, access to health care, and access to insurance.

AGE

Adolescent mothers are at a high risk of obtaining late or no prenatal care, with the greatest risk being among mothers <15 years of age (for more information, see the Pregnancy in Adolescents chapter).

EDUCATION

In studies of mothers with live-born infants, timing of the first prenatal visit is strongly associated with educational attainment. In 1988, 92% of mothers with at least some college education began care early in pregnancy, compared with 53% of mothers who had less than a high school education *(25)*. The probability that a pregnant woman will obtain care late or not at all decreases steadily as her educational level increases.

BIRTH ORDER

The more children a woman has had, the more likely she is to obtain insufficient care or none at all.

MARITAL STATUS

In 1988, among women with live-born infants, unmarried mothers were more than three times as likely as married mothers to obtain late or no prenatal care (13.2% vs. 3.7%) *(30)*. Unmarried white mothers were almost four times as likely as married black mothers to obtain late or no care; and unmarried black mothers were twice as likely as married black mothers to obtain late or no care.

POVERTY

Low income is one of the most important predictors of insufficient prenatal care. Women with incomes below the federal poverty level consistently show higher rates of late or no prenatal care and lower rates of early care than women with larger incomes.

GEOGRAPHIC LOCATION

Insufficient prenatal care is concentrated in certain geographic areas, most often inner cities and isolated rural areas. States vary in their rates of early and late entry into prenatal care, and great diversity in use of prenatal care can exist within states, counties, and cities *(27,31–33)*.

TIME TRENDS

The most detailed analysis of national time trends available from NCHS is for 1970–1990 *(29,32)*. Using birth certificate data of live-born infants, researchers examined national trends in prenatal care use among white and black mothers separately. The proportion of black mothers with early prenatal care (in the first trimester) increased each year during the 1970s, but the average annual percentage point increase for 1976–1980 (1.2) was smaller than that for 1970–1975 (2.3). The proportion of black mothers with early care declined from 62.4% in 1980 to 60.6% in 1990. For white mothers, average annual increases in the proportion with early care were similar for 1970–1975 and 1976–1980 (0.8 and 0.6 percentage points). The proportion of white mothers receiving early care remained stable at about 79% between 1980 and 1990 (Figure 1).

Barriers to Care

The Institute of Medicine report reviewed a great deal of literature on barriers to prenatal care and classified the known barriers into three groups: socioeconomic, system-related, and attitudinal (Table 1) (22,23). This literature has also been reviewed in detail by Goldenberg et al. (34) and Perez-Woods (35). National surveys of women's use of prenatal care can be another rich source of information on barriers to care:

- Analyses of data from the 1980 NNS revealed that patterns of prenatal care among mothers of live-born infants varied widely among population subgroups (36). Mothers <18 years of age and unmarried mothers were the least likely to obtain first trimester care (49% and 56%) and the most likely to

obtain care only in the third trimester or not at all (about 12% in each group). Women aged 18–19 years, blacks, Hispanics, poor women and women with little education also had disproportionately high levels of late or no care (7%–9%). In contrast, women who were married, white, and not poor obtained the most timely prenatal care. Compared with this subgroup of women, the population as a whole had twice the risk of obtaining inadequate prenatal care. Unmarried women ran the highest relative risk (five times the risk for women who were married, white, and not poor), followed by adolescents, Hispanic women, women with little education, poor women, and blacks (who had three to four times the risk for the comparison group).

- An analysis of NSGF data collected in 1982 and 1983 revealed that three groups of women were more likely to begin prenatal care after the first trimester: women with no health insurance; women on public assistance (including Medicaid and state and local

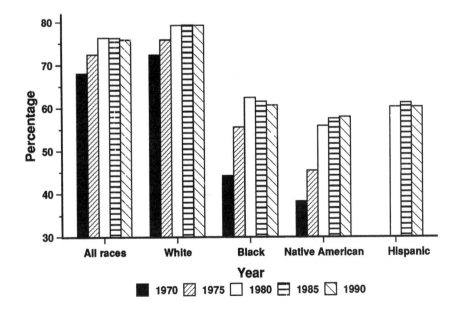

FIGURE 1. Percentage of live-born infants whose mothers received early prenatal care, by race-ethnicity and years* — United States, 1970–1990

* Separate data on Hispanic births were not available for 1970 and 1975.

Source: NCHS, CDC. National natality files.

TABLE 1. Barriers to the use of prenatal care

I. Sociodemographic

Poverty

Inner-city or rural residence

Minority status

Age of <18 years

High parity

Non-English speaking

Unmarried

Less than high school education

II. System-related

Inadequacies in private insurance policies (waiting periods, coverage limitations, coinsurance and deductibles, requirements for up-front payments)

Absence of either Medicaid or private insurance coverage of maternity services

Inadequate or no maternity care providers for Medicaid-enrolled, uninsured, and other low-income women (long wait to get appointment)

Complicated, time-consuming process to enroll in Medicaid

Poorly advertised availability of Medicaid

Inadequate transportation services, long travel time to service sites, or both

Difficulty obtaining child care

Weak links between prenatal services and pregnancy testing

Inadequate coordination among such services as WIC and prenatal care

Inconvenient clinic hours, especially for working women

Long wait to see physician

Language and cultural incompatibility between providers and clients

Poor communication between clients and providers, exacerbated by short interactions with providers

Negative attributes of clinics, including rude personnel, uncomfortable surroundings, and complicated registration procedures

Limited information on exactly where to get care (phone numbers and addresses)

III. Attitudinal

Pregnancy unplanned, viewed negatively, or both

Ambivalence

Signs of pregnancy not known or recognized

Prenatal care not valued or understood

Fear of doctors, hospitals, procedures

Fear of parental discovery

Fear of deportation or problems with the Immigration and Naturalization Service

Fear that certain health habits will be discovered and criticized (smoking, eating disorders, drug or alcohol abuse)

TABLE 1. Barriers to the use of prenatal care — continued

III. Attitudinal — continued

Attitudes related to selected lifestyles (drug abuse, homelessness)

Attitudes related to inadequate social supports and personal resources

Excessive stress

Denial or apathy

Concealment

Source: Institute of Medicine *(27,28).*

government assistance); and women with less than a high school education *(21).*[†]

- In 1986 and 1987, the U.S. General Accounting Office conducted a survey of 1,157 women who were uninsured or receiving Medicaid benefits, questioning them about their experience with prenatal care, including the number of visits, their timing, and the barriers and problems encountered. A multivariate analysis, which used the Kessner Index as the measure of accessibility of prenatal care, revealed the following findings *(37):*[†]

Enrollment in Medicaid and participation in state outreach programs increased women's access to prenatal care. Moreover, participants in state outreach programs had substantially better access to prenatal care than did Medicaid enrollees.

Six barriers to care were significantly related to the Kessner Index: financial problems, transportation problems, time conflicts, ambivalent feelings about pregnancy, the belief that prenatal care is not important, and a lack of knowledge about prenatal care.

Even after surveyors controlled for individual circumstances and attitudes, black and Hispanic women still had substantially worse access to prenatal care than other women participating in the survey.

- The National Maternal and Infant Health Survey (NMIHS) was a nationally representative sample of 9,953 women who had live births, 3,309 who had late fetal deaths (≥28 weeks of gestation), and 5,332 who had infant deaths in 1988 *(22).* Mothers were mailed questionnaires based on information from certificates of live birth, reports of fetal death, and certificates of infant death. Information supplied by the mother, prenatal care providers, and hospitals of delivery was linked with vital records data. Little has been published on the use of prenatal care from the NMIHS; however, an abundance of information on prenatal care is available from both the NMIHS Mothers' Questionnaire and the Prenatal Care Provider Questionnaire. According to data from the mothers' questionnaire, more than a third of live-born infants were born to women who received no prenatal care advice on smoking, alcohol, or drug use, and about half of these infants were born to women who received no information on breast-feeding. The amount of advice given differed by race, maternal age, and site of care *(38).*

The Case-Control Approach

In a recent study conducted in Cleveland, Ohio, investigators deliberately sought out 120 women giving birth who had received inadequate prenatal care (case group) and compared them with a sample of 120 women who had received adequate prenatal care (control group) at the same inner-city hospital *(39).* Using logistic regression analyses of the women's medical records, the

---

[†] Findings are based on all pregnant women.

111

researchers discovered that higher parity, an age of <30 years, an unmarried status, smoking, drug abuse, and residing in an area of low-socioeconomic status were independently associated with increased odds of not receiving adequate prenatal care. A similar case-control study design was used in a much larger investigation conducted by the Missouri Department of Health *(40)* (for details, see the Interpretation Issues section that follows).

INTERPRETATION ISSUES

The validity of prenatal care indexes depends on the accuracy with which gestational age and pre-natal care variables are reported on the birth certificate *(41–43)*. Several reports have demonstrated inconsistencies for those items between the birth certificate information and the information provided by the mother after delivery *(44–46)*. Although those researchers have not determined the validity of the information on the birth certificate, the discrepancies raise concerns regarding the accuracy of prenatal care information recorded on the birth certificate.

In a recent NCHS study, analysts compared the reporting of variables related to prenatal care from the birth certificate and the 1988 NMIHS *(46)*. They compared information from the NMIHS questionnaires, completed by mothers 6–30 months after delivery, with vital certificate data for the same births. Agreement ranged from 85% for the trimester of prenatal care among white women to 40% for the number of prenatal visits among black women. Approximately 60% of women recorded as initiating prenatal care during the second or third trimester on the birth certificate reported receiving earlier care in the survey. Women in high-risk groups (receiving late or little prenatal care and having a low level of education) had the lowest agreement rates.

Birth certificate information is often used in the surveillance of the use of prenatal care. The analysis just described raises questions regarding the accuracy of two variables often used in the creation of prenatal care indexes: the number of prenatal visits and the trimester of prenatal care initiation. In general, women reported on the maternal questionnaire receiving earlier prenatal care and more prenatal visits than were recorded on the birth certificate. Several previous studies have demonstrated potential problems in the calculation and recording of gestational age *(41,47,48)*, another variable that is commonly used in the creation of indexes of prenatal care. The validity of epidemiologic surveillance depends on the accuracy of the data being analyzed. Of great concern is that groups of women with delayed or small amounts of prenatal care are the least likely to have birth certificate data that correspond with information supplied by the mother. The differences described in the 1988 NMIHS study should be considered when performing analyses of prenatal care using vital statistics data *(46)*.

A second potential limitation of using vital statistics data to examine the effects of the use of prenatal care is that the regular methods of surveillance provide information only on the quantity of care received rather than the content of prenatal care. Many of the studies examining the relationship between the use of prenatal care and birth outcomes were based on summary utilization measures, such as the Kessner Index. Few researchers had the opportunity to examine the content of prenatal care. Peoples-Sheps *(49)*, among others, recognized that a significant shortcoming in studying the relationship between prenatal care and birth outcomes was the lack of information on the content of prenatal care.

In a 1989 report entitled *Caring for Our Future: The Content of Prenatal Care (50)*, panel members of the Public Health Service Expert Panel on the Content of Prenatal Care went beyond what the published literature had covered by delineating which components should be included in providing the most effective prenatal care. Among their recommendations was a detailed listing of the components of prenatal care that included guidelines for physical examination, laboratory tests for risk assessments, information to gather for a health history, and health promotion activities such as the provision of advice. The panelists also included details on when, during pregnancy, each individual component should be provided. They noted that many prenatal care practices have not been studied and that many practices that were studied were not evaluated rigorously or with an adequate research design.

In a recent review of prenatal programs, Fink et al. indicated that much more progress in measuring the effectiveness of the content of prenatal care needs to be achieved *(51)*. The authors noted that the criteria for determining the appropriate content of prenatal care remains an unsolved and major public health issue, one that is currently inadequately covered in literature on the prenatal care program.

The NMIHS included information on women's reports of initial prenatal procedures received and health behavior advice received throughout pregnancy, among mothers of live-born infants. An examination of the NMIHS data indicated that advice on prenatal health behavior is not a uniform feature of all prenatal care (38). Disparities by race, maternal age, and site of care are evident. Moreover, one third or more of the women surveyed reported receiving no prenatal advice on alcohol, tobacco, or drug use, and approximately 50% received no prenatal information on breast-feeding.

A second investigation using NMIHS data examined how receiving initial prenatal procedures and health behavior advice affected the risk of low birth weight *(Kogan, Alexander, Kotelchuck, Nagey, unpublished data, 1994)*. The findings, based on mothers of live-born infants only, suggest that women who received sufficient health behavior information, as part of their prenatal care were less likely to deliver a low-birth-weight infant. In addition, females who were at a greater risk—such as teenagers or women with lower incomes—showed the greatest beneficial effects. Therefore, the quality of prenatal care services has an apparent effect independent of the quantity of prenatal services received. In the future, periodic surveillance surveys such as the NMIHS, will attempt to obtain more detailed information on the content of women's prenatal care.

In reviewing these findings, we must recognize that attempts to investigate the relationship between prenatal care and perinatal outcomes can have serious methodologic problems because women who receive adequate prenatal care differ greatly from those who receive inadequate care (Table 1). For example, in an analysis of the 1980 NNS data of mothers of live-born infants, Kleinman found that after adjusting the data for race, age, parity, and education, married mothers who began care in the first trimester were 20% less likely to have smoked before pregnancy, 36% less likely to have had heavy alcohol consumption before pregnancy, and 60% more likely to have planned their pregnancies than married mothers who received late or no care *(42)*. These differences result in serious **selection bias** in all evaluations of the association between prenatal care and pregnancy outcomes. Women who receive adequate prenatal care are a self-selected group. In evaluations of the effects of prenatal care, the factors associated with inadequate prenatal care—smoking, alcohol consumption, unplanned pregnancy, higher income and education, adolescent pregnancy—must be considered as potential confounding variables, because they are related to the receipt of prenatal care and to outcome measures such as low birth weight and perinatal mortality. However, the problem of self-selection involves more than just confounding, because self-selection cannot be fully measured and analytically controlled *(43)*. The ways in which recipients and nonrecipients of prenatal care differ are not fully known *(34)*. Even if we control for basic social and demographic variables, the two groups will probably differ in respects that have not been measured.

Another biasing factor that must be considered in evaluations of the effects of prenatal care on pregnancy outcomes is pregnancy curtailment *(41,43)*. Women whose pregnancies are shortened by preterm delivery or induction of labor will have less of an opportunity to have prenatal visits. These women also have a greater risk of low-birth-weight births and perinatal mortality. Prenatal care indexes such as the Kessner Index were developed to control for this bias.

EXAMPLES OF USING DATA

States, cities, and local health departments have often used data on the use of prenatal care for program and policy planning. In this section, we describe several examples of such analyses.

New York City

In a multivariate analysis of 1981 live births in New York City, researchers studied the effects of financial coverage (Medicaid vs. third-party insurance), maternal education, race, maternal age, and marital status on the start of prenatal care (52). Late or no prenatal care was found to be associated with both Medicaid coverage and an education of <12 years. For the most part, the association of race and age with late or no prenatal care could be explained by Medicaid coverage and education. In other words, Hispanics, blacks, and adolescents were more likely to have incomplete education and Medicaid insurance, and this resulted in their greater risk of receiving late or no prenatal care.

In another New York City study, conducted in 1992, investigators assessed the many barriers to prenatal care that involve deficiencies in the maternity care system, rather than the characteristics of individual women. The New York City Department of Health's Bureau of Maternity Services and Family Planning conducted a telephone survey to document whether or not prenatal health care providers were accessible by telephone (53). Bureau staff posed as women in their first trimester of pregnancy (with a positive pregnancy test) seeking prenatal care. Speaking in either English or Spanish, the bureau staff telephoned >115 providers and asked four questions:

- Can I get a prenatal care appointment? (If not, why not?)

- How soon can I get the appointment?

- Do I get to see a doctor at that time? (If not, how soon?)

- I do not have any health insurance. Is that OK?

The results of this study clearly demonstrated that women who rely on public services in New York City face grave inconveniences. The survey was conducted over a 2-week period with available bureau staff and equipment. This is a relatively inexpensive method for evaluating a prenatal care system, and health departments in other cities and states may want to consider carrying out similar surveys.

Missouri

Postpartum interviews with 1,484 primarily low-income women were conducted during 1987–1988 in three areas of Missouri with the highest rates of inadequate prenatal care. In this study, carried out by the Missouri Department of Health, women with live-born infants who received inadequate prenatal care were more likely to be black and unmarried, to have a higher parity, and to have less education than those who received adequate care (40). These women were also more likely to be poor and Medicaid-eligible, to have an unwanted pregnancy, to experience more stress and problems during pregnancy, and to have less social support than women receiving adequate care. In a multivariate analysis, race and marital status lost their statistical importance. The strongest predictor of inadequate prenatal care was not being aware of the pregnancy in the first four months. The investigators concluded that to improve the rate of adequate prenatal care, society must address poverty and wantedness of pregnancy.

Arizona

Mexican-Americans' use of prenatal care was the focus in an analysis of Arizona birth certificates of live-born infants issued in 1986 and 1987 (54). The adequacy of prenatal care was evaluated using the index designed by Alexander and Corneley (20). Mexican-Americans were much more likely to have inadequate or no care than were non-Hispanic whites. Moreover, Mexico-born Mexican-Americans tended to have less adequate care than United States-born Mexican-Americans.

North Carolina

The North Carolina Center for Health and Environmental Statistics studied data on approximately 45,000 North Carolina women with live-born infants who gave birth in 1989 and 1990 and received prenatal care in public health facilities; the study's purpose was to assess the effects of prior family planning services on adequacy of prenatal care in a low-income population (55). Women who had used family planning services in the 2 years before conception were more likely to receive early and adequate prenatal care and to be involved in a food supplement program and maternity care coordination. The investigators advised that these findings must be interpreted with caution because of self-selection into family planning programs, but they concluded that family planning services may improve the use of prenatal health services among low-income women.

Tennessee

To investigate the effects of a 1985 Tennessee Medicaid regulatory change that expanded eligibility for pregnant women, investigators linked birth certificate files with Medicaid enrollment files (56). The findings based on women with live-born infants only, show the greatest Medicaid coverage increase occurred among white married women <25 years of age with <12 years of education; their enrollment increased 18%. However, in that group of mothers, as well as among all mothers studied, the authors observed no concomitant improvements in the use of early prenatal care. Analysis of the timing of enrollment relative to the beginning of pregnancy revealed that more than two thirds of the women who enrolled in Medicaid did so after the first trimester.

California

Beginning in 1989, California officials amended their birth certificates to include confidential information on the principal source of payment for prenatal care. This allowed analysts to use 1990 birth certificate data to study whether a lack of financial access was a significant barrier to prenatal care following major expansions of Medicaid eligibility (57). The findings, based on women with live-born infants only, show that compared with women who had private fee-for-service coverage, uninsured women were at an elevated risk of receiving no prenatal care, late care (after the first trimester), and too few visits. Women with Medi-Cal coverage had a high risk of receiving late care. The investigators concluded that, in spite of major Medicaid coverage expansions,

access to prenatal care was limited for women without private insurance.

Hawaii

The Institute of Medicine's report on prenatal care (27) suggested that the identification of geographic **hot spots**, where a high proportion of women had insufficient prenatal care, would be a fruitful avenue of future research. Hawaiian data have recently been used to address this issue. Patterns and predictors of the use of prenatal care in Hawaii were examined to identify census tracts with high levels of inadequate use of prenatal care services (33). Data were drawn from 1980 census reports and from 1979–1987 live birth files. The area-level methods used in this report may be useful to health-care planners in other areas.

FUTURE ISSUES

The year 2000 objective for prenatal care is to "increase to at least 90% the proportion of all pregnant women who receive prenatal care in the first trimester of pregnancy." This objective of 90% is meant to encompass mothers of all racial and ethnic groups, including black, Native American, Alaska Native, and Hispanic women. Clearly substantial progress still needs to be made if this goal is to be reached (Table 2) (58).

Data from birth certificates in 1989 and subsequent years will be particularly useful for analyzing prenatal care. Questions about tobacco use, drinking, and weight gain during pregnancy have been added to the revised birth certificates. The new item on clinical estimate of gestation also may improve the data on gestational age. The item on the birth attendant now differentiates between lay and certified nurse-midwives, and the place of delivery is more fully delineated to provide more data on when care begins. Also, timing of the initiation of prenatal care can be analyzed in relation to weight gain, complications of labor and delivery, obstetric procedures performed, and abnormal conditions of the newborn. The revised birth certificate also contains information on prenatal technologies, including amniocentesis, tocolysis, and ultrasound. Indeed,

TABLE 2. Progress toward meeting the year 2000 national health objective for prenatal care in the first trimester

Race/ethnicity	Proportion of pregnant women receiving early prenatal care who deliver a live birth		
	1987 (baseline)*	1990*	2000 (target)*
All women	76.0	75.8	90
Black women	60.8	60.6	90
American Indian and Alaska Native women	57.6	57.9	90
Hispanic women	61.0	60.2	90

*From *Healthy People 2000 Review (58)*.

an analysis of the 1990 national natality file has already been conducted to investigate black-white differences in the use of these prenatal technologies *(59)*. We also anticipate that future national surveys, such as the next NMIHS, will attempt to obtain more detailed information on the various components of prenatal care.

Prenatal care will continue to provide invaluable monitoring and support functions for pregnant women. Information obtained from state and national vital records as well as state and national surveys will help us to examine trends in prenatal care utilization and to delineate the prenatal procedures that are most effective for increasing a woman's chances for a healthy pregnancy.

REFERENCES

1. Thompson JE, Walsh LV, Merkatz IR. The history of prenatal care: cultural, social, and medical contexts. In: Merkatz IR, Thompson JE, Mullen PD, Goldenbert RL, eds. New perspectives on prenatal care. New York: Elsevier Science Publishing Co., 1990.

2. Institute of Medicine. Preventing low birthweight. Washington, DC: National Academy Press, 1985.

3. US Congress, Office of Technology Assessment. Healthy Children: investing in the future, Washington, DC: US Government Printing Office, 1988; OTA-H-345

4. Gortmaker SL. The effects of prenatal care upon the health of the newborn. Am J Public Health 1979;69: 653–60.

5. Sokol RJ, Woolf RB, Rosen MG, Weingarden K. Risk, antepartum care, and outcome: impact of a maternity and infant care project. Obstet Gynecol 1980;56: 150–56.

6. Quick JD, Greenlick MR, Roghmann KJ. Prenatal care and pregnancy outcome in an HMO and general population: a multivariate cohort analysis. Am J Public Health 1981;71:381–90.

7. Peoples MD, Siegal E. Measuring the impact of programs for mothers and infants on prenatal care and low birth weight: the value of refined analyses. Medical Care 1983;21:586–608.

8. Greenberg RS. The impact of prenatal care in different social groups. Am J Obstet Gynecol 1983;145: 797–801.

9. Showstack JA, Budetti PP, Minkler D. Factors associated with birthweight: an exploration of the roles of prenatal care and length of gestation. Am J Public Health 1984;74:1003–8.

10. Fisher ES, LoGerfo JP, Daling JR. Prenatal care and pregnancy outcomes during the recession: the Washington State Experience. Am J Public Health 1985; 75:866–9.

11. Shiono PH, Klebanoff MA, Graubard BI, Berendes HW, Rhoads GG. Birth weight among women of different ethnic groups. JAMA 1986;255:48–52.

12. Moore TR, Origel W, Key TC, Resnik R. The perinatal and economic impact of prenatal care in a low-socioeconomic population. Am J Obstet Gynecol 1986;154:29–33.

13. Lieberman E, Ryan KJ, Monson RR, Schoenbaum SC. Risk factors accounting for racial differences in the rate of premature birth. N Engl J Med 1987;317:743–8.

14. Koonin LM, Atrash HK, Lawson HW, Smith JC. Maternal mortality surveillance, United States, 1979–1986. In: CDC Surveillance Summaries, MMWR 1991;40(SS-1):1–13.

15. Poland ML, Ager JW, Sokol RJ. Prenatal care: a path (not taken) to improved perinatal outcome. J Perinat Med 1991;19:427–33.

16. McLaughlin FJ, Altemeier WA, Christensen MJ, Sherrod KB, Dietrich MS, Stern DT. Randomized trial of comprehensive prenatal care for low-income women: effect on infant birth weight. Pediatrics 1992;89:128–32.

17. Buekens P, Kotelchuck M, Blondel B, Kristensen FB, Chen J-H, Masuy-Stroobant G. A comparison of pre-natal care use in the United States and Europe. Am J Public Health 1993;83:31–6.

18. Miller CA. Prenatal care outreach: an international perspective [appendix B]. In: Brown SS, ed. Prenatal care: reaching mothers, reaching infants. Washington, DC: National Academy Press, 1988:210–28.

19. Kessner DM, Singer J, Kalk CE, Schlesinger ER. Infant death: an analysis by maternal risk and health care. In: Contrasts in health status. Vol. I. Washington, DC: Institute of Medicine, National Academy of Sciences, 1973.

20. Alexander GR, Corneley DA. Prenatal care utilization: its measurement and relationship to pregnancy outcome. Am J Prev Med 1987;3:243–53.

21. Fingerhut LA, Makuc D, Kleinman JC. Delayed pre-natal care and place of first visit: differences by health insurance and education. Fam Plann Perspect 1987;19:212–4, 234.

22. Sanderson M, Placek PJ, Keppel KG. The 1988 national maternal and infant health survey: design, content, and data availability. BIRTH 1991;18:26–32.

23. Adams MM, Shulman HB, Bruce C. Hogue C, Brogan D, and the PRAMS Working Group. The Pregnancy Risk Assessment Monitoring System: design, questionnaire, data collection and response rates. Paediat Perinat Epidemiol 1991;5:333-46.

24. NCHS. Advance report of final natality statistics, 1991. Hyattsville, Maryland: US Department of Health and Human Services, Public Health Service, CDC, 1993. (Monthly vital statistics report; vol.42, no. 3, suppl.)

25. NCHS. Vital Statistics of the United States, 1988. Vol. 1, natality. Hyattsville, Maryland: US Department of Health and Human Services, Public Health Service, CDC, 1990;DHHS Publication no.(PHS)90-1100.

26. Kogan MD, Kotelchuck M, Johnson S. Racial differ-ences in late prenatal care visits. J Perinatol 1993;XIII:14–21.

27. Institute of Medicine. Prenatal care: reaching mothers, reaching infants. Washington, DC: National Academy Press, 1988.

28. Brown SS. Drawing women into prenatal care. Fam Plann Perspect 1989;21:73–80.

29. NCHS. Health, United States, 1992. Hyattsville, Maryland: US Department of Health and Human Services, Public Health Service, CDC, 1993;DHHS publication no.(PHS)93-1232.

30. CDC. Trends in fertility and infant and maternal health—United States, 1980–1988. MMWR 1991;40:381–3, 389–90.

31. Kalmuss D. Darabi KF. Lopez I. Caro FG. Marshall E. Carter A. Barriers to prenatal care: an examination of use of prenatal care among low-income women in New York City. New York: Community Service Society, 1987.

32. Ingram DD, Makuc D, Kleinman JC. National and state trends in use of prenatal care, 1970–83. Am J Public Health 1986;76:415–23.

33. Kieffer E, Alexander GR, Mor J. Area-level predictors of use of prenatal care in diverse populations. Public Health Rep 1992;107:653–8.

34. Goldenberg RL, Patterson ET, Freese MP. Maternal demographic, situational and psychosocial factors and their relationship to enrollment in prenatal care: a review of the literature. Women Health 1992;19:133–51.

35. Perez-Woods RC. Barriers to the use of prenatal care: critical analysis of the literature 1966–1987. J Perinatol 1990;10:420–34.

36. Singh S, Torres A, Forrest JD. The need for prenatal care in the United States: evidence from the 1980 National Natality Survey. Fam Plann Perspect 1985;17:118–24.

37. Schlesinger M, Kronebusch K. The failure of prenatal care policy for the poor. Health Aff 1990;9:91–111.

38. Kogan MD, Kotelchuck M, Alexander GR, Johnson WE. Racial disparities in reported prenatal care advice from health care providers. Am J Public Health 1994 (in press).

39. Melnikow J, Alemagno SA, Rottman C, Zyzanski SJ. Characteristics of inner-city women giving birth with little or no prenatal care: a case-control study. J Fam Pract 1991;32:283–8.

40. Sable MR. Stockbauer JW, Schramm WF, Land GH. Differentiating the barriers to adequate prenatal care in Missouri, 1987–88. Public Health Rep 1990; 105:549–55.

41. Alexander GR, Tompkins ME, Petersen DJ, Weiss J. Source of bias in prenatal care utilization indices: impli-cations for evaluating the Medicaid expansion. Am J Public Health 1991;81:1013–6.

42. Kleinman JC. Methodologic issues in the analysis of vital statistics. In: Kiely M., ed. Reproductive and peri-natal epidemiology. Boca Raton, Florida: CRC Press, 1991:447–68.

43. Liberatos P, Kiely JL. Selected issues in the evaluation of prenatal care. In: Kiely M, ed. Reproductive and perinatal epidemiology. Boca Raton, Florida: CRC Press, 1991:79–97.

44. Forrest JD, Singh S. Timing of prenatal care in the United States: how accurate are our measurements? Health Serv Res 1987;22:235–53.

45. Fingerhut LA, Kleinman JC. Comparability of reporting between the birth certificate and the 1980 National Natality Survey. Hyattsville, Maryland: US Department of Health and Human Services, Public Health Service, NCHS, 1985. (Vital and health statistics; series 23, no.99);DHHS publication no.(PHS)86-1373.

46. Schoendorf KC, Parker JD, Batkhan LZ, Kiely JL. Comparability of the birth certificate and 1988 Maternal and Infant Health Survey. Hyattsville, Maryland: US Department of Health and Human Services, Public Health Service, CDC, NCHS, 1993. (Vital and health statistics, series 2, no.116);DHHS publication no.(PHS)93-1390.

47. Kramer MS, McLean FH, Boyd ME, Usher RH. The validity of gestational age estimation by menstrual dating in term, preterm, and postterm gestations. JAMA 1988;260:3306–8.

48. David RJ. The quality and completeness of birthweight and gestational age data in computerized birth files. Am J Public Health 1980;70:964–73.

49. Peoples-Sheps MD, Kalsbeek WD, Siegal E. Why we know so little about prenatal care nationwide: an assessment of required methodology. Health Serv Res 1988;23:359–79.

50. National Institute of Health. Caring for our future: the content of prenatal care. US Department of Health and Human Services, Public Health Service, 1989;NIH publication no.90-3182.

51. Fink A, Yano EM, Goya D. Prenatal programs: what the literature reveals. Obstet Gynecol 1992;80:867–72.

52. Cooney JP. What determines the start of prenatal care? Prenatal care, insurance, and education. Med Care 1985;23:986–97.

53. Christmas JJ, Pirani S, Heagarty MA, Schwartz L. Prenatal care appointment study: a survey by the infant mortality work group of the Mayor's Advisory Council on Child Health. Bull Acad Med 1993;70:87–94.

54. Balcazar H, Cole G, Hartner J. Mexican-Americans' use of prenatal care and its relationship to maternal risk factors and pregnancy outcome. Am J Prev Med 1992;8:1–7.

55. Jamieson DJ, Buescher PA. The effect of family planning participation on prenatal care use and low birth weight. Fam Plann Perspect 1992;24:214–8.

56. Piper JM, Ray WA, Griffin MR. Effects of Medicaid eligibility expansion on prenatal care and pregnancy outcome in Tennessee. JAMA 1990;264:2219–23.

57. Braveman P, Bennett T, Lewis C, Egerter S, Showstack J. Access to prenatal care following major Medicaid eligibility expansions. JAMA 1993;269: 1285–9.

58. NCHS. Healthy people 2000 review. In: Health, United States, 1992. Hyattsville, Maryland: US Department of Health and Human Services, Public Health Service, CDC, 1993; DHHS publication no. (PHS)93–1232.

59. Brett KM, Schoendorf KC, Kiely JL. Black-white differences in the use of prenatal care technologies. Am J Obstet Gynecol 1994 (in press).

Pregnancy-Related Nutrition

Geraldine S. Perry, Dr.P.H., R.D.,[1] Colette L. Zyrkowski, M.P.H., R.D.,[1]
Linda D. Clark, M.P.H., R.D.,[1] and Stella Yu, Sc.D., M.P.H., R.D.[2]

PUBLIC HEALTH IMPORTANCE

Birth outcomes are affected by many socio-demographic and physiologic variables, including ethnicity (1–3), socioeconomic status (4), maternal age (5,6), and nutritional risk factors such as prepregnancy weight (7–10), gestational weight gain (7–9), alcohol consumption (11–13), and anemia (14–16). The risk of infant mortality is directly related to birth weight and increases as birth weight decreases. Low birth weight is also associated with an increased risk of neuro-developmental conditions, congenital anomalies, and lower respiratory tract infections (17).

One of the national *Healthy People 2000* objectives for infant health is to "reduce low birth weight to an incidence of no more than 5% of all live births and very low birth weight to no more than 1% of live births." To reach this objective, we need additional data on the many risk factors for low birth weight that have been identified in previous studies. Such information will allow states to monitor and examine the interrelationship of these variables in pregnant women and will assist health care workers in the early identification of women who are at risk of delivering low-birth-weight infants.

Although numerous risk factors for low birth weight have been identified, this chapter addresses only those risk factors that are nutrition-related, including prepregnancy weight, weight gain during pregnancy, maternal anemia (as defined by CDC hemoglobin or hematocrit criteria for anemia), and alcohol consumption.

Prepregnancy Weight

Prepregnancy weight is a major factor affecting birth weight. An association between prepreg-nancy underweight and low birth weight was documented as early as the 1950s and has been confirmed in more recent studies (6–9). A significant linear relationship has been shown between prepregnancy weight (expressed as body mass index or BMI. BMI = weight in kilograms/[height in meters]^2) and birth weight, independent of gestational weight gain (7). Additionally, prepregnancy overweight has a significant independent effect on birth weight, with the incidence of macrosomia (high birth weight, >4,000 g) increasing with prepregnancy weight (18). High-birth-weight infants have an increased risk of perinatal morbidity and mortality.

Gestational Weight Gain

Total gestational weight gain in full-term pregnancies is an important determinant of low birth weight (6,8), and adequate weight gain is even more beneficial among women who are underweight before pregnancy (7). The latest National Academy of Sciences prenatal weight gain recommendations are higher for women with a low prepregnancy BMI than for women with a high prepregnancy BMI (19). The risk of low birth weight is increased among infants born to women with inadequate weight gain during pregnancy. About 14% of low-birth-weight births in the United States can be attributed to inadequate gestational weight gain (19). Adequate weight gain during pregnancy is affected by many variables including socioeconomic factors. Income

[1] Division of Nutrition
National Center for Chronic Disease Prevention
and Health Promotion
Centers for Disease Control and Prevention
Atlanta, Georgia

[2] Office of Vital and Health Statistics Systems
National Center for Health Statistics
Centers for Disease Control and Prevention
Hyattsville, Maryland

status is an independent predictor of low birth weight *(4)* and may also be related to gestational weight gain *(8)*. The prevalence of low gestational weight gain is higher among women with <12 years of education than among women with ≥13 years of education *(20)*. The risk of low birth weight decreases among women with at least 12 years of education *(8)*.

Maternal Anemia

Anemia, often related to iron deficiency, is very common during pregnancy. During the third trimester, approximately 33% of all pregnant low-income women *(21)* and 41% of low-income black women aged 15–44 years are anemic *(22)*. Anemia during pregnancy has been associated with adverse pregnancy outcomes such as low birth weight and preterm delivery *(14,15)*; however, this is a controversial issue, and a causal relationship has not been established *(16)*. Although anemia during pregnancy often reflects inadequate iron intake, the decreases in hemoglobin levels observed in pregnancy may also be related to normal blood volume expansion (hemodilution). Additionally, in the third trimester, the demand for iron is increased because of the increased fetal growth rate. These normal physiologic demands are reflected in the CDC trimester-specific reference criteria for anemia during pregnancy *(23)*.

Alcohol Consumption

Alcohol consumption is associated with poor fetal outcome throughout pregnancy. Although the exact mechanism by which alcohol produces adverse pregnancy outcome is not well understood, alcohol consumption clearly may lead indirectly to poor consumption of nutritious foods, thereby affecting maternal nutritional status *(24)*. However, studies have not shown that alcohol consumption causes poor gestational weight gain *(20)* (for additional information about related topics and surveillance activities, see the Behavioral Risk Factors Before and During Pregnancy, Prenatal Care, Low Birth Weight and Intrauterine Growth Retardation, and Infant Mortality chapters).

HISTORY OF DATA COLLECTION

CDC began the Pregnancy Nutrition Surveillance System (PNSS) in 1979. The PNSS collects data on risk factors for low birth weight (<2,500 g or <5 lbs 8 oz) to furnish states with timely information that will help them identify and monitor the prevalence of prenatal nutrition problems and behavioral risk factors related to adverse pregnancy outcomes (i.e., infant mortality and low birth weight) among low-income women.

When the PNSS was established, it included only five states—Arizona, California, Kentucky, Louisiana, and Oregon. By 1990, the number of states reporting data to the system had increased to 18 plus the District of Columbia and Puerto Rico. Currently, 22 states, the District of Columbia, Puerto Rico, and American Samoa report data to the PNSS. The number of surveillance records increased from <10,000 in 1979 to >378,500 in 1991. Although the system has grown, no state has consistently participated in the system every year. The surveillance system was enhanced in 1989 to collect more quantitative information on smoking behavior, alcohol consumption, weight gain, infant feeding practices, income, and federal program participation.

Another source of data on nutrition during pregnancy is the 1980 National Natality Survey *(8)*. These data were used by the Institute of Medicine's Subcommittee on Nutritional Status and Weight Gain During Pregnancy, to "determine the independent effects of maternal characteristics on total weight gain" (results and recommendations of the committee can be found in *Nutrition During Pregnancy: Weight Gain, Nutrient Supplements) (19)*.

The 1988 National Maternal and Infant Health Survey (NMHS) and the 1991 (NMIHS) Longitudinal Followup also provide information on a wide range of nutrition-related variables observed from preconception to early infancy. These variables include the mother's height, gestational weight gain, hemoglobin and hematocrit levels, blood pressure, urine glucose and protein measurements, maternal vitamin and mineral supplementation, receipt of nutrition advice, dietary habits, and participation in the Special Supplemental Food Program for Women, Infants and Children (WIC). Information on the infant's birth weight, length, head circumference, vitamin and mineral supplementation, and feeding practices is also collected.

The CDC Pregnancy Risk Assessment Monitoring System is a state-specific, population-based survey of women who have recently given birth to live infants. It is conducted on an ongoing basis and represents about one third of U.S. births. This system includes questions on maternal height and weight, maternal weight gain during pregnancy, alcohol consumption, and prenatal nutritional counseling.

CDC SURVEILLANCE ACTIVITIES

The PNSS is designed as a state-based surveillance system. State and territorial health departments and Indian health agencies collect data on pregnant women participating in publicly funded, health, nutrition, and food assistance programs such as the WIC program, prenatal clinics funded by Maternal and Child Health Program block grants, and Commodity Supplemental Food Programs. The data are therefore collected on a convenience population. The WIC program has been the primary source of data for the surveillance system, providing >99% of the records in 1990 (no data are collected from private practices providing prenatal care to high-risk women). Because participation in these programs is based on income, women are eligible for benefits only if their family income is 185% of the poverty level as established by the state and/or federal governments. Therefore, the PNSS includes data on low-income women only.

Data

The state and territorial health departments and Indian health agencies participating in the PNSS collect information using standard questions at the time of women's enrollment into the program and at the postpartum visit. The information is recorded on the program's intake forms and stored in a state master file. Records are submitted quarterly to CDC on computer tapes and diskettes.

Data collected on women include height, weight, and hemoglobin or hematocrit level at enrollment, self-reported prepregnancy weight, total weight gain during pregnancy, parity, and trimester of initiation of prenatal care. Additionally, quantitative information is collected on smoking behavior and alcohol consumption 3 months before pregnancy and at enrollment. Information on smoking behavior and alcohol consumption during the last 3 months of pregnancy is collected on those women who are enrolled in the program at postpartum. Information on income and federal food and medical assistance program participation (e.g., food stamps, Medicaid) is also collected.

Data collected at postpartum include the infant's date of birth, birth weight, sex, status at birth and at postpartum visit, and feeding practices (e.g., breast-feeding and formula feeding), and whether the birth was singleton or multiple.

Variables

PREPREGNANCY WEIGHT

Self-reported prepregnancy weight and measured height are used to calculate prepregnancy BMI. Women are classified into one of four weight categories according to their prepregnancy BMI. The weight categories are based on the criteria recommended by the Institute of Medicine (19): underweight, BMI <19.8 kg/m^2; normal weight, BMI 19.8 to 26.0 kg/m^2; overweight, BMI >26.0 to ≥29.0 kg/m^2; and very overweight, BMI >29.0 kg/m^2. These criteria correspond with <90%, 90%–120%, >120%–135%, and >135% of the Metropolitan Life Insurance Company's 1959 weight-for-height standards. In this chapter, we have combined data on women in the overweight and very overweight categories.

GESTATIONAL WEIGHT GAIN

Total gestational weight gain is based on self-reported prepregnancy weight and maximum weight reached during pregnancy. Women are grouped into total gestational weight gain categories at, below, or above the Institute of Medicine's recommended levels (19). The recommended weight gain ranges for term gestations (based on prepregnancy weight) are 28–40 lbs for underweight women, 25–35 lbs for normal weight women, 15–25 lbs for overweight women, and at least 15 lbs for very overweight women *(19)*.

MATERNAL ANEMIA

CDC criteria, which take into account trimester of pregnancy, smoking status, and altitude, are used to define anemia *(23)*. In the first and third trimesters, a hemoglobin level of <11.0 g/dL or a hematocrit level of <33.0% is used to define anemia in nonsmokers residing at altitudes of <3,000 ft, and a hemoglobin level of <10.5 g/dL or a hematocrit level of <31.5% is used in the second trimester.

ALCOHOL CONSUMPTION

In 1989, the system began collecting more quantitative information on the number of days per week pregnant women drank alcoholic beverages and the number of drinks they consumed per day.

BIRTH WEIGHT

Birth weight is reported by mothers at the first postpartum visit or at WIC enrollment for their infants. A validity study of maternally reported birth weights among WIC participants showed that very little misclassification of low birth weight occurred in the PNSS when the maternally reported birth weight was verified by birth certificate birth weight data *(25)*.

Data Analysis and Reports

CDC generates agency-specific annual summary tables on nutrition-related problems and behavioral risk factors by age and race/ethnicity for each participating state or agency in the system. States also receive a summary table for each reporting county. Participating agencies are encouraged to distribute the reports to the appropriate counties, clinics, and programs for use in planning, management, evaluation, and improvement of maternal health programs. States and agencies are provided assistance in interpreting the data if needed. CDC also aggregates state data to produce a national data set in order to permit national estimates for the PNSS

population. Annual reports of national and state estimates are produced. The total number of records in the total data set is used as the denominator to calculate prevalence rates.

GENERAL FINDINGS

In this chapter, we use the PNSS 1990 national data set to discuss general findings concerning the surveillance system population. Trends in prepregnancy weight and anemia are based on the 1979–1990 national data set.

Demographics

In 1990, the median age of women in the PNSS was 23 years, which was approximately the same between 1979 and 1990. About 25% of these mothers were teenagers, 34% were aged 20–24 years, 24% were aged 25–29 years, and 17% were aged 30–44 years. The racial/ethnic distribution of participants in the system was 45% white, 28% black, 21% Hispanic, 2% Asian, 1% Native American, and 3% of unknown racial or ethnic backgrounds. Of the participants who reported educational level, 25% had completed a high school education or greater (18% 12 grades, 7% >12 grades), 15% had completed grades 8–11, and 5% had completed <8 grades. The ethnic and educational makeup of the population probably indicates the income eligibility requirement of the programs that make up the surveillance system. The racial/ethnic and age distribution of the analytical samples may differ from the demographic makeup of the general surveillance population because of missing information on certain variables.

Alcohol Consumption

Approximately 14% of participants in the PNSS in 1990 reported that they consumed alcohol 3 months before pregnancy, whereas only 4% reported that they consumed alcohol during pregnancy *(21)*. Mothers who were younger (12–19 years), Hispanic, and Asian had the lowest prevalence of alcohol consumption 3 months before and during pregnancy, whereas Native American and white mothers were more likely to report alcohol consumption during these periods. Although overall estimates were lower than the prevalence of 20% reported by the 1988 Behavioral Risk Factor Surveillance System (26), drinking before and during pregnancy is still a public health problem for the PNSS population, especially Native American (29%) and white (19%) women. Note, however, that not all states collect information on alcohol consumption, and the response rates for those states that do collect information is low. The 1990 PNSS estimates of alcohol consumption before pregnancy were based on only 36% of the records, and estimates of alcohol consumption during pregnancy were based on only 26% of the records.

The 1990 crude incidence of low birth weight among infants born to women who consumed alcohol during pregnancy was 7.1% compared with 6.2% among nondrinkers (21). Further, within racial/ethnic groups, infants born to women who drank during pregnancy had a higher incidence of low birth weight than infants born to nondrinkers in the same racial/ethnic group (14.9% vs. 10% for blacks and 6.6% vs. 5.7% for whites). Drinking had a greater effect on low birth weight among black women than among white women. Older women who consumed alcohol during pregnancy were also at a greater risk of having a low-birth-weight infant (11.2%) than their younger counterparts. Note that these comparisons were not adjusted for other factors that may affect birth weight, such as cigarette smoking.

Maternal Risk Factors

PREPREGNANCY WEIGHT

Estimates from the 1990 data indicate that 51% of women in the system were classified as having a normal weight according to their prepregnancy BMI whereas about 20% were underweight and 29% were overweight (21). Only 6% of the women were classified as being very underweight (BMI <18 kg/m^2,) but 19% were classified as being very overweight (BMI >29 kg/m^2). The percentage of women in the underweight and normal weight prepregnancy weight categories decreased as age increased. The highest prevalence of underweight was observed in younger women and Asian women, whereas older women and Native American women were most likely to be overweight. Overall, the prevalence of prepreg-

nancy overweight has increased steadily among low-income black, Hispanic, and white women in the United States. This finding is consistent with the overall U.S. trend of increases in the mean BMI of young women (27). Although the difference in the prevalence of overweight between these three ethnic groups was very small between 1979 and 1990, blacks have had the highest prevalence of overweight before pregnancy since 1983 (21).

GESTATIONAL WEIGHT GAIN

Calculations based on the Institute of Medicine's recommendations for gestational weight gain (19) indicate that approximately 39% of women in the PNSS in 1990 gained less than the recommended weight during their pregnancy (21). Overall, the percentages of women who gained the recommended amount of weight (28%) or more (33%) were slightly below the national estimates for married women in 1980 (22). Asian and Native American women were most likely to gain less than the recommended weight, and Asians were least likely to gain more than the recommended amount of weight. Blacks (34.8%) and Hispanics (34.2%) were equally likely to gain more than the recommended amount of weight. Age did not appear to affect the attainment of recommended weight.

A greater percentage of women who were underweight before pregnancy had a low-birth-weight infant than did normal-weight or overweight women (10.4% for underweight women, 6.8% for normal-weight women, and 5.5% for overweight women) (Table 1). This was true regardless of racial/ethnic group or age-group. The incidence of low birth weight was greatest for infants born to black women who were underweight before pregnancy and was lowest for infants born to normal-weight and overweight Native American women.

Overall, infants born to women who gained less than the recommended amount of weight during pregnancy were at greater risk for low birth weight (10.0%) than were infants born to women who gained the recommended weight (5.9%) or more (3.5%) (Table 1). The incidence of low birth weight was highest for infants born to black women who gained less than the recommended amount of weight and was lowest for infants born

TABLE 1. Incidence of low birth weight (%), by prepregnancy weight status and gestational weight gain — Pregnancy Nutrition Surveillance System, 1990

	Prepregnancy weight status (%)				Gestational weight gain (%)			
	N	Underweight	Normal	Overweight	N	Less	Recommended	More
Race/ethnicity								
White	87,975	9.9	6.1	4.5	59,974	9.7	5.4	3.3
Black	43,732	13.4	10.2	8.3	24,679	15.8	9.7	5.2
Hispanic	22,173	10.5	6.4	5.8	12,067	9.4	4.9	3.4
Native American	1,719	7.2	4.2	3.7	1,405	5.1	5.4	2.6
Asian and other	2,706	7.4	5.1	4.5	1,924	7.1	3.7	2.5
Age (years)								
12–19	44,940	10.7	7.3	5.9	27,541	11.7	6.9	3.7
20–24	54,972	9.8	6.3	4.9	35,621	9.6	5.0	3.1
25–29	35,929	10.3	6.1	5.6	22,762	8.9	5.6	3.3
30–44	23,722	11.7	7.8	6.0	14,064	10.0	7.0	4.5
All	159,563	10.4	6.8	5.5	100,049	10.0	5.9	3.5

to Asian and Native American mothers who gained more than the recommended amount. Younger women were at a greater risk for delivering a low-birth-weight infant than older women only if they gained less than the recommended amount of weight during pregnancy. Adequate weight gain is important in all women; however, the difference in the incidence of low birth weight among infants born to women who gained less than the recommended amount of weight and those gaining the recommended weight or more was more pronounced in black women. These differences are not likely related to race per se but to socioeconomic, geographic, and other factors. Although gaining more than the recommended amount of weight appeared to be beneficial, gaining too much weight during pregnancy may pose other risks, such as fetal macrosomia (18), delivery complications, and excess weight retention after pregnancy (28).

Use caution when interpreting gestational weight gain data, because prepregnancy weight and gestational weight gain are based on self-reported prepregnancy weight, which can be biased by a woman's current BMI. Overweight women are more likely to underreport their prepregnancy weight (29).

ANEMIA

In 1990, the percentage of women who were anemic increased as the trimester of pregnancy at enrollment increased (9.8% in the first trimester, 13.8% in the second trimester, and 33.0% in the third trimester) (Table 2). This pattern indicates decreasing iron stores as pregnancy progresses. The prevalence of anemia was highest for black women at each trimester. Recent evidence suggests that factors other than iron nutrition may contribute to higher rates of anemia among black women (30).

Women who were severely anemic during the first and second trimesters of pregnancy were at a greater risk (data were not adjusted for other factors) of having a low-birth-weight infant than their nonanemic counterparts, regardless of race/ethnicity or age (Table 3). Overall, women who were severely anemic in the third trimester were at no greater risk of having a low-birth-weight infant than nonanemic women. This was not true among black, Hispanic, and younger women who were anemic in the third trimester. Although the incidence of low birth weight was lower among women who were anemic in the third trimester than it was among those who were anemic in the first and second trimesters, the high prevalence of third-trimester anemia for women, especially black women (46%), is of definite concern.

TABLE 2. Prevalence of anemia in women who enrolled in participating clinics at first, second, and third trimesters, by race/ethnicity and age — Pregnancy Nutrition Surveillance System, 1990

	First trimester		Second trimester		Third trimester	
	N	(%)	N	(%)	N	(%)
Race/ethnicity						
White	32,659	6.1	39,337	9.3	24,398	24.6
Black	17,174	16.9	32,015	21.4	17,603	45.8
Hispanic	12,194	9.6	22,791	11.4	11,323	31.9
Native American	439	8.4	687	11.9	399	32.8
Asian and other	1,800	10.8	2,425	11.8	1,271	26.8
Age (years)						
12–19	16,176	10.8	26,182	15.9	14,281	36.7
20–24	21,484	8.9	33,090	13.5	19,520	32.8
25–29	16,334	10.0	23,048	12.7	12,972	31.5
30–44	11,623	10.0	17,115	12.8	9,307	30.2
All	65,617	9.8	99,538	13.8	56,144	33.0

TABLE 3. Incidence of low birth weight (%) among women who were severely anemic* in the first, second, and third trimesters of pregnancy — Pregnancy Nutrition Surveillance System, 1990

	First trimester		Second trimester		Third trimester	
	Anemic	Nonanemic	Anemic	Nonanemic	Anemic	Nonanemic
Race/ethnicity						
White	10.3	5.9	9.0	6.5	6.7	5.6
Black	12.1	10.1	11.7	9.9	7.8	8.4
Hispanic	9.6	6.6	8.0	6.7	4.4	5.3
Native American	†	4.2	†	5.0	†	2.5
Asian and other	†	5.1	†	6.0	†	3.4
Age (years)						
12–19	10.7	7.9	8.6	8.4	6.2	7.3
20–24	10.3	6.4	8.8	6.8	6.6	5.6
25–29	12.6	6.6	12.0	7.1	6.7	5.5
30–44	9.1	7.3	14.3	7.9	8.2	6.5
All	10.7	7.0	10.2	7.5	6.7	6.1

* Hemoglobin and hematocrit cutoff points that are 1 g/dL and 3% lower, respectively, than the CDC criteria.
† Sample size is too small to be reliable.

INTERPRETATION ISSUES

One of the most important issues to consider when using and interpreting PNSS data is that we cannot generalize these data. The surveillance data are collected from a convenience population of pregnant women and not a random sample of the general population. Therefore, the generalizability is limited to the PNSS population. Further, the data are not representative of the total state population because the PNSS is mainly composed of low-income women. The generalizability will vary by state, and in many cases, by county. Within a state, perhaps the most important issue of concern is the total number of records submitted and accepted to the system

125

in a given year. In general, data are not used in analyses for any state reporting <100 records. Other issues of concern include the enrollment eligibility criteria used and the number of counties and clinics reporting to the system. Often states may change their eligibility criteria because of budgetary constraints. For example, women who have an inadequate dietary intake without anemia may not be enrolled in the program. In such cases, the prevalence of anemia for the population may be lower because of this change in eligibility criteria.

Other limitations include changes in the number of states reporting data to the system; changes in a state's counties and clinics participating in the PNSS; changes in program eligibility criteria within a given county or state; differences in states' eligibility criteria; and increases in the number of records submitted by states.

Despite these limitations, the PNSS is a unique data set in that it is the largest, most diverse (racially, ethnically, and geographically) data set available on low-income pregnant women in the nation.

EXAMPLES OF USING DATA

Overall, PNSS data have enabled states to revise their existing data systems or to develop new data systems that provide more comprehensive and accessible data at the state and local levels. States have also used PNSS data to support legislative recommendations, make budget decisions, and develop program and policy planning activities. State staff supported by the PNSS grant provide other state and local health departments with training about how to use the surveillance data.

Georgia

Georgia used its PNSS grant to help develop and train staff for the new data system for the WIC program. The new data system provides local health departments with immediate information they can use to monitor the health status and behaviors of women enrolled in their health programs. The incidence of specific risk factors for poor pregnancy outcome, such as prenatal weight gain, are reviewed for all local clinics to identify those with a higher-than-expected incidence. As a result, appropriate intervention programs can be developed more rapidly. Also, the data system can assist clinic staff in coordinating services to increase accessibility and therefore improve the continuity of care received by clients.

Massachusetts

Massachusetts is using its PNSS data to conduct quality assurance and outreach programs and to develop smoking cessation interventions. Local agencies in Massachusetts use PNSS data to identify medical charts for audit as part of their clinical quality assurance program. A western Massachusetts prenatal clinic uses PNSS data annually to identify women who deliver low-birth-weight babies. The medical records for these women are audited to determine if the women were identified as being at risk and, if so, whether appropriate health and nutrition services were provided. To increase participation in both the prenatal clinics and the WIC program, agencies match the prenatal clinic records with WIC program records. Clients with medical records that do not indicate participation in both programs are contacted and offered the services they were lacking. PNSS data are also used by state and local staff to plan, develop, and evaluate smoking cessation programs in Massachusetts. The characteristics of women who quit smoking during pregnancy and those who continue to smoke are being examined to identify key risk factors and to more effectively target interventions. In addition, state staff are using PNSS smoking data to identify local prenatal clinics with a high percentage of smokers. These clinics are provided assistance with planning a smoking cessation program at their sites. State and local staff will use PNSS data to evaluate the effectiveness of smoking cessation strategies.

Indiana

Indiana uses PNSS data in various state and local planning activities. At the state level, the PNSS data are included in the Indiana Department of Health's year 2000 health objectives plan to increase to at least 75% the proportion of mothers who breast-feed their babies in the early postpartum period and to increase to at least 85% the proportion of mothers who achieve the minimum recommended weight gain during their pregnancies. The PNSS demographic, health status, behavior, and pregnancy outcome data are included in the prenatal needs assessment information submitted in the Indiana Department of Health state plan, the WIC state plan and the Maternal and Child Health Block Grant application. PNSS data are also used in other grant applications. Future activities planned include a comparison of the pregnancy outcomes of women participating in health department programs with the pregnancy outcomes of all women in the state.

North Carolina

North Carolina uses PNSS data primarily for program planning and evaluation. State and county PNSS reports are prepared annually and are sent to all public health agencies, county boards of health, universities, the Governor's Commission on the Reduction of Infant Mortality, and other state and community groups. PNSS data are also used by the North Carolina Department of Environment, Health, and Natural Resources to conduct needs assessments for various state plans and grant applications; the department's Nutrition Services Section has used PNSS breast-feeding data to make decisions about competitive breast-feeding promotion grants to county health departments. Presentations on special studies using PNSS data have been given at various national meetings; topics have ranged from the influence of maternal weight gain on birth weight among overweight and obese pregnant women to racial differences in the effects of maternal cigarette smoking on infant birth weight among the low-income women.

FUTURE ISSUES

CDC will continue to serve as the major source for national data on nutrition-related problems and behavioral risk factors that are associated with adverse pregnancy outcomes among high-risk, low-income women. These data are needed to help states and federal programs identify and target interventions for women at risk of delivering low-birth-weight infants. Such interventions are needed to meet the following year 2000 health objectives related to pregnancy nutrition:

- Objective 2.10: Reduce iron deficiency to <3% among children aged 1 to 4 years and among women of childbearing age.

- Objective 2.11: Increase to at least 75% the proportion of mothers who breast-feed their babies in the early postpartum period and to at least 50% the proportion who continue breast-feeding until their babies are 5 to 6 months old.

- Objective 14.6: Increase to at least 85% the proportion of mothers who achieve the minimum recommended weight gain during their pregnancies.

Future developments will continue to increase states' capacity to conduct nutrition surveillance and thus meet these objectives. Presently, only 22 states, the District of Columbia, Puerto Rico, and American Samoa report data to the PNSS. To increase the quality and quantity of data available to help states and other federal agencies reach these national year 2000 health objectives, we must encourage more states to participate in the PNSS. Future efforts should also include expanding pregnancy nutrition surveillance to encompass non-WIC pregnant women (both low-income and all other women) and to collect data on other important risk factors for poor pregnancy outcome, such as gestational diabetes and dietary intake information. These needs could be meet through collaborative surveillance efforts among a number of divisions within CDC.

REFERENCES

1. Kessel SS, Villar J, Berendes HW, Nugent RP. The changing pattern of low birth weight in the United States: 1970 to 1980. JAMA 1984;251:1978–82.

2. Kleinman JC, Kessel SS. Racial differences in low birth weight: trends and risk factors. N Engl J Med 1987;317:749–53.

3. Shiono PH, Klebanoff MA, Graubard BI, Berendes HW, Rhoads GG. Birth weight among women of different ethnic groups. JAMA 1986;255:48–52.

4. Stein A, Campbell EA, Day A, McPherson K, Cooper PJ. Social adversity, low birth weight, and preterm delivery. BMJ 1987;295:291–3.

5. Haiek L, Lederman SA. The relationship between maternal weight for height and term birth weight in teens and adult women. J Adolesc Health Care 1988;10:16–22.

6. Kramer MS. Determinants of low birth weight: methodologic assessment and meta-analysis. Bull World Health Organ 1987;65:663–737.

7. Abrams BF, Laros RK. Prepregnancy weight, weight gain, and birth weight. Am J Obstet Gynecol 1986; 154:503–9.

8. Taffel S. Maternal weight gain and the outcome of pregnancy: United States, 1980. Washington, DC: US Department of Health and Human Services, Public Health Service, NCHS, 1986. (Vital and health statistics; series 21, no. 44, DHHS publication no. (PHS)86-1922.)

9. Gormican A, Valentine J, Satter E. Relationships of maternal weight gain, prepregnancy weight, and infant birthweight. J Am Diet Assoc 1980;77:662–7.

10. Naeye RL. Maternal body weight and pregnancy outcome. Am J Clin Nutr 1990;52:273–9.

11. Council on Scientific Affairs. Fetal effects of maternal alcohol use. JAMA 1983;249:2517–21.

12. Mills JL, Graubard BI, Harley EE, Rhoads GG, Berendes HW. Maternal alcohol consumption and birth weight. JAMA 1984;252:1875–9.

13. Little RE, Asker RL, Sampson PD, Renwick JH. Fetal growth and moderate drinking in early pregnancy. Am J Epidemiol 1986;123:270–8.

14. Garn SM, Ridella SA, Petzold AS, Falkner F. Maternal hematologic levels and pregnancy outcomes. Semin Perinatol 1981;5:155–62.

15. Murphy JF, O'Riordan J, Newcombe RG, Coles EC, Pearson JF. Relation of haemoglobin levels in first and second trimesters to outcome of pregnancy. Lancet 1986;1:992–5.

16. Klebanoff MA, Shiono PH, Berendes HW, Rhoads GG. Facts and artifacts about anemia and preterm delivery. JAMA 1989;262:511–5.

17. National Academy of Sciences. Preventing low birthweight: report of the Committee to Study the Prevention of Low Birthweight. Washington, DC: National Academy Press, 1985.

18. Larsen CE, Serdula MK, Sullivan KM. Macrosomia: influence of maternal overweight among a low-income population. Am J Obstet Gynecol 1990;162:490–4.

19. Institute of Medicine. Nutrition during pregnancy: part I, weight gain, part II, nutrient supplements. Washington, DC: National Academy Press, 1990.

20. Kleinman JC. Maternal weight gain during pregnancy: determinants and consequences. Hyattsville, Maryland: US Department of Health and Human Services, Public Health Service, NCHS, 1990. (Working paper; series no. 33.)

21. Kim I, Hungerford DW, Yip R, Kuester SA, Zyrkowski C, Trowbridge FL. Pregnancy Nutrition Surveillance System—United States, 1979–1990. In: CDC Surveillance Summaries, November 21, 1992. MMWR 1992;41(No. SS-7):25–41.

22. Public Health Service. Healthy people 2000: national health promotion and disease prevention objectives—full report, with commentary. Washington, DC: US Department of Health and Human Services, Public Health Service, 1991; DHHS publication no. (PHS)91-50212.

23. CDC. CDC criteria for anemia in children and childbearing-aged women. MMWR 1989;38:400–4.

24. Sokol RJ, Miller SI, Debanne S, et al. The Cleveland NIAAA Prospective Alcohol-in-Pregnancy Study: the first year. Neurobehav Toxicol Teratol 1981;3:203–9.

25. Gayle HD, Yip R, Frank MJ, Nieburg P, Binkin NJ. Validation of maternally reported birth weights among 46,637 Tennessee WIC program participants. Public Health Rep 1988;103:143–7.

26. Serdula M, Williamson DF, Kendrick JS, Anda RF, Byers T. Trends in alcohol consumption by pregnant women: 1985 through 1988. JAMA 1991;265:876–9.

27. Flegal KM, Harlan WR, Landis JR. Secular trends in body mass index and skinfold thickness with socioeconomic factors in young adult women. Am J Clin Nutr 1988;48:535–43.

28. Keppel KG, Taffel SM. Pregnancy-related weight gain and retention: implications of the 1990 Institute of Medicine Guidelines. A J Public Health 1993;83: 1100–3.

29. Stevens-Simon C, McAnarney ER, Coulter MP. How accurately do pregnant adolescents estimate their weight prior to pregnancy? J Adolesc Health Care 1986;7:250–4.

30. Perry GS, Byers T, Yip R, Margen S. Iron nutrition does not account for the hemoglobin differences between blacks and whites. J Nutr 1992;122:1417–24.

Pregnancy-Related Morbidity

Audrey F. Saftlas, Ph.D., M.P.H.,[1] Herschel W. Lawson, M.D.,[2]
and Hani K. Atrash, M.D., M.P.H.[3]

PUBLIC HEALTH IMPORTANCE

The **tip of the iceberg** is a term often used to describe the estimated 300 pregnancy-related deaths that occur in the United States each year (1). The rest of the iceberg represents the large pool of surviving women who have experienced complications related to pregnancy and childbirth in a given year. Until recently, we had no estimates of the burden of total pregnancy-related morbidity* for this country. In 1992, Franks and colleagues assessed 1986–1987 data from the National Hospital Discharge Survey (NHDS) and estimated that 22.2 of every 100 hospitalizations involving a birth were nondelivery hospitalizations of pregnant women (14.6 hospitalizations involving a pregnancy complication and 7.6 involving a pregnancy loss) (2). The investigators established that hospitalization for pregnancy-related complications is a surprisingly frequent event, which required an average of >2 million hospital days of care per year and cost >1 billion dollars annually. As high as these figures may seem, they are an underestimate of the total burden of pregnancy morbidity because pregnancy complications that arose during the intrapartum and postpartum period were not considered. Moreover, the researchers were unable to ascertain directly the burden of hospitalization on women and their families in terms of lost productive days, family disruption, emotional anguish, and financial strain. Although predelivery hospitalization was the primary focus, this study also provides the only recent nationwide estimation of serious pregnancy-related morbidity following

childbirth; 62,400 readmissions occurred during the postpartum period, yielding an average annual rate of 8.1 readmissions per 1,000 deliveries (3).

Ectopic pregnancy, an important cause of pregnancy morbidity and mortality in the United States, is the leading cause of pregnancy-related death during the first trimester of pregnancy; it accounted for 12% of all such deaths from 1979 through 1986 (4). Although U.S. case-fatality rates have decreased by 90% since 1970, incidence has increased steadily by nearly fourfold from 4.5 to 16.8 ectopic pregnancies per 1,000 during the first 17 years of surveillance. These increases also have been observed in several European countries, including the United Kingdom and Sweden (5). Data on ectopic pregnancy incidence in developing countries are limited, though some estimates are available. For example, rates derived from hospital-based African studies have ranged from 4.8 to 23.2 ectopic pregnancies per 1,000 deliveries (5).

Women in developing countries have up to 200 times the risk of maternal death as do women in the United States, and the burden of pregnancy morbidity is thought to be extremely high (6). Unfortunately, we have no reliable estimates of

---

* Except in quotations and titles, this report uses the terms **pregnancy morbidity** and **pregnancy-related morbidity** instead of **maternal morbidity** because the terms are more inclusive and semantically correct.

[1] Yale School of Medicine
   Department of Epidemiology and Public Health
   New Haven, Connecticut

[2] Division of Cancer Prevention and Control
   National Center for Chronic Disease Prevention
      and Health Promotion
   Centers for Disease Control and Prevention
   Atlanta, Georgia

[3] Division of Reproductive Health
   National Center for Chronic Disease Prevention
      and Health Promotion
   Centers for Disease Control and Prevention
   Atlanta, Georgia

total morbidity from acute and long-term conditions related to pregnancy and childbirth in the developing world because few methodologically sound, community-based studies have been conducted. In 1989, the World Health Organization convened a technical working group to review what is known about the extent of reproductive morbidity and to provide guidelines on how to improve research in this area (7). This working group concluded that the long-term consequences of pregnancy and childbirth are particularly understudied and that future research should use prospective community-based designs and attempt to validate diagnoses and to define clearly the conditions under study.

Surveillance of both acute and long-term pregnancy-related morbidity is needed to monitor trends over time and within population subgroups and to provide public health practitioners with information to formulate effective interventions for improving maternal and infant health. Ectopic pregnancy is the only maternal complication regularly monitored in the United States; other pregnancy complications are reported from time to time. For additional information about related topics and surveillance activities, see the Sexually Transmitted Diseases, Behavioral Risk Factors Before and During Pregnancy, Pregnancy-Related Nutrition, Pregnancy-Related Mortality, and Infant Mortality chapters.

HISTORY OF DATA COLLECTION

Conducted annually since 1965 by CDC's National Center for Health Statistics (NCHS), the NHDS abstracts and weights data from about 200,000 patient records from approximately 400 hospitals, representing the >30 million hospitalizations that occur each year nationwide.

In 1970, CDC began using NHDS data to conduct ongoing, annual surveillance of ectopic pregnancy in the United States. In addition, CDC has used the NHDS data set to conduct special studies of selected complications of pregnancy—such as preeclampsia, abruptio placentae, and placenta previa—and to evaluate trends in operative procedures for delivery and treatment of ectopic pregnancy.

NCHS has conducted periodic National Natality Surveys since 1963. The most recent of these surveys, conducted in 1988, was called the National Maternal and Infant Health Survey (NMIHS). The NMIHS is a stratified probability sample of live births, fetal deaths, and infant deaths corresponding to 1988 births in the 50 states. In addition, for >6 years, CDC has collaborated with several state health departments to collect data on pregnancy morbidity through the Pregnancy Risk Assessment Monitoring System (PRAMS), a state-based probability sample of live births (8).

One of the oldest systems of data collection is national birth registration, established in 1915 when 10 states and the District of Columbia began participating in surveillance. By 1933, all states and the District of Columbia were participating (9). The revised U.S. Standard Certificates of Live Birth (1991) and Fetal Death (1989) provide a check-box format to collect information on maternal risk factors, complications of labor and delivery, and obstetric procedures. These data can be used for surveillance purposes (10,11); however, validation studies involving reviews of hospital delivery records indicate low sensitivity of birth certificates as a data source for evaluating the occurrence of complications of labor and delivery (12,13). Little information is available to confirm whether fetal death certificates are a valid data source for evaluating pregnancy-related complications of mothers.

Within the past three decades, some states have established their own hospital discharge databases, collecting information on demographic characteristics, discharge diagnoses, and operative procedures for all hospital admissions for a given year. States use these data for estimating the incidence of pregnancy morbidity and for monitoring trends. Despite the availability of these data, they are often used solely for internal purposes. A lack of analytic capacity and other priorities may result in the apparent absence of widely disseminated information from these databases. A recent Healthcare Cost and Utilization Project feasibility study, supported by the Agency for Health Care Policy and Research, identified 38 states that collect hospital discharge data through a state data organization, a state hospital association, or some other private organization *(14)* (Figure 1).

Health officials in the State of Washington recently established a valuable linked database comprised of information from birth certificates, infant death certificates, and information abstracted from the mother's and the infant's hospital delivery records. This system is known as the Birth Events Records Database. Analysis of these data provide state health officials with reliable annual estimates of the incidence of various pregnancy complications for research and planning purposes.

In Tennessee, researchers at Vanderbilt University are currently developing a statewide surveillance system for monitoring serious pregnancy morbidity among the state's Medicaid population (Piper protocol) *(3)*. Serious pregnancy morbidity is defined as illness of the mother that results in a hospital stay for delivery that is more than two standard deviations longer than the mean length of stay, or that results in the readmission of the mother within 28 days following the delivery discharge. This proposed system uses Tennessee's Medicaid enrollment files linked to birth certificates to identify women whose delivery was reimbursed by Medicaid (38.5% of births in 1989). This surveillance system is designed to identify the magnitude of serious pregnancy

morbidity, risk factors for prolonged hospital stays following childbirth and for readmission of the mothers, and the responsible pregnancy-related complications. Preliminary findings indicate that 2.2% of women whose deliveries were funded by Medicaid had prolonged hospital stays for delivery, and 2.4% of these were readmitted within 28 days of delivery.

CDC SURVEILLANCE ACTIVITIES

National Hospital Discharge Survey

The NHDS is a nationally representative sample of discharge records from nonfederal short-stay hospitals (average length of stay <30 days) in the United States. Before 1988, hospitals in the National Master Facility Inventory comprised the sampling frame. Since 1988, the sampling frame has consisted of nonfederal short-stay hospitals listed in the April 1987 SMG Hospital Market Tape. All such hospitals with at least 1,000 beds or 40,000 discharges annually are selected. The remaining hospitals are selected according to a three-stage sampling design *(15)*.

Data abstracted from the discharge summaries include up to seven discharge diagnoses and four

FIGURE 1. State hospital discharge databases, 1992

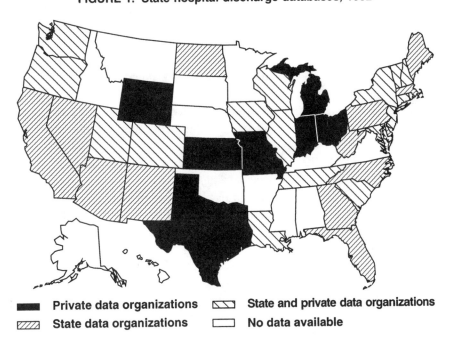

- ■ **Private data organizations**
- ▨ **State data organizations**
- ◲ **State and private data organizations**
- ▭ **No data available**

Source: Agency for Health Care Policy and Research, Hospital Cost Data Base Feasibility Study, 1992.

131

operative procedures coded according to the *International Classification of Diseases, 9th Revision, Clinical Modification (ICD-9-CM) (16)*. Additional abstracted variables include the patient's date of birth, admission and discharge dates, dates of coded procedures, sex, marital status, expected source of payment for hospitalization, and geographic region of residence. Medical record number, hospital number, and patient ZIP code are collected but are not available on public use tapes to ensure patient confidentiality.

CDC has used the NHDS as its data source for ectopic pregnancy surveillance since reporting was initiated. For the years 1970–1978, an ectopic pregnancy was identified when the diagnostic code 631 appeared on the discharge summary. Since the introduction of the *ICD-9-CM* in 1979, all records with a code of 633 met the case definition for ectopic pregnancy. Ectopic pregnancy surveillance reports are published every 1–2 years in the *Morbidity and Mortality Weekly Report*. Reports in the *MMWR Surveillance Summaries* series are also published every 2 years, providing estimates of the number of ectopic pregnancies, number of ectopic pregnancy deaths, and case-fatality and incidence per 1,000 pregnancies (sum of live births, legally induced abortions, and ectopic pregnancies) stratified by period, race, age, and geographic region of the country.

The NHDS can also be used to monitor demographic risk factors for other pregnancy-related conditions such as preeclampsia, abruptio placentae, antepartum pregnancy morbidity, and placenta previa as well as trends in the surgical treatment of ectopic pregnancy and operative procedures for delivery.

National Maternal and Infant Health Survey

The NMIHS mails questionnaires to mothers to obtain information about any antepartum and postpartum hospitalizations. The medical records for the delivery hospitalization and any additional hospitalizations are abstracted to obtain an objective determination of the associated diagnoses. Information on antenatal complications are also obtained from women's prenatal care providers.

Pregnancy Risk Assessment Monitoring System

State health departments participating in CDC's PRAMS request information from mothers via a mailed questionnaire on antepartum and post-partum complications of pregnancy that required hospitalization. These data are not verified by medical record reviews, however, and may lack accuracy and reliability.

GENERAL FINDINGS

Ectopic Pregnancy Surveillance

Analyses of the NHDS data for 1970–1987 indicate that the risk of ectopic pregnancy varies considerably by age, race, and region of the country *(4)*. Rates of ectopic pregnancy rose steadily with increasing age. As is the case with most data collection systems, the NHDS continues to employ race and ethnicity as variables that serve as convenient markers for a variety of potential risk factors. Women of all races aged 35–44 years had more than a threefold greater risk of ectopic pregnancy than did females aged 15–25 years. Rates of ectopic pregnancy increased almost threefold for black women and women of other minority races and almost fourfold for white women during the 18-year surveillance period, though the racial gap decreased slightly (Figure 2). The average annual rate for white women of all ages was 9.7 per 1,000 pregnancies compared with a rate of 14.2 for black women and women of other minority races (rate ratio [RR] = 1.46). Case fatality rates were also consistently higher for black women and women of other minority races, although the racial gap has decreased dramatically over the surveillance period. In the early 1970s, case fatality was three to five times higher among black women and women of other minority races than it was among white women; by 1987, the rate ratio had decreased to 1.8.

In an analysis of 1970–1987 NHDS data, Young and colleagues examined national trends in the management of ectopic pregnancy and determined that operative procedures that attempt to

FIGURE 2. Ectopic pregnancy rates, by race and year — United States, 1970–1987

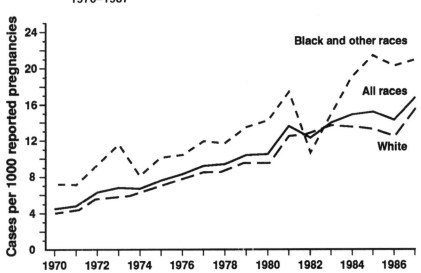

preserve the function of the fallopian tube (conservative surgery) increased from 2% in 1970–1978 to 12% in 1984–1987 (17). Moreover, conservative procedures were more than twice as common among women with private insurance than among women without it. No significant age, race, marital status, or regional differences in the rate of conservative surgery were found. Whereas the rate of diagnostic laparoscopy use had increased from 10% to 33% of tubal pregnancies by the second half of the study period, the rate of diagnostic laparotomy use had decreased from 24% to 2%.

Special Studies of the Causes of Pregnancy Morbidity

In a 1986–1987 study of nondelivery hospitalizations for complications of pregnancy, Franks et al. found that black women had hospitalization ratios (i.e., number of antenatal or pregnancy-loss admissions per number of delivery admissions) that were 40% higher than those for white women (2). They also identified risk factors for antenatal hospitalization by race and found that black females aged 15–19 years had a significantly decreased ratio of antenatal hospitalization than did black women aged 35–44 years (Table 1). In contrast, white teens had significantly higher antenatal hospitalization ratios than did white women aged 35–44 years. No substantial differences in hospitalization ratios, by marital

status or insurance coverage were observed among black women; however, white women who were unmarried or who did not have private insurance had significantly elevated ratios.

The leading diagnoses for antenatal hospitalizations were preterm labor (31%), genitourinary infection (10%), early pregnancy hemorrhage (9%), excessive vomiting (9%), pregnancy-induced hypertension (7%), and diabetes mellitus (6%). Mean length of stay was longest for women hospitalized with diabetes mellitus (4.4 days for whites and 5.5 days for blacks) and shortest for those diagnosed with preterm labor (1.8 days for whites and 2.4 days for blacks).

PREECLAMPSIA AND ECLAMPSIA

Preeclampsia and eclampsia comprise the second leading cause of pregnancy-related death in the United States and the leading cause in many developing nations (1). Saftlas et al. reported the first nationally-based estimate of the incidence of preeclampsia and eclampsia using the NHDS database (18). The average annual incidence of preeclampsia for the years 1979–1986 was 26.1 per 1,000 deliveries, with annual rates showing little variation over time. The rate decreased (trend test: p = 0.06) for black women and women of other minority races; by 1986 their rate was approximately the same as that for white women. Eclampsia occurred much less frequently

TABLE 1. Antenatal hospitalization, by race, age, marital status, and insurance status — National Hospital Discharge Survey, 1986 and 1987

	White				Black			
	No. of hospitali-zations	Hospitali-zation ratio*	Relative ratio[†]	95% confidence interval	No. of hospitali-zations	Hospitali-zation ratio	Relative ratio	95% confidence level
Age (years)[§]								
15–19	105,800	20.7	1.8	1.4–2.2	42,700	17.7	0.7	0.5–0.9
20–34	530,900	13.3	1.1	0.9–1.4	156,400	19.6	0.8	0.5–1.0
35–44	42,400	11.6	1.0	referent	12,700	25.4	1.0	referent
Marital status[¶]								
Married	398,000	12.2	1.0	referent	63,000	18.9	1.0	referent
Unmarried	134,900	19.5	1.6	1.3–1.9	113,400	19.1	1.0	0.5–1.3
Private insurance[**]								
Yes	418,200	12.5	1.0	referent	69,900	18.1	1.0	referent
No	240,500	17.6	1.4	1.1–1.7	136,400	20.6	1.1	0.9–1.4

* Hospitalization ratio is the number of antenatal or pregnancy-loss admissions per 100 delivery admissions.
[†] Relative ratio is the ratio of the antenatal hospitalization ratio in one category of women vs. the ratio in another category of women.
[§] Excluded are 2,000 hospitalizations of white women and 900 hospitalizations of black women with age unknown and 1,400 hospitalizations of white females and 2,500 of black females aged <15 or >44 years.
[¶] Excluded are 148,900 hospitalizations of white women and 38,900 hospitalizations of black women with marital status unstated.
[**] Excluded are 23,800 hospitalizations of white women and 9,000 hospitalizations of black women with unclassifiable insurance status.

Source: Franks et al. (2).

over the 8-year study period, affecting an average of 2,000 deliveries annually, or 0.56 women per 1,000 births. The eclampsia rate decreased by 36% over the years 1979–1982 and 1983–1986.

The rate of preeclampsia was lowest for women aged 30–34 years (19.8 per 1,000 deliveries) and highest for females aged 15–17 years (50.9 per 1,000 deliveries) (RR = 2.6; 95% Confidence Interval [CI] = 2.1,3.1). Women ≥35 years of age had a 30% greater risk of preeclampsia than did women 30–34 years of age—a difference that was of borderline statistical significance. Black and other minority women ≥35 years of age had a significantly (70%) greater risk of preeclampsia than did their counterparts 30–34 years of age. Also at increased risk were unmarried women (RR = 1.3; 95% CI = 1.2,1.5). Among women of all races, the investigators observed little geographic variation and no significant differences by expected source of payment for the birth.

ABRUPTIO PLACENTAE AND PLACENTA PREVIA

Abruptio placentae and placenta previa are two leading causes of third-trimester bleeding. Both conditions can result in serious pregnancy morbidity and an increased risk of pregnancy-related and perinatal mortality. Data from the NHDS indicate that the rate of abruptio placentae increased significantly between 1979 and 1987 for women of all racial groups: the rate increased from 8.2 per 1,000 deliveries in 1979–1980 to 11.5 cases per 1,000 deliveries in 1987 (test for trend: p = 0.02) (19). Rates increased most sharply for black women and women of other minority races. The increased incidence occurred mainly among women <25 years of age, unmarried women, and women on Medicaid compared with those who had private insurance. The increased prevalence of poverty and use of crack cocaine in the 1980s may have contributed to the increased rates that were observed (19).

Risk factor analyses for 1983–1987 indicate that white women in the extreme age-groups (<20 years and ≥35 years) had a 60% increased risk of abruptio placentae (p <0.05) than did women aged 20–24 years; however, black and other minority women showed little variation in risk by age. In addition, unmarried women and women on Medicaid (relative to women on private insurance) had a 50% increased risk (p <0.05). No significant regional variations were noted.

Certain adverse obstetric problems that occurred significantly more often among women with abruptio placentae included coagulopathy (RR = 54.1), stillbirth (RR = 11.1), preterm labor (RR = 7.5), and chorioamnionitis (RR = 2.5).

Iyasu and colleagues found that placenta previa complicated 4.8 per 1,000 deliveries annually during 1979–1987 (20). Whereas rates for white women remained fairly constant, rates for black and other minority women increased and exceeded the rate for white women after 1980. The researchers observed no significant associations by marital status, region of residence, or expected payment source for the delivery. The risk of placenta previa was strongly associated with increased age among white, black, and other minority women; women aged ≥35 years had almost five times the rate as women aged <20 years. Placenta previa has also been associated with increased parity. Unfortunately, the contribution of age, independent of parity, could not be assessed because data on parity are not collected by the NHDS. Several studies have evaluated the independent effects of age and parity, with some recent studies suggesting that parity has a greater effect on risk than age does (21,22).

TRENDS IN OPERATIVE DELIVERY PROCEDURES

NCHS has recently started using the NHDS data to track trends in the rate of primary and repeat cesarean sections and vaginal births after cesarean sections (VBAC) (23). This analysis documented the rise in the rate of cesarean section from 4.5% in 1965 to 23.5% in 1991, with the rate remaining fairly stable since 1986. Although the VBAC rate increased from <1% in 1970 to 24.2% of all women with a previous cesarean section in 1991, this increase had only a small effect on the overall rate of cesarean section, suggesting that substantial reductions in the cesarean section rate must accompany increases in the VBAC rate if we are to reach the year 2000 national health objective of 15 cesarean sections per 100 deliveries.

Although the rising rates of cesarean deliveries in the United States are a major public health concern, very little has been reported about the rate of other obstetric surgical procedures.

Zahniser et al. recently analyzed 1980–1987 NHDS data to examine trends and risk factors associated with cesarean sections, the use of forceps, and vacuum extraction procedures (24). They found that the number of operative procedures increased from 1.2 million to 1.4 million during the study period; by 1987, 35.7% of all deliveries involved an operative procedure compared with 31.6% in 1980. The cesarean section rate increased by 48% over the 8-year period, while a concomitant 43% decrease in the use of forceps was observed. This finding is consistent with the hypothesis that the increase in cesarean section rates is responsible in part for a decrease in forceps-assisted births. Vacuum extraction procedures increased from 0.6% to 3.3% of all deliveries.

The rate of cesarean section increased significantly with the mother's age; women aged 35–44 years had a 30% higher rate than did women aged 20–34 years. Women with private insurance were significantly more likely to have any of the three operative procedures than were women without private insurance. Although white women had a similar rate of cesarean section as did black and other minority women, the risk of forceps procedures was significantly higher among white women. After the investigators controlled for insurance status, however, this racial difference disappeared, suggesting that race was serving as a proxy for insurance status. Analyses by geographic region revealed significantly higher cesarean section rates in the Northeast and the South and higher rates of forceps delivery in the South.

INTERPRETATION ISSUES

The NHDS is a valuable resource that can be used to estimate the national incidence of selected pregnancy-related conditions and obstetric procedures, track trends over time, and compare rates across geographic areas and other population subgroups. The recent study of the national burden of pregnancy morbidity has drawn national attention to this important problem by quantifying its magnitude in the population as a whole and in selected populations such as racial and ethnic groups (2). Such analyses signal the importance of studying pregnancy morbidity and conducting more detailed studies, and they often guide the direction of future research. State-based

135

analyses, however, are not possible because revealing an individual's state of residence would compromise the strict confidentiality guidelines adhered to by the NHDS.

As valuable as the NHDS database has been for nationally based analyses, it has several limitations that can affect case ascertainment efforts, influence case definitions, and restrict the level of detail of the studies that use it. For instance, sampling design changes introduced into the NHDS in 1988 may limit trend analyses to periods before and after 1988 primarily because data collected under the new design may not be comparable with data obtained under the previous sampling design. As is true of other hospital discharge databases, case ascertainment requires that the individual be hospitalized for the condition and that the condition be coded accurately on the hospital discharge face sheet. For example, although underascertainment of ectopic pregnancy is unlikely because untreated ectopic gestations result in bleeding and possibly death, other conditions are known to be underreported on the hospital discharge face sheet. In a recent epidemiologic study of preeclampsia among Navajo Indians, chart reviews revealed that hospital discharge data underestimated the rate of preeclampsia by 25% (25). In addition, the hospital face sheet may contain incorrect diagnoses that should be excluded from analysis (26). For example, the study by Iyasu et al. found that women with placenta previa were 14 times more likely to have abruptio placentae (20). The authors doubted the strength of this association and concluded it may have resulted from including abruptio placentae in the differential diagnosis on admission; this inclusion, in turn may have been transcribed inadvertently onto the discharge summary.

The introduction of diagnosis-related groups (DRGs) in 1984 may have led to more accurate reporting of discharge diagnoses—particularly diagnosis of the more severe complications of pregnancy and procedures most likely to prolong hospital stays. DRGs also have led to substantial decreases in the length of hospital stays of women admitted for pregnancy complications and childbirth as well as increases in outpatient procedures and management of care. Thus, in recent years, hospital discharge databases have become less sensitive in the surveillance of

certain obstetric procedures and conditions such as preterm labor, which used to be treated exclusively in the hospital. Although most ectopic pregnancies still require hospitalization, there is a trend toward outpatient laparoscopy and chemotherapy of early ectopic gestations, which makes surveillance of this condition more challenging.

Another limitation of hospital discharge databases, in general, relates to the fact that diagnoses are determined from codes on the discharge face sheet; thus, applying standardized case definitions is impossible without access to the original medical records. Moreover, measures to ensure confidentiality by the NHDS and state-based surveys often prohibit researchers from referring back to the medical records. Related to this problem is the inability to evaluate and conduct analyses stratified by severity of the disease or condition.

Confidentiality measures also frequently prevent hospital discharge surveys from providing personal identifiers that would enable analysts to identify multiple admissions of the same patient. For example, NHDS analysts must use hospitalizations rather than individuals as the unit of analysis. Therefore, making reliable estimates of the incidence of conditions or procedures that can result in multiple hospitalizations in a given year is difficult. In the national analysis of pregnancy morbidity (2), the authors were unable to determine if their finding of a racial difference in the antenatal hospitalization ratio was related to a higher rate of multiple hospitalizations among black and other minority women or if it reflected a true racial difference in hospitalization rates. This limitation is, fortunately, not quite as restrictive for some analyses of pregnancy morbidity, such as those that focus on the number of deliveries as the analytic unit; only rarely will a woman have two deliveries within a year.

Because the NHDS is a national complex probability sample of hospitalizations, sample size problems may result, sometimes restricting analyses of time trends or population subgroups, particularly for relatively infrequent conditions such as eclampsia or placenta previa. The sampling design also requires the use of sophisticated survey analytic methods to obtain the appropriate standard errors on estimated numbers, rates, and ratios.

NHDS has been a good data source overall for ectopic pregnancy surveillance and estimating the national incidence of selected obstetric conditions and procedures; however, several categories of data that would enhance such analytic efforts are not available. For instance, the survey would be more useful if it provided data on income, education, and state of residence; reproductive history variables such as parity and length of gestation at time of admission; and a medical history, including information on sexually transmitted diseases and behavioral risk factors such as smoking, alcohol, and drug use. Before 1986, data on race were coded according to several categories: white, black and other races, and unknown race. Since 1986, more detailed racial and ethnic breakdowns have been available, including a category for Hispanic origin. Racial and ethnic designations such as white, black, and Hispanic may be given unintended significance, however. Although phenotypic racial markers are not related to genetic susceptibility to disease, such markers have been used in the past as convenient surrogates for potential biological, social, cultural, and environmental risk factors that are not genetically linked to race. The current epidemiologic challenge is to explore beyond these markers.

EXAMPLES OF USING DATA

Surveillance of ectopic pregnancy trends over the past several years has led to increased awareness that rates of ectopic pregnancy have risen to epidemic proportions. This increased awareness may have resulted in a higher rate of early diagnosis of this life-threatening condition. Surveillance data have also spurred numerous studies aimed at identifying etiologic factors for this condition. National-, state-, or locality-specific data allow for the development of interventions that further increase providers' and patients' awareness of this condition and facilitate access to services that permit early detection and treatment, reducing personal suffering and economic loss.

The findings of various analyses of NHDS data have been used to form national year 2000 objectives for the health of mothers and should be used to measure our progress toward meeting these objectives (27). The study of the burden of pregnancy morbidity was used as the basis of the year 2000 objective to reduce severe complications of pregnancy from 22 to no more than 15 antenatal and pregnancy-loss hospitalizations per 100 deliveries (2). For many years, data from the NHDS have been used to track trends in cesarean births and have guided the development of national health objectives in this area of great public health concern. The year 2000 objective for cesarean delivery is to reduce the rate to no more than 15 cesarean births per 100 deliveries.

FUTURE ISSUES

The continued use of NHDS as the sole data source for ectopic pregnancy surveillance has been debated because of an emerging trend toward outpatient management of this condition. NCHS recently initiated the Ambulatory Care Survey, which collects information from outpatient treatment facilities. Data collected from this new survey will supplement the NHDS data on ectopic pregnancy and other conditions for which initial outpatient treatment occurs.

In general, few risk reduction objectives for pregnancy morbidity are included in the year 2000 national health objectives, and none of the objectives specifically addresses a reduction in rates of ectopic pregnancy. In addition to objectives for reducing pregnancy morbidity and cesarean section, other pregnancy-related health objectives focus on reducing low birth-weight births and improving appropriate weight gain among pregnant women.

Although numerous studies attest to the safety of legal induced abortions performed by skilled medical providers, no nationally representative data about legal abortion-related morbidity have been available or collected since the 1970s. Since then, numerous changes have occurred in the methodology used for performing abortions, without any data—other than abortion mortality data—being available to assess the effects of those changes. Although current surveillance efforts are not directed at this outcome, such efforts would provide continuously updated information about the complications associated with legal induced abortions and would enhance our ability to determine whether the year 2000 objective of reducing pregnancy-related morbidity is being met.

Although the NHDS has provided the first national estimates of the burden of pregnancy morbidity and the incidence of selected major complications of pregnancy, wider dissemination of information from state-based pregnancy morbidity surveillance systems is needed to identify regional pregnancy-related health problems. Such surveillance data can guide clinicians and health departments in the planning of relevant programs and policies affecting the health and medical care management of pregnant women.

REFERENCES

1. Atrash HK, Koonin LM, Lawson HW, Franks AL, Smith JC. Maternal mortality in the United States, 1979–1986. Obstet Gynecol 1990;76:1055–60.

2. Franks AL, Kendrick JS, Olson DR, Atrash HK, Saftlas AF, Moien M. Hospitalization for pregnancy complications, United States, 1986 and 1987. Am J Obstet Gynecol 1992;166:1339–44.

3. Piper JM. Maternal morbidity following childbirth in the Tennessee Medicaid population. Vanderbilt University School of Medicine, Department of Preventive Medicine, Division of Pharmacoepidemiology, 1992; study protocol submitted to CDC.

4. Nederlof KP, Lawson HW, Saftlas AF, Atrash HK, Finch EL. Ectopic pregnancy surveillance, United States, 1970–1987. In: CDC Surveillance Summaries. MMWR 1990;39(no. SS-4):9–17.

5. Liskin LS. Maternal morbidity in developing countries: a review and comments. Int J Gynecol Obstet 1992; 37:77–87.

6. Maine D. Safe motherhood programs: options and issues. New York: Columbia University, Center for Population and Family Health, 1991.

7. World Health Organization. Measuring reproductive morbidity. Report of a technical working group: Geneva, 30 August–1 September 1989. Geneva: World Health Organization, 1989.

8. Adams MM, Shulman HB, Bruce C, Hogue C, Brogan D, the PRAMS Working Group. The Pregnancy Risk Assessment Monitoring System: design, questionnaire, data collection and response rates. Pediatr Perinat Epidemiol 1991;5:333–46.

9. NCHS. Vital statistics of the United States, 1988. Vol. 1, natality. Hyattsville, Maryland: US Department of Health and Human Services, Public Health Service, CDC, 1990; DHHS publication no. (PHS)90-1100.

10. NCHS. Advance report of maternal and infant health data from the birth certificate, 1990. Hyattsville, Maryland: US Department of Health and Human Services, Public Health Service, CDC, 1993. (Monthly vital statistics report; vol. 42, no. 2, suppl.)

11. NCHS. Advance report of new data from the 1989 birth certificate. Hyattsville, Maryland: US Department of Health and Human Services, Public Health Service, CDC, 1992. (Monthly vital statistics report; vol. 40, no. 12, suppl.)

12. Piper JM, Mitchel EF, Snowden M, Hall C, Adams M, Taylor P. Validation of 1989 Tennessee birth certificates using maternal and newborn hospital records. Am J Epidemiol 1993;137:758–68.

13. Carucci PM. Reliability of statistical and medical information reported on birth and death certificates. Albany, New York: New York State Department of Health, 1979; monograph no. 15.

14. Agency for Health Care Policy and Research. Final report of AHCPR Hospital Cost Data Base Feasibility Study, Santa Barbara, California: SysteMetrics/ McGraw-Hill, 1992.

15. Graves EJ. 1990 Summary: National Hospital Discharge Survey. Hyattsville, Maryland: US Department of Health and Human Services, Public Health Service, CDC, 1992. (Advance data from vital and health statistics; no. 210.)

16. Public Health Service. International classification of diseases, ninth revision, clinical modification. Washington, DC: US Department of Health and Human Services, Public Health Service, Health Care Financing Administration, 1991; DHHS publication no. (PHS) 91-1260.

17. Young PL, Saftlas AF, Atrash HK, Lawson HW, Petrey FF. National trends in the management of tubal pregnancy, 1970–1987. Obstet Gynecol 1991;78: 749–52.

18. Saftlas AF, Olson DR, Franks AL, Atrash HK, Pokras R. Epidemiology of preeclampsia and eclampsia in the United States, 1979–1986. Am J Obstet Gynecol 1990;163:460–5.

19. Saftlas AF, Olson DR, Atrash HK, Rochat R, Rowley D. National trends in the incidence of abruptio placentae, 1979–1987. Obstet Gynecol 1991;78: 1081–6.

20. Iyasu S, Saftlas AF, Rowley DL, Koonin LM, Lawson HW, Atrash HK. The epidemiology of placenta previa in the United States, 1979 through 1987. Am J Obstet Gynecol 1993;168:1424–9.

21. Spellacy WN, Miller SJ, Winegar A. Pregnancy after 40 years of age. Obstet Gynecol 1986;68:452–4.

22. Clark SL, Koonings PP, Phelan JP. Placenta previa/ accreta and prior cesarean section. Obstet Gynecol 1985;66:89–92.

23. CDC. Rates of cesarean delivery—United States, 1991. MMWR 1993;42:285–9.

24. Zahniser SC, Kendrick JS, Franks AL, Saftlas AF. Trends in obstetric operative procedures, 1980 to 1987. Am J Public Health 1992;82:1340–4.

25. Saftlas AF, Atrash HK, Olson DR, Franks AL, Pokras R. Epidemiology of preeclampsia and eclampsia: reply [Letter]. Am J Obstet Gynecol 1991;165:238.

26. Ales KL, Charlson ME. Epidemiology of preeclampsia and eclampsia [Letter]. Am J Obstet Gynecol 1991; 165:238.

27. Public Health Service. Healthy people 2000: national health promotion and disease prevention objectives— full report, with commentary. Washington, DC: US Department of Health and Human Services, Public Health Service, 1991; DHHS publication no. (PHS) 91-50212.

Pregnancy-Related Mortality

Hani K. Atrash, M.D., M.P.H.,[1] Herschel W. Lawson, M.D.,[2]
Tedd V. Ellerbrock, M.D.,[3] Diane L. Rowley, M.D., M.P.H.,[1]
and Lisa M. Koonin, M.N., M.P.H.[1]

PUBLIC HEALTH IMPORTANCE

Each year, 300–500 pregnancy-related deaths*
are reported in the United States. This number
represents outcomes of only the most severe of
pregnancy-related complications. For every
pregnancy-related death, >3,600 admissions to
hospitals are for pregnancy-related complications
not associated with delivery. Understanding the
characteristics of women who die as a result of
pregnancy complications and the risk factors for
pregnancy-related death is essential if we are to
develop strategies to prevent both mortality and
severe morbidity associated with pregnancy
complications.

In 1990, the U.S. Department of Health and
Human Services identified pregnancy-related
mortality as a high-priority public health area in
which further improvement is needed to achieve
the national year 2000 health goals. The *Healthy
People 2000* objective for pregnancy-related mortality is to "reduce the maternal mortality ratio to
no more than 3.3 [pregnancy-related deaths] per
100,000 live births" *(1)*. Alternatively, because
these ratios differ depending on the source of
data used, the objective further states that "if
other sources of maternal mortality data (besides
vital statistics) are used, a 50% reduction in maternal mortality is the intended target." We must
overcome two main obstacles to achieve further
reductions in pregnancy-related mortality: the
slow decline in pregnancy mortality ratios since
1980 and the continuing gap between rates for
various racial and ethnic groups.

The reported pregnancy mortality ratio dropped
56% from 1970 to 1980. Since 1981, however,
the reported pregnancy mortality ratio has
remained relatively stable, declining by only 3.5%
between 1981 and 1990 *(2)*. Moreover, black
women continue to have a greater risk of
pregnancy-related death than do white women.
In 1960, black women had a pregnancy mortality ratio 4.1 times that of white women; in 1970,
this relative risk increased to 4.4; in 1980, it
dropped to 3.5; and in 1990, it increased again
to 4.2 *(2,3)* (for additional information about
related topics and surveillance activities, see the
Legal Induced Abortion, Prenatal Care, and
Pregnancy-Related Morbidity chapters).

HISTORY OF DATA COLLECTION

National vital statistics have served as our only
national source of information on numbers, ratios,
and causes of pregnancy-related deaths in the
United States. State and local pregnancy mortality information has been obtained from state vital
statistics reports and from publications based on
vital records linkage, review of death certificates,

---

* Except in quotations and titles, this report uses the term
pregnancy-related death rather than **maternal death** because
it is more accurate (see definitions in the CDC Surveillance
Activities section of this chapter). See discussion later in this
chapter on mortality rates and ratios.

[1] Division of Reproductive Health
National Center for Chronic Disease Prevention
   and Health Promotion
Centers for Disease Control and Prevention
Atlanta, Georgia

[2] Division of Cancer Prevention and Control
National Center for Chronic Disease Prevention
   and Health Promotion
Centers for Disease Control and Prevention
Atlanta, Georgia

[3] Division of HIV/AIDS
National Center for Infectious Diseases
Centers for Disease Control and Prevention
Atlanta, Georgia

medical records, or autopsy reports or from reports by state-based Maternal Mortality Review Committees. In fact, pregnancy death investigation was one of the first areas of regular death investigation, with widespread participation by practitioners and the public health community. In recent years, however, the number of Maternal Mortality Review Committees has declined dramatically *(4)*. Today, national estimates and most state estimates of pregnancy mortality ratios are based on published vital statistics reports.

For more than 20 years, CDC has conducted nationwide surveillance and investigation of abortion-related deaths. CDC's abortion mortality surveillance has relied on multiple reporting sources for case identification and on multiple data sources for case classification and ascertainment. Most abortion deaths have been identified through four main sources: state health departments, national vital statistics, Maternal Mortality Review Committees, and reports by individuals *(5,6)*. Multiple sources have improved the completeness of the reporting. For example, CDC investigated 538 possible abortion-related deaths in 1972–1982. If we had relied solely on state health departments, only 63% of these deaths would have been included. Nineteen percent were first reported by individuals, 6% were identified from national vital statistics, and 13% were reported by other sources *(5,6)*.

The sources of information on abortion mortality surveillance include death certificates, autopsy reports, hospital records, case summaries, personal contacts, and reports from Maternal Mortality Review Committees. The availability of information from multiple sources made possible a more accurate classification of the deaths. Of the 538 possible abortion-related deaths reported to CDC in 1972–1982, 402 (75%) were found to be abortion-related (186 related to legal induced abortions, 84 related to illegal induced abortions, and 132 related to spontaneous abortions). Twenty percent of the 337 cases reported to CDC from state health departments and 37% of the additional 30 cases identified from national vital statistics were classified as not being abortion-related on the basis of information collected from multiple sources *(5,6)*.

In 1987, CDC collaborated with the Maternal Mortality Special Interest Group of the American College of Obstetricians and Gynecologists (ACOG), the Association of Vital Records and Health Statistics (AVRHS), and state and local health departments to initiate the National Pregnancy Mortality Surveillance System. This surveillance was designed to be similar to the abortion mortality surveillance, established in 1972. A CDC/ACOG Maternal Mortality Study Group was established to provide continuing advice to CDC on the implementation of the National Pregnancy Mortality Surveillance System. This study group includes representatives from CDC and other federal agencies, ACOG, state health departments, and other provider organizations with a broad interest and expertise in maternal health. The group meets annually during the clinical meeting of ACOG.

CDC SURVEILLANCE ACTIVITIES

At its inception, the National Pregnancy Mortality Surveillance System had two major components: 1) a retrospective component based on linked vital records (death certificates of all identified pregnancy-related deaths that occurred in the United States during 1979–1986 were linked to records of their associated pregnancy outcomes); and 2) a prospective component based on ongoing investigation of all pregnancy-related deaths identified through the individual state systems and other sources of reporting, starting with deaths in 1987. Both components attempt to identify all pregnancy-related deaths in the United States, starting with pregnancy-related deaths reported through the vital statistics systems, and to more appropriately classify causes of death into meaningful clinical categories. In addition, the CDC/ACOG Maternal Mortality Study Group introduced new definitions and coding procedures for use in conducting pregnancy mortality surveillance.

The most commonly used definition of a pregnancy-related (maternal) death is that developed by the World Health Organization (WHO) *(7)*:

> A **maternal death** is defined as the death of a woman while pregnant or within 42 days of termination of pregnancy, irrespective of the duration and the site of the pregnancy, from

any cause related to or aggravated by the pregnancy or its management but not from accidental or incidental causes.

Maternal deaths should be subdivided into two groups:

- **Direct obstetric deaths:** those resulting from obstetric complications of the pregnant state (pregnancy, labor, and puerperium), from interventions, omissions, incorrect treatment, or from a chain of events resulting from any of the above.

- **Indirect obstetric deaths:** those resulting from previous existing disease that developed during pregnancy and which was not due to direct causes, but which was aggravated by physiologic effects of pregnancy.

The WHO's definition is used for estimating pregnancy mortality ratios at the national level; however, many states have modified the interval between pregnancy termination and death and used intervals ranging from 42 days to a year or more (Table 1) (3,8–18).

The CDC/ACOG Maternal Mortality Study Group introduced two new terms that are being used by CDC and increasingly by some states and researchers. The study group differentiates between pregnancy-associated and pregnancy-related deaths, defining them as follows (6):

A **pregnancy-associated death** is the death of any woman, from any cause, while pregnant or within 1 calendar year of termination of pregnancy, regardless of the duration and the site of pregnancy.

A **pregnancy-related death** is a pregnancy-associated death resulting from 1) complications of the pregnancy itself, 2) the chain of events initiated by the pregnancy that led to death, or 3) aggravation of an unrelated condition by the physiologic or pharmacologic effects of the pregnancy that subsequently caused death.

The term **pregnancy-associated death** is preferred to **maternal death** because some of these

deaths may not be **related** to pregnancy. Moreover, some pregnancies result in abortions, ectopic pregnancies, and gestational trophoblastic neoplasias. Because maternal means **pertaining to the mother** (19), its use is semantically inaccurate in describing these pregnancy outcomes. In comparison, the term **pregnancy-associated** is nonspecific and includes all pregnancy outcomes. In addition to introducing these new terms, the CDC/ACOG definitions also extend the interval between termination of pregnancy and death from 42 days to 1 year.

With the advent of intensive care units and advanced life-support systems, a limitation of 42 days or even 90 days does not include all pregnancy-associated deaths. For instance, in Georgia during the period 1974–1975, 22 of 78 (29%) deaths related to pregnancy occurred after 42 days of the termination of pregnancy (20). In the same study, 6% of deaths due to causes clearly related to the pregnancy occurred >90 days postpartum.

Case Finding and Data Collection

The National Pregnancy Mortality Surveillance System is designed to rely on multiple reporting sources for case identification and on multiple information sources for data collection. As in the case of abortion mortality surveillance, multiple sources are expected to improve the completeness of the reporting, improve the accuracy of case ascertainment, and result in more accurate classification of these deaths. The system is designed to collect information from death certificates, matching birth or fetal death records, autopsy reports, hospital records of women, case summaries, personal contacts, Maternal Mortality Review Committee reports, and hospital records of newborns.

To allow for more accurate classification and better understanding of the risk factors associated with pregnancy-related deaths, the National Pregnancy Mortality Surveillance System, in classifying deaths, takes into account the interaction of five main factors (6):

- The outcome of pregnancy (e.g., abortion, ectopic pregnancy, live birth).

TABLE 1. Overview of selected maternal mortality studies, United States and Puerto Rico*

Author	Place/dates	Number of deaths	Definition of interval[†]	MMR[§] Study	MMR[§] Vital stats	Sources of data and method of review
Hansen (9)	New Jersey, 1988	40	NR[¶]	34	NR	Review of maternal deaths by the maternal mortality subcommittee
May (10)	North Carolina, 1988–1989	48	1 year	24	9.5	Enhancement of vital records by computer-matching of birth and fetal death records with death certificates
Comas (11)	Puerto Rico, 1989	22	1 year	33	19.5	Use of question on death certificate that asked whether a decedent was pregnant within the past year
Comas (12)	Puerto Rico, 1982	28	90 days	40.4	11.5	Review of medical records of women whose cause of death was likely to be related to pregnancy
Kirshon (13)	Jefferson Davis Hospital. Houston, Tex, 1981–1987	21	90 days	21.9	NR	Review of medical records of all women of reproductive age who died at the hospital
Rumbolz (14)	Nebraska, 1987–1989	30	90 days	11.1	NR	Review of maternal deaths by the maternal child health committee
Allen (15)	New York City, 1983–1984	58 / 37	6 months / 6 months	51.6 / 32.6	40.8 / 24.1	Enhanced ongoing surveillance activity by manual examination of death certificates; linkage of birth and fetal death files with death files; review of autopsy reports of death to women whose cause of death was likely to be related to pregnancy
Dorfman (16)	New York City, 1981–1983	120	6 months	36.1	NR	Ongoing surveillance; review of all death certificates
Syverson (17)	New York City, 1981–1984	224	1 year	40.2	NR	Ongoing surveillance
Koonin (18)	United States, 1979–1986	2,644	1 year	9.1	NR	Review of vital records
NCHS** (3)	United States, 1988	330	42 days	NA[††]	8.4	Routine reporting of deaths

* Abstracted from Atrash HK, Rowley D, Hogue CJR (8).
† Internal from pregnancy termination to death.
§ Maternal mortality ratio; maternal deaths per 100,000 live births.
¶ NR, not reported.
** National Center for Health Statistics.
†† Not applicable.

- The method of pregnancy termination (e.g., normal vaginal delivery, cesarean section, suction curettage).

- The time of death in relation to pregnancy termination (e.g., during pregnancy, during labor and delivery, or postpartum).

- The cause of death (e.g., hemorrhage, sepsis, embolism).

- The underlying obstetric or medical condition that precipitated the cause of death (e.g., placenta previa, chorioamnionitis, diabetes).

The CDC/ACOG Maternal Mortality Study Group has also designed a new system of classifying pregnancy-related deaths. This system differentiates between the immediate and underlying causes of death as stated on the death certificate, associated obstetrical and medical conditions or complications, and the outcome of pregnancy. For example, if a woman died of a hemorrhage that resulted from a ruptured ectopic pregnancy, the immediate cause of death would be classified as hemorrhage, the associated obstetrical condition would be classified as ruptured fallopian tube, and the outcome of pregnancy would be ectopic pregnancy. This classification scheme allows us to analyze the chain of events that led to death.

The study group also designed an abstract form and coding manual for data collection, coding and entry (Table 2) (21). The coding manual is available from CDC on request. The abstract form and coding manual were used as the basis for developing menu-driven, Epi Info-based personal computer software for data entry and analysis of pregnancy mortality data (22). The software is being pilot-tested and will soon be available for distribution to state and local health departments, Maternal Mortality Review Committees, and individual researchers.

Data Analysis and Interpretation

To facilitate comparisons and identify groups at special risk, CDC analyzes information from the National Pregnancy Mortality Surveillance System using three statistical measures of pregnancy-related mortality: pregnancy mortality ratio, pregnancy mortality rate, and outcome-specific pregnancy mortality rate.

The **pregnancy mortality ratio** (equivalent to the term **maternal mortality rate**) is defined as the number of pregnancy-related deaths per 100,000 live births. The word **ratio** is used instead of **rate** because the numerator is not a portion of the denominator. **Pregnancy mortality rate** is defined as the number of pregnancy-related deaths per 100,000 pregnancies (pregnancies include all live births, stillbirths, induced and spontaneous abortions, ectopic pregnancies, and molar pregnancies). **Outcome-specific pregnancy mortality rate** is defined as the number of deaths due to a pregnancy outcome per 100,000 pregnancies with the same outcome (e.g., ectopic pregnancy, induced abortion, live birth). This rate is used to determine the risk of death associated with specific pregnancy outcomes.

Each death is reviewed to confirm whether it is pregnancy-related. Classification by immediate cause of death, associated conditions, and outcome of pregnancy is made after the review of each death. After each death has been investigated, data are abstracted and input into computerized files. To ensure confidentiality, individual identifiers are removed from all records, and access to the surveillance data is restricted to CDC staff members responsible for analyzing the data. All data and results of analysis are disseminated in a manner that preserves the anonymity of each individual.

GENERAL FINDINGS

Analysis of data on all pregnancy-related deaths for 1979–1986 has been completed; analysis methods are described elsewhere (18,23). When reviewing these findings, keep in mind that the National Pregnancy Mortality Surveillance System has not been fully implemented, and data for 1979–1986 are based on reports from state health departments. Most states have identified their pregnancy-related deaths from vital statistics; some have identified additional deaths through linkages of birth and death records or through other sources. As a result, the numbers and ratios reported here are not substantially different than numbers and ratios reported through national vital statistics. However, this chapter includes more information about the characteristics of the women who died because we had, in addition to death certificates, matching birth and fetal death records for most women who died following a live birth or stillbirth (18,23).

Overall, 2,726 deaths during 1979–1986 were reported to CDC. After reviewing available records, we determined that 2,644 were pregnancy-related deaths. Of these deaths, 1,363 (51.6%) occurred after live births, 343 (13.0%) were associated with ectopic pregnancies, 263 (9.9%) occurred after stillbirths, 146 (5.5%) deaths occurred before delivery, 124 (4.7%) were related to abortions (induced legal, induced illegal, and spontaneous), and 14 (0.5%) were associated with molar pregnancies. The outcome of pregnancy was unknown for 391 (14.8%) deaths. Matching records were available for 95% of pregnancies that resulted in live births and 86% of pregnancies that resulted in stillbirths.

TABLE 2. National pregnancy mortality surveillance code sheet, developed by the CDC/ACOG Maternal Mortality Study Group

1. Case number (1-8) __ __ __ __ __ __ __ __

2. Death certificate number (9-16) __ __ __ __ __ __ __ __

3. Date of death (17-22) __ __/__ __/__ __

4. Initial date case reported (23-26)__ __/__ __

5. Initial source of notification (27) __

6. Death certificate in case file (28) __

7. Matching live birth or fetal death certificate in case file (29) __

8. Pregnancy status indicated on death certificate (30) __

9a. State of death (31-32) __ __

9b. County of death (33-35) __ __ __

10a. State of residence (36-37) __ __

10b. County of residence (38-40) __ __ __

11. SMSA county of residence (41) __

12. Age (42-43) __ __

13. Date of birth (44-49) __ __/__ __/__ __

14a. Race/ethnicity (50) __

14b. Hispanic origin (51) __

15. Marital status (52) __

16. Occupation (53) __

17. Educational level (54-55) __ __

18. Place of death (56) __

19. Month prenatal care began (57-58) __ __

20. Number of prenatal visits (59-60) __ __

21. Birth weight (61-64) __ __ __ __ gms.

22. Sex of infant (65) __

23. Autopsy report in case file (66) __

24. Hospital record in case file (67) __

25. Report of personal contact with attending M.D. in case file (68) __

26. Maternal Mortality Study Committee report in case file (69) __

27. Newborn hospital record in case file (70) __

TABLE 2. National pregnancy mortality surveillance code sheet, developed by the CDC/ACOG Maternal Mortality Study Group — continued

28. Place of initial event/acute illness (71) __

29. Woman's height (72-73) __ __ inches

30a. Prepregnancy weight (74-76) __ __ __pounds

30b. Weight at time of death (77-79) __ __ __pounds

31a. Total number of pregnancies (gravidity) (80-81) __ __

31b. Outcome of previous pregnancies (if twins, count each separately)
Live births (82-83) __ __
Stillbirths (84) __
Induced abortion (85) __
Spontaneous abortion (86) __
Abortion, type unknown (87) __
Ectopic pregnancy (88) __
Molar pregnancy (89) __

32. Outcome of pregnancy (90-91) __ __

33. Procedure for termination of pregnancy (92-93) __ __

34. Gestational age in weeks at termination of pregnancy (94-95) __ __

35. Date of termination of pregnancy (96-101) __ __/__ __/__ __

36. Type of obstetrical anesthesia/analgesia (102-103) __ __

37. Other operative procedure (104) __

38. Type of anesthesia/analgesia for other operative procedure (105) __

39. Days between termination of pregnancy and other operative procedure (106-108) __ __ __

40. CDC immediate (precipitating) cause of death (110-111) __ __

41. #1 Associated condition leading to death (112-114) __ __ __
#2 Associated condition leading to death (115-117) __ __ __
#3 Associated condition leading to death (118-120) __ __ __

42. Concurrent medications (yes = 1, no = 2, unknown = 9)
Anticonvulsants (125) __
Anticoagulants (126) __
Antibiotics (127) __
Antineoplastics (128) __
Antihypertensives (129) __
Corticosteroids (130) __
Hormones (OCPs, estrogens) (131) __
Insulin (132) __
Narcotics (Rx only) (133) __
Sedatives/hypnotics/anxiolytics (134) __
Tocolytics (135) __
Thyroid/antithyroid medications (136) __

43. If death due to injury, list type of injury (140-141) __ __

147

TABLE 2. National pregnancy mortality surveillance code sheet, developed by the CDC/ACOG Maternal Mortality Study Group — continued

44. Selected risk factors present:
    Alcohol abuse (142) __
    Drug abuse
       Heroin, intravenous (IV) (143) __
       Cocaine, IV (144) __
       Crack cocaine (145) __
       Cocaine, not IV/not specified (146) __
       Narcotics, other/not specified, IV (147) __
       Narcotics, not IV (148) __
       Amphetamines (149) __
       Barbiturates, sedatives, or anxiolytics (150) __
       Marijuana (151) __
       Other drug abuse/not specified (152) __
    Obesity (153) __
    Smoking (154) __
    Refused medical therapy or treatment (155) __
    Other (156) __

45. Date case file closed (158-161) __ __/__ __

46. Final classification of death (162) __

47. Coder initials (163-164) __ __

48. State ICD code (165-168) __ __ __ __

49. Conditions of special interest (169-170) __ __

The interval between the time of birth or pregnancy termination and death of the mother was known in 66% of the deaths. About 69% of these deaths occurred during pregnancy or within the first week after delivery or pregnancy termination; 25% occurred 8–42 days after delivery; and 6% occurred between 43 days and 1 year after the pregnancy (Figure 1).

The overall pregnancy mortality ratio for the 8-year study period was 9.1 deaths per 100,000 live births; the ratio dropped steadily from 10.9 in 1979 to 7.4 in 1986 (Figure 2). The ratio decreased from 7.1 in 1979 to 5.1 in 1986 for white women and from 27.2 in 1979 to 16.6 in 1986 for black women and women of other minority races (Figure 2). For each of the 8 years, the pregnancy mortality ratio for black women and women of other minority races was higher than that for white women, with risk ratios ranging from 2.5 to 3.8. Age-specific mortality ratios were also higher for black women and women of other minority races than for white women in each age-group (Figure 3). For all racial groups,

the pregnancy mortality ratio increased with age and was highest for women aged ≥40 years (Figure 3).

The age-adjusted pregnancy mortality ratio was 7.1 per 100,000 live births for married women and 20.7 for unmarried women. Unmarried white women had an age-adjusted ratio 2.7 times that for married white women (15.6 vs. 5.8), whereas unmarried black women had an age-adjusted pregnancy mortality ratio only 1.2 times that for married black women (24.7 vs. 20.5).

For deaths associated with live births, the age-adjusted pregnancy mortality ratio by live birth order was 5.8 per 100,000 live births for women following their first live birth. The risk decreased to 4.1 for women following their second live birth and then increased with increasing live birth order.

Under CDC's new classification system—which differentiates between causes of death, associated (obstetric and medical) conditions, and outcomes of pregnancy—each pregnancy outcome

FIGURE 1. Percentage of pregnancy deaths, by number of days from time of termination of pregnancy to death — United States, 1979–1986

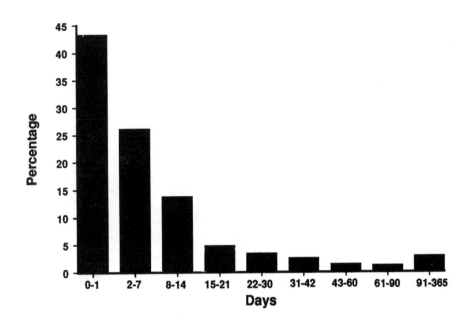

FIGURE 2. Pregnancy mortality ratios, by race — United States, 1979–1986

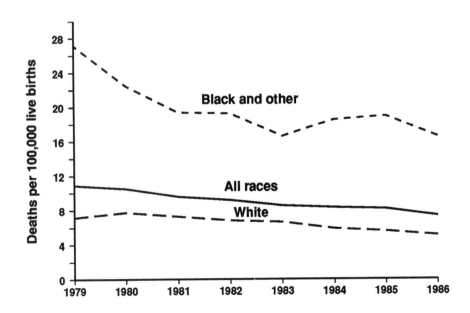

149

FIGURE 3. Pregnancy mortality ratios, by age and race — United States, 1979–1986

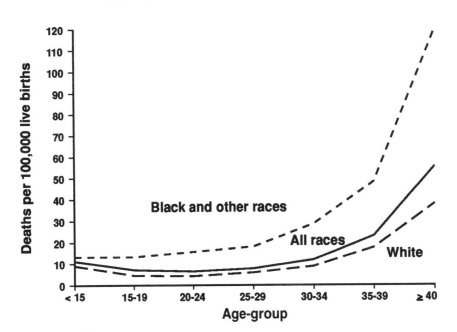

was associated with a specific leading cause of death (Table 3). The leading causes of pregnancy-related death after a live birth were thrombotic pulmonary embolism, pregnancy-induced hypertension complications, hemorrhage (primarily postpartum uterine bleeding), and infection. More than half of the deaths were attributed to these four causes. Women with preeclampsia succumbed to a variety of conditions, whereas those with eclampsia died primarily of central nervous system insults. For women whose pregnancies ended in stillbirths, the leading causes of death were hemorrhage (largely from abruptio placentae), pregnancy-induced hypertension complications, and amniotic fluid pulmonary embolism. Almost 90% of women whose deaths were associated with ectopic pregnancies died of hemorrhage from rupture of the ectopic site. The leading causes of death for women whose pregnancies ended in a spontaneous or induced abortion were hemorrhage from uterine bleeding, generalized infection, and thrombotic pulmonary embolism. Women who had a molar pregnancy died of a variety of causes and conditions, whereas most women who died before delivery died of thrombotic and amniotic fluid embolism, hemorrhage from uterine rupture or laceration, and central nervous system complications related to eclampsia.

Overall, 5.5% of women in the United States who had a live birth during the study period had inadequate prenatal care (defined as no care or care starting in the third trimester) (24). In comparison, 15% of women who had a live birth and subsequently died had inadequate prenatal care.

INTERPRETATION ISSUES

Pregnancy mortality surveillance based only on vital statistics reports has serious limitations as a source of numbers, ratios, and causes of pregnancy-related death (25). Vital records are not designed to be used in investigating pregnancy-related deaths, and the information available from these records is limited. Moreover, because pregnancy-related death definitions are based on causes of death, and because clinical information listed on death certificates is often inadequate, numbers of pregnancy-related deaths based on vital statistics are usually underestimates of the true number of pregnancy-related deaths (8). Furthermore, the published causes of pregnancy-related death are a mixture of outcomes of pregnancy, immediate causes of death, and underlying obstetric conditions (3). In-depth investigations of pregnancy-related deaths

TABLE 3. Cause of pregnancy-related death, by outcome of pregnancy, United States,* 1979–1986†

Cause of death	Live birth		Stillbirth		Ectopic		Abortion§		Molar		Undelivered		Unknown		Total	
	No.	%	No.	%	No.	%	No.	%	No.	%	No.	%	No.	%	No.	%
Hemorrhage	249	18.3	89	33.9	305	88.9	43	34.8	2	14.3	30	20.5	81	20.7	799	30.2
Pulmonary embolism	370	27.1	47	17.9	10	2.9	24	19.4	2	14.3	60	41.1	106	27.1	619	23.4
Pregnancy-induced hypertension	307	22.5	59	22.4	1	0.3	1	0.8	2	14.3	17	11.6	92	23.5	479	18.1
Infection	101	7.4	22	8.4	6	1.7	35	28.2	2	14.3	8	5.5	28	7.2	202	7.6
Cardiomyopathy	53	3.9	4	1.5	0	0.0	1	0.8	0	0.0	2	1.4	30	7.7	90	3.4
Anesthesia complications	65	4.8	3	1.1	4	1.2	11	8.9	0	0.0	0	0.0	3	0.8	86	3.3
Other	218	16.0	39	14.8	17	5.0	9	7.3	6	43.0	29	19.9	51	13.0	369	14.0
Total maternal deaths	1,363	100.0	263	100.0	343	100.0	124	100.0	14	100.0	146	100.0	391	100.0	2,644	100.0

* Including Puerto Rico.
† From Koonin LM, Atrash HK, Lawson HW, Smith JC (18).
§ Includes spontaneous and induced abortions.

published over the last decade have reported pregnancy mortality ratios two to six times higher than ratios in vital statistics reports (Table 1) (8). Therefore, the true national pregnancy mortality ratio is most likely higher than the reported ratio. We have a clear need for pregnancy mortality surveillance activities that identify all pregnancy-related deaths and collect adequate information to characterize these deaths. Other approaches used to better identify and classify pregnancy-related deaths include matching death records with pregnancy outcome records, reviewing medical records and autopsy reports, reviewing death certificates, and reviewing reports from Maternal Mortality Review Committees. Although each of these sources has some advantages, each has been found to have serious limitations as well (25).

The National Pregnancy Mortality Surveillance System, when fully implemented, will provide information about national numbers and ratios of pregnancy mortality and will identify clusters of pregnancy-related deaths by age, geographic location, cause, and other factors. However, because every death is unique, we must learn lessons from each death and carry out appropriate and relevant interventions at the local level to prevent future morbidity and mortality caused by similar chains of events. Therefore, pregnancy-related death review should be an ongoing process conducted by professionals and program decision makers at the local level. Pregnancy-related death review should include not only medical contributing factors but also any other possible contributors such as quality of care, access to and use of services, socioeconomic circumstances, and behaviors during pregnancy. Active, state-based pregnancy mortality surveillance that relies on multiple sources for identifying and classifying pregnancy-related deaths historically has been conducted by Maternal Mortality Review Committees. The number of states with Maternal Mortality Review Committees has decreased dramatically over the past decade, primarily for two reasons: the decreasing number of pregnancy-related deaths and the medicolegal climate of today's practice of medicine (4). Optimally, state-based Maternal Mortality Review Committees will be reestablished in all states to investigate and learn from each pregnancy-related death.

In conjunction with the National Pregnancy Mortality Surveillance System and the legal advisors at CDC and ACOG, the CDC/ACOG Maternal

Mortality Study Group commissioned Ronald F. Wright, J.D., assistant professor of law at Wake Forest University School of Law, to study legal protection afforded medical review processes at the state level. He found that "in all but a few states, the legal risk of participating in expert review is negligible. Most states have statutes that protect information involved in the review process from disclosure or use in subsequent litigation. Laws in most states also protect participants in the review process . . . from civil liability" (26). A state-by-state annotation of statutes regarding the protection of expert review committees was published by ACOG and is available on request (27).

EXAMPLES OF USING DATA

Despite the limitations of the National Pregnancy Mortality Surveillance System mentioned above, the large numbers of deaths collected through such a system allow for analyses that are not possible to conduct using state and local data. For example, the retrospective study of pregnancy-related deaths for 1979–1986 includes 90 deaths caused by cardiomyopathies, 86 deaths caused by anesthesia complications, >350 deaths among Hispanic women, and about 300 deaths among teenagers. Furthermore, a national system is needed to provide national rates for monitoring trends, identifying clusters, allowing comparisons with state and international rates, and tracking our progress in achieving national goals such as the year 2000 health objectives (1).

Numerous reports of pregnancy-related deaths include findings from different approaches to identifying and investigating pregnancy-related deaths (3,8–18). To better describe and understand the pregnancy mortality problem, we cannot rely on vital statistics alone as a source of information and numbers (Table 1). Every state needs an active surveillance system to monitor pregnancy-related deaths, using multiple sources of information to identify and characterize such deaths.

FUTURE ISSUES

With improving technology and advanced medical skills, the causes of pregnancy-related death have changed dramatically over the past 50 years. The triad of infection, bleeding, and toxemia—which in the past accounted for >90% of all pregnancy-related deaths—now accounts for <60% of such deaths. New causes of death are emerging; for instance, anesthesia complications, embolism, and cardiomyopathy were responsible for 30% of all pregnancy-related deaths during 1979–1986.

Another emerging cause of pregnancy-related death is AIDS. During the last decade, the incidence of AIDS among women of reproductive age has increased dramatically, with the number of deaths ranging from 92 in 1983 to 1,016 in 1987 and 2,645 in 1991 (28,29). In 1991, AIDS became the seventh leading cause of death among females aged 15–24 years and the fifth leading cause of death among women aged 25–45 years (29). With >6 million pregnancies in the United States every year, and with the increasing incidence of AIDS among women of reproductive age, we can also expect to see a concurrent increase in the number of deaths among pregnant women with AIDS. Nationally, 26 pregnancy-associated deaths due to AIDS were reported for 1981–1988 (30). This accounted for about 1% of all pregnancy-related deaths for the period. In New York City, 2 of 224 (0.9%) pregnancy-related deaths caused by AIDS were reported for 1982–1984 (17), whereas in New Jersey, 6 of 40 (15%) pregnancy-related deaths reported for 1988 were caused by AIDS (9).

At the 1991 CDC/ACOG Maternal Mortality Study Group meeting, members noted that pregnancy-related mortality and serious pregnancy-related morbidity are increasingly associated with emerging technology and practices; in particular, they noted an increasing prevalence of pregnancy-related mortality associated with adult respiratory distress syndrome (ARDS). Members reported several pregnancy-related deaths resulting from ARDS associated with preeclampsia and upper urinary tract infection (pyelonephritis). Our review of the literature revealed that 5 of 40 pregnancy-related deaths reported by Hansen and Chez (9), and 10 of 21 pregnancy-related deaths reported by Kirshon et al. (13) resulted from ARDS; most of these deaths were associated with preeclampsia (13).

These findings highlight the importance of active, ongoing surveillance of pregnancy-related deaths and the investigation of each such death to ensure an up-to-date understanding of the rapidly changing circumstances that contribute to serious pregnancy-related morbidity and mortality. Without this detailed knowledge, we will have extreme difficulty formulating strategies to achieve further reductions in pregnancy-related mortality and morbidity.

The National Pregnancy Mortality Surveillance System encourages and supports state-based intensive investigations of pregnancy-related deaths to supplement information and numbers obtained through vital statistics. However, to reduce the health risks associated with pregnancy, we should direct our attention toward reducing pregnancy morbidity. Pregnancy mortality is only the tip of the iceberg. CDC estimates that >800,000 women are discharged from hospitals every year for pregnancy complications *(31)*. This does not include complications during labor and delivery, complications during the postpartum period, or complications treated on an ambulatory basis.

The ultimate objective of the National Pregnancy Mortality Surveillance System is to contribute to the reduction of pregnancy morbidity and mortality in the United States. Toward that end, we must develop a close partnership between CDC, ACOG, other public health agencies (local and federal), and professional organizations of clinical providers, particularly those caring for pregnant women. Any recommendations for preventing pregnancy morbidity and mortality can be effective only if health-care providers follow them. CDC and ACOG's collaboration in developing and carrying out the National Pregnancy Mortality Surveillance System is just the first step in developing this partnership.

REFERENCES

1. Public Health Service. Healthy people 2000: national health promotion and disease prevention objectives—full report, with commentary. Washington, DC: US Department of Health and Human Services, Public Health Service, 1991:366–90; DHHS publication no. (PHS)91-50212.

2. Public Health Service. Health, United States, 1991. Hyattsville, Maryland: US Department of Health and Human Services, Public Health Service, CDC, NCHS, 1992:172; DHHS publication no. (PHS)92-1232.

3. National Center for Health Statistics. Vital statistics of the United States, 1988; vol. II, mortality, part A. Washington, DC: US Department of Health and Human Services, Public Health Service, CDC, 1991: (sec. 1) 69, (sec. 4) 1.

4. Entman SS, Atrash HK, Koonin LM, Smith JC. Maternal mortality surveillance [Letter]. Am J Public Health 1988;78:1499–1500.

5. Atrash HK, Lawson HN, Smith JC. Legal abortion in the US: trends and mortality. Contemp Obstet Gynecol 1990;35:58–69.

6. Ellerbrock TV, Atrash HK, Hogue CJR, Smith JC. Pregnancy mortality surveillance: a new initiative. Contemp Obstet Gynecol 1988;31:23–34.

7. AbouZahr C, Royston E. Maternal mortality: a global factbook. Geneva: World Health Organization, 1991:17.

8. Atrash HK, Rowley D, Hogue CJR. Maternal and perinatal mortality. Curr Opin Obstet Gynecol 1992;4:61–71.

9. Hansen GF, Chez RA. Maternal deaths in New Jersey: 1988. N J Med 1990;87:995–8.

10. May WJ, Buescher PA, Murray MA. Enhanced maternal mortality surveillance—North Carolina, 1988 and 1989. MMWR 1991;40:469–71.

11. Comas A, Navarro A, Carrera A, et al. Maternal mortality surveillance—Puerto Rico, 1989. MMWR 1991; 40:521–3.

12. Comas A, Navarro A, Conde J, Blasini I, Adamsons K. Misreporting of maternal mortality in Puerto Rico. Bol Assoc Med P Rico 1990;82:343–6.

13. Kirshon B, Hinkley CM, Cotton DB, Miller J. Maternal mortality in a maternal-fetal medicine intensive care unit. J Reprod Med 1990;35:25–8.

14. Rumbolz WL. A report of maternal deaths in Nebraska for the years 1987, 1988, and 1989. Nebraska Med J February 1991:31–4.

15. Allen MH, Chavkin W, Marinoff J. Ascertainment of maternal deaths in New York City. Am J Public Health 1991;81:380–2.

16. Dorfman SF. Maternal mortality in New York City, 1981–1983. Obstet Gynecol 1990;76:317–23.

17. Syverson CJ, Chavkin W, Atrash HK, Rochat RW, Sharp ES, King GE. Pregnancy-related mortality in New York City, 1980 to 1984: causes of death and associated risk factors. Am J Obstet Gynecol 1991; 164:603–8.

18. Koonin LM, Atrash HK, Lawson HW, Smith JC. Maternal mortality surveillance, United States, 1979–1986. In CDC Surveillance Summaries, July 1991: MMWR 1991;40(no. ss-2):1–13.

19. Taylor EJ, Anderson DM, Patwell JM, Plaut K, McCullough K, eds. Dorland's illustrated medical dictionary, 27th ed. Philadelphia: W.B. Saunders Company, 1988.

20. Rubin G, McCarthy B, Shelton J, Rochat RW, Terry J. The risk of childbearing re-evaluated. Am J Public Health 1981;71:712–6.

21. National Center for Chronic Disease Prevention and Health Promotion. National pregnancy mortality surveillance coding manual. Atlanta: US Department of Health and Human Services, Public Health Service, CDC, 1992.

22. Dean AG, Dean JA, Burton AH, Dicker RC. Epi info, version 5: a word processing, database, and statistics program for epidemiology on microcomputers. Atlanta: CDC, 1990.

23. Atrash HK, Koonin LM, Lawson HW, Franks AL, Smith JC. Maternal mortality in the United States, 1979–1986. Obstet Gynecol 1990;76:1055–60.

24. Public Health Service. Health, United States, 1988. Hyattsville, Maryland: US Department of Health and Human Services, Public Health Service, CDC, NCHS, 1989; DHHS publication no. (PHS)89-1232.

25. Atrash HK, Ellerbrock TV, Hogue CJR, Smith JC. The need for national pregnancy mortality surveillance. Fam Plann Perspect 1989;21:25–6.

26. Wright RF, Smith JC. State level expert review committees—are they protected? Public Health Rep 1990;105:13–23.

27. Wright RF, Smith JC. Are expert review committees protected? An annotation of relevant state statutes. Washington, DC: American College of Obstetricians and Gynecologists, 1990.

28. Chu SY, Buehler JW, Berkelman RL. Impact of the human immunodeficiency virus epidemic on mortality in women of reproductive age, United States. JAMA 1990;264:225–9.

29. NCHS. Advance report of final mortality statistics, 1991. Hyattsville, Maryland: US Department of Health and Human Services, Public Health Service, CDC, 1993. (Monthly vital statistics report; vol. 42, no. 2, suppl.)

30. Koonin LM, Ellerbrock TV, Atrash HK, et al. Pregnancy-associated deaths due to AIDS in the United States. JAMA 1989;261:1306–9.

31. Franks AL, Kendrick JS, Olson DR, Atrash HK, Saftlas AF, Moien M. Hospitalization for pregnancy complications, United States, 1986 and 1987. Am J Obstet Gynecol 1992;166:1339–44.

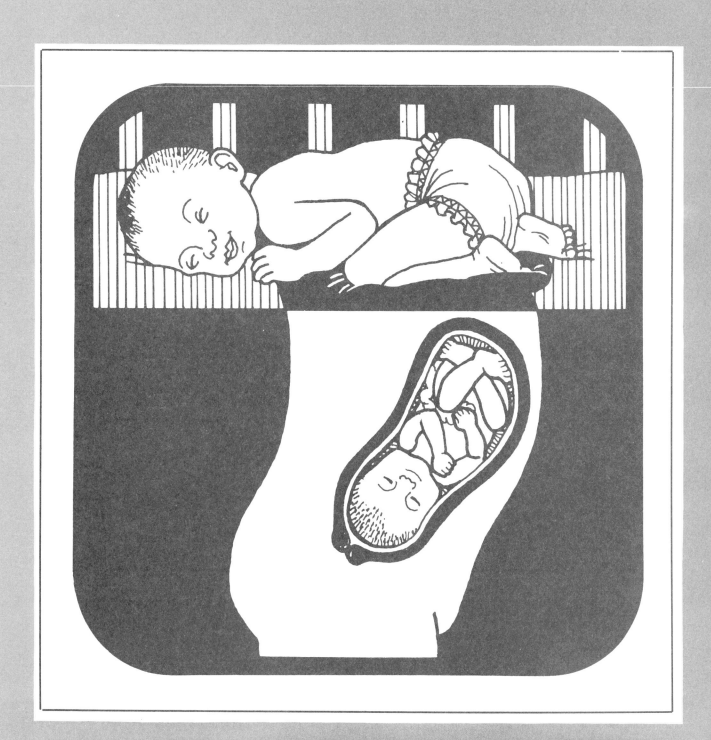

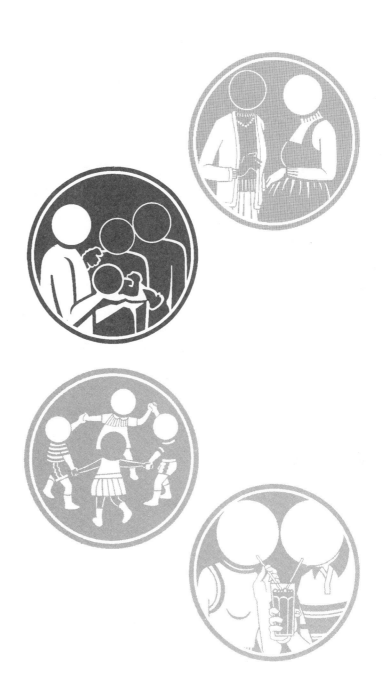

Commentary

on Birth Outcomes
from the Rhode Island Department of Health

The birth of a baby is a milestone, a marker, and a blessed event for a family and the community. For millennia, births have been memorable, noted, and, therefore, countable life events. In the last three centuries, we've also counted infant deaths, and the infant mortality rate has become one of the few truly universal public health indicators. The births and deaths of infants are common, easily counted, intuitively relevant, and important measures. The infant mortality rate is what it says—a measure of bad outcomes for infants. The infant mortality rate is also what we have learned about it over centuries—a measure of women's health, reproductive success, and health services. In addition, the infant mortality rate is what we have made it—a marker for the health of children and families, or a whole health system, or a whole society.

As leaders in public health, we are expected to know our numbers. We must answer the question, "How are we doing?" whether it comes from neighbors, colleagues, the mayor's office, or the media. In many places, the infant mortality rate is a big story, with press releases, interviews, and even leaks. But as health leaders, we know that infant deaths are merely the tip of an iceberg, the most visible point of the much larger and more important issues of maternal and child health (MCH). The numbers we need to know are the measures of all the pregnancies and all the infants: Who? What? Where? Did we know the needs? Did we do the right things, and did we do them right?

In a series of recent conferences and publications, we have learned some of the data concerns of state and local MCH leaders. To address the MCH mandate, to assess MCH needs, to develop an effective system of family-centered, community-based care, and to report on the system performance and outcomes for mothers and children, MCH leaders need information that is—

- **Relevant**, reflecting good measures of the major problems of this population.

- **Credible**, both scientifically and intuitively.

- **Responsive** to the current concerns of public health leaders and the public.

- **Timely**, for practical and political reasons.

- **Local**, reflecting a direct measure of the problem in the community of concern, or being obviously generalizable there too.

- **Comparable** with other jurisdictions or populations relevant to the discussion.

- **Stable**, allowing repeated measurements to detect time trends.

- **Sustainable**, having technical, leadership, and financial costs that are reasonable.

The chapters in the Birth Outcomes section address several of these important issues related to the collection of good information for MCH leadership and the ways in which CDC can help, with expertise and data on birth outcomes. Most state and local leaders are in constant need of data for management of programs, for their Title V responsibilities, and for the many other dimensions of public health leadership. We all, however, face the tense scenario, described in the Overview by Wilcox and Marks, in which we have difficulty supporting data-gathering and data-analysis activities while services needs remain unmet. In fact, a challenge of leadership is to move beyond that tension, to a synthesis, which is often found at the local or family level of analysis. *Mrs. M.A.'s* wonderful letter to the Children's Bureau (described in the Overview) captures the elements of education, optimism, resilience, and advocacy that are at the heart of the ongoing MCH agenda. In this monograph, surveillance is defined as the monitoring of diseases and conditions—their frequency, risk factors, consequences, and service requirements. To provide leadership for an effective system of family-centered care, we need to adopt these tools and adjust them to help us estimate unmet needs, track and manage problems, detect vulnerabilities, improve resistance to risks, and support the resilience of *Mrs. M.A.* and all the other successful parents in America.

In these chapters on birth outcomes, the authors review CDC activities that produce traditional population measures of poor birth outcomes—preterm births, intrauterine growth retardation, fetal losses, and measures of infant morality. When we pull all of these measures together, we can see that our most important challenge is to find the solution to America's recalcitrant problems of birth weight distribution, especially among vulnerable minority groups. At the state and local levels, which interventions should we make, for whom, and what effects can we expect? For example, should we alter the content of prenatal care, placing more emphasis on nutrition, on effective interventions against tobacco and alcohol use, or on the control of occult infections? Which recent advances may have perverse secondary effects, as has occurred with fertility interventions? In the Low Birth Weight and Intrauterine Growth Retardation chapter, Kiely and colleagues highlight some of our most promising opportunities, ephasizing that prenatal care must become much more than the ritual documentation of a few risks—it needs to become a much richer, more flexible portfolio of effective maternity interventions. The authors also suggest several ways in which state and local MCH programs can apply these data, and they present Massachusetts, Illinois, and Missouri as examples of states that have used birth outcomes data to improve the public health system.

In the Neonatal and Postneonatal Mortality chapter, Rowley and colleagues emphasize the relative costs of the preventable losses of early childhood. They note the false dichotomy between medical and social factors. Public health leaders have always known that health and social factors need to be addressed together, both to assess needs and to evaluate the effectiveness of various interventions. With the advent of health-care reform in the United States, this worry is especially apropos—because universal coverage may help with access to medical care but may actually diminish our effective attention to the social and behavioral dimensions of MCH. In the context of health-care reform and cost-containment, the attention to perinatal regionalization, one of our stunning successes in birth outcomes surveillance, is also helpful. Maintaining surveillance—as in South Carolina and Puerto Rico—will be important to ensure that regional system effectiveness does not deteriorate. Rowley and colleagues also give us a useful discussion of birth weight-specific analysis, which is critical for informed leadership. However, they also warn us that our obsession with the huge and complex problem of low birth weight may divert us from more specific opportunities and effective points of intervention. The trick to good public health leadership is to identify specific practical points of public health action and to achieve small gains against preventable components of big, complicated problems.

In the Infant Mortality chapter, MacDorman and colleagues raise more methodological issues, but they also address one of the overriding concerns of state and local leadership. In the final analysis, **all** public health is **local** public health. How are we to measure unmet needs and opportunities in small areas with small numbers and follow local time trends? Many of us have lived with the dilemmas of aggregation. Combining data from several years, or combining data from various neighborhoods, may diminish precision, but such analyses are often more useful than adjusted national rates or simple anecdotes— the usual alternatives.

The two chapters on birth defects surveillance address another epidemiologic tradition—one that is based on the surveillance of unusual specific conditions. New surveillance is driven by public concerns about birth defects, pregnancy outcomes, and local exposures. The authors point out that prenatal and perinatal surveillance as well as childhood tracking are mushrooming (because of improved technology, both in diagnoses and data management), but our established mechanisms of birth defects surveillance, such as hospital discharge data systems, are becoming less effective.

In fact, both the justification and the resources for birth outcomes surveillance may be shifting away from epidemiology and etiologic investigations and moving toward program entitlements and assurance of care. At the state and local levels, new foundations for monitoring and tracking are rapidly arising—from early childhood initiatives, from the entitlement mandate in Part H of the Individuals with Disabilities Education Act, and from the expanded MCH responsibilities for children eligible for Supplemental Security Income. These mandates may provide more stable long-term tracking as part of a coordinated system of care, but they will also force some shifting away from the familiar ground of biologic diagnoses to focus on functional and behavioral/social indicators of vulnerability. **Major disabilities** and **special health needs** include acquired and idiopathic conditions as well as canonical birth defects. At the state and local levels, family and community nurturing capacities are often more powerful predictors of long-term child development than infant diagnoses.

In this monograph, the Maternal and Child Health Bureau and Special Projects of Regional and National Significance are suggested as possible resources for birth outcomes surveillance activities. In fact, birth outcomes analyses originated from the earliest mandate of the Children's Bureau (to study and report on infant health) and its successor, the Maternal and Child Health Bureau (to assess needs; to plan and support a family-centered, community-based, culturally competent coordinated system of care; and to report the status of women and children's health and the effectiveness of interventions according to the measures outlined in the *Healthy People 2000* objectives).

Federal, state, and local MCH leaders benefit from these surveillance tools—tools that help us to know our numbers and address the four Ps of MCH leadership:

- **Policy**. Are we addressing the right problems?

- **Politics**. Do we have the right support for action?

- **Program**. Are we serving the right people?

- **Practice**. Are we doing the right things right?

Past surveillance has offered us important guidance, which will need to be adjusted to circumstances of managed care, new program constraints, and new definitions of maternal and child health programs. But beyond surveillance itself, some more specific changes must be addressed for effective MCH leadership. We need a core common MCH data set, with the same definitions in Title V, Title X, Title XIX, the Special Supplemental Food Program for Women, Infants, and Children, Part H of the Individuals with Disabilities Education Act, and elsewhere. We need better, more timely, and more consistent vital statistics data. We need to make use of morbidity measures—hospital discharge or other critical event markers for preventable but not mortal childhood losses. We need effective childhood tracking systems so that we can combine the proliferation of health and development monitoring mandates we now face. We need simple protocols and support for direct child mortality reviews, akin to current maternal mortality reviews. Finally, we need a broad renewal of state and local leadership capacity—a new cadre of sophisticated MCH leaders from many disciplines with quantitative and analytic skills and with interests extending well beyond the traditional purview of the health professions to include the behavioral sciences, community organizations, integrated family support networks, and a broad vision of the issues that will govern the health and development of children in the twenty-first century.

William H. Hollinshead, M.D., M.P.H.
Medical Director
Division of Family Health
Rhode Island Department of Health
Providence, Rhode Island

Fetal Deaths

James A. Gaudino, Jr., M.D., M.S., M.P.H.,[1]
Donna L. Hoyert, Ph.D.,[2] Marian F. MacDorman, Ph.D.,[2]
Julie A. Gazmararian, Ph.D., M.P.H.,[1] Melissa M. Adams, Ph.D., M.P.H.,[1]
and John L. Kiely, Ph.D.[3]

PUBLIC HEALTH IMPORTANCE

In 1989, fetal deaths* represented a substantial portion of pregnancy losses in the United States, accounting for 54.8% of perinatal deaths. For every 1,000 live births, 7.5 fetal deaths occurred, compared with 6.2 neonatal deaths. Whether measured by numbers or by the anguish of affected families, fetal deaths are an important public health concern. Historically, however, the factors contributing to fetal mortality have been less researched than those contributing to infant mortality, and fewer prevention efforts have been initiated because of our limited understanding of the etiology of many fetal diseases, problems of measuring fetal well-being in utero, and the poorer quality of fetal mortality data relative to infant mortality data. Consequently, the public and public health professionals have a limited awareness of fetal mortality as a public health problem and are less likely to use fetal mortality surveillance in prevention efforts.

We have observed numerous changes in fetal death trends since 1950, when the United States adopted the World Health Organization's (WHO) definition of fetal death (1):

Death prior to the complete expulsion or extraction from its mother of a product of conception, irrespective of the duration of pregnancy; the death is indicated by the fact that after such separation, the fetus does not breathe or show any other evidence of life such as beating of the heart, pulsation of the umbilical cord, or definite movement of voluntary muscles.

This definition emphasizes the absence of signs of life at delivery regardless of gestational age. Since the WHO definition was adopted, we have made improvements in diagnosis and intervention that have resulted in decreases in the risks for fetal death. For example, some investigators have reported a decline in the proportion of fetal deaths occurring during labor to those occurring before labor (2). With these clinical advances, the leading etiologies of infant mortality have changed as well. To address such shifts in the epidemiology of perinatal outcomes, we need to better understand the predisposing factors, such as type I diabetes and birth defects. Prevention efforts that address these factors may differ greatly from interventions involving improved obstetrical procedures. Therefore, we need to shift our emphasis in perinatal mortality research from intervention to

---

* The term **fetal death** as used here refers to death at ≥20 weeks of gestation. This description is a portion of the definition used in current U.S. reporting requirements. **Perinatal death** as used here refers to death occurring from ≥20 weeks of gestation through the first 28 days of life. **Neonatal death** refers to death occurring from birth through the first 28 days of life. **Infant mortality** refers to death within the first year of life.

[1] Division of Reproductive Health
National Center for Chronic Disease Prevention
 and Health Promotion
Centers for Disease Control and Prevention
Atlanta, Georgia

[2] Division of Vital Statistics
National Center for Health Statistics
Centers for Disease Control and Prevention
Hyattsville, Maryland

[3] Division of Health and Utilization Analysis
National Center for Health Statistics
Centers for Disease Control and Prevention
Hyattsville, Maryland

prevention and from infancy to **pregnancy**, focusing on the prevention of poor pregnancy outcomes such as preterm delivery, very low birth weight, and birth defects (3,4).

One major goal, then, of the surveillance of fetal deaths is to monitor our progress toward preventing these pregnancy losses. Another goal for surveillance is to collect fetal mortality data that, in combination with data on births and neonatal deaths, will provide a more complete picture of pregnancy outcomes and their risks. Because some etiologies cause both fetal and neonatal deaths, the evaluation of interventions targeted at these etiologies must be based on the surveillance of all perinatal deaths. A final goal is to collect data that will provide a sensitive enough pregnancy health indicator to allow more timely assessments of prevention efforts.

Despite these goals, our current data collection systems have major limitations. For example, fetal mortality statistics understate the magnitude of total fetal loss because most states require the reporting of only fetal deaths at $\geq$20 weeks, even though fetal deaths at <20 weeks of gestation are much more frequent (5). Moreover, not all of these reportable fetal deaths are reported (6).

To gain a better perspective on the magnitude of and the potential for prevention of these pregnancy losses, international comparisons can be useful. However, U.S. fetal mortality rates cannot be compared meaningfully with those of many other countries because of differences in fetal death reporting requirements and reporting completeness. Instead, the perinatal mortality rate is more informative for these comparisons, because it takes into account inconsistencies in international classifications of fetal and infant deaths. In 1989, the United States was ranked 18th internationally in perinatal mortality (fetal deaths at $\geq$28 weeks of gestation plus infant deaths occurring <7 days after birth) (*NCHS, unpublished data, 1993*) (for additional information about related topics and surveillance activities, see the Behavioral Risk Factors Before and During Pregnancy, Prenatal Care, Prevalence of Birth Defects, Infant Mortality, and Neonatal and Postneonatal Mortality chapters).

HISTORY OF DATA COLLECTION

Vital statistics on stillbirths were first collected by the Bureau of the Census in 1918. Beginning in 1922, the bureau began annually collecting and tabulating these statistics from the states in the birth-registration area. At that time, states had variations in their legal definitions of stillbirth and how stillbirths were reported (7). By 1933, all states were admitted into the birth-registration area, and this allowed the national compilation of state-specific statistics. Although the first standard fetal death certificate was developed in 1930 (8), until 1939, the nationally recommended procedure for fetal death registration required the filing of both a live birth and a death certificate. Since 1939, the filing of a separate fetal death certificate has been recommended (9). In 1946, the responsibility for maintaining vital statistics for the entire nation moved to the Public Health Service (10); this responsibility now rests with CDC's National Center for Health Statistics (NCHS).

Since 1950, the term **fetal death** has been used in preference to other terms to reflect the adoption of the WHO's recommended definition and to end confusion between the terms **stillbirth**, **abortion**, and **miscarriage**. Most states individually have adopted the WHO or comparable definitions over time. After the legalization of induced abortions, separate reporting for spontaneous fetal deaths and induced terminations was begun in 1970 (9).

CDC SURVEILLANCE ACTIVITIES

U.S. fetal death registration is based on state law, and reports are filed and maintained in state vital statistics offices. Fetal mortality data from the National Vital Statistics System are cooperatively produced by NCHS and state vital statistics offices under a joint agreement known as the Vital Statistics Cooperative Program.

Key Variables Available

About every 10 years, NCHS works with states to develop a recommended U.S. Standard

Report of Fetal Death to serve as the model for state reports (for the most recent revision in 1989, see Figure 1). Although conforming closely with the standard report, state reports continue to differ from or lack certain items included in the U.S. standard report, often because of unique state needs or state vital statistics laws *(8)*.

The 1978 revision of the standard fetal death report recommended that state reports include data on the delivering hospital; parents' names and basic demographic data; maternal pregnancy history; basic clinical information about the fetus; and fill-in lines for causes of death, congenital malformations, significant conditions, maternal conditions, and complications of pregnancy, labor, and delivery *(11)*. The 1989 revision added these new items: parental occupations, parental Hispanic origin, maternal smoking and alcohol use history, and maternal weight gain. Also, check-box items replaced most fill-in lines, offering the potential to improve reporting *(12)*.

Reporting Requirement Differences

Reporting requirements for fetal deaths vary according to state laws *(13)*. While continuing to promote standard reporting, the 1977 revision of the *Model State Vital Statistics Act and Regulations* recommended reporting of all spontaneous losses occurring at ≥20 weeks or weighing ≥350 g *(14)* rather than continuing to recommend the reporting of deaths at all gestations *(15)*. Currently, nine states have adopted this reporting requirement. An additional 27 states have adopted the very similar requirement of reporting deaths ≥20 weeks of gestation. Three states require the reporting of deaths of fetuses weighing ≥500 g, whereas four states use different gestational age or birth-weight requirements or a combination of both. Over time, some states have modified their requirements to accommodate state needs in light of NCHS recommendations (see the Technical Appendix in NCHS, 1991 [11]). In addition, although eight states and several territories require reports for all spontaneous losses regardless of gestation *(13)*, as of 1989, only five states were sending

these reports to NCHS. Specific reporting differences are described elsewhere (see the Technical Appendix in NCHS, 1991 [11]).

Data Collection and Processing

Medical information on the fetal death report, including the cause of death, is generally provided by the attending physician, medical examiner, or coroner. Generally, the funeral director completes the report's demographic portion, using information from the family, and files the report with the state. However, when a funeral director is not involved, physicians or medical records personnel complete and file the entire report. Although the cooperation of medical personnel in filling out the fetal death report is required, the extent of their input varies by state, and this may affect the quality of the data. Currently, medical personnel complete about half of all state reports.

NCHS promotes uniformity in the collection and processing of fetal death data in a number of ways, such as by issuing periodic updates to the standard report. NCHS also periodically updates the *Model State Vital Statistics Act and Regulations* to assist states in developing and revising state vital statistics laws, provides training and technical assistance to state vital statistics offices, and provides states with annually updated instruction manuals that contain information on standard coding and data processing procedures.

Beginning in 1989, NCHS initiated a special project to code data on the underlying cause of fetal death. Although cause-of-death information using ICD coding standards was available before 1989, it was not coded by NCHS. Data on the underlying cause of fetal death will be available on the fetal death data tape in the future. In the meantime, state-specific information on the underlying causes of fetal deaths can be obtained from some state vital statistics offices (see discussion on cause-of-death coding in the Infant Mortality chapter).

Once fetal death reports are filed and processed in state vital statistics offices, states send NCHS

FIGURE 1.

U.S. STANDARD
REPORT OF FETAL DEATH   STATE FILE NUMBER

TYPE/PRINT IN PERMANENT BLACK INK FOR INSTRUCTIONS SEE HANDBOOK

1. FACILITY NAME (If not institution, give street and number)

2. CITY, TOWN, OR LOCATION OF DELIVERY   3. COUNTY OF DELIVERY   4. DATE OF DELIVERY (Month, Day, Year)   5. SEX OF FETUS

PARENTS

6a. MOTHER'S NAME (First, Middle, Last)   6b. MAIDEN SURNAME   7. DATE OF BIRTH (Month, Day, Year)

8a. RESIDENCE STATE   8b. COUNTY   8c. CITY, TOWN, OR LOCATION   8d. STREET AND NUMBER

8e. INSIDE CITY LIMITS? (Yes or no)   8f. ZIP CODE   9. FATHER'S NAME (First, Middle, Last)   10. DATE OF BIRTH (Month, Day, Year)

11. OF HISPANIC ORIGIN? (Specify No or Yes—If yes, specify Cuban, Mexican, Puerto Rican, etc.)	12. RACE—American Indian, Black, White, etc. (Specify below)	13. EDUCATION (Specify only highest grade completed)		14. OCCUPATION AND BUSINESS/INDUSTRY (Worked during last year)	
		Elementary/Secondary (0-12)	College (1-4 or 5+)	Occupation	Business/Industry

MOTHER

11a. ☐ No ☐ Yes Specify   12a.   13a.   14a.   14b.

FATHER

11b. ☐ No ☐ Yes Specify   12b.   13b.   14c.   14d.

15. PREGNANCY HISTORY (Complete each section)   16. MOTHER MARRIED? (At delivery, conception, or any time between) (Yes or no)   17. DATE LAST NORMAL MENSES BEGAN (Month, Day, Year)

MULTIPLE BIRTHS Enter State File Number for Mate(s) LIVE BIRTH(S)

LIVE BIRTHS   OTHER TERMINATIONS (Spontaneous and induced at any time after conception)

15a. Now Living Number ____ ☐ None
15b. Now Dead Number ____ ☐ None
15d. (Do not include this fetus) Number ____ ☐ None

18. MONTH OF PREGNANCY PRENATAL CARE BEGAN—First, Second, Third, etc. (Specify)   19. PRENATAL VISITS—Total Number (If none, so state)

20. WEIGHT OF FETUS (Specify Unit)   21. CLINICAL ESTIMATE OF GESTATION (Weeks)

FETAL DEATH(S)

15c. DATE OF LAST LIVE BIRTH (Month, Year)   15e. DATE OF LAST OTHER TERMINATION (Month, Year)

22a. PLURALITY—Single, Twin, Triplet, etc. (Specify)   22b. IF NOT SINGLE BIRTH—Born First, Second, Third, etc. (Specify)

MEDICAL AND HEALTH INFORMATION

23a. MEDICAL RISK FACTORS FOR THIS PREGNANCY (Check all that apply)

Anemia (Hct. < 30/Hgb. < 10) .... 01 ☐
Cardiac disease .... 02 ☐
Acute or chronic lung disease .... 03 ☐
Diabetes .... 04 ☐
Genital herpes .... 05 ☐
Hydramnios/Oligohydramnios .... 06 ☐
Hemoglobinopathy .... 07 ☐
Hypertension, chronic .... 08 ☐
Hypertension, pregnancy-associated .... 09 ☐
Eclampsia .... 10 ☐
Incompetent cervix .... 11 ☐
Previous infant 4000 + grams .... 12 ☐
Previous preterm or small-for-gestational-age infant .... 13 ☐
Renal disease .... 14 ☐
Rh sensitization .... 15 ☐
Uterine bleeding .... 16 ☐
None .... 00 ☐
Other ____ 17 ☐
(Specify)

23b. OTHER RISK FACTORS FOR THIS PREGNANCY (Complete all items)

Tobacco use during pregnancy ...... Yes ☐ No ☐
  Average number cigarettes per day ____
Alcohol use during pregnancy ...... Yes ☐ No ☐
  Average number drinks per week ____
Weight gained during pregnancy ____ lbs.

24. OBSTETRIC PROCEDURES (Check all that apply)

Amniocentesis .... 01 ☐
Electronic fetal monitoring .... 02 ☐
Induction of labor .... 03 ☐
Stimulation of labor .... 04 ☐
Tocolysis .... 05 ☐
Ultrasound .... 06 ☐
None .... 00 ☐
Other .... 07 ☐
(Specify)

25. COMPLICATIONS OF LABOR AND/OR DELIVERY (Check all that apply)

Febrile (>100°F. or 38°C.) .... 01 ☐
Meconium, moderate/heavy .... 02 ☐
Premature rupture of membrane (>12 hours) .... 03 ☐
Abruptio placenta .... 04 ☐
Placenta previa .... 05 ☐
Other excessive bleeding .... 06 ☐
Seizures during labor .... 07 ☐
Precipitous labor (<3 hours) .... 08 ☐
Prolonged labor (>20 hours) .... 09 ☐
Dysfunctional labor .... 10 ☐
Breech/Malpresentation .... 11 ☐
Cephalopelvic disproportion .... 12 ☐
Cord prolapse .... 13 ☐
Anesthetic complications .... 14 ☐
Fetal distress .... 15 ☐
None .... 00 ☐
Other .... 16 ☐
(Specify)

26. METHOD OF DELIVERY (Check all that apply)

Vaginal .... 01 ☐
Vaginal birth after previous C-section .... 02 ☐
Primary C-section .... 03 ☐
Repeat C-section .... 04 ☐
Forceps .... 05 ☐
Vacuum .... 06 ☐
Hysterotomy/Hysterectomy .... 07 ☐

27. CONGENITAL ANOMALIES OF FETUS (Check all that apply)

Anencephalus .... 01 ☐
Spina bifida/Meningocele .... 02 ☐
Hydrocephalus .... 03 ☐
Microcephalus .... 04 ☐
Other central nervous system anomalies (Specify) .... 05 ☐
Heart malformations .... 06 ☐
Other circulatory/respiratory anomalies (Specify) .... 07 ☐
Rectal atresia/stenosis .... 08 ☐
Tracheo esophageal fistula/Esophageal atresia .... 09 ☐
Omphalocele/Gastroschisis .... 10 ☐
Other gastrointestinal anomalies (Specify) .... 11 ☐
Malformed genitalia .... 12 ☐
Renal agenesis .... 13 ☐
Other urogenital anomalies (Specify) .... 14 ☐
Cleft lip/palate .... 15 ☐
Polydactyly/Syndactyly/Adactyly .... 16 ☐
Club foot .... 17 ☐
Diaphragmatic hernia .... 18 ☐
Other musculoskeletal/integumental anomalies (Specify) .... 19 ☐
Down's syndrome .... 20 ☐
Other chromosomal anomalies (Specify) .... 21 ☐
None .... 00 ☐
Other .... 22 ☐
(Specify)

CAUSE OF FETAL DEATH

28.
PART I. Fetal or maternal condition directly causing fetal death.
IMMEDIATE CAUSE
a. ____   Specify Fetal or Maternal
DUE TO (OR AS A CONSEQUENCE OF):

Fetal and/or maternal conditions, if any, giving rise to the immediate cause(s), stating the underlying cause last.
b. ____   Specify Fetal or Maternal
DUE TO (OR AS A CONSEQUENCE OF):
c. ____   Specify Fetal or Maternal

Enter only one cause per line for a, b, and c.

PART II. Other significant conditions of fetus or mother contributing to fetal death but not resulting in the underlying cause given in Part I.

29. FETUS DIED BEFORE LABOR, DURING LABOR OR DELIVERY, UNKNOWN (Specify)

30. ATTENDANT'S NAME AND TITLE (Type/Print)
Name ____
☐ M.D. ☐ D.O. ☐ C.N.M. ☐ Other Midwife
☐ Other (Specify) ____

31. NAME AND TITLE OF PERSON COMPLETING REPORT (Type/Print)
Name ____
Title ____

DEPARTMENT OF HEALTH AND HUMAN SERVICES — PUBLIC HEALTH SERVICE — NATIONAL CENTER FOR HEALTH STATISTICS — 1989 REVISION

PHS-T-007
REV 1/89

state-coded computer tapes and microfilm copies of the original fetal death reports, which are then coded by NCHS. Beginning with data from 1992, NCHS will use state-coded data in the national fetal death file for selected states while continuing to use data coded from the microfilm copies for the remaining states and registration areas. NCHS develops special rules to handle state variations in data collection and processing. Personal identifiers are not included in the fetal death data file.

Quality control of fetal death data takes place in a number of ways. Some states have their own procedures and regularly query reports with problem data back to the original data source. NCHS encourages these state efforts and provides guidelines for such queries (16). Fetal death data are subject to NCHS quality control procedures at several processing stages to check for the completeness, coding validity, and consistency of data items. First, problems or inconsistencies are checked against the original source and are corrected if possible. A list of coding inconsistencies is returned to the states for information and corrective action. Second, a quality control sample of records is dual-coded, and both microfilm copies and state-coded files are compared. Third, for each state, the percentages of nonresponses for each item are compared with the state's previous year percentages and the U.S. average percentages. States are contacted when very high percentage or large changes in nonresponses are noted. Counts and percentages of records with impossible or out-of-range codes are also reviewed and compared with the previous year's performance. Finally, according to written procedures, invalid or inconsistent values may be modified or assigned as **unknowns**. Selected missing items may be imputed, either by using data from a previous record or other report items, or by assigning a standard value (e.g., the modal value 1 for missing plurality). Imputed values are flagged. Also, numeric values such as gestational age are computed.

Fetal mortality data are generally available about 2 years after the close of a data year. Tables of these data are published annually in *Vital Statistics of the United States, Volume II, Mortality, Part A (17)*, as well as in periodic NCHS reports.

Also, a number of unpublished tables are produced annually and are available from NCHS on request. NCHS also produces public-use data tapes containing individual record information on all registered fetal deaths; data for 1982–1988 are currently available. The tape contents, file characteristics, and cost are described in NCHS's *Catalog of Electronic Data Products (18)*.

Additional sources of fetal death data include the National Fetal Mortality Survey of 1980 and the National Maternal and Infant Health Survey of 1988, which are nationally sampled surveys produced periodically with a wider range of variables than the annual vital statistics data files (19). Birth defects surveillance programs may also report data on fetal deaths (see the Prevalence of Birth Defects chapter).

GENERAL FINDINGS

In this section, we present important findings from U.S. national surveillance activities and other studies that help highlight important issues for the prevention of fetal deaths.

Global measurements of the numbers of and risks for the approximately 60,000 fetal deaths reported in U.S. fetal death statistics are available from NCHS (see the CDC Surveillance Activities section) and are highlighted here. Most of the data reported by NCHS focus primarily on the estimated 30,000 U.S. deaths occurring at ≥20 weeks of gestation and include frequency counts according to several characteristics. Also, fetal death ratios (defined in the Interpretation Issues section) were formerly provided by gestation, maternal characteristics, race, sex, birth weight, residence, and other items. However, more recently, fetal death rates are provided instead of ratios (see discussion later in this chapter concerning rates and ratios). In 1989, new tables on Hispanic origin and prenatal care were included in NCHS's fetal death reports.

Nationally, overall fetal mortality rates have declined by more than half since 1960, from 15.8 in 1960 to 7.5 in 1989, continuing to drop even after the 1977 change in reporting requirements (Figure 2)(also see Table 3-2 in NCHS, 1994 [17]). The fetal mortality rate did not decline between 1960 and 1965. From 1965 to 1970, however, the rate declined by an average of 2.5% per year. From 1970 to 1980 the rate declined more rapidly, averaging 4.2% per year. From 1980 to 1989, the velocity of the decline in the fetal mortality rate again slowed to an average of 2.1% per year. Various factors may have contributed to these declines, including the better management of maternal complications, such as hypertension, pregnancy-associated diabetes, and Rh isoimmunization, which may have reduced the incidence of antepartum fetal deaths, and improvements in obstetrical management of labor, such as electronic fetal monitoring, which may have reduced the incidence of intrapartum fetal deaths (20–24).

Although fetal mortality rates have declined for all race groups, the gap between black and white fetal mortality rates has widened since 1970. In 1970, the fetal mortality rate for blacks was 23.2—1.90 times the rate of 12.3 for whites. By 1989, the fetal mortality rate for blacks was 13.1—2.05 times the rate of 6.4 for whites. These rates, which are not adjusted for other factors such as maternal age and medical risks, may indicate differences in socioeconomic resources and access to care between comparison groups (see discussion of this topic in the Infant Mortality chapter). For example, NCHS data on the month in which prenatal care began indicate that 63% of white mothers compared with 45% of African-American mothers who experienced a fetal death had begun prenatal care in the first 3 months of the pregnancy (see Table 3-18 in NCHS, 1994 [17]). In addition, 7% of white mothers compared with 18% of black mothers experiencing fetal deaths received no prenatal care. Other populations with apparently higher fetal death rates than whites include Native Americans and Hawaiians, each of whom have a rate of 7.6. In contrast, rates were substantially lower for Asian subgroups—3.2 for Chinese, 3.1 for Japanese, 5.6 for Filipinos, and 5.6 for other Asian and Pacific Islanders.

Besides varying by race and ethnic origin, fetal mortality rates also differ with respect to numerous other demographic factors. Similar to infant mortality rates, fetal mortality rates in the 43 areas where marital status is adequately reported are also substantially higher for unmarried than for married mothers, although the magnitude of the difference is reduced when maternal race is controlled (Table 1). The risk of fetal death also varies by the age of the mother, with the youngest and oldest mothers experiencing the greatest risk (Table 1). Data on the differences in fetal mortality rates by state are available from NCHS but should be interpreted with caution (see the Interpretation Issues section).

Fetal deaths are etiologically heterogeneous with respect to the timing and causes of death, and we must carefully distinguish between **intrapartum** fetal deaths, occurring **during labor**, and **antepartum** fetal deaths, occurring **before labor**. Despite the lack of national cause-of-death data, major causes of fetal deaths identified in the literature include maternal conditions, preterm labor, asphyxia, abruptio placentae, infection, proteinuric hypertension, and birth defects (20,25,26). However, because of limitations with cause-of-death information and variations in study design (see Interpretation Issues section), studies have reported different distributions of the causes of fetal deaths. For example, the proportion of deaths caused by birth defects has ranged from 10%–15% (20,27,28) to as high as 30% (29). Although the distribution of gestations for the fetal deaths may differ, most of the studies cited above include gestational ages of ≥20 weeks in their case definitions. One of the few consistencies is the large percentage (ranging from 23% to 52%) of reports with an unknown cause of death (20,25). In a recent Canadian study, Fretts et al. demonstrated temporal changes in cause-specific fetal death rates from the 1960s to 1980s (24). They found that fetal deaths caused by intrapartum asphyxia and Rh isoimmunization had almost disappeared, with significant declines occurring in unexplained antepartum deaths and in those caused by fetal growth retardation. However, they observed no significant changes in deaths due to intrauterine infection or abruptio placentae. In contrast to the 1960s—when the risk was elevated for women with hypertension, diabetes, or a history of stillbirth—during the 1980s, only women with a history of insulin-dependent diabetes were at detectable risk. After 28 weeks of gestation, fetal deaths were most often attributed to fetal growth retardation or abruptio placentae, although many were still unexplained.

FIGURE 2. Fetal and neonatal mortality rates* — United States, 1942–1989

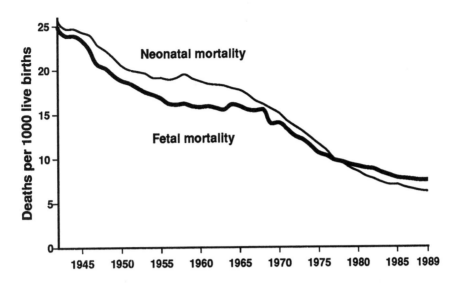

* Fetal mortality rates are per 1,000 live births and fetal deaths. Neonatal mortality rates are per 1,000 live births.

Source: NCHS, 1994 *(17).*

TABLE 1. Fetal mortality rates,* by race, marital status, and age of mother — United States, 1989

	Race		
	All races[†]	**White**	**Black**
Marital status[§]			
Total	7.6	6.4	13.3
Married	6.3	5.9	11.6
Unmarried	11.1	8.7	14.2
Age (years)[¶]			
Total	7.5	6.4	13.1
<15	14.4	12.4	16.3
15–19	8.6	7.4	11.6
20–24	7.4	6.2	12.0
25–29	6.6	5.7	13.1
30–34	7.1	6.1	15.5
35–39	9.4	8.4	17.7
40–44	13.5	12.0	25.0
45–49	23.8	24.8	**

* Per 1,000 live births and fetal deaths.
[†] Includes races other than white and black.
[§] Rates by marital status are for 42 states and the District of Columbia.
[¶] Rates by age are for all states and the District of Columbia.
**Rate does not meet standards of reliability or precision (<20 fetal deaths).

Source: NCHS, 1994 *(17).*

In the United States, as in other developed countries, most fetal deaths occur during the antepartum period, before the onset of labor *(25)*. In comparing antepartum fetal deaths (between 24 weeks of gestation and before labor), intrapartum fetal deaths, and neonatal deaths among all single births that occurred in New York City in 1976–1978, Kiely, Paneth, and Susser found that 12.8% of deaths occurred during labor, 72.6% occurred before labor, but for 14.6% of deaths, the time of death was unknown *(30)*.

Unlike the risk factors for antepartum deaths, most risk factors for intrapartum stillbirths are related to labor and delivery problems *(2,21,22,25)*. The most striking finding in the New York City studies is the clear association between less available perinatal technology (as measured by the level of the hospital or facility) and an increased risk for intrapartum fetal death— an association that does not occur in late antepartum fetal deaths *(2,22,29)*. In contrast, after controlling for prior fetal loss, type of service (public vs. private), race, marital status, and mother's educational attainment, the investigators found that increasing maternal age was strongly associated with antepartum fetal deaths but not with intrapartum fetal deaths and that high parity was strongly associated with intrapartum deaths but not to antepartum deaths. More recently, Little and Weinberg found similar results for maternal age, but they also discovered that overweight women had differentially higher risks for intrapartum vs. antepartum fetal deaths at ≥28 weeks of gestation *(31)*.

In addition, health-care professionals and researchers recognize that the risk of fetal death declines as gestation advances. Also, several studies have shown that the risk increases with younger and older maternal age, high parity, prior fetal loss, morbidity conditions, inadequate prenatal care, smoking, lower socioeconomic status, and reproductive tract infections *(20,22,26,32–38)*. A few studies have displayed an increased risk among older smokers than among younger smokers *(32,33)*. In contrast, for intrapartum deaths, no increased risks have been found for social, demographic, or antenatal care variables such as maternal age, parity, adverse obstetric history, and the level of the delivery hospital *(25)*. Although risks for fetal death associated with illegal drug use have been less frequently studied,

some researchers have identified an increased risk due either to direct toxicity or an indirect effect on other high risk conditions such as abruptio placentae *(39)*.

INTERPRETATION ISSUES

Registration Completeness

DIFFERENCES IN THE INTERPRETATION OF STANDARD DEFINITIONS

Fetal deaths, especially those involving preterm fetuses, can be misclassified as live births because of either individual difficulties with or differences in the clinical interpretation of the WHO fetal death definition. To help practitioners distinguish between fetal deaths and live births, the American Academy of Pediatrics and the American College of Obstetricians and Gynecologists have clarified the WHO's fetal death definition as follows *(13,40)*: "Heartbeats are to be distinguished from transient cardiac contractions, respirations are to be distinguished from fleeting respiratory efforts or gasps."

Despite these guidelines, which are endorsed by NCHS, distinguishing between fetal deaths and live births in practice depends on such factors as the skill and experience of the hospital's clinical and registrar's staff, differences between individual physicians and hospitals in the application of definitions, and changes in medical practice over time. For example, Kleinman attributed some of the notable changes in both the incidence of live births and the proportion of deaths among infants weighing <500 g from 1981–1985 to changes that had occurred in reporting classifications of pregnancy outcomes *(41)*. In addition, trend analyses for fetal deaths may be difficult to interpret because of the increased reporting of deliveries of infants weighing <500 g at birth. Kleinman attributed these increases to practice and reporting changes *(41)*. He found that in 1970–1985, not only were these increases notable, but they differentially increased by 39% for whites and by 78% for blacks.

Other possible factors that might bias the classification of outcomes include financial incentives to classify outcomes as live births in ambivalent cases or legal disincentives to classify early neonatal demises as fetal deaths (e.g., deaths related to intrapartum fetal distress).

These classification problems occur for fetal and infant death statistics worldwide. These problems are the reason for the development of perinatal mortality measures that bypass inconsistencies in classifying deaths that occur very near the time of delivery by incorporating various combinations of later fetal deaths and neonatal infant deaths (11,40,42). Analyses using such measures have an advantage because late fetal deaths and neonatal deaths often share the same etiologies and, to examine the full impact of these risks with respect to outcomes, combining such losses makes good sense.

Early fetal deaths at <20 weeks of gestation, however, may have substantially different etiologies than late fetal or neonatal deaths, and they should be assessed separately. Although NCHS has procedures to adjust these perinatal measures for unknown gestations, perinatal mortality measurements cannot help us assess these earlier fetal death risks, deal with the underreporting of fetal deaths (especially earlier deaths), or fully account for fetal deaths with unknown gestations (6.7% in 1989).

REPORTING REQUIREMENTS

State differences in reporting requirements, as described previously, pose difficulties in the interpretation of both national trends and state comparisons (13). Because most states require reports for fetal deaths at ≥20 weeks of gestation, NCHS addresses the comparability problem by presenting most fetal death tables in the annual publication, *Vital Statistics of the United States*, based on reports of deaths at ≥20 weeks of gestation (see the Technical Appendix in NCHS, 1991 [11]). However, this approach does not address the problem of age-dependent underreporting resulting from the different reporting requirements used.

UNDERREPORTING

Substantial evidence indicates that not all fetal death reports for which reporting is required are filed (6,43,44). Greb and colleagues compared Wisconsin reports to hospital referrals to the Wisconsin Stillbirth Service Project and found that 17.8% of fetal deaths evaluated at the project were never reported to the state (6). Furthermore, Goldhaber found that the completeness of reporting from Northern California Kaiser Foundation hospitals depended on how close the estimated gestational age of the deceased fetus at delivery was to the state reporting minimum of age of ≥20 weeks, with approximately 10% of deaths at 20–27 weeks being reported compared with 79% of deaths at ≥28 weeks (43). Reporting also depended on whether hospitalization was required for delivery or whether physicians classified the event as a fetal death. Thus, underreporting of fetal deaths is most likely to occur in the earlier part of the required reporting period for each state (43,44).

National evidence of underreporting was found in a recent NCHS comparison of 1989 fetal mortality rates, similar to work previously reported by Kleinman (45). The overall fetal death rate (≥20 weeks) of 9.9 for the five states reporting fetal deaths at all gestations was 39% higher than the rate of 7.1 for all other states combined. In contrast, the neonatal mortality rate for these five states was 18% higher than the rate for all other states combined. The magnitude of these percentage differences strongly suggests that higher underreporting occurs in states reporting fetal deaths at ≥20 weeks than in states reporting deaths at all gestations.

Completeness of reports for deaths at the shortest gestations in states reporting all gestational ages has also been questioned. Complete reporting at these ages could depend on the mothers' experience with and knowledge of the possibility of pregnancy, access to pregnancy testing before a loss, and health beliefs and attitudes about when to seek care as well as providers' attitudes about the significance of the loss and need for reporting.

Although we have no better solutions to underreporting other than improved reporting, some researchers have limited their analyses to late fetal deaths at ≥28 weeks to avoid underreporting. However, this solution still ignores the problem of earlier losses, because at least one third of deaths at ≥20 weeks fall in the 20–27 week category, and losses at <20 weeks account for 80% of all losses in states that report them (45). The apparent dependency of reporting completeness on the earliest gestational age for registration suggests that if we are to adequately measure fetal losses at ≥20 weeks, we might be able to determine minimum reporting ages to maximize completeness and address concerns about adequate ascertainment and burdensome costs of very early loss reports.

Data Quality

ITEM-SPECIFIC NONRESPONSE

In comparison with other vital statistics records, fetal death records generally have more not-stated responses to individual items. Item non-response in fetal death records reflects both difficulty in ascertaining early death data, such as cause of death, sex, or birth defects, and limitations in access to necessary information, such as funeral directors' lack of access to medical charts. Even the physician or medical records staff may have difficulty obtaining information, for example, if the death occurs before the onset of clinical prenatal assessment or if important clinical data are only in another providers' records. In addition, important information such as birth weight may be missed if the delivery occurred out of the hospital or was attended by emergency room providers not aware of requirements or not accustomed to collecting this information. This latter reason was given by a number of hospitals that missed gestational ages and birth weights in a recent study of fetal deaths at ≥20 weeks in Georgia (46). In contrast to data on live births, missing birth weights were a larger problem than missing gestational ages. Among the 40% of the selected problem records that were missing data, most were missing data on birth weights. As the result of active hospital follow-up of these problem records, 48% of the missing weights were obtained, and important corrections were made to data on gestational age and birth weight. Additional factors contributing to item nonresponse may include the lower priority given to the fetal death system than to other vital statistics systems and fewer resources available for follow-up.

Nationally, in records on fetal deaths at ≥20 weeks, the percentage of not-stated responses for items varies widely (Table 2). Reporting is virtually complete for some items, such as the place of delivery (0.1% stated in 1989). Reporting for other items, particularly new items such as maternal weight gain, reflects a high non-response percentage (46.9% not stated in 1989). Yet the overall quality of fetal death records has been improving. Further improvements are expected in the national data file after NCHS shifts to using selected state-coded data tapes rather than microfilm copies of reports. These state-coded files will contain the results of queries received after the microfilm copies are sent to NCHS.

GESTATIONAL AGE MEASUREMENTS

Because risks for poor pregnancy outcomes of fetuses differ across gestational periods, the accuracy of gestational age estimates is important to the interpretation and further analysis of these data. At NCHS, the gestational age of the fetus is computed by subtracting the date of delivery from the date of last menstrual period (LMP). The physician's estimate of gestation is used if the calculated estimate is missing, is outside of an acceptable range, or is inconsistent with reported birth weight but the physician's estimate meets these criteria. Some inaccuracies have been reported in the use of both the physician's estimate and LMP measures of gestational age. Problems with the use of the physician's estimate include clustering of responses on even-numbered weeks of gestation and a pronounced clustering at 40 weeks of gestation (47). Problems with gestational age estimates computed from LMP include substantial reporting inaccuracies for postterm pregnancies (47). The physician's estimate of gestational age can be made by using methods such as ultrasound, clinical assessments, calculation of dates, or a combination of these approaches; biases may be introduced by the lack of uniform measurement methods. For LMP gestation, calculated estimates may also be misleading when a fetal death has occurred days or weeks before the fetus is delivered. Therefore, without better standardized measurements, the problem of gestational age ascertainment will remain an issue, especially among at-risk

TABLE 2. Percentage of nonresponses for selected items on records of fetal deaths at ≥20 weeks of gestation — United States, 1989

	Percentage of fetal death records
Place of delivery	0.1
Hispanic origin*	3.6
Marital status†	5.8
Total-birth order	6.6
Birth weight	11.5
Month prenatal care began	13.4
Method of delivery§	13.4
Maternal education¶	19.2
Weight gain**	46.9

* Total of 31 states.
† Total of 42 states and the District of Columbia.
§ Total of 39 states and New York City.
¶ Total of 48 states and New York City.
**Total of 38 states and New York City.

Source: NCHS, 1994 (17).

pregnancies in which minimal or no prenatal ascertainments were made.

CAUSE AND TIMING OF DEATH

Because fetal deaths are heterogeneous events with respect to causes, cause-of-death analyses are important for examining preventable risks (see the General Findings section). However, both the uniformity and plausibility of these data have been and will continue to be important issues, especially in the new national data on underlying cause of fetal death that will be available in the future. Despite the lack of national data, four specific points addressing these issues have been raised in reviews of state-specific data:

- A major drawback to uniformity is that many fetuses who die are not autopsied or otherwise evaluated. For example, in a recent review of fetal deaths in Kansas, Cowles et al. found that only 37% of the 243 reports indicated an autopsy was obtained (23). Factors that may affect whether such evaluations occur are the wishes of the family during this sensitive time, the costs of evaluations, who will

pay these costs, the perception that finding the cause of a fetal death is less important than finding the cause of an infant death, and the availability of skilled pathologists and technicians. Cost may be less of an issue because an increasing number of third-party payers will pay for placental examinations—a necessary component of the pathologic review of fetal deaths (48).

- Cause-of-death determinations also depend on the adequacy and completeness of the postmortem workup and the condition of the fetus. Highlighting one of the most distressing facts about fetal death cause-specific analyses, Pitkin showed that all known and suspected causes and associated conditions combined accounted for no more than 50% of observed fetal deaths, leaving half or more undiagnosed (49). Moreover, this incomplete determination of causes limits the assessment of risks. For example, Yudkin et al. found that death rates for unexplained postterm deaths were four times higher than rates for postterm deaths with known causes, indicating that risk factors may be differentially distributed by cause category and

173

could be missed in cause-specific analyses not accounting for undetermined causes (50). However, Pitkin points out the need for further examinations with careful pathologic assessments that could provide additional information on more than half of the deaths with no apparent cause (49).

- Implausible or misclassified causes of death have also been identified as a problem. Although various factors may increase the risk of death, some factors may not be important in the cascade of events that caused the death, yet they can be presumed and reported to be the cause without careful assessments by knowledgeable reviewers such as clinicians and certifiers. In a recent review of cause-of-fetal-death reporting by five states, Kirby questioned the plausibility of reported causes of deaths (51). Both Kirby's review and an accompanying editorial by Atkinson agreed that improvements in these data are needed (51,52). Consistent with other studies mentioned above, he found that 24.2%–33.7% of these deaths had unspecified causes. Comparing causes on 112 state reports with causes derived by using an extensive protocol, Greb et al. found marked discrepancies. For example, 23 of the 35 placenta- or cord-related deaths were reclassified with an unknown cause because of the lack of confirmation of a placenta- or cord-related injury (6). Also, they found that many of the "appropriately" categorized reported diagnoses were wrong.

- As we mentioned in the General Findings section, the distinction between intrapartum fetal deaths and late antepartum fetal deaths should be made. Because the causes of these two groups of fetal deaths are clearly different, public health implications and methods of prevention are different for them.

As a result of these problems with the quality of cause and timing data, analysts using these data collection systems have had limited ability to classify causes in meaningful ways for public health decision making about resource allocations and interventions. Golding describes several major classification schemes for fetal and perinatal mortality (53). Although most schemes require more extensive clinical evaluation, one scheme proposed by Wigglesworth was designed to be simpler and reliable and, with improvements in the data, could be used to provide important general information to target areas for prevention. This scheme requires information on the presence or absence of a congenital abnormality and specific conditions described on the fetal death certificate, such as the timing of the demise. Other schemes demand even better, more specific clinical information; should such information become available, these schemes could provide even greater insight into the causes of fetal deaths, especially those related to antepartum deaths.

The lack of adequate cause-of-death information and the difficulties in developing and applying more refined classifications related to the etiologic heterogeneities among fetal deaths (e.g., antepartum vs. intrapartum) are substantial barriers in the identification of preventable risks for fetal deaths, especially when surveillance data are being used.

RISK MEASURES AND OTHER ANALYTIC TECHNIQUES

In addition to fetal death frequency counts, a number of fetal or perinatal death risk measures are in use. For example, before 1989, fetal death ratios—the number of fetal deaths divided by the number of live births—were used in national report tables. Beginning with 1989 fetal death data, fetal mortality rates—the number of fetal deaths divided by the number of live births plus fetal deaths—were selected to replace death ratios because this denominator provides a better indication of the population at risk of fetal death (i.e., pregnancies). Also, various perinatal mortality rate formulas are available, and several are in use by NCHS (11,40). Additional measures and types of analyses, which may be useful, are detailed elsewhere (35,54–56).

EXAMPLES OF USING DATA

The analysis of fetal death surveillance data to address prevention needs is still a relatively new concept and has not been conducted in-depth by many states. We hope that this chapter will encourage public health departments to improve their fetal death surveillance data collection, analysis, and application to develop and monitor prevention efforts.

FUTURE ISSUES

Two of the national health objectives for the year 2000 address fetal deaths (57):

- Reduce the fetal death rate (≥20 weeks of gestation) to no more than 5 per 1,000 live births plus fetal deaths. (Baseline: 7.6 per 1,000 live births plus fetal deaths in 1987.)

- Reduce the fetal death rate for blacks to 7.5 per 1,000 live births plus fetal deaths. (Baseline: 12.8 per 1,000 live birth plus fetal deaths in 1987.)

To meet the first objective for the entire U.S. population, we need to maintain the 3.2% annual decline in fetal mortality observed in 1981–1986. The objective for blacks calls for accelerating the annual decline in fetal mortality from 2.3% in 1981–1986 to 3.6% in the 1990s.

The likelihood of achieving these goals depends on the availability and use of interventions to avert fetal deaths. Given that the causes of many fetal deaths are unknown, the prospects for prevention are unclear. Although a large percentage of fetal deaths are attributed to lethal malformations (20), only a small proportion of these malformations may be prevented by changes in maternal behaviors (e.g., increasing periconceptional multivitamin use and decreasing periconceptional and antenatal alcohol and drug use), and prevention remains a problem because the causes of most malformations are unknown. In addition, because prior fetal death associated with certain malformations can be a risk for subsequent fetal demise—perhaps because of the increased risk for a subsequent malformation (58)—better medical evaluation of fetal deaths with genetic screening and counseling may also lead to prevention and enhanced surveillance (59).

Interventions to address other known causes of fetal death include improved prenatal diagnosis and treatments of maternal morbidities, such as hypertension and maternal-fetal infections, and efforts to reduce maternal cigarette smoking and the use of illegal drugs. Such improvements in access to and the quality of prenatal care may decrease fetal mortality.

Future needs for the improvement of fetal death surveillance include increased completeness of reporting, increased scope and accuracy of routinely reported data, and modified approaches to analysis. Whereas in the short-term, improved reporting may cause either a modest increase in fetal death rates or a leveling off of declines in these rates; in the long-term better reporting will support prevention efforts and could lead to a rate decline.

The 1989 revisions of the fetal death report and live birth certificate—which contain information on maternal smoking, drinking, and use of prenatal care—may help to assess how changes in these factors affect the rate of fetal death. In addition, wider use of early ultrasound for determination of gestational age as well as improved access to and earlier initiation of prenatal care may improve the accuracy of fetal gestational age data.

Currently, the etiologic heterogeneity and the lack of adequate cause-of-death information are substantial barriers in the identification of preventable risks. In fact, more rapid declines in fetal death rates may be possible if we promote and conduct effective research into the unknown causes and the primary prevention of malformations and low birth weight (26). Furthermore, the cause of death according to the timing of death (antepartum or intrapartum) must be further examined.

Therefore, we should focus on improving physicians' ascertainment of the initiating and contributing causes of fetal death. Improvements in the quality and availability of national reporting can help us to address the problems of unknown, inappropriately classified, and inconsistent cause reporting. Kirby recently raised these issues and proposed several ways to improve the data, challenging us to establish public health priorities supporting cause reporting that will improve our ability to monitor and prevent fetal deaths *(51)*. With such improvements, NCHS's plans to compile and soon make available national cause-specific data will help public health professionals and researchers better quantify the causes of and risks for fetal death and will allow better tracking of changing cause-specific trends. We also will be able to use appropriate cause-of-death classification schemes that provide meaningful information for public health decision making and better understanding of the initiating causes of such deaths. Knowing these causes will permit us to better target our intervention efforts.

From an analytic viewpoint, analyses of perinatal mortality data can overcome inconsistencies among demographic groups and across geographic areas in the classification of birth outcomes as fetal or infant deaths. Etiologically, the analysis of perinatal mortality data makes sense because late fetal and neonatal deaths share many of the same etiologies. To assess the effects of public health interventions, the analysis of perinatal mortality is preferable, because we would expect these interventions to reduce both fetal and neonatal deaths. To better understand and prevent fetal deaths that occur earlier in pregnancy, we need to conduct separate analyses of early fetal deaths to measure risks affecting fetal outcomes before the perinatal period, with better clinical risk and outcome markers.

Compared with the wide range of analyses conducted on live birth data, far fewer analyses have focused on fetal death data. The availability of more complete and accurate fetal mortality data and the combined analysis of fetal and neonatal mortality will help direct our future efforts to reduce adverse pregnancy outcomes.

REFERENCES

1. Public Health Service. International recommendations on definitions of live birth and fetal death. Washington, DC: US Department of Health, Education, and Welfare, 1950.

2. Kiely JL, Paneth N, Susser M. Fetal death during labor: an epidemiologic indicator of level of obstetric care. Am J Obstet Gynecol 1985;153:721–7.

3. McCormick MC. The contribution of low birth weight to infant mortality and childhood morbidity. N Engl J Med 1985;312:82–90.

4. Institute of Medicine. Preventing low birthweight. Washington, DC: National Academy Press, 1985.

5. Abramson FD. Spontaneous fetal death in man. Soc Biol 1973;20:375–403.

6. Greb AE, Pauli RM, Kirby RS. Accuracy of fetal death reports: comparison with data from an independent stillbirth assessment program. Am J Public Health 1987;77:1202–6.

7. Bureau of the Census. Vital statistics of the United States, 1937. Part I. Natality and mortality data for the United States tabulated by place of occurrence with supplemental tables for Hawaii, Puerto Rico, and the Virgin Islands. Washington, DC: US Government Printing Office, 1939.

8. Tolson GC, Barnes JM, Gay GA, Kowaleski JL. The 1989 revision of the U.S. standard certificates and reports. Hyattsville, Maryland: US Department of Health and Human Services, Public Health Service, CDC, NCHS, 1991. (Vital and health statistics; Series 4, no. 28.)

9. NCHS. Vital statistics of the United States, 1976. Vol. II. Mortality, part A. Hyattsville, Maryland: US Department of Health and Human Services, Public Health Service, 1980.

10. Public Health Service. Vital statistics of the United States, 1950. Vol. I. Analysis and summary tables with supplemental tables for Alaska, Hawaii, Puerto Rico, and Virgin Islands. Washington, DC: US Government Printing Office, 1954.

11. NCHS. Vital statistics of the United States, 1988. Vol. II. Mortality, part A. Hyattsville, Maryland: US Department of Health and Human Services, Public Health Service, CDC, 1991.

12. Freedman MA, Gay GA, Brokert JE, Potrzebowski PW, Rothwell CJ. The 1989 revisions of the US Standard Report of Fetal Death. Am J Public Health 1988;78:168–72.

13. Kleinman JC, Kiely JL. Infant mortality. Hyattsville, Maryland: US Department of Health and Human Services, Public Health Service, CDC, NCHS, 1991. (Healthy people 2000 statistical notes; vol. 1, no. 2.)

14. NCHS. Model state vital statistics act and model state vital statistics regulations. Hyattsville, Maryland: US Department of Health, Education, and Welfare, Public Health Service, 1978; DHEW publication no. (PHS)78-1115.

15. Shapiro S, Bross D. Risk factors for fetal death in studies of vital statistics data: inference and limitations. In: Porter IH, Hook EB, eds. Human embryonic and fetal death. New York: Academic Press, 1980:89–105.

16. NCHS. Guidelines for implementing field and query programs for registration of births and deaths, 1993. Hyattsville, Maryland: US Department of Health and Human Services, Public Health Service, CDC, 1993. (NCHS instruction manual; part 18.)

17. NCHS. Vital statistics of the United States, 1989. Vol. II. Mortality, part A. Washington, DC: US Department of Health and Human Services, Public Health Service, CDC, 1994 (in press).

18. NCHS. Catalog of electronic data products. Hyattsville, Maryland: US Department of Health and Human Services, Public Health Service, CDC, 1992; DHHS publication no. (PHS)92-1213.

19. Sanderson M, Placek PJ, Keppel KG. The 1988 National Maternal and Infant Health Survey: design, content, and data availability. BIRTH 1991;18; 1:26–31.

20. Lammer EJ, Brown LE, Anderka MT, Guyer B. Classification and analysis of fetal deaths in Massachusetts. JAMA 1989;261:1757–62.

21. Kiely JL, Paneth N. Susser M. An assessment of the effects of maternal age and parity in different components of perinatal mortality. Am J Epidemiol 1986;123:444–54.

22. Albers LL, Savitz DA. Hospital setting and fetal death during labor among women at low risk. Am J Obstet Gynecol 1991;164:868–73.

23. Cowles TA, Ryan RK, Bennett TL, Evans J, Finley BE. Stillbirth is not a cause of fetal death. Kans Med January 1992:22–8.

24. Fretts RC, Boyd ME, Usher RH, Usher HA. The changing pattern of fetal death, 1961–1988. Obstet Gynecol 1992;79:35–9.

25. Alessandri LM, Stanley FJ. A case-control study of intrapartum stillbirths. Br J Obstet Gynaecol 1992; 99:719–23.

26. Alessandri LM, Stanley FJ, Waddell VP, Newnham J. Stillbirths in Western Australia 1980–83: influence of race, residence and place of birth. Aust NZ J Obstet Gynaecol 1988;28:284–93.

27. Dommisse J. The causes of perinatal deaths in the Greater Cape Town area. Satr Med J 1991;80: 270–5.

28. Morrison I, Olsen J. Weight-specific stillbirths and associated causes of death: an analysis of 765 stillbirths. Am J Obstet Gynecol 1985;152:975–80.

29. Kalter H. Five-decade international trends in the relation of perinatal mortality and congenital malformations: stillbirth and neonatal death compared. Int J Epidemiol 1991;20:173–9.

30. Kiely JL, Paneth N, Susser MW. Preventability of fetal death during labor: epidemiologic studies and ongoing surveillance using New York City vital records. In: Proceedings of the 1985 Public Health Conference on Records and Statistics. Hyattsville, Maryland: US Department of Health and Human Services, Public Health Service, NCHS, 1985; DHHS publication no. (PHS)86-1214:201–3.

31. Little RE, Weinberg CR. Risk factors for antepartum and intrapartum stillbirth. Am J Epidemiol 1993; 137:1177–89.

32. Cnattinguis S, Haglund B, Meirik O. Cigarette smoking as risk factor for late fetal and early neonatal death. BMJ 1988;297:258–61.

33. Ferraz EM, Gray RH. A case-control study of stillbirths in Northeast Brazil. Int J Gynecol Obstet 1990;34:13–9.

34. Gaudino J, Blackmore C, Rochat R, Atrash H. Fetal death: a forgotten pregnancy loss. In: Meeting abstracts of the 121st annual meeting of the American Public Health Association, abstract 1021. Presented at the 121st annual meeting of the American Public Health Association, San Francisco, California, October 24–28, 1993.

35. Feldman GB. Prospective risk of stillbirth. Obstet Gynecol 1992;79:547–53.

36. Casterline, JB. Maternal age, gravidity, and pregnancy spacing effects on spontaneous fetal mortality. Soc Biol 1989;36:186–212.

37. Källén B. Epidemiology of human reproduction. Boca Raton, Florida: CRC Press, 1988.

38. Schulz KF, Schulte JM, Berman SM. Maternal health and child survival: opportunities to protect both women and children from the adverse consequences of reproductive tract infections. In: Reproductive tract infections: global impact and priorities for women's reproductive health. New York, New York: Plennum Press, 1992.

39. Robins LN, Mills VL, Krulewitch C, Herman AA. Effects of in utero exposure to street drugs. Am J Public Health 1993;83:Suppl,1–32.

40. American Academy of Pediatrics, American College of Obstetricians and Gynecologists. Standard terminology for reporting of reproductive health statistics in the United States. Public Health Rep 1988;103: 464–71.

41. Kleinman JC. Methodological issues in the analysis of vital statistics. In: Kiely M, ed. Reproductive and perinatal epidemiology. Boca Raton, Florida: CRC Press, 1991.

42. Hartford RB. Definitions, standards, data quality, and comparability. In: Proceedings of the international collaborative effort on perinatal and infant mortality, volume III. Hyattsville, Maryland: US Department of Health and Human Services, Public Health Service, CDC, NCHS, 1992.

43. Goldhaber MK. Fetal death ratios in a prospective study compared to state fetal death certificate reporting. Am J Public Health 1989;79:1268–70.

44. Harter L, Starzyk P, Frost F. A comparative study of hospital fetal death records and Washington State fetal death certificates. Am J Public Health 1986; 76:1333–4.

45. Kleinman JC. Underreporting of infant deaths: then and now [Editorial]. Am J Public Health 1986;76: 365–6.

46. Gaudino J, Blackmore C, Yip R, Rochat R. Quality assessment of Georgia fetal death records: evidence for room for improvement. Presented at the 120th annual meeting of the American Public Health Association, Washington, DC, November 8–12, 1992.

47. Alexander GR, Petersen DJ, Powell-Griner EP, Tompkins ME. A comparison of gestational age reporting methods based on physician estimate and date of last normal menses from fetal death reports. Am J Public Health 1989;79:600–2.

48. Travers H, Schmidt WA. College of American Pathologists Conference XIX on the Examination of the Placenta: introduction. Arch Pathol Lab Med 1991; 115:660–2.

49. Pitkin RM. Fetal death: diagnosis and management. Am J Obstet Gynecol 1987;157:583–9.

50. Yudkin PL, Wood L, Redman CWG. Risk of unexplained stillbirth at different gestational ages. Lancet 1987;8543:1192–4.

51. Kirby RS. The coding of underlying cause of death from fetal death certificates: issues and policy considerations. Am J Public Health 1993;83:1088–91.

52. Atkinson D. Improving cause-of-death statistics: the case of fetal deaths [Editorial]. Am J Public Health 1993;83:1084–5.

53. Golding J. Epidemiology of perinatal death. In: Kiely M, ed. Reproductive and perinatal epidemiology. Boca Raton, Florida: CRC Press, 1991.

54. French FE, Bierman JM. Probabilities of fetal mortality. Public Health Rep 1962;77:10:835–47.

55. Raymond E, Clemens JD. Prospective risk of stillbirth [Letter]. Obstet Gynecol 1992;80:473–4.

56. Kiely JL. Some conceptual problems in multivariable analyses of perinatal mortality. Paediat Perinat Epidemiol 1991;5:243–57.

57. Public Health Service. Healthy people 2000: national health promotion and disease prevention objectives—full report, with commentary. Washington, DC: US Department of Health and Human Services, Public Health Service, 1991; DHHS publication no. (PHS)91-50212.

58. Little J, Elwood JM. Epidemiology of neural tube defects. In: Kiely M, ed. Reproductive and perinatal epidemiology. Boca Raton, Florida: CRC Press, 1991.

59. Wigglesworth JS. Role of pathology in modern perinatal medicine. In: Textbook of fetal and perinatal pathology. Wigglesworth JS, Singer DB, eds. Boston: Blackwell Scientific Publications, 1991.

Preterm Birth

Cheryl A. Blackmore, Ph.D., M.P.H., M.S.N.,[1]
Diane L. Rowley, M.D., M.P.H.,[1] and John L. Kiely, Ph.D.[2]

PUBLIC HEALTH IMPORTANCE

Preterm delivery, the termination of pregnancy before completion of 37 weeks of gestation, is one of the predominant proximate causes of low birth weight and, together with low birth weight, is the third leading cause of infant mortality in the United States (1). According to CDC's National Center for Health Statistics (NCHS), 440,082 preterm births (10.8% of all live births with a known period of gestation) occurred in the United States in 1991 (1).

In addition to its causal relationship to increased rates of neonatal mortality, preterm delivery also is associated with increased neonatal morbidity. Other neonatal consequences of preterm delivery include necrotizing enterocolitis, hyaline membrane disease, severe respiratory distress syndrome, and intraventricular hemorrhage (2–4). Perinatal sepsis risks are also significantly higher among preterm infants than among term infants (5,6). For additional information about related topics and surveillance activities, see the Behavioral Risk Factors Before and During Pregnancy, Prenatal Care, Pregnancy-Related Nutrition, Low Birth Weight and Intrauterine Growth Retardation, Infant Mortality, and Neonatal and Postneonatal Mortality chapters.

HISTORY OF DATA COLLECTION

Through the National Vital Statistics System, managed by NCHS, CDC collects and publishes data on births in the United States (7). Preterm delivery primarily is determined by assessing length-of-gestation data collected on birth certificates, which each state provides to NCHS. Since 1933, NCHS has obtained information on births from the registration offices of all states, New York City, the District of Columbia, Puerto Rico, the U.S. Virgin Islands, and Guam (7). Additional national surveillance data on the estimated prevalence of preterm delivery in the United States have been provided by the National Natality Followback Surveys—conducted in 1963, 1964–1966, 1967–1969, 1972, and 1980—and the 1988 National Maternal and Infant Health Survey (NMIHS) (8,9). All of these surveys provide data for estimating the length of pregnancy, although the agreement between the birth certificate and the survey data on the prevalence of preterm vs. term delivery has been variable (10,11).

Over the past four decades, refinements in the birth certificate have helped to improve estimations of the length of pregnancy. In 1949, the Standard Certificate of Live Birth was revised to request the length of pregnancy in weeks, and in the 1956 revision, the certificate was refined to ask for "completed weeks of gestation" (12). In a 1972 publication (12), NCHS refined the World Health Organization's definition of prematurity by distinguishing a difference between preterm births and low-birth-weight births as follows: "Infants who are premature because of curtailed gestation (gestational age of <37 completed weeks) are designated 'preterm.'. . . Infants who are premature by virtue of birth weight (2,500 grams or less at birth) are designated 'low birth weight' infants."

[1] Division of Reproductive Health
National Center for Chronic Disease Prevention
　　and Health Promotion
Centers for Disease Control and Prevention
Atlanta, Georgia

[2] Office of Analysis, Epidemiology and Health Promotion
National Center for Health Statistics
Centers for Disease Control and Prevention
Hyattsville, Maryland

CDC SURVEILLANCE ACTIVITIES

The registration of births is a local and state function, but uniform registration practices and use of the records for national statistics have been established over the years through co-operative agreements between the states and NCHS *(13)*. The civil laws of every state provide for a continuous and permanent birth registration system. In general, the local registrar of a town, city, county, or other geographic location collects the records of births occurring in the area; inspects, queries, and corrects these records, if necessary; maintains a local copy, register, or index; and transmits the records to the state health department. There the vital statistics office inspects the records for promptness of filing and for completeness and consistency of information; queries the data, if necessary; numbers, indexes, and processes the statistical information for state and local use; and binds the records for permanent reference and safe-keeping. Microfilm copies of the individual records or machine-readable data are transmitted to NCHS for use in compiling the final annual national vital statistics volume *(13)*.

The surveillance of preterm births depends on 100% registration of births from all states and the District of Columbia. The data are provided to NCHS through the Vital Statistics Cooperative Program. The length of gestation is measured from the first day of the mother's last normal menstrual period (LMP) to the date of birth. The LMP is used as the initial date because it can be more accurately determined than the date of conception, which usually occurs 2 weeks after the LMP. When the length of gestation as computed from the LMP is inconsistent with the reported birth weight or is incompletely reported, the **clinical estimate of gestation**—an item added to the 1989 revision of the birth certificate—is used *(1)*.

The period of gestation is often reported in terms of weeks or months of pregnancy. When months are reported, they are converted to gestation intervals in weeks as follows *(14)*:

- ≤3 months to "not stated."

- 4 months to 17 weeks.

- 5 months to 22 weeks.

- 6 months to 26 weeks.

- 7 months to 30 weeks.

- 8 months to 35 weeks.

- 9 months to 40 weeks.

- 10 months to 44 weeks.

Births occurring before 37 weeks of gestation are considered **preterm** for purposes of classification. At 37–41 weeks of gestation, births are considered **term**, and at ≥42 weeks, they are considered **postterm**. These distinctions are according to the *International Classification of Diseases, Ninth Revision* definitions *(15)*.

Before 1981, NCHS only computed the period of gestation when a valid month, day, and year of LMP were reported on the birth certificate. However, length of gestation could not be determined from a substantial number of live birth certificates each year because the day of LMP was missing. From 1968–1978, 12.0%–16.4% of records reported to NCHS by states had day only missing from the LMP date *(16)*. Therefore, in 1981, NCHS began imputing weeks of gestation for records missing the day of LMP when a valid month and year were provided. Each such record is assigned the gestational period in weeks of the preceding record that has a complete LMP date with the same computed months of gestation and the same 500 g birth-weight interval. The effect of the imputation procedure is to increase slightly the proportion of preterm births and to lower the proportion of births at 39, 40, 41, and 42 weeks of gestation *(15,16)*.

Because of postconception bleeding or menstrual irregularities, the presumed date of LMP may be in error. In these instances, the computed gestational period may be longer or shorter than the true gestational period, but the extent of such errors is unknown *(15,16)*.

GENERAL FINDINGS

The preterm delivery rate has been increasing gradually from 9.4% of live births in 1981 to

10.8% in 1991. Of the 438,905 preterm births with stated weights reported by NCHS in 1991, 180,218 (41.1%) of the infants were also classified as low birth weight because they weighed <2,500 g. Risk factors for preterm delivery include low socioeconomic status, low prepregnancy weight, inadequate weight gain during the pregnancy, previous preterm delivery, a history of infertility problems, vaginal spotting or light bleeding during pregnancy, antepartum hemorrhage and abnormal placental implantation, alcohol consumption before the third trimester of pregnancy, negative attitude about the pregnancy, smoking, multiple gestation, cervical factors, myometrial factors, problems with the fetal membranes, and decreased uteroplacental blood flow (17–21).

For more than a decade, black women have experienced twice the risk of preterm delivery as white women. In 1991, 18.9% of black infants compared with 9.1% of white infants were born before completing 37 weeks of gestation (1). The reasons for this disparity are largely unexplained (22–25). To further understand why black women are disproportionately represented among all women who experience a preterm birth, Lieberman and colleagues evaluated economic, demographic, and behavioral predictors of preterm delivery among a hospital-based cohort of black women in Massachusetts (24). The presence of any one of the following conditions significantly increased black women's risk of a preterm birth: being <20 years of age, being single, receiving welfare, and not having graduated from high school. These socioeconomic differences accounted for a major portion (77%) of the discrepancy in risks of preterm delivery between blacks and whites, but they did not explain the total gap or suggest proximate interventions to reduce this racial disparity (24).

INTERPRETATION ISSUES

Preterm delivery rates are somewhat imprecise because of the difficulty in ascertaining gestational age with certainty. Thus, the actual incidence of preterm delivery is difficult to estimate. In a recent review, Savitz et al. report the incidence of preterm births as varying from 4.4% to 21.5%, depending on the population studied and the criterion used to define prematurity (26). Whereas multiple gestation has been associated with preterm delivery, many studies focus on singleton preterm births, which results in a slight underestimation of the true number of preterm births. The wide range in risks is partially accounted for by a tendency to equate prematurity with low birth weight.

A few analyses have been conducted at the state level to assess the quality of birth certificate data specifically for the accuracy of reported gestational ages. In a 1980 study of North Carolina vital records, David found that targeting the 10 hospitals reporting the most inaccuracies and incomplete records might decrease the missing data by almost 50% (27). This intervention would improve the state's ability to accurately estimate rates of neonatal mortality, intrauterine growth retardation, and other adverse perinatal outcomes. More recently, several investigators compared data from Tennessee birth certificates with data from delivery hospital medical records as part of a case control study (28). They found that gestational age concordance ranged from 41.6% to 84.8% depending on whether exact agreement or agreement within 2 weeks was sought. Moreover, when the Kessner Index of prenatal care was applied to this population, the investigators found that birth certificate data overestimated the adequacy of prenatal care when compared with the medical records data. These findings could have implications during evaluations of the adequacy of health-care delivery systems for pregnant women in a state.

EXAMPLES OF USING DATA

Several investigators have observed a disproportionately increased risk of preterm delivery for black women at the shortest gestations (25,29,30). Others have noted that preterm delivery is associated with the highest mortality rates among infants weighing <1,500 g (31). Few states have conducted the surveillance of birth certificate data to address local issues relevant to preterm delivery. Most analyses have been at the national level. Nevertheless, monitoring these rates locally while implementing intervention strategies could allow for the early recognition of improvements in the health status of women and their infants.

FUTURE ISSUES

Several of the year 2000 objectives for improving maternal and infant health will depend on decreasing the rate of preterm births. Thus, using vital records data to examine preterm delivery rates is an important approach to developing appropriate prevention strategies. Reducing the infant mortality rate to no more than 7 per 1,000 live births, the incidence of low birth weight to no more than 5% of live births, and the incidence of very low birth weight to no more than 1% of live births will require a marked reduction in the prevalence of preterm delivery (32). Moreover, separating the prevalence of preterm delivery from the prevalence of intrauterine growth retardation is an important distinction to make when planning effective interventions.

To further understand what risk factors may predispose women to experience preterm births, we must investigate the heterogeneity of preterm delivery. Preterm delivery is an adverse reproductive outcome initiated primarily by one of three situations: idiopathic preterm labor, preterm premature rupture of membranes, or intentional medical/surgical intervention. Hence, treating three different processes as if they were a single entity may not be appropriate.

Despite the diversity in the initial circumstances that can lead to preterm birth, epidemiologic studies of preterm delivery rarely differentiate among the etiologic pathways. When studies that do examine the etiology of preterm delivery are examined, marked differences are found from study to study in the frequency of each etiologic pathway. However, geographic locations of the studies, periods of data collection, and racial and socioeconomic distributions of the populations also differ from study to study (26).

To begin understanding which risk factors are most amenable for intervention, basic information is needed on the descriptive epidemiology of preterm delivery. With minimal data

quantifying the frequency of either idiopathic preterm labor or preterm premature rupture of membranes, it is difficult to estimate the effectiveness of strategies aimed at either condition. If a particular exposure is a risk factor for only one etiologic pathway for preterm delivery, it may not be identified in studies that aggregate preterm birth as a single, homogenous, adverse reproductive outcome (26). Given the differences in the risks of preterm birth between black and white women, examining preterm delivery by its heterogeneous components may shed light on the reasons for this racial disparity.

REFERENCES

1. National Center for Health Statistics. Advance report of final natality statistics, 1991. Hyattsville, Maryland: US Department of Health and Human Services, Public Health Service, CDC, 1993. (Monthly vital statistics report; vol. 42, no. 3, suppl.)

2. Arias F, Tomich P. Etiology and outcome of low birth weight and preterm infants. Obstet Gynecol 1982; 60:277–81.

3. Daikoku NH, Kaltreider F, Johnson TRB Jr, Johnson JWC, Simmons MA. Premature rupture of membranes and preterm labor: neonatal infection and perinatal mortality risks. Obstet Gynecol 1981;58: 417–25.

4. Johnson JWC, Daikoku NH, Niebyl JR, Johnson TRB Jr, Khouzami VA, Witter FR. Premature rupture of the membranes and prolonged latency. Obstet Gynecol 1981;57:547–56.

5. Buetow KC, Klein SW, Lane RB. Septicemia in premature infants. Am J Dis Child 1965;110:29–41.

6. Klein JO, Marcy SM. Bacterial sepsis and meningitis. In: Remington JS, Klein JO, eds. Infectious diseases of the fetus and newborn infant. Philadelphia: W.B. Saunders Company, 1990:601–56.

7. Kovar MG. Data systems of the National Center for Health Statistics. Hyattsville, Maryland: US Department of Health and Human Services, Public Health Service, CDC, NCHS, 1989; DHHS publication no. (PHS)89-1325. (Vital and health statistics; series 1, no. 23.)

8. Schoendorf KC, Parker JD, Batkhan LZ, Kiely JL. Comparability of the birth certificate and 1988 Maternal and Infant Health Survey. Hyattsville, Maryland: US Department of Health and Human Services, Public Health Service, CDC, NCHS, 1993; DHHS publication no. (PHS)93-1390. (Vital and health statistics; series 2, no. 116.)

9. Sanderson M, Placek PJ, Keppel KG. The 1988 National Maternal and Infant Health Survey: design, content, and data availability. BIRTH 1991;18: 26–32.

182

10. Fingerhut LA, Kleinman JC. Comparability of reporting between the birth certificate and the 1980 National Natality Survey. Hyattsville, Maryland: US Department of Health and Human Services, Public Health Service, NCHS, 1985; DHHS publication no. (PHS)86-1373. (Vital and health statistics; series 2, no. 99.)

11. Querec LJ. Comparability of reporting between the birth certificate and the National Natality Survey. Hyattsville, Maryland: US Department of Health, Education, and Welfare, Public Health Service, NCHS, 1980: DHEW publication no. (PHS)80-1357. (Vital and health statistics; series 2, no. 83.)

12. Chase HC, Byrnes ME. Trends in "prematurity": United States: 1950–67. Rockville, Maryland: US Department of Health, Education, and Welfare, Public Health Service, Health Services and Mental Health Administration, NCHS, 1972; DHEW publication no. (HSM)72-1030. (Vital and health statistics; series 3, no. 15.)

13. Pearce ND. Data systems of the National Center for Health Statistics. Hyattsville, Maryland: US Department of Health and Human Services, Public Health Service, Office of Health Research, Statistics, and Technology, NCHS, 1981; DHHS publication no. (PHS)82-1318. (Vital and health statistics; series 1, no. 16.)

14. Instruction Manual, Part 3a—Classification and Coding Instructions for Live Birth Records, 1993. Section V—Data Classification and Machine Entry, p. 28. Hyattsville, Maryland: US Department of Health and Human Services, Public Health Service, CDC, NCHS, 1993.

15. NCHS. Vital statistics of the United States, 1988. Vol. I, natality, Hyattsville, Maryland: US Department of Health and Human Services, Public Health Service, CDC, NCHS, 1990.

16. Taffel S, Johnson D, Heuser R. A method of imputing length of gestation on birth certificates. Hyattsville, Maryland: US Department of Health and Human Services, Public Health Service, Office of Health Research, Statistics, and Technology, NCHS, 1982; DHHS publication no. (PHS)82-1367. (Vital and health statistics; series 2, no. 93.)

17. Berkowitz GS. An epidemiologic study of preterm delivery. Am J Epidemiol 1981;113:81–92.

18. Harger JH, Hsing AW, Tuomala RE, et al. Risk factors for preterm premature rupture of fetal membranes: a multicenter case-control study. Am J Obstet Gynecol 1990;163:130–7.

19. Williams MA, Mittendorf R, Stubblefield PG, Lieberman E, Schoenbaum SC, Monson RR. Cigarettes, coffee, and preterm premature rupture of the membranes. Am J Epidemiol 1992;135:895–903.

20. Gazaway P, Mullins CL. Prevention of preterm labor and premature rupture of the membranes. Clin Obstet Gynecol 1986;29:835–49.

21. Naeye RL. Pregnancy hypertension, placental evidences of low uteroplacental blood flow, and spontaneous premature delivery. Hum Pathol 1989;20:441–4.

22. Behrman RE. Premature births among black women [Editorial]. N Engl J Med 1987;317:763–5.

23. Hogue CJR, Yip R. Preterm delivery: can we lower the black infant's first hurdle? JAMA 1989;262:548–50.

24. Lieberman E, Ryan KJ, Monson RR, Schoenbaum SC. Risk factors accounting for racial differences in the rate of premature birth. N Engl J Med 1987;317:743–8.

25. Shiono PH, Klebanoff MA. Ethnic differences in preterm and very preterm delivery. Am J Public Health 1986;76:1317–21.

26. Savitz DA, Blackmore CA, Thorp JM. Epidemiologic characteristics of preterm delivery: etiologic heterogeneity. Am J Obstet Gynecol 1991;164:467–71.

27. David RJ. The quality and completeness of birth weight and gestational age data in computerized birth files. Am J Public Health 1980;70:964–73.

28. Piper JM, Mitchel EF Jr, Snowden M, Hall C, Adams M, Taylor P. Validation of 1989 Tennessee birth certificates using maternal and newborn hospital records. Am J Epidemiol 1993;137:758–68.

29. Adams MM, Read JA, Rawlings JS, Harlass FB, Sarno AP, Rhodes PH. Preterm delivery among black and white enlisted women in the United States Army. Obstet Gynecol 1993;81:65–71.

30. Blackmore CA, Savitz DA, Edwards L, Harlow S, Bowes W. Racial differences in the rates of idiopathic preterm labor, preterm rupture of membranes, and medically indicated preterm delivery in central North Carolina. Am J Epidemiol 1992;136:980.

31. Iyasu S, Becerra JE, Rowley DL, Hogue CJR. Impact of very low birth weight on the black-white infant mortality gap. Am J Prev Med 1992;8:271–7.

32. Public Health Service. Healthy people 2000: national health promotion and disease prevention objectives—full report, with commentary. Washington, DC: US Department of Health and Human Services, Public Health Service, 1991; DHHS publication no. (PHS) 91-50212.

Low Birth Weight and Intrauterine Growth Retardation

John L. Kiely, Ph.D.,[1] Kate M. Brett, Ph.D.,[1]
Stella Yu, Sc.D., M.P.H., R.D.,[2] and
Diane L. Rowley, M.D., M.P.H.[3]

PUBLIC HEALTH IMPORTANCE

Low birth weight (LBW) is defined as a birth weight of <2,500 g (5 lb, 8 oz). LBW is of public health importance because of the strong relationship between birth weight and infant mortality and morbidity. Studies using linked birth/infant death files have reported that infants weighing <2,500 g at birth are at a considerably increased risk of neonatal mortality. Neonatal death is 40 times more likely among LBW infants and 200 times greater among very-low-birth-weight infants (infants weighing <1,500 g at birth) than it is among infants of normal birth weight. The 7% of U.S. infants born weighing <2,500 g account for two thirds of the nation's neonatal deaths.

Infant and childhood morbidity are also associated with low birth weight. LBW infants are at an increased risk of neurological problems such as cerebral palsy and seizure disorders, severe mental retardation, lower respiratory tract conditions, and general morbidity.

Reducing the prevalence of LBW deliveries in the United States has been difficult. The proportion of LBW infants has remained fairly constant over the past 30 years. The reported prevalence of LBW infants born in the United States was 7.5% of live births in 1950 and 7.0% in 1990. In 1990, the prevalence of LBW deliveries was more than twice as high among black women (13.3%) as it was among white women (5.7%). This difference in LBW deliveries between black and white women also has been fairly consistent over time.

The best available global estimates of the prevalence of low birth weight produced were by the World Health Organization (WHO) in the 1980s (1,2). The highest rates were reported for Asia, with LBW rates ranging from 30% to 40% in the Indian subcontinent to 5% to 6% in China and Japan. In West Africa, the LBW rates were 10%–20%, whereas in North Africa the rates were 5%–15%. The ranges of LBW rates were 10%–18% in Central America and 9%–12% in South America. The lowest LBW rates were reported for North America and Europe, with rates in the range of 4%–8%. In developing countries, most LBW is related to intrauterine growth retardation (IUGR), whereas in developed countries most LBW is related to preterm birth (3,4). (See the History of Data Collection section for definitions of IUGR and preterm birth; for additional information about related topics and surveillance activities, see the Behavioral Risk Factors Before and During Pregnancy, Prenatal Care, Pregnancy-Related Nutrition, Preterm Birth, Infant Mortality, and Fetal Alcohol Syndrome chapters.)

HISTORY OF DATA COLLECTION

The definition of LBW as infants weighing <2,500 g was originally chosen by Arvo Ylppö in 1919

---

[1] Division of Health and Utilization Analysis
National Center for Health Statistics
Centers for Disease Control and Prevention
Hyattsville, Maryland

[2] Division of Vital Statistics
National Center for Health Statistics
Centers for Disease Control and Prevention
Hyattsville, Maryland

[3] Division of Reproductive Health
National Center for Chronic Disease Prevention
   and Health Promotion
Centers for Disease Control and Prevention
Atlanta, Georgia

(5) as a means to differentiate preterm infants from term infants. Hence, LBW was a surrogate measure for short gestational age. The blur between birth weight, gestational age, immaturity, and prematurity continued well into the second half of this century.

Today, obstetricians and pediatricians accept without question the concept that birth weight is determined by both gestational age at delivery and fetal growth rate. In a perusal of research reports published between the 1920s and the 1970s, however, one is struck by the common use of **prematurity** as an entity defined by birth weight alone. In most historical accounts, this practice originated with Ylppö's proposal that prematurity be defined by a birth weight of ≤2,500 g *(5)* and became entrenched in 1950, when the WHO published its official recommendation *(6)*. A major advance in the measurement of prematurity occurred when researchers and clinicians began to appreciate that birth weight and gestation are far from perfectly correlated and that both pieces of data are useful in assessing newborn prognosis. This was first demonstrated in the 1940s by McKeown and associates in an epidemiologic study of perinatal mortality in Birmingham, England *(7)*, in which they used the interval from the date of the last menstrual period to the date of delivery as their measure of gestation. The use of these data was in itself an advance, because in the preultrasound era, gestation based on the date of the last menstrual period proved to have greater biological validity than gestation based on a physician's estimates.

In the 1950s and 1960s, epidemiologists and perinatal clinicians began to recognize that LBW babies consist of two major groups—preterm infants and intrauterine growth retarded infants. Preterm infants are those born at <37 weeks of gestation. IUGR has been more difficult to define. Obstetric and pediatric clinicians have preferred to use the 10th percentile of birth weight for gestational age as the criterion for IUGR *(8,9)*. The need for IUGR standards based on percentiles of birth weight for gestation has led to the use of state birth certificate files. Vital data from both California *(10)* and North Carolina *(11)* have been used to construct percentiles of birth weight within each week of gestation. Indeed, the Cali-

fornia IUGR standards are still used in both clinical practice and epidemiologic research *(9,12)*.

In a simpler definition, intrauterine growth retarded infants are considered those who are gestationally full-term (≥37 weeks) but of a low birth weight (<2,500 g) *(13–17)* (Figure 1). When an investigator does not have birth weight-for-gestation percentiles for a population similar to the one being studied, this definition of IUGR is quite useful. Studies that distinguish between preterm and full-term LBW infants may provide us with new clues about how to prevent different types of low birth weight.

CDC SURVEILLANCE ACTIVITIES

Data on birth weight are collected on birth certificates filed in each of the states through their vital registration systems. Although vital registration is a state activity, CDC's National Center for Health Statistics (NCHS), promotes uniformity in the data collected through recommended standard certificates. These standard certificates are developed in cooperation with state vital statistics offices as well as providers and users of the information. They are revised about every 10 years. In 1949, birth weight was added to the U.S. Standard Certificate of Live Birth.

State data are provided on computer tape to NCHS, which compiles the information into national data and disseminates it annually. The primary vehicles for dissemination are 1) the *Advance Report of Final Natality Statistics (18)*, which contains summary tabulations; 2) *Vital Statistics of the United States, Volume I, Natality (19)*, which contains detailed tabulations; 3) public-use computer tapes; and 4) periodic analytic reports. Generally, the computerized national natality files are available within 18–24 months of the end of the data year. State-level data are available from all of these files. With only a few exceptions, all characteristics are shown by state in the published annual natality volumes, *Vital Statistics of the United States, Volume I, Natality.*

Investigations of IUGR require data on both birth weight and gestational age. (For details about birth certificate data on gestational age, *see* the Preterm Birth chapter.)

FIGURE 1. Suggested classification scheme for birth weight and gestational age — CDC, 1994

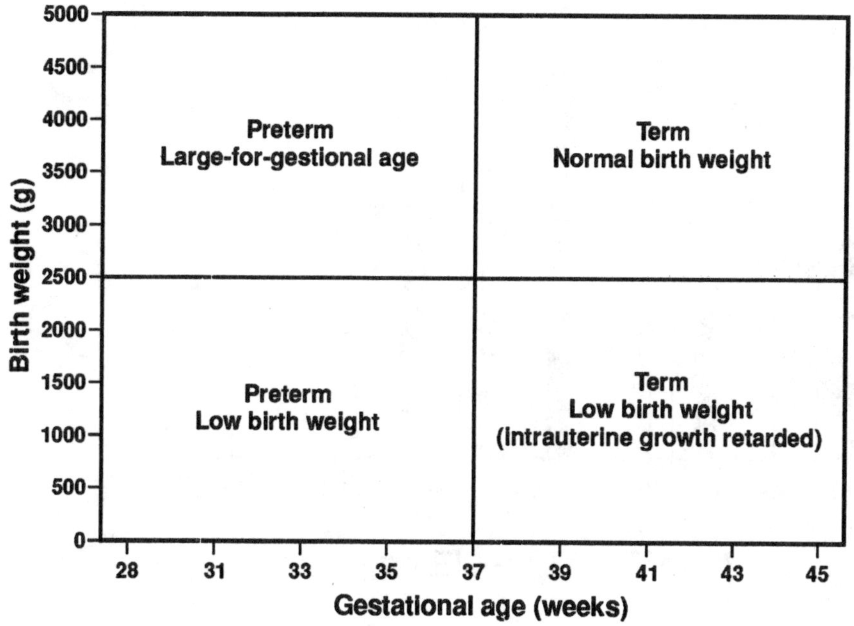

GENERAL FINDINGS

Time Trends

In the United States, the low-birth-weight rate (the proportion of live-born infants* weighing <2,500 g) has changed little in the last few decades (Figure 2). The low-birth-weight rate for the United States was 7.93% in 1970 and 6.75% in 1985—a decline of 15%. The rate then rose slightly to 6.97% in 1990. Among infants of black women, the rate was 13.90% in 1970 and 12.65% in 1985—a decline of 9%. The rate then rose to 13.25% in 1990. Among infants of Native Americans and Alaska Natives, we observed a striking decrease in low birth weight between 1970 and 1975, when the rate declined by 20%, from 7.97% to 6.41%. The rate continued to

decline, although at a much slower pace, and reached a nadir of 5.86% in 1985. The rate then increased slightly to 6.11% in 1990. Among infants of Hispanics, the low-birth-weight rate remained quite stable between 1980 and 1990. (In 1970 and 1975, national natality files did not include information on Hispanic origin.)

The proportion of live-born infants weighing <1,500 g (categorized as "very-low-birth-weight infants") for the United States increased from 1.17% to 1.27% between 1970 and 1990 (Figure 3). This increase was owed entirely to the 22% rise in very-low-birth-weight births among black women. Among infants of black women, the very-low-birth-weight rate increased from 2.40% in 1970 to 2.92% in 1990. For infants of white, Native American or Alaska Native, and Hispanic women, the very-low-birth-weight rate has remained fairly stable.

Major Risk Factors

Numerous researchers have studied the possible determinants of LBW. Many of these studies lacked methodologic soundness, or the investigators did not control for other risk factors in their analyses. However, for any one factor, at least a

---

* A live birth is "the complete expulsion or extraction from the mother of a product of human conception, irrespective of the duration of pregnancy, which after expulsion or extraction, breathes or shows any other evidence of life, such as beating of the heart, pulsation of the umbilical cord, or definite movement of voluntary muscles, whether or not the umbilical cord has been cut or the placenta is attached. Heartbeats are to be distinguished from transient cardiac contractions; respirations are to be distinguished from fleeting respiratory efforts or gasps" (20).

187

FIGURE 2. Time trends in low birth weight (<2,500 g), by race/ethnicity* — United States, 1970–1990

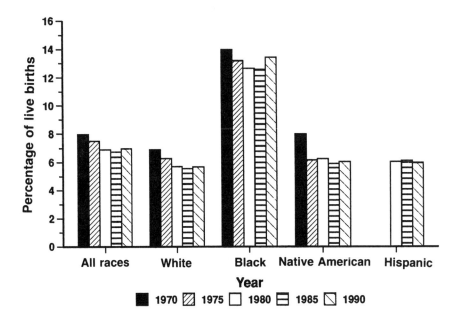

* Separate data on Hispanic births were not available for 1970 or 1975.

Source: NCHS national natality files.

FIGURE 3. Time trends in very low birth weight (<1,500 g), by race/ethnicity* — United States, 1970–1990

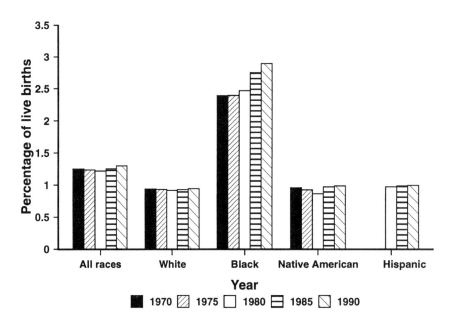

* Separate data on Hispanic births were not available for 1970 or 1975.

Source: NCHS national natality files.

few good studies provide data that can be used to make generalizations.

Several review articles and books on the etiology of LBW exist *(21–25)*. Our discussion here will be limited to the most important risk factors for which some consensus exists regarding probable causal influence (Table 1) *(22,23)*. Some of these factors are more specifically related to preterm delivery and others are related more to IUGR.

Demographic Risk Factors

MATERNAL AGE

Females <17 years of age and women >34 years of age are at an increased risk of LBW delivery *(22,26,27)*. A great deal of debate has focused on whether increased maternal age is an independent risk factor or only acts as a risk factor in the presence of other factors *(27)*. With regard to

---

TABLE 1. Principal maternal risk factors associated with delivering low-birth-weight infants *(22,23)*

Demographic risks

Mother's age of ≤16 or ≥35 years

Black race

Low socioeconomic status

Unmarried

Low level of education

Medical risks predating pregnancy

Parity of 0 or ≥5

Low weight-for-height

Genitourinary anomalies/surgery

Selected diseases such as diabetes or chronic hypertension

Nonimmune status for selected infections such as rubella

Poor obstetric history, including:
    Previous intrauterine growth retarded infants
    Previous preterm deliveries
    Multiple spontaneous abortions

Maternal genetic factors such as low weight at their own births

Medical risks in current pregnancy

Multiple pregnancy

Poor weight gain

Short interpregnancy interval

Hypotension

Hypertension/preeclampsia/toxemia

Selected infections such as symptomatic bacteriuria, rubella, and cytomegalovirus

Bleeding in the first or second trimester

Placental problems such as placenta previa or abruptio placentae

Hyperemesis

Oligohydramnios/polyhydramnios

TABLE 1. Principal maternal risk factors associated with delivering low-birth-weight infants *(22,23)* — continued

Anemia/abnormal hemoglobin

Isoimmunization

Fetal anomalies

Incompetent cervix

Spontaneous rupture of membranes

Behavioral and environmental risks

Smoking

Poor nutritional status

Heavy alcohol consumption

Illicit drug use

Diethylstilbestrol (DES) exposure and other toxic exposures, including occupational hazards

High altitude

Health-care risks

Absent or inadequate prenatal care

Iatrogenic prematurity

adolescent childbearing, we must remember that adolescent mothers come disproportionately from disadvantaged and minority populations. Therefore, the relationship between adolescent pregnancy and LBW may be confounded by poverty and other social factors *(28)*.

RACE AND ETHNICITY

Almost all studies of LBW's association with race and ethnicity have found that black women have about twice the risk of LBW delivery as whites *(17,21–25,29–31)*. The racial gap in very-low-birth-weight rates is even wider, with a risk about three times higher among blacks than among whites *(31,32)*. The relationship between black race and LBW has been found even when potential socioeconomic and behavioral mediators such as income, education, and harmful habits are controlled. The adjusted relative risk of IUGR in blacks is 1.39, according to the results of a metaanalysis of numerous well-executed studies *(24)*. Some researchers have questioned whether the criterion for LBW should be differ-

ent for blacks and whites *(33)*. Because blacks may be exposed to many social risks that have not been well described, creating separate standards has not been generally acceptable *(21,25)*.

LBW rates among Mexican-Americans, Asians, and Native Americans are not much higher than rates among non-Hispanic whites *(31,34,35)*. LBW rates among Puerto Ricans, on the other hand, are about 60% higher than rates among non-Hispanic whites *(31,36)*. The intrauterine growth patterns of Chinese infants have been the special focus of two studies that can serve as models for readers interested in using natality files to investigate intrauterine growth patterns *(37,38)*.

MARITAL STATUS

About twice as many infants born to single mothers weigh <2,500 g at birth than infants of married mothers *(22)*. However, in some studies in which race, maternal age, and socioeconomic status have been held constant, birth weight was not significantly different between the infants of married and unmarried women (39,40). Therefore, some controversy exists as to whether this variable is an independent risk factor.

SOCIOECONOMIC STATUS

Socioeconomic status (SES) incorporates three major avenues by which an individual can obtain societal position: class, status, and political power. SES is usually measured as some combination of education, income, and occupation because these three variables add unique information about a person's status (41). British studies have consistently found an association between their social class scale and birth weight (42), but these findings may not be directly applicable to the U.S. population. The most readily available marker of SES in most U.S. perinatal data sets, including birth certificate files, is maternal educational level. In the 1980 National Natality Survey, maternal education was associated with LBW delivery even after investigators controlled for smoking and other demographic risk factors (43). In most studies, the influence of SES on LBW is not explained by other factors. Therefore, the general consensus in the literature is that low SES is an independent risk factor for LBW delivery.

Parker et al. recently compared associations between five indicators of socioeconomic status (maternal education, paternal education, maternal occupation, paternal occupation, and family income) and LBW among women in the 1988 National Maternal and Infant Health Survey. Nearly all socioeconomic indicators were associated with LBW among both black and white women. Maternal and paternal education were the best overall predictors (44).

Toxic Exposure Risk

CIGARETTE SMOKING

Cigarette smoking has been well established as a risk factor for LBW and IUGR (22–24,43,45). A dose-response curve has been established in some of the larger, more accurate studies. The relative risk for LBW among smokers compared with nonsmokers has been estimated to be about 2.42 (24). The Institute of Medicine considered cigarette use to be the clearest risk factor for LBW delivery (22,23).

ALCOHOL CONSUMPTION

Strong evidence suggests that heavy use of alcohol can lead to IUGR (24). IUGR has been reported to be associated with heavy drinking, even in the absence of signs of fetal alcohol syndrome (see the chapter on Fetal Alcohol Syndrome).

ILLICIT DRUG USE

We have little evidence that marijuana use is associated with LBW. The association between cocaine use and LBW appears to be strong, however (46,47). In maternity patients in urban hospitals, a history of using several drugs during pregnancy is not uncommon, and this is probably related to LBW.

Pregnancy Risk Factors

MATERNAL HEIGHT AND WEIGHT

Maternal height, prepregnancy weight, and weight-for-height are all closely connected. All three factors have been found to be associated with birth weight (43,48).

REPRODUCTIVE HISTORY

The relationship between reproductive history and LBW is clearly established. Primiparous women have a 23% greater risk of IUGR than multiparous women, according to data from four studies of 142,259 births (24). The risk of delivering an infant with IUGR is 2.75 times greater for women with one or more previous LBW infants than for women with no history of LBW deliveries (24).

WEIGHT GAIN DURING PREGNANCY

Pregnancy weight gain is a variable incorporating the laying down of fat stores, growth of breast and uterine tissues, increased plasma volume, growth of the fetus and placenta, and amniotic fluid. Several studies have found correlations between poor weight gain and LBW, especially in adolescent pregnancies (49–51).

191

PRENATAL CARE

A great deal of evidence suggests an association between reduced incidence of LBW and prenatal care, especially first-trimester prenatal care that continues at regular intervals until delivery (52). Computerized birth certificate files contain information on both the timing of the first prenatal care visit and the number of visits. Thus, studies of the relationship of prenatal care to LBW can easily be conducted by using state vital statistics files.

Medical Risks

Hypertension of all types is the one medical factor most strongly associated with IUGR. According to the review by the Institute of Medicine (22), the relative risk for IUGR among women with preexisting high systolic blood pressure ranges from 1.9 to 4.2. The relative risk for IUGR among women with preeclampsia ranges from 6.2 to 40.4.

Severe anemia also appears to increase the risk of low birth weight, as do hyperemesis, isoimmunization, and fetal anomalies (22). The frequency of IUGR in infants with congenital malformations is almost three times higher than in nonmalformed infants (53).

INTERPRETATION ISSUES

User-Friendly Perinatal Databases

The NCHS and most states use computer-based systems for birth certificate files, with records listed by date of filing on a mainframe computer-based magnetic tape. Accessing birth certificate files is often difficult, slow, and cumbersome. Therefore, analysts sometimes feel discouraged before they begin. However, with the advent of modern computer technology, especially the microcomputer or personal computer, analysis of natality data no longer needs to be such a cumbersome process. For example, Wartenberg et al. (54) have described their construction of a user-friendly microcomputer-based database of all 735,000 singleton births in Massachusetts during 1975–1984. They point out, "implementing similar systems for state registries on births . . .

potentially offers investigators easy access to vast stores of information and would enable public health officials to produce timely reports [and] initiate a variety of surveillance activities" (54). Another user-friendly data system, designed for the analysis of perinatal outcomes in California, has been described by Gould et al. (55).

One approach that can ease the statistical analysis of natality files is to use a **synthetic** case-control design (56) that allows the analysis of a data set consisting of all LBW infants (cases) and a sample (say, 10%) of normal-birth-weight infants (controls). This design was used in a recent birth certificate study of the association between waterborne chloroform and IUGR in Iowa (12).

Maternal Recall of Child's Birth Weight

When evaluating prenatal health-care programs, collecting data on birth weight by interviewing the mother often is easier than using a computer to link program records with birth certificates. The question arises: when birth weight information is obtained by maternal recall, are these data valid? The results of a recent CDC study, conducted in collaboration with the Tennessee Department of Health and Environment, sheds light on this question (57). When comparing birth weights reported by mothers in the Tennessee Special Supplemental Food Program for Women, Infants, and Children (WIC) with birth weights recorded on the corresponding Tennessee birth certificate file, the investigators found that only 1.1% of birth weights reported by mothers would have been incorrectly classified into low- or normal-birth-weight categories. These results suggest that maternally reported birth weights are sufficiently accurate for research and programmatic purposes when birth certificate information is not readily available.

Measuring Intrauterine Growth Retardation

In our discussion of IUGR standards, we mentioned the construction of birth-weight-for-gestation percentiles from computerized birth certificate data (10,11). Three issues should be considered by anyone contemplating the development or use of such IUGR standards. First, in vital statistics data based on the data of the last menstrual period, a substantial number of births reported at gestations of <37 weeks have gestational ages that are off by 4–20 weeks (10,11). We must develop a procedure to eliminate these erroneous birth records when developing birth-weight-for-gestation percentiles (10,11). Second, in the development of IUGR standards, we must use as recent data as possible because birth-weight distributions in the United States have shifted upward in the last 25 years. Third, when using percentiles of birth-weight-for-gestation in studies of risk factors for IUGR or in evaluations of the effect of public health interventions on the incidence of IUGR, we should use percentiles that were derived from a population of infants similar to the population being studied (8,58). For example, the California standards (10) might not be useful in a study of IUGR among infants in Washington, D.C.

When measurements of newborns' length and head circumference are available, a common clinical practice is to classify infants with IUGR according to body proportionality based on measurements of length and head circumference. Thus, **disproportionally** or **asymmetrically** growth-retarded infants have relatively normal length and head circumference for gestational age but low weight-for-length (i.e., they are thin). **Proportionally** growth-retarded infants have symmetric reductions in weight, length, and head circumference (i.e., they are small but normally proportioned for size) (59–61).

Villar and Belizan (60) and others have identified three different types of IUGR based on the period when supplies to the fetus are diminished. With **chronic** IUGR, well-proportioned but small infants result from reductions in sustenance that began early in the first trimester and continued through the rest of gestation. With **subacute** and **acute** IUGR, newborns show weight reduction but a less marked damage in length growth. According to Villar and Belizan's hypothesis, with subacute IUGR, growth is adversely affected by a process beginning some time between 27 and 30 weeks of gestation, whereas with acute IUGR, growth is adversely affected in the last month of gestation.

To our knowledge, only two states—Missouri and Wisconsin—record crown-heel length and head circumference on the birth certificate. Studies

using Missouri and Wisconsin vital statistics data, in which analysts will be able to classify growth-retarded newborns as symmetric and asymmetric, may provide new clues about how to prevent different types of IUGR.

Prenatal Care and Low Birth Weight

Vital statistics have been used frequently to analyze the relationship between prenatal care and LBW (22,52). However, a number of methodologic and interpretive problems must be considered when vital statistics are used to assess this association (24,42,62,63). First, we must consider the problem of self-selection bias. Important differences exist between women who begin care early and those who begin late. Many of these differences pertain to variables that are not available from birth certificates. See the Prenatal Care chapter for more details.

A second pitfall relates to the fact that a large proportion of LBW cases are associated with short gestation. This shortened gestation implies that women with preterm LBW deliveries have less time to receive prenatal care. Prenatal care utilization indexes, such as the Kessner Index, have been developed to control for the fact that women with short gestations have less time in which to receive care and consequently have fewer prenatal care visits. These indexes classify adequacy of care according to the month care began, number of visits, and gestational age. However, Kleinman has shown that the Kessner Index's dependence on gestation can produce a seriously biased overestimate of the relationship between inadequate prenatal care and LBW (63). This bias occurs because the index was created for a data set that truncated all prenatal care visits over nine as being nine or more. Thus, adequate care is defined as nine or more visits even when gestation is at >36 weeks. The usual recommendation by the American College of Obstetricians and Gynecologists is to have a visit every week after 36 weeks.

Following this rule, the recommended number of visits for a woman 42 weeks pregnant is 16, whereas the Kessner Index still considers nine visits as adequate. As a result, the Kessner Index artificially induces a relationship between **less-than-adequate care** and LBW. The arbitrary cutoff of nine visits for **adequate care** introduces a large bias in the association between prenatal care and LBW because the proportion of women classified as having **less than adequate care** is smaller among women with long gestations than it is among women with short gestations simply because the former women had more time in which to obtain nine visits (63). Analyses that use the newer indexes of prenatal care use developed by Kotelchuck (64) and by Alexander and Cornely (65) are not subject to this bias.

This bias in analyses using the Kessner Index occurs even when gestation is well measured. However, another problem with all prenatal care use indexes is that errors of measurement in gestation result in bias that artifactually increases the strength of the association between adequacy of care and birth weight. This bias has also been demonstrated by Kleinman using the following example (63):

> If the birth certificate gestation is ≥37 weeks but the true gestation is <37 weeks, a woman's probability of being classified as having **adequate care** will be low because the number of prenatal care visits required is greater than it should be. On the other hand, if the true gestation is ≥37 weeks and the birth certificate gestation is <37 weeks, the opposite occurs because the number of visits required to be classified as **adequate** is too low.

This example shows how some infants who are truly preterm are classified as having inadequate care and some infants who are full-term are misclassified as having adequate care. Both of these errors would artificially increase the association between prenatal care and low birth weight. This bias should be a serious concern in analyses of the association between prenatal care and LBW because substantial measurement error is known to occur in gestational ages based on last menstrual period (66), especially those recorded on birth certificates (67). Note that **all** prenatal care use indexes, including the newer versions developed by Kotelchuck (64) and Alexander and Cornely (65), are subject to this bias.

Another problem is that researchers who use birth certificate data can examine the timing of prenatal care and the quantity of prenatal visits, but

neither of these variables are measures of the **quality** of prenatal care. Few studies have actually attempted to investigate the relationship between the **content** of prenatal care and perinatal outcome. One notable exception is a study by Kogan et al. (unpublished data, 1993). (See the Prenatal Care chapter.) In that study, recommendations from Caring for Our Future: The Content of Prenatal Care (68) were used as guidelines to develop a measure of quality of care.

Lastly, in most studies of the association between prenatal care and LBW, separate analyses of IUGR have not been conducted. A biological rationale appears to support the hypothesis that routine prenatal care—with its emphasis on advice about nutrition, weight gain, and smoking—would have some effect on preventing IUGR. However, because most studies have grouped together all LBW infants, only a few studies have been able to evaluate this hypothesis. The few studies that have separately analyzed preterm and term LBW suggest that prenatal care may have a stronger protective association with term LBW than with preterm LBW (62). We know of no published studies in which percentiles of birth-weight-for-gestation have been examined in relation to adequacy of prenatal care. In the future, we recommend that evaluations of the effects of prenatal care include separate analyses of term LBW (≥37 weeks of gestation; <2,500 g) as an outcome.

Gestational Weight Gain and Birth Weight

Now that birth certificates in most states include a question on weight gain during pregnancy, the relationship of gestational weight gain to perinatal outcome will undoubtedly be considered in state and national evaluations of maternal and infant health status. Analyzing the relationship of weight gain during pregnancy to birth weight requires consideration of a number of complex methodologic issues (69), which have been discussed in detail in the Institute of Medicine report titled Nutrition During Pregnancy (49). First, it is crucial that **intrauterine growth** be analyzed as a separate outcome because gestational weight gain affects intrauterine growth and preterm birth through entirely different biological mechanisms. Indeed, most evidence indicates that weight gain during pregnancy has no effect on gestational duration *(24)*.

Second, the Institute of Medicine report recommends that prepregnancy weight-for-height should be considered in all analyses of gestational weight gain because desirable weight gain among normal weight women is higher than it is among overweight women and lower than it is among thin women *(49)*. Unfortunately, data on prepregnancy weight and height are not available from birth certificates in most states. Third, although maternal prepregnancy weight and height are the most important potential confounders in any analysis of the perinatal effects of gestational weight gain, investigators must also control for age, parity, racial and ethnic origin, socioeconomic status, cigarette smoking, alcohol use, and prenatal care *(24,49)*.

Fourth, the Institute of Medicine report strongly emphasized that the use of total weight gain leads to overstatements of the association of gestational weight and intrauterine growth *(49)*. That is, if birth weight is not subtracted from the mother's weight gain, the association will be biased. We can avoid this problem by using **net gain**, subtracting the baby's weight from the mother's weight.

Time Trends in LBW Before 1970

Reported national rates of LBW for persons of races other than white apparently increased between 1950 and 1970. Analysts should be aware, however, that reported U.S. LBW rates for African-Americans before 1970 have serious validity problems.

According to the *Vital Statistics of the United States*, in 1950, >6% of births among persons of races other than white were unregistered and, in 1960, almost 3% of these births were unregistered (Table 2) *(19)*. A special study *(70)* by the National Office of Vital Statistics in 1950 found that these unregistered births occurred primarily in the South, occurred primarily in rural areas, and were usually out-of-hospital births. Although no definitive statistical evidence supports this point, we have good reason to believe that a

TABLE 2. Proportion of live births that were registered, by race — United States, 1950, 1960, and 1970

Year	White	Other races
1950	98.6%	93.6%
1960	99.4%	97.3%
1970	99.5%	98.5%

large number of these unregistered births involved LBW infants.

Therefore, the apparent increase in the reported LBW rate for African-Americans between 1950 and 1970 is probably an artifact of the underreporting of LBW babies born to African-Americans in 1950 and 1960 *(71)*. The **true** rate of LBW among African-Americans probably either decreased or remained stable during 1950–1970. Unfortunately, we will never know because we are unable to estimate the number of LBW infants whose births were unregistered in this period.

EXAMPLES OF USING DATA

Birth-weight data from computerized natality files have been a rich resource for program and policy planning. In addition, health departments have often gone beyond birth certificate data and conducted special studies of low birth weight. Examples of both types of studies are described in this section.

Racial and Ethnic Differences

Evaluations of racial and ethnic differences in LBW have been a prime concern in many analyses of state natality files. For example, in a study that uses Illinois vital records to compare black and white births in Chicago, investigators used the median income of each mother's census tract as an ecologic variable *(72)*. Maternal age, education, marital status, poverty level, parity, and prior infant deaths were considered as risk factors. The black/white relative risk for LBW was lower among high-risk mothers from the lower-income areas than it was among mothers from higher-income areas. Low-risk blacks did not fare as well as low-risk whites. Thus, traditional risk factors did not completely explain racial differences in LBW. In another analysis using the same data, biracial infants were compared with white infants (73). When poverty and other socio demographic factors were controlled, the adjusted odds ratio of LBW for infants born to black mothers and white fathers was 1.4. The adjusted odds ratio for infants born to white mothers and black fathers was 1.0. LBW rates among infants of biracial couples have also been studied by using natality data from Washington State and from NCHS national files (74,75).

Few in-depth investigations have focused on pregnancy outcomes among Native Americans, a situation that has been improved by a recent study using birth certificates from Upstate New York (35). Compared with white infants, Native American infants had a high-risk maternal profile: their mothers were younger, were a higher parity, had lower educational levels, and delayed initiating prenatal care more often. Despite this high-risk maternal profile, Native American infants had LBW rates similar to rates among white infants.

Since the mid-1970s, we have experienced a large influx of Southeast Asian refugees into the United States. Local and federal agencies have been concerned with the health status of these people because most of them have undergone severe hardships. State birth certificate files have been used in a number of creative ways to assess maternal and child health in the community of Southeast Asian immigrants. Li et al. analyzed Washington State births in 1980–1986 to Southeast Asian parents whose birthplace was coded as being outside the United States (76). The LBW rate decreased from 7.2% in 1980–1981 to 5.4% in 1986. Because the father's and mother's occupations were coded on the state birth files, investigators were able to ascertain that changes in paternal occupational status (from student to employed) was associated with 27% of the reduction in the LBW rate. A similar temporal change in birth weight was not observed among infants of United States-born Asian mothers, however.

Hmong immigrants were the subject of a study using California birth certificates from Merced and San Joaquin counties (77). The Hmong are an agricultural population living in relatively remote villages in the mountainous regions of southwestern China and northern Southeast Asia. In this study, the names of both parents were inspected, and Hmong ethnicity was assigned by using protocols designed with the help of members of the Hmong community. Despite a high-risk sociodemographic profile, the LBW rate was only slightly higher among infants of Hmong women (4.6%) than among infants of non-Hispanic whites (3.9%).

Perhaps the most detailed study of the maternal and infant health status of Asians is a recent report from the Massachusetts Department of Public Health, entitled *Chinese and Southeast Asian Births in Massachusetts (78)*. In 1987–1990, Chinese infants were less likely (4.2%) and Southeast Asian infants were substantially more likely (7.6%) to have low birth weights than were non-Hispanic white infants (5.0%). Within Southeast Asian ethnic subgroups in Massachusetts, LBW rates were 6.8% among Vietnamese infants, 8.1% among Cambodian infants, and 7.8% among Laotian infants.

Few investigators have used computerized birth files to study racial and ethnic differences in intrauterine growth (rather than LBW). One notable exception is a study of California natality data, in which researchers plotted median birth-weight-for-gestation values for non-Hispanic white, Hispanic white, black, Chinese, and Japanese infants (79). This is another study that should be referred to as a model by anyone interested using vital statistics data to analyze intrauterine growth patterns.

Smoking and LBW

Now that questions about cigarette smoking during pregnancy have been added to most states' birth certificates, studies of the effects of smoking on pregnancy outcomes should be conducted **and publicized** often. In a recent report from the Massachusetts Department of Public Health, IUGR was defined as a birth weight below the 10th percentile at each week of gestation (80). The growth standards used to identify IUGR were derived from a file of Massachusetts live births for 1987–1991. In Massachusetts in 1990, women who smoked during pregnancy had more than double the risk of LBW than women who did not smoke (8% vs. 3.9%). The authors attributed about 18% of LBW births among smokers to maternal smoking during pregnancy. Smokers were 2.43 times more likely to deliver an intrauterine growth-retarded infant than were nonsmokers. The authors calculated that about 22% of infants with IUGR born to smokers could be attributed to smoking during pregnancy. They observed a dose-response relationship between the number of cigarettes consumed daily during pregnancy and both LBW and IUGR.

Illinois is one of the states that participates in the CDC's Pregnancy Nutrition Surveillance System (PNSS), which tracks nutritional status during pregnancy and pregnancy outcome information on low-income women in the WIC program (see the Pregnancy-Related Nutrition chapter). In a report based on PNSS tabulations for Illinois, the data show that low prepregnancy weight, advanced age, and smoking increased the risk of LBW (81). Women >30 years who smoked and entered pregnancy while underweight were at greatest risk of delivering LBW babies.

Observations of women who have changed their maternal smoking behavior over time also are of great epidemiologic interest. Recently, investigators from the Missouri Department of Health (82) reported some intriguing findings from time trend analyses of Missouri live birth certificates. From 1978 to 1990, the percentage of black teenagers who smoked decreased from 35.8% to 7.2%. During the same period, the LBW rate among infants of black teenagers declined from 15.4% to 13.3% (a 13.6% decrease). The authors point out that we need to develop a better understanding of the reasons behind this drastic change in the smoking behavior of pregnant black teenagers to improve smoking cessation and other health promotion efforts and, thus, decrease the prevalence of LBW (82).

Environmental Exposures

The possibility that exposure to environmental toxins might increase the prevalence of LBW and IUGR has long been a concern of public health officials. Therefore, in eastern Missouri, soil contamination with 2,3,7,8-tetrachlorodibenzo-ρ-dioxin (TCDD) led the Missouri Department of

Health, in collaboration with the CDC, to conduct a retrospective cohort study of adverse reproductive outcomes in the region (83). Data on birth weight, gestational age, sociodemographic characteristics, smoking, and previous reproductive history were obtained from birth certificates. IUGR was defined as a case in which a live-born infant who weighed <2,500 g and had a gestational age of >36 weeks. The TCDD-exposed group had an increased risk of LBW, but the relationship was not statistically significant. The investigators concluded that statistically significant adverse reproductive effects may not have been detected because of the small size of the population.

Investigators from the CDC and the University of Iowa have recently reported results from their case-control study of the association between waterborne chloroform and IUGR (12). Data on birth weight, gestational age, sociodemographic characteristics, and smoking were obtained from birth certificates. IUGR was defined as a case in which a live-born infant had a birth weight below the fifth percentile for a particular gestational age, as determined from the California standards for non-Hispanic whites (10). Investigators randomly selected 187 cases of IUGR and 935 control subjects from Iowa birth certificate data for 1989–1990. Exposures to chloroform and other trihalomethanes were ecologic variables based on maternal residence and a 1987 municipal water survey. After adjusting for potential confounding variables, researchers concluded that residence in municipalities with chloroform concentrations of ≥10 μg/L was associated with an increased risk of IUGR.

Prenatal Care and Birth Weight

Many researchers have analyzed the effects of prenatal care on LBW. Several of the classic investigations of this issue have used state birth certificate files. These studies, which usually involve comparisons of women with and without adequate prenatal care, have been reviewed in detail elsewhere (22,52). Additionally, over the last decade, maternal and child health researchers have compared the different **types** of prenatal care women receive. Investigators at the North Carolina Center for Health and Environmental Statistics, pioneers in this research effort, linked

197

birth certificates to records from the Northwest North Carolina Prematurity Prevention Project *(84)*. They were then able to compare births to women in the project to nonproject births in the same 20-county region. A logistic regression analysis—in which race, marital status, age, and other sociodemographic factors were controlled— revealed that women not in the project were 1.32 times as likely as project participants to have LBW deliveries.

In another North Carolina study, conducted in collaboration with the Guilford County Public Health Department, records of women in the county health department's prenatal care pro- gram and records of Medicaid-paid claims were linked to birth certificates *(85)*. Researchers could then evaluate the effect of the county's compre- hensive prenatal care program on LBW among infants born to low-income women. Medicaid- eligible women, who received care primarily from private practice physicians, had a LBW rate more than twice as great as women in the health department's program, even after the investiga- tors controlled for race, marital status, WIC participation, quantity of prenatal care, and other risk factors.

This study design was later expanded to link pub- lic health department program files and Medicaid- paid claim files to birth certificate files for all of North Carolina and Kentucky *(86)*. Again, women enrolled in Medicaid who received prenatal care outside public health departments were more likely than those who received care at health departments to have LBW babies. A recent study of low-income mothers in inner-city Chicago has reported similar findings *(87)*.

Using Both Birth Certificate and Census Data

Because birth certificates are not meant to be detailed questionnaires, the information on com- puterized birth files is limited. The only indicators of social or economic status on the U.S. Stan- dard Certificate of Live Birth are the mother's and father's race, ethnicity, and education and the mother's marital status. A great deal of infor- mation can be added to evaluations of maternal and infant health when birth certificate data on the mother's place of residence are used in

conjunction with data from the U.S. census. In the Chicago studies of racial differences in LBW *(72,73)*, investigators appended the income char- acteristics of each mother's census tract to records from birth files. In a study in Los Angeles County, researchers used a similar approach to investi- gate the relationship between median family income of the census tract of maternal residence and LBW rates *(88)*. In an analysis of LBW rates in Hawaii, census tract information on unem- ployment, crowding, and poverty was examined along with birth certificate data on sociodemo- graphic characteristics and prenatal care *(89)*. The advantages and disadvantages of studies in which individual-level data (such as birth certificates) are linked to census tract data have recently been discussed by Krieger *(90)*.

FUTURE ISSUES

The year 2000 objectives include two goals related to birth weight:

- To reduce low birth weight to an incidence of no more than 5% of live births and very low birth weight to no more than 1% of live births.

- To reduce low birth weight among blacks to an incidence of no more than 9% of live births and very low birth weight to no more than 2% of live births.

Clearly substantial reductions in LBW still need to occur between now and year 2000 if these goals are to be reached (Table 3). The fact that

TABLE 3. **Progress toward meeting the year 2000 objective for low birth weight and very low birth weight (percentage of live births)**

	1987 baseline	1990	2000 target
Low birth weight (all races)	6.9	7.0	5
Low birth weight (black)	13.0	13.3	9
Very low birth weight (all races)	1.2	1.3	1
Very low birth weight (black)	2.8	2.9	2

rates actually **increased** slightly between 1987 and 1990 is alarming.

Data from birth certificates in 1989 and subsequent years will be particularly useful for analyzing low birth weight. The *Medical risk factors for this pregnancy* item includes questions on *Anemia and Previous preterm or small-for-gestational age infant.* Also added were questions on tobacco and alcohol use and on weight gain during pregnancy. Additionally, the new item *Clinical estimate of gestation* may improve the data on gestational age.

Because birth certificate data are used extensively to evaluate maternal and infant health programs, we must closely monitor the quality of the new information. Already, several validation studies have compared post-1988 birth certificate data with hospital medical record data *(91–93)*. The findings suggest that investigators should be cautious in using birth certificate data to evaluate associations with maternal medical risk factors, complications of labor and delivery, abnormal conditions of newborns, and congenital anomalies.

As we have stressed several times throughout this chapter, one of the most pressing data needs in future evaluations of maternal and infant health status is to develop a better understanding of the distinctive etiologies and epidemiologies of IUGR and preterm birth. Because the means of prevention may be different for these two components of LBW, we strongly recommend that the two outcomes be analyzed separately. The classification of infants by birth weight and gestational age need not be a complex task because term LBW ($\geq$37 weeks of gestation, <2,500 g) is generally considered an acceptable definition of IUGR (Figure 1). An added benefit of separately analyzing IUGR and preterm birth is that this approach will improve communication between public health researchers and clinical practitioners.

REFERENCES

1. World Health Organization. The incidence of low birth weight: a critical review of available information. World Health Stat Q 1980;33:197–224.

2. World Health Organization. The incidence of low birth weight: an update. Wkly Epidemiol Rec 1984; 59:205–11.

3. Villar J, Belizan JM. The relative contribution of prematurity and fetal growth retardation to low birth weight in developing and developed societies. Am J Obstet Gynecol 1982;143:793–8.

4. Pérez-Escamilla R, Pollitt E. Causes and consequences of intrauterine growth retardation in Latin America. Bull Pan Am Health Organ 1992;26:128–47.

5. Ylppö A. Zur physiologie, klinik, zum schicksal der frühgeborenen. Zeitschrift für kinderheilkunde 1919;24:1–110.

6. World Health Organization. Expert Group on Prematurity. Final report. Technical report, series 27. Geneva: World Health Organization, 1950.

7. McKeown T, Gibson JR. Observations on all births (23,970) in Birmingham, 1947. II. Birth weight. Br J Soc Med 1951;5:98–112.

8. Forbes JF, Smalls MJ. A comparative analysis of birth weight for gestational age standards. Br J Obstet Gynaecol 1983;99:297–303.

9. Goldenberg RL, Cutter GR, Hoffman HJ, et al. Intrauterine growth retardation: standards for diagnosis. Am J Obstet Gynecol 1989;161:271–7.

10. Williams RL, Creasy RK, Cunningham GC, Hawes WE, Norris FD, Tashiro M. Fetal growth and perinatal viability in California. Obstet Gynecol 1982;59:624–32.

11. David RJ. Population-based intrauterine growth curves from computerized birth certificates. South Med J 1983;76:1401–6.

12. Kramer MD, Lynch CF, Isacson P, Hanson JW. The association of waterborne chloroform with intrauterine growth retardation. Epidemiology 1992;3:407–13.

13. Yerushalmy J. The classification of newborn infants by birth weight and gestational age. J Pediatr 1967; 71:164–72.

14. Hoffman HJ, Lundin FE Jr, Bakketeig LS, Harley EE. Classification of births by weight and gestational age for future studies of prematurity. In: Reed DM, Stanley FJ, eds. The epidemiology of prematurity. Baltimore: Urban & Schwarzenberg, 1977:297–325.

15. Adelstein P, Fedrick J. Antenatal identification of women at increased risk of being delivered of a low birthweight infant at term. Br J Obstet Gynaecol 1978;85:8–11.

16. Michielutte R, Ernest JM, Moore ML, et al. A comparison of risk assessment models for term and preterm low birthweight. Prev Med 1992; 21:98–109.

17. Kallan JE. Race, intervening variables, and two components of low birth weight. Demography 1993; 30:489–506.

18. NCHS. Advance report of final mortality statistics, 1991. Hyattsville, Maryland: US Department of Health and Human Services, Public Health Service, CDC, 1993. (Monthly vital statistics report; vol. 42, no. 3, suppl.)

19. NCHS. Vital statistics of the United States, 1988. Vol. I, natality. Hyattsville, Maryland: US Department of Health and Human Services, Public Health Service, CDC, 1990.

20. American Academy of Pediatrics, American College of Obstetricians and Gynecologists. Standard terminology for reporting of reproductive health statistics in the United States. Public Health Rep 1988; 103:464–71.

21. Stein ZA, Susser M. Intrauterine growth retardation: epidemiological issues and public health significance. Semin Perinatol 1984;8:5–14.

22. Institute of Medicine. Preventing low birthweight. Washington, DC: National Academy Press, 1985.

23. Brown SS. Can low birth weight be prevented? Fam Plann Perspect 1985;17:112–8.

24. Kramer MS. Determinants of low birth weight: methodological assessment and meta-analysis. Bull World Health Organ 1987;65:663–737.

25. Kline J, Stein Z, Susser M. Conception to birth: epidemiology of prenatal development. New York: Oxford University Press, 1989.

26. US Congress, Office of Technology Assessment. Adolescent health—volume II: background and the effectiveness of selected prevention and treatment services. Washington, DC: US Government Printing Office, 1991:323–427; publication no. OTA-H-466.

27. Berendes HW, Forman MR. Delayed childbearing: trends and consequences. In: Kiely M, ed. Reproductive and perinatal epidemiology. Boca Raton, Florida: CRC Press, 1991.

28. Geronimus AT, Korenman S. Maternal youth or family background? On the health disadvantages of infants with teenage mothers. Am J Epidemiol 1993; 137:213–25.

29. Kleinman JC, Kessel SS. Racial differences in low birth weight: trends and risk factors. N Engl J Med 1987;317:749–53.

30. Kessel SS, Kleinman JC, Koontz AM, Hogue CJR, Berendes HW. Racial differences in pregnancy outcomes. Clin Perinatol 1988; 15:745–54.

31. NCHS. Health, United States, 1992. Hyattsville, Maryland: US Department of Health and Human Services, Public Health Service, CDC, 1993; DHHS publication no. (PHS)93-1232.

32. Iyasu S, Becerra JE, Rowley DL, Hogue CJR. Impact of very low birthweight on the black-white infant mortality gap. Am J Prev Med 1992;8:271–7.

33. Wilcox A, Russell I. Why small black infants have a lower mortality rate than small white infants: the case for population-specific standards for birth weight. J Pediatr 1990;116:7–10.

34. Balcazar H, Aoyama C, Cai X. Interpretative views on Hispanics' perinatal problems of low birth weight and prenatal care. Public Health Rep 1991;106:420–6.

35. Buck GM, Mahoney MC, Michalek AM, Powell EJ, Shelton JA. Comparison of Native American births in Upstate New York with other race births, 1980–86. Public Health Rep 1992;107:569–75.

36. Mendoza FS, Ventura SJ, Valdez RB, et al. Selected measures of health status for Mexican-American, Mainland Puerto Rican, and Cuban-American children. JAMA 1991;265:227–32.

37. Lin C-C, Emanuel I. A comparison of American and Chinese intrauterine growth standards. Are American babies really smaller? Am J Epidemiol 1972; 95:418–30.

38. Yip R, Li Z, Chong W-H. Race and birth weight: the Chinese example. Pediatrics 1991;87:688–93.

39. Kennedy ET, Gershoff S, Reed R, Austin JE. Evaluation of the effect of WIC supplemental feeding on birth weight. J Am Diet Assoc 1982;80:220–7.

40. Horon IL, Strobino DM, MacDonald HM. Birth weights among infants born to adolescent and young adult women. Am J Obstet Gynecol 1983;146:444–9.

41. Liberatos P, Link BG, Kelsey JL. The measurement of social class in epidemiology. Epidemiol Rev 1988;10:87–121.

42. Illsley R. The sociological study of reproduction and its outcome. In: Richardson SA, Guttmacher AF, eds. Childbearing: its social and psychological aspects. Baltimore, Maryland: Williams and Wilkins, 1967.

43. Kleinman JC, Madans JH. The effects of maternal smoking, physical stature, and educational attainment on the incidence of low birth weight. Am J Epidemiol 1985;121:843–55.

44. Parker JD, Schoendorf KC, Kiely JL. Associations between measures of socioeconomic status and low-birthweight, small for gestational age, and premature delivery in the United States. Am J Epidemiol 1994 (in press).

45. Floyd RL, Rimer BK, Giovino GA, Mullen PD, Sullivan SE. A review of smoking in pregnancy: effects on pregnancy outcomes and cessation efforts. Annu Rev Public Health 1993;14:379–411.

46. Handler A, Kristin N, Davis F, Ferré C. Cocaine use during pregnancy: perinatal outcomes. Am J Epidemiol 1991;133:818–25.

47. Robins LN, Mills JL, Krulewitch C, Herman AA. Effects of in utero exposure to street drugs. Am J Public Health 1993;83(suppl):1–32.

48. Arbuckle TE, Sherman GJ. Comparison of the risk factors for pre-term delivery and intrauterine growth retardation. Paediatr Perinat Epidemiol 1989; 3:115–29.

49. Institute of Medicine. Nutrition during pregnancy. Washington, DC: National Academy Press, 1990.

50. Rees JM, Engelbert-Fenton KA, Gong EJ, Bach CM. Weight gain in adolescents during pregnancy: rate-related to birth-weight outcome. AM J Clin Nutr 1992;56:868–73.

51. Scholl TO, Hediger ML, Khoo C-S, Healey MF, Rawson NL. Maternal weight gain, diet and infant birth weight: correlations during adolescent pregnancy. J Clin Epidemiol 1991;44:423–8.

52. US Congress, Office of Technology Assessment. Healthy children: investing in the future. Washington, DC: US Government Printing Office, 1988; publication no. OTA-H-345.

53. Khoury MJ, Erickson JD, Cordero JF, McCarthy BJ. Congenital malformations and intrauterine growth retardation: a population study. Pediatrics 1988; 82:83–90.

54. Wartenberg D, Agamennone VJ, Ozonoff D, Berry RJ. A microcomputer-based vital records data base with interactive graphic assessment for states and localities. Am J Public Health 1989;79:1531–6.

55. Gould JB, Mahajan N, Lucero M. Improving perinatal outcome through data management: the design of the small area analysis system. J Perinat Med 1988; 16:305–14.

56. Mantel N. Synthetic retrospective studies and related topics. Biometrics 1973;29:479–86.

57. Gayle HD, Yip R, Frank MJ, Nieburg P, Binkin NJ. Validation of maternally reported birth weights among 46,637 Tennessee WIC program participants. Public Health Rep 1988;103:143–7.

58. Sloan CT, Lorenz RP. Importance of locally derived birth weight nomograms. J Reprod Med 1991; 36:598–602.

59. Rosso P, Winick M. Intrauterine growth retardation: a new systematic approach based on the clinical and biochemical characteristics of the condition. J Perinat Med 1974;2:147–60.

60. Villar J, Belizan JM. The timing factor in the pathophysiology of the intrauterine growth retardation syndrome. Obstet Gynecol Surv 1982;37:499–506.

61. Khoury MJ, Berg CJ, Calle EE. The ponderal index in term newborn siblings. Am J Epidemiol 1990; 132:576–83.

62. Liberatos P, Kiely JL. Selected issues in the evaluation of prenatal care. In: Kiely M, ed. Reproductive and perinatal epidemiology. Boca Raton, Florida: CRC Press, 1991:79–97.

63. Kleinman JC. Methodological issues in the analysis of vital statistics. In: Kiely M, ed. Reproductive and perinatal epidemiology. Boca Raton, Florida: CRC Press, 1991:447–68.

64. Kotelchuck M. The mismeasurement of prenatal care adequacy in the U.S. and a proposed two-part index. Am J Public Health 1994 (in press).

65. Alexander GR, Cornely DA. Prenatal care utilization: its measurement and relationship to pregnancy outcome. Am J Prev Med 1987;3:243–53.

66. Kramer MS, McLean FH, Boyd ME, Usher RH. The validity of gestational age estimation by menstrual dating in term, preterm, and postterm gestations. JAMA 1988;260:3306–8.

67. David RJ. The quality and completeness of birthweight and gestational age data in computerized birth files. Am J Public Health 1980;70:964–73.

68. Public Health Service Expert Panel on the Content of Prenatal Care. Caring for our future: the content of prenatal care. Washington, DC: US Department of Health and Human Services, Public Health Service, 1989; NIH publication no. 90-3182.

69. Susser M. Maternal weight gain, infant birth weight, and diet: causal sequences. Am J Clin Nutr 1991; 53:1384–96.

70. National Office of Vital Statistics. Test of birth registration completeness for 1950. In: US Department of Health, Education, and Welfare. Vital Statistics of the United States, 1950. Vol. I: analysis and summary tables with supplemental tables for Alaska, Hawaii, Puerto Rico, and Virgin Islands. Washington, DC: United States Government Printing Office, 1954:108–27.

71. David RJ. Did low birthweight among US blacks really increase? Am J Public Health 1986;76:380–4.

72. Collins JW Jr, David RJ. The differential effect of traditional risk factors on infant birthweight among blacks and whites in Chicago. Am J Public Health 1990; 80:679–81.

73. Collins JW Jr, David RJ. Race and birthweight in biracial infants. Am J Public Health 1993;83:1125–9.

74. Migone A, Emanuel I, Mueller B, Daling J, Little RE. Gestational duration and birthweight in white, black and mixed-race babies. Paediatr Perinat Epidemiol 1991;5:378–91.

75. Parker JD, Schoendorf KC. Influence of paternal characteristics on the risk of low birth weight. Am J Epidemiol 1992;136:399–407.

76. Li D-K, Ni H, Schwartz SM, Daling JR. Secular change in birthweight among Southeast Asian immigrants to the United States. Am J Public Health 1990;80:685–8.

77. Helsel D, Petitti DB, Kunstadter P. Pregnancy among the Hmong: birthweight, age, and parity. Am J Public Health 1992;82:1361–4.

78. Massachusetts Department of Public Health. Chinese and Southeast Asian births in Massachusetts. Boston: Massachusetts Department of Public Health, 1993.

79. Williams RL. Intrauterine growth curves: intra- and international comparisons with different ethnic groups in California. Prev Med 1975;4:163–72.

80. Massachusetts Department of Public Health. The burden of smoking on mothers and infants in Massachusetts. Boston: Massachusetts Department of Public Health, 1993.

81. Nandi C, Nelson MR. Maternal pregravid weight, age, and smoking status as risk factors for low birth weight births. Public Health Rep 1992;107:658–62.

82. Land GH, Stockbauer JW. Smoking and pregnancy outcome: trends among black teenage mothers in Missouri. Am J Public Health 1993;83:1121–4.

83. Stockbauer JW, Hoffman RE, Schramm WF, Edmonds LD. Reproductive outcomes of mothers with potential exposure to 2,3,7,8-tetrachlorodibenzo-ρ-dioxin. Am J Epidemiol 1988;128:410–9.

84. Buescher PA, Meis PJ, Ernest JM, Moore ML, Michielutte R, Sharp P. A comparison of women in and out of a prematurity prevention project in a North Carolina perinatal care region. Am J Public Health 1988;78:264–7.

85. Buescher PA, Smith C, Holliday JL, Levine RH. Source of prenatal care and infant birth weight: the case of a North Carolina county. Am J Obstet Gynecol 1987;156:204–10.

86. Buescher PA, Ward NI. A comparison of low birth weight among Medicaid patients of public health departments and other providers of prenatal care in North Carolina and Kentucky. Public Health Rep 1992;107:54–9.

87. Handler A, Rosenberg D. Improving pregnancy outcomes: public versus private care for urban low-income women. BIRTH 1992;19:123–30.

88. Gould JB, LeRoy S. Socioeconomic status and low birth weight: a racial comparison. Pediatrics 1988;82:896–904.

89. Kieffer EC, Alexander GR, Lewis ND, Mor J. Geographic patterns of low birth weight in Hawaii. Soc Sci Med 1993;36:557–64.

90. Krieger N. Overcoming the absence of socioeconomic data in medical records: validation and application of a census-based methodology. Am J Public Health 1992;92:703–10.

91. Piper JM, Mitchel EF, Snowden M, Hall C, Adams M, Taylor P. Validation of 1989 Tennessee birth certificates using maternal and newborn hospital records. Am J Epidemiol 1993;137:758–68.

92. Buescher PA, Taylor KP, Davis MH, Bowling JM. The quality of the new birth certificate data: a validation study in North Carolina. Am J Public Health 1993;83:1163–5.

93. Parrish KM, Holt VL, Connell FA, Williams B, LoGerfo JP. Variations in the accuracy of obstetric procedures and diagnoses on birth records in Washington State, 1989. Am J Epidemiol 1993;138:119–27.

Prevalence of Birth Defects

Levy M. James, M.S.,[1] J. David Erickson, D.D.S., Ph.D.,[1]
and Anne B. McClearn, B.A.[1]

PUBLIC HEALTH IMPORTANCE

The prevalence of birth defects varies considerably with respect to type of defect, time, place, and other demographic, genetic, and environmental factors. In this chapter, we describe the prevalence of birth defects as determined by two CDC surveillance systems, the Birth Defects Monitoring Program (BDMP) and the Metropolitan Atlanta Congenital Defects Program (MACDP). For additional information about related topics and surveillance activities, see the State Use of Birth Defects Surveillance, Infant Mortality, Neonatal and Postneonatal Mortality, and Fetal Alcohol Syndrome chapters.

HISTORY OF DATA COLLECTION

In the early 1950s, the fact that rubella can cause birth defects became clear. A decade later came the discovery that maternal use of thalidomide had caused an epidemic of limb reduction deformities. Thus, in the 1960s, the realization emerged that infectious and other environmental factors could cause birth defects, and this realization resulted in the establishment of birth defects surveillance programs in a number of countries.

CDC was an early participant in this surveillance activity, starting the MACDP in 1967 and the BDMP in 1974. The New York State Health Department also began an early surveillance program, based on birth certificates. In 1974, CDC and representatives from nine other surveillance programs, primarily from Europe, formed the International Clearinghouse for Birth Defects Monitoring Systems (ICBDMS). Today, the ICBDMS comprises 24 programs. Many of these programs are based in Europe, and

some programs are from Australia, China, New Zealand, and Japan. Over the past decade, several state health departments have begun their own birth defects surveillance systems (these state-based activities are described in detail in the State Use of Birth Defects Surveillance chapter).

CDC SURVEILLANCE ACTIVITIES

CDC's two systems for assessing the prevalence of birth defects—the BDMP and the MACDP—are both overseen by CDC's National Center for Environmental Health (NCEH) *(1)*.

The BDMP, a national program to monitor congenital malformations, uses hospital discharge data on newborns gathered by the Commission on Professional and Hospital Activities (CPHA), based in Ann Arbor, Michigan. Data from this system cover both live-born and stillborn infants in participating member hospitals from 1970 to the present. The database includes information on >17 million births occurring in 1,200 predominately midsized community hospitals across the United States. The system covers approximately 405,000 births annually—>10% of all births occurring in the nation—although the coverage proportion varies considerably by state. Because participation is voluntary, the sampling is not random; thus, the degree of representativeness is an issue to be considered in interpreting the data. The data are derived from newborn discharge information provided to CPHA by participating member hospitals. CPHA processes these data, conducting range

---

[1] Division of Birth Defects and Developmental Disabilities
National Center for Environmental Health
Centers for Disease Control and Prevention
Atlanta, Georgia

and consistency edit checks for input accuracy. Diagnoses made for readmissions are not included, because to do so could introduce duplicate counting of infants. Semiannually, CPHA provides CDC with data tapes that include the following information: state and county of birth occurrence, year and month of birth, live-born/stillborn status, race, sex, birth weight, up to 31 *International Classification of Diseases, Ninth Revision, Clinical Modification (ICD-9-CM)* procedure codes, and up to 31 *ICD-9-CM* diagnostic codes *(2)*.

Because the BDMP is a surveillance system with passive case ascertainment based on hospital discharge summaries of newborns, the proportion of cases it detects depends on the severity of the specific defect; less severe defects can be overlooked in the newborn period, whereas more severe defects are more likely to result in prompt and accurate diagnoses. An additional problem is the declining number of participating hospitals. CDC researchers are investigating new avenues for national birth defects surveillance, including collaboration among state birth defects monitoring programs.

The MACDP is one of the oldest birth defects surveillance systems in the country *(1)*. This population-based birth defects surveillance system was founded by the Georgia Mental Health Institute, Emory University School of Medicine, and CDC. Day-to-day program operations are the responsibility of NCEH.

The MACDP monitors all births—approximately 38,000 births a year—occurring in the five-county metropolitan Atlanta area. The program collects information on all stillborn and live-born infants diagnosed with at least one major birth defect within the first year of life, with diagnoses ascertained within the first 5 years of life.

The MACDP has served as a prototype for numerous birth defects surveillance systems. MACDP researchers have encouraged the development of uniform methods of birth defects surveillance, developed a more defect-specific coding system and a uniform set of variables for data collection, and provided a focus for collaborative studies between surveillance systems with active case ascertainment.

MACDP researchers gather data using an in-house coding form (Figure 1). They use the precise diagnosis and written description of defects collected and classified according to the six-digit MACDP code, which permits improved classification of birth defects and improves researchers' ability to study specific types of malformations. Case ascertainment includes a review of maternal and infant medical records in multiple sources, including birth hospitals, pediatric referral hospitals, cytogenetic laboratories, specialty clinics, and vital statistics from the Georgia Department of Human Resources. Multiple sources of ascertainment are used to identify potential cases. Hospital records reviewed include obstetric, nursery, pediatric, surgery, autopsy, and laboratory logs as well as cardiac catheterization records and disease indexes. MACDP staff review charts of all infants who are stillborn, die shortly after birth, weigh <2,500 g, or are born before 37 weeks of gestational age. Similar data from pediatric referral hospitals are reviewed as are laboratory service records. In addition, birth and death certificates are reviewed to search for previously unidentified cases.

MACDP case records include basic demographic information (identification of the case infant, case mother, and case father as well as the infant's race, sex, plurality, live-born/stillborn status, date of birth, birth weight, hospital of birth, and date of first diagnosis), laboratory examination results, specific written diagnoses, six-digit MACDP codes, cytogenetic data, complications of birth, prenatal data, pregnancy history, family history, and other birth-related and risk factor information.

These data are computer processed in monthly batches that undergo a variety of edit checks. From 1968 to the present, the MACDP has ascertained the occurrence of birth defects for approximately 725,000 births. MACDP staff monitor birth defects rates and trends by conducting quarterly reviews and analysis of data, and they make temporal and geographic comparisons to search for significant changes in birth defects rates.

GENERAL FINDINGS

In this chapter, we focus on the prevalence of a selected set of 26 birth defects reported through

FIGURE 1.

U.S. DEPARTMENT OF HEALTH AND HUMAN SERVICES
Public Health Service
Centers for Disease Control and Prevention (CDC)
Atlanta, Georgia 30093

REPRODUCTIVE OUTCOMES CASE RECORD

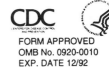

FORM APPROVED
OMB No. 0920-0010
EXP. DATE 12/92

(1-) ROCR

| STATE (5-) 11 | I.D. No.(7-) _ _ _ _ _ _ | INFORMATION RECORDED: Mo   Da   Yr |
| | | INITIALS(13-) _ _ _   DATE(16-) _ _ - _ _ - _ _   HOSP.(22-) _ _ _ _ |

PATIENT NAME: (26-) LAST FIRST MIDDLE | MOTHER'S NAME (50-) LAST FIRST (MAIDEN) | AGE AT BIRTH (74-) _ _

RESIDENCE AT BIRTH (76-) | FATHER'S NAME:(108-) LAST FIRST MIDDLE | AGE AT BIRTH (132-) _ _

CITY (134-) | COUNTY (150-) _ _ _ | ZIP(153-) _ _ _ _ _ | CENSUS TRACT (158-) _ _ _ _ | HOME PHONE (164-) _ _ _ / _ _ _ - _ _ _ _

MOTHER'S BIRTH DATE (174-) _ _ - _ _ - _ _ (MDY) | MOTHER'S SSN (180-) _ _ _ - _ _ - _ _ _ _ | FATHER'S BIRTH DATE (189-) _ _ - _ _ - _ _ (MDY) | FATHER'S SSN (195-) _ _ _ - _ _ - _ _ _ _

MOTHER'S RACIAL OR ETHNIC GROUP (204)
☐ 1 WHITE, NOT HISP   ☐ 3 HISPANIC   ☐ 5 ASIAN OR PACIFIC ISLANDER
☐ 2 BLACK, NOT HISP   ☐ 4 AMERICAN INDIAN OR ALASKAN NATIVE   ☐ 9 NOT STATED

PENDING (206)   ☐ 1 YES   ☐ 2 NO

SEX (214)
☐ 1 MALE   ☐ 3 AMBIGUOUS
☐ 2 FEMALE   ☐ 9 NOT STATED

PLURALITY (215)
☐ 1 SINGLE   ☐ 3 OTHER MULTIPLE BIRTH
☐ 2 TWIN   ☐ 9 NOT STATED

OUTCOME OF DELIVERY (216)
☐ 1 LIVE BORN   ☐ 3 INDUCED AB
☐ 2 STILLBORN   ☐ 9 NOT STATED

CO-TWIN SEX (217)
☐ 1 MALE   ☐ 3 AMBIGUOUS
☐ 2 FEMALE   ☐ 9 NOT STATED

CO-TWIN CONCORDANCE (218)
☐ 1 CO-TWIN NORMAL   ☐ 3 CO-TWIN WITH OTHER DEFECT
☐ 2 CO-TWIN WITH SAME DEFECT   ☐ 9 NOT STATED

CO-TWIN LB/SB (219)
☐ 1 CO-TWIN LB   ☐ 9 NOT STATED
☐ 2 CO-TWIN STILL BORN

DX CODE	DIAGNOSIS
(258-) _ _ _ . _ _ _	
(264-) _ _ _ . _ _ _	
(270-) _ _ _ . _ _ _	
(276-) _ _ _ . _ _ _	
(282-) _ _ _ . _ _ _	
(288-) _ _ _ . _ _ _	

APGAR SCORE   1 MIN   5 MIN
(220-) _ _   (222-) _ _

DATE OF BIRTH   Mo   Da   Yr
(224-) _ _ - _ _ - _ _

BIRTH WEIGHT
(230-) _ _ _ _ GRAMS
OR
(234-) _ _ LBS. _ _ OZS.

HOSPITAL OR PLACE OF FIRST DIAGNOSIS
(238-) _ _ _

DATE OF FIRST DIAGNOSIS   Mo   Da   Yr
(242-) _ _ - _ _ - _ _

HEAD CIRCUMFERENCE (251) ☐ 1 CM ☐ 2 IN
(248-) _ _ . _

LENGTH (255) ☐ 1 CM ☐ 2 IN
(252-) _ _ . _

GEST. AGE BY NEONATAL EXAM (294-) _ _ WKS.

DUBOWITZ EXAM (296)
☐ 1 YES   ☐ 3 NOT APPLICABLE
☐ 2 NO   ☐ 9 NOT STATED

ULTRASOUND DATE   Mo   Da   Yr
(297-) _ _ - _ _ - _ _

ULTRASOUND DATING (303-) _ _ WKS.

DATE OF   Mo   Da   Yr
LMP (305-) _ _ - _ _ - _ _

MOTHER'S HEMATOCRIT (256-) _ _ _

EDC (311-) _ _ - _ _ - _ _

SYNDROME (317-) _ - _ _ _ _ _ _

CYTOGENETICS: (323)
☐ 1 NORMAL   ☐ 4 NOT DONE
☐ 2 ABNORMAL   ☐ 9 NOT STATED
☐ 3 PENDING

LABORATORY (324-) _ _ _ _

DIAGNOSIS (328) _ _ - _ _ _ _ _

TO BE INTERVIEWED (334)
☐ 1 YES   ☐ 2 NO

ACTION CODE (335)
☐ 1 ORIG.   ☐ 3 CORR.
☐ 2 CONT.   ☐ 4 DELE.

CDC 84.1A REV. 11-92

(SEE REVERSE)

FIGURE 1. — continued

PRENATAL DX TEST (336)

☐1 DONE   ☐2 NOT DONE   ☐9 NOT STATED

TYPE TEST (337-) __ __

       Mo   Da   Yr

DATE (339-) __ __ - __ __ - __ __

PLACE   (345-) __ __ __ __

COMPLICATIONS OF BIRTH

    YES NO NS
     1   2   9
(349) ☐ ☐ ☐RLF
     1   2   9
(350) ☐ ☐ ☐TORCH
     1   2   9
(351) ☐ ☐ ☐NEONATAL SEPSIS/MENINGITIS
     1   2   9
(352) ☐ ☐ ☐NEONATAL SEIZURES

EXPIRED (362)

☐1 YES   ☐2 NO   ☐9 NOT STATED

DATE OF DEATH   Mo   Da   Yr

    (363-) __ __ - __ __ - __ __

PLACE OF DEATH

    (369-) __ __ __ __

AUTOPSY

(373) ☐1 YES, REVIEWED   ☐3 YES, PENDING

    ☐2 NO   ☐9 NOT STATED

         Mo   Da   Yr

DATE (374-) __ __ - __ __ - __ __

PLACE (380-) __ __ __ __

TOTAL NUMBER OF PREVIOUS PREGNANCIES (Present not Included)   (384-) __ __

NUMBER OF LIVE BIRTHS   (386-) __ __

NUMBER OF STILL BIRTHS   (388-) __ __

NUMBER OF INDUCED AB   (390-) __ __

NUMBER OF SPONTANEOUS AB (392-) __ __

NUMBER OF UNSPECIFIED TYPE AB   (394) __

HOSPITAL OF BIRTH

    (395-) __ __ __ __

CHART NUMBER: MOTHER

    (399-) __ __ __ __ __ __ __ __ __ __

CHART NUMBER: INFANT

    (409-) __ __ __ __ __ __ __ __ __ __

HOSPITAL OF SECOND ADMISSION

    (419-) __ __ __ __

CHART NUMBER: INFANT

    (423-) __ __ __ __ __ __ __ __ __ __

(433) ☐1 READMISSION   ☐2 TRANSFER

SECOND ADMISSION DATE   Mo   Da   Yr

    (434-) __ __ - __ __ - __ __

HOSPITAL OF LABOR

    (440-) __ __ __ __

CHART NUMBER: MOTHER

    (444-) __ __ __ __ __ __ __ __ __ __

LABOR ADMISSION DATE   Mo   Da   Yr

    (454-) __ __ - __ __ - __ __

NAMES OF PHYSICIANS (LAST FIRST INIT.)

OBSTETRICIANS _____
    (460-)   (490-)

PEDIATRICIANS _____
    (519-)   (543-)   (567-)

OTHERS _____
    (591-)   (615-)   (639-)

PRESENT PREGNANCY INFORMATION (663-)

PREVIOUS PREGNANCY AND MEDICAL HISTORY (743-)

FAMILY HISTORY (823-)

INFANT HISTORY, OTHER INFORMATION (903-962)

the BDMP and 25 birth defects reported through the MACDP (Rh hemolytic disease is not reported through the MACDP) (Tables 1 and 2). These defects were chosen to reflect a variety of organ systems and the wide range of occurrence rates for individual birth defects.

Many of the overall birth defects rates mask important temporal trends, as is evident in the BDMP prevalence rates for 1970–1971 and 1990–1991 as well as the mean annual percent change in rates between these two periods (Table 1). MACDP data for 1968–1970 and 1989–1991 reveal important trends (Table 2).

BDMP data indicate that the four birth defects with the largest mean annual percentage declines in 1970–1991 were anencephalus, spina bifida without anencephalus, anophthalmos/ microphthalmos, and Rh hemolytic disease. According to the MACDP, the four birth defects with the largest declines in 1968–1991 were anencephalus, spina bifida without anencephalus, hydrocephalus without spina bifida, and clubfoot without central nervous system (CNS) defects. Both reporting systems found that the two central nervous system defects, anencephalus and spina bifida without anencephalus, declined substantially; anencephalus declined the most, averaging approximately 7% per year, whereas spina bifida declined a mean of 3%–5% per year. BDMP data reveal that the prevalence of combined anophthalmos and microphthalmos

declined an average of 1.8% per year from 1970 to 1991, but virtually all of the decrease occurred before 1975. According to the BDMP, Rh hemolytic disease of the newborn declined on average approximately 6% per year between 1970 and 1991 (Table 1), and almost all of the decline occurred before 1980. MACDP data indicate that the prevalence of hydrocephalus declined a mean of 2.6% and the prevalence of clubfoot without CNS defects fell a mean 3.5% per year (Table 2).

The four birth defects with the largest increases in prevalence in 1970–1991 were endocardial cushion defect, patent ductus arteriosus, pulmonary artery anomaly, and lung agenesis and hypoplasia, according to BDMP data. In comparison, MACDP findings indicate that the four birth defects with the largest increases in prevalence in 1968–1991 were atrial septal defect, endocardial cushion defect, patent ductus arteriosus, and pulmonary artery anomaly. Three of these birth defects are common to both reporting systems: endocardial cushion defect, patent ductus arteriosus, and pulmonary artery anomaly. Atrial septal defect, another cardiovascular defect, was among the four birth defects with the largest increases, according to MACDP data, and it also increased by a substantial 8.9% according to the BDMP findings. These data clearly show that birth defects with the largest increases in prevalence over these two periods are concentrated in the cardiovascular organ system (Tables 1 and 2).

TABLE 1. Reported prevalence of selected birth defects and mean annual percentage change in prevalence — Birth Defects Monitoring Program, 1970–1991*

Birth defect	Rate			Mean annual percentage change
	1970–1991	1970–1971	1990–1991	
CNS				
Anencephalus	3.6	5.48	1.19	−7.4
Spina bifida without anencephalus	5.4	7.55	4.31	−2.8
Hydrocephalus without spina bifida	4.9	4.81	5.01	0.2
Encephalocele	1.2	1.20	0.88	−1.5
Eye				
Anophthalmos/microphthalmos	0.7	0.97	0.67	−1.8
Congenital cataract	0.8	0.64	1.09	2.7

TABLE 1. Reported prevalence of selected birth defects and mean annual percentage change in prevalence — Birth Defects Monitoring Program, 1970–1991* — continued

Birth defect	Rate			Mean annual percentage change
	1970–1991	1970–1971	1990–1991	
Cardiovascular				
Common truncus	0.3	0.28	0.40	1.8
Transposition of great arteries	1.1	0.76	2.23	5.5
Tetralogy of Fallot	1.0	0.57	2.49	7.7
Ventricular septal defect	12.1	4.45	23.78	8.7
Atrial septal defect	2.5	1.91	10.48	8.9
Endocardial cushion defect	0.5	0.08	1.40	15.4
Patent ductus arteriosus	20.2	3.96	52.10	13.8
Coarctation of aorta	0.7	0.42	1.46	6.4
Pulmonary artery anomaly	1.3	0.38	3.52	11.8
Respiratory				
Lung agenesis and hypoplasia	1.9	0.17	3.71	16.7
Orofacial				
Cleft palate without cleft lip	5.2	5.05	5.32	0.3
Cleft lip with or without cleft palate	9.1	9.91	8.54	−0.7
Gastrointestinal				
Tracheoesophageal anomalies	1.9	1.67	2.60	2.2
Rectal and intestinal atresia	3.5	3.75	3.72	−0.0
Genitourinary				
Renal agenesis and dysgenesis	1.4	0.71	2.54	6.6
Bladder exstrophy	0.3	0.35	0.29	−0.9
Musculoskeletal				
Clubfoot without CNS defects	25.5	27.49	23.85	−0.7
Limb reduction deformity	3.5	3.16	3.69	0.8
Chromosomal				
Down's syndrome	8.3	8.17	9.93	1.0
Other				
Rh hemolytic disease	20.6	42.28	12.01	−6.1
Number of births	17,736,971	1,730,257	816,496	

* Rates per 10,000 total births.

TABLE 2. Reported prevalence of selected birth defects and mean annual percentage change in prevalence — Metropolitan Atlanta Congenital Defects Program, 1968–1991*

Birth defect	Rate			Mean annual percentage change
	1968–1991	1968–1970	1989–1991	
CNS				
Anencephalus	5.0	9.69	2.26	−6.7
Spina bifida without anencephalus	7.2	11.96	4.26	−4.8
Hydrocephalus without spina bifida	8.2	10.05	5.73	−2.6
Encephalocele	1.9	1.56	1.22	−1.2
Eye				
Anophthalmos microphthalmos	3.4	2.39	3.04	1.2
Congenital cataract	2.1	0.72	1.74	4.3
Cardiovascular				
Common truncus	0.8	0.48	0.78	2.3
Transposition of great arteries	4.3	3.47	3.91	0.6
Tetralogy of Fallot	3.4	2.51	4.34	2.6
Ventricular septal defect	21.1	12.08	26.15	3.7
Atrial septal defect	19.4	5.26	41.53	10.3
Endocardial cushion defect	3.0	1.56	4.00	4.6
Patent ductus arteriosus	44.6	10.89	39.79	6.4
Coarctation of aorta	3.9	3.47	4.69	1.4
Pulmonary artery anomaly	5.1	1.44	9.21	9.2
Respiratory				
Lung agenesis and hypoplasia	5.1	2.63	4.69	2.8
Orofacial				
Cleft palate without cleft lip	5.4	3.95	4.78	0.9
Cleft lip with or without cleft palate	10.4	10.53	9.12	−0.7
Gastrointestinal				
Tracheoesophageal anomalies	2.2	2.03	1.74	−0.7
Rectal and intestinal atresia	4.0	4.78	3.91	−1.0
Genitourinary				
Renal agenesis and dysgenesis	3.3	2.27	3.65	2.3
Bladder exstrophy	0.3	0.24	0.17	−1.6
Musculoskeletal				
Clubfoot without CNS defects	27.7	32.78	14.33	−3.5
Limb reduction deformity	5.5	7.54	4.60	−2.3

TABLE 2. Reported prevalence of selected birth defects and mean annual percentage change in prevalence — Metropolitan Atlanta Congenital Defects Program, 1968–1991* — continued

Birth defect	Rate			Mean annual percentage change
	1968–1991	1968–1970	1989–1991	
Chromosomal				
Down's syndrome	10.0	8.85	10.95	1.0
Number of births	**696,057**	**83,599**	**115,105**	

* Rates per 10,000 live births.

According to the BDMP, the prevalence of lung agenesis and hypoplasia rose 6.6% per year on average.

Geographic differences in the prevalence of birth defects were evaluated by using data for 1970–1987. Because of the rarity of these conditions, the data had to be smoothed by aggregating groups of counties. The groups were aggregated by superimposing a grid of squares—each representing approximately 40 miles per side—over a U.S. map (Figures 2 and 3). Data from counties whose population centers fell within the same square were combined, resulting in greater stability of prevalence estimates. After indirect adjustment for the year of birth and race, the observed and expected numbers of cases within each square were compared for statistically significant differences under the Poisson assumption. The two birth defects with the most striking geographic clustering were anencephalus and spina bifida without anencephalus, both of which tended to occur more frequently in the eastern part of the country in a band roughly corresponding with the Appalachian mountain region. The clustering of high-prevalence squares in this area was particularly striking for spina bifida without anencephalus. Concomitantly, most of the significantly low-prevalence squares for these birth defects were located in the western states.

The prevalence of many birth defects vary markedly according to race (Table 3). Rates of almost all CNS defects were lowest for Asians, with the exception of anencephalus rates, which were lowest for blacks. Hispanics had the highest rates of anencephalus and spina bifida without anencephalus, whereas Native Americans had the highest prevalence of hydrocephalus and encephalocele. Compared with other races, Asians were at a decreased risk of the two eye birth defects—anophthalmos/microphthalmos and congenital cataract. Hispanics had the lowest rates of all but three of the nine cardiovascular defects followed; and, among these three conditions, only coarctation of the aorta showed a substantial elevation. For the two orofacial defects, rates were lowest for blacks and highest for Native Americans. Native Americans had the highest rates of the two genitourinary defects—renal agenesis/dysgenesis and bladder exstrophy—whereas Asians had the lowest rates.

The strong relationship between Down's syndrome and maternal age is reflected by MACDP data for 1968–1991 (Table 4). The age-specific rates began to increase substantially after the age of 29 years and attained levels in the range of 1%–2% for women >40 years of age.

INTERPRETATION ISSUES

The diagnosis and reporting of birth defects is rarely perfect, and problems of sensitivity and specificity of ascertainment abound. Thus, completeness and accuracy of birth defects reporting must be considered in the interpretation of nominal rates. For example, the birth prevalences of externally apparent malformations such as

FIGURE 2.

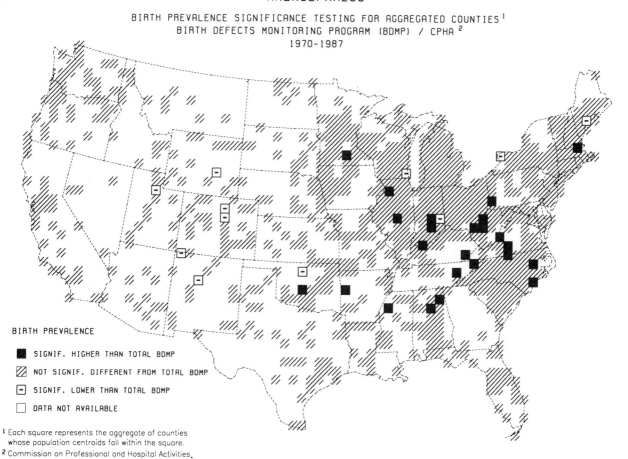

ANENCEPHALUS

BIRTH PREVALENCE SIGNIFICANCE TESTING FOR AGGREGATED COUNTIES [1]
BIRTH DEFECTS MONITORING PROGRAM (BDMP) / CPHA [2]
1970-1987

BIRTH PREVALENCE

■ SIGNIF. HIGHER THAN TOTAL BDMP

▨ NOT SIGNIF. DIFFERENT FROM TOTAL BDMP

⊡ SIGNIF. LOWER THAN TOTAL BDMP

☐ DATA NOT AVAILABLE

[1] Each square represents the aggregate of counties
whose population centroids fall within the square.
[2] Commission on Professional and Hospital Activities.

anencephalus, spina bifida, and cleft lip are more secure than those for birth defects of the cardio-vascular system, which may not be manifest during the newborn period or which require sophisticated techniques for diagnosis. In addition, birth defects reporting through the MACDP, which uses multiple ascertainment methods, is more complete than reporting through the BDMP, which relies on passive reporting of newborn hospital discharge diagnoses. Often the more relevant occurrence statistic is the change in prevalence over time or geographic-based differences in birth defects rates. Even though the absolute levels in reported prevalence may be highly questionable in certain instances, we may judge that changes or differences in rates are fairly reliable.

The finding that maternal intake of folic acid decreases the risk of anencephalus and spina

bifida (3–6) suggests that increasingly better nutrition during the past two decades has contributed to the decline in prevalence of these neural tube defects. Although the increasing use of prenatal diagnosis and pregnancy termination may have introduced a downward bias in the birth prevalences of anencephalus and spina bifida, the decline in reported prevalence began, in the 1980s, before these procedures were used significantly. The halving of the prevalence of combined anophthalmos and microphthalmos between 1970 and 1976, followed by subsequent stability of rates, is striking, but we have no explanation for this pattern of rates. An explanation for the marked decline in the prevalence of Rh hemolytic disease is easy to find—the introduction of Rh immunoglobulin in the late 1960s was the undoubted preventive agent. We have no good explanations for

FIGURE 3.

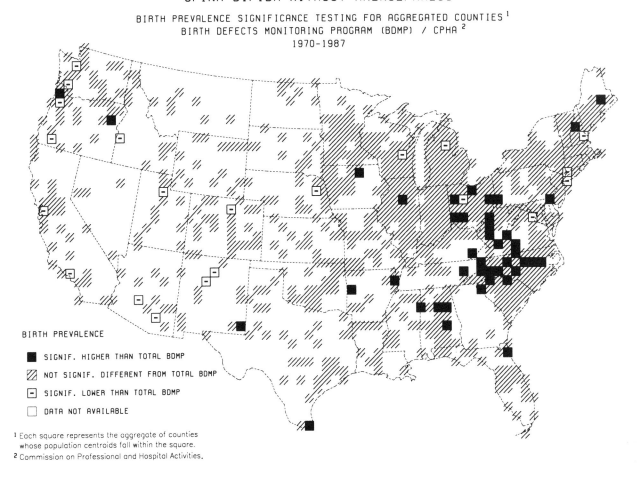

SPINA BIFIDA WITHOUT ANENCEPHALUS

BIRTH PREVALENCE SIGNIFICANCE TESTING FOR AGGREGATED COUNTIES [1]
BIRTH DEFECTS MONITORING PROGRAM (BDMP) / CPHA [2]
1970-1987

BIRTH PREVALENCE

■ SIGNIF. HIGHER THAN TOTAL BDMP

▨ NOT SIGNIF. DIFFERENT FROM TOTAL BDMP

⊟ SIGNIF. LOWER THAN TOTAL BDMP

☐ DATA NOT AVAILABLE

[1] Each square represents the aggregate of counties
whose population centroids fall within the square.
[2] Commission on Professional and Hospital Activities.

**TABLE 3. Prevalence of selected birth defects, by race, and race-specific rate ratios — Birth Defects
Monitoring Program, 1981–1991***

Birth Defect	White		Black		Hispanic		Asian		Native American	
	Rate	Ratio	Rate	Ratio	Rate	Ratio	Rate	Ratio	Rate	Ratio
CNS										
Anencephalus	2.6	1.36	*1.9*	*1.00*	**3.7**	**1.95**	3.5	1.84	2.8	1.49
Spina bifida without anencephalus	4.8	3.49	3.4	2.49	**5.2**	**3.78**	*1.4*	*1.00*	4.0	2.90
Hydrocephalus without spina bifida	5.4	1.37	8.4	2.13	4.5	1.14	*4.0*	*1.00*	**11.7**	**2.95**
Encephalocele	1.0	1.04	1.1	1.14	1.3	1.27	*1.0*	*1.00*	**4.0**	**4.06**
Eye										
Anophthalmos microphthalmos	0.8	1.54	0.9	1.80	0.6	1.16	*0.5*	*1.00*	**2.0**	**4.06**
Congenital cataract	1.0	2.06	**1.5**	**2.96**	0.8	1.59	*0.5*	*1.00*	0.8	1.63

TABLE 3. Prevalence of selected birth defects, by race, and race-specific rate ratios — Birth Defects Monitoring Program, 1981–1991* — continued

Birth Defect	White Rate	White Ratio	Black Rate	Black Ratio	Hispanic Rate	Hispanic Ratio	Asian Rate	Asian Ratio	Native American Rate	Native American Ratio
Cardiovascular										
Common truncus	0.3	1.67	0.3	1.37	*0.2*	*1.00*	**0.4**	**2.16**	0.0	0.00
Transposition of great arteries	1.4	1.79	*0.8*	*1.00*	0.9	1.11	1.0	1.27	**1.6**	**2.07**
Tetralogy of Fallot	1.4	1.35	1.3	1.28	*1.0*	*1.00*	**1.8**	**1.70**	1.6	1.54
Ventricular septal defect	19.1	1.28	15.7	1.05	*15.0*	*1.00*	**19.9**	**1.33**	18.9	1.26
Atrial septal defect	3.7	1.73	4.4	2.06	*2.1*	*1.00*	6.3	2.01	**5.2**	**2.47**
Endocardial cushion defect	0.9	1.09	0.9	1.10	*0.8*	*1.00*	1.0	1.22	**1.6**	**1.98**
Patent ductus arteriosus	31.2	1.19	**58.9**	**2.24**	*26.2*	*1.00*	31.8	1.21	41.9	1.60
Coarctation of aorta	0.9	2.39	0.8	2.05	0.9	2.25	*0.4*	*1.00*	**1.2**	**3.05**
Pulmonary artery anomaly	1.7	1.04	**5.6**	**3.50**	1.8	1.14	2.2	1.35	*1.6*	*1.00*
Respiratory										
Lung agenesis and hypoplasia	3.3	1.36	3.4	1.38	*2.5*	*1.00*	3.1	1.25	**4.8**	**1.96**
Orofacial										
Cleft palate without cleft lip	5.8	1.56	*3.7*	*1.00*	4.4	1.18	5.2	1.38	**8.5**	**2.27**
Cleft lip with or without cleft palate	9.6	2.17	*4.4*	*1.00*	8.8	1.97	12.0	2.71	**16.9**	**3.82**
Gastrointestinal										
Tracheoesophageal anomalies	**2.5**	**1.91**	*1.3*	*1.00*	1.9	1.50	1.5	1.15	2.0	1.56
Rectal and intestinal atresia	3.7	1.28	3.0	1.01	*2.9*	*1.00*	3.6	1.22	**5.2**	**1.78**
Genitourinary										
Renal agenesis and dysgenesis	2.1	2.39	1.5	1.72	1.7	1.94	*0.9*	*1.00*	**2.4**	**2.71**
Bladder exstrophy	0.3	3.32	0.2	1.62	0.2	1.59	*0.1*	*1.00*	**0.8**	**8.13**
Musculoskeletal										
Clubfoot without CNS defects	**26.9**	**1.91**	19.4	1.38	19.7	1.40	*14.1*	*1.00*	14.5	1.03
Limb reduction deformity	**3.8**	**1.91**	3.7	1.83	3.2	1.60	2.8	1.38	*2.0*	*1.00*
Chromosomal										
Down syndrome	8.9	1.29	*6.9*	*1.00*	11.7	1.70	**11.8**	**1.72**	8.9	1.29
Other										
Rh hemolytic disease	15.3	3.36	13.8	3.02	**19.1**	**4.18**	*4.6*	*1.00*	10.9	2.39
Number of births	4.887.008		872.816		381.603		100.882		24.821	

* Rates per 10,000 total births. Rates are computed with respect to the smallest race-specific rate greater than zero (italics). Maximum rate ratios for each defect are shown in boldface type.

**TABLE 4. Prevalence of Down's syndrome, by maternal age —
Metropolitan Atlanta Congenital Defects Program, 1968–1991***

Maternal age (years)	No. cases	No. births	Rate
<20	81	112,112	7.2
20–24	138	206,003	6.7
25–29	159	210,276	7.6
30–34	176	122,902	14.3
35–39	89	38,120	23.3
40–44	49	5,436	90.1
45+	5	223	224.2
Unknown	6	985	60.9
Total, all ages	703	696,057	10.1

* Rates per 10,000 live births.

declines in the occurrence of hydrocephalus and clubfoot, but physicians' tightening of the diagnostic criteria for these conditions during this period may have contributed to these reductions. Substantial increases in the occurrence of most cardiovascular malformations raise the question of whether these increases may have been related to improvements in case ascertainment. Technological advances in diagnostic techniques, such as in the field of echocardiography, are likely responsible for some portion of these increases. In addition, better survival of affected infants over time increases the probability of a diagnosis being made. However, it would be premature to discount the existence of underlying true increases in the occurrences of these defects. Increases in the prevalence of lung agenesis and hypoplasia between 1970 and 1991 can be attributed partly to 1974 and 1979 coding changes that included additional conditions in this diagnostic category. Continued increases after 1979, however, point to other unknown factors that influence the rates.

The decreasing prevalence of spina bifida from eastern to western states (Figure 3) is consistent with the finding by Hewitt of a similar gradient in infant mortality caused by this birth defect (7). Given the embryologic connection between anencephalus and spina bifida, it is not surprising that anencephalus has a similar geographic gradient in prevalence, although not quite as striking. Whether these patterns of rates are related to genetic or environmental factors is not known.

Given the previously mentioned finding that dietary folic acid reduces the risk of these neural tube defects, nutritional differences associated with geography quite possibly may play a role.

The variations in birth defect occurrence according to race could result from differences in risk-related exposures or to race-specific susceptibility (Table 3). We now lack the data needed to judge which of these two possibilities are operative for particular birth defects. We may reasonably surmise that, at least for some defects, both factors could have contributed to the observed differences.

The increased risk of Down's syndrome among women over the age of 30 years has been long recognized. These data underscore the need for increased awareness of this risk among the relevant population and the availability of prenatal testing procedures for detecting affected fetuses.

EXAMPLES OF USING DATA

Birth defects surveillance systems provide current and baseline data that allow investigators to monitor changes in the prevalence of specific malformations on a national or local level. Exploring the occurrence patterns of these birth defects can generate etiologic hypotheses, descriptive epidemiologic studies, follow-up studies, family studies, case-control studies, and cluster investigations.

As a national, hospital-based system, the BDMP has provided researchers, policymakers, and the lay public with time- and place-specific prevalence data. These data have helped to dispel unwarranted concerns about the possibility of increased birth defects risks in a particular area. They have also generated investigations of seemingly unexplained increases in birth defects occurrence. The ability to evaluate geographic differences in rates is especially important in areas that do not have a local birth defects surveillance system. Public health officials can often use this information to help them make decisions and establish policies.

The MACDP is an intensive, population-based system that has served as a prototype for other state and local birth defects surveillance systems. Consistent and systematic surveillance procedures—which include detailed coding, uniform variables, and standard data collection methods—have been developed and enhanced through MACDP and have facilitated collaborative birth defects studies across the country.

Birth defects registries can also help to identify children who may be eligible for special programs or services. This role can lead to the expansion of surveillance programs to incorporate prevention, intervention, and evaluation components into their systems.

FUTURE ISSUES

During the next decade we can expect to see tremendous increases in the ability to make prenatal diagnoses of birth defects. This change in capability will necessitate changes in the methods and data sources used for birth defects surveillance.

Over the past two decades, chromosomal analysis of amniotic fluid cells has become widely available for pregnant women aged 35 years and older, primarily because these women are at increased risk of having a fetus affected by Down's syndrome. Alpha-fetoprotein screening of maternal serum is also widely used, mainly to detect fetuses affected by neural tube defects. More recently, prenatal diagnoses of neural tube defects and other types of malformations have been made by fetal ultrasonographic examination. As prenatal ultrasonography becomes more commonly used, and as instrumentation and techniques improve, we can expect to see a greater proportion and variety of malformations diagnosed prenatally. Advances in the analysis of DNA (i.e., the new genetics) should also increase the numbers of prenatally diagnosed congenital malformations.

Many women who discover that they are carrying a fetus with a defect elect to have their pregnancy terminated. Most current birth defects surveillance programs, including the MACDP and the BDMP, make use of records created in hospitals at the time of birth. Understanding variations observed in the frequency of birth defects at birth will increasingly require a knowledge of the effects of pregnancy terminations that are done as the result of prenatal diagnoses of birth defects.

Methods of collecting birth defects data will also need to change to adapt to revisions in hospital data processing methods. The BDMP was started at a time when, for convenience and economical reasons, small- and medium-sized hospitals had computer service organizations handle their data processing. The advent of more accessible and affordable data processing equipment has reduced the number of hospitals that use these organizations. Therefore, the CPHA, the source of BDMP hospital discharge abstract data, no longer services the large number of hospitals that it once did, and the number of hospitals available for the BDMP has dropped from 1,264 in 1974 to 464 in 1991.

These changes will force us to seek new sources of data. We hope that the much discussed healthcare reform brings changes that will improve our prospects for having more accessible data for national birth defects surveillance and thus, for achieving our year 2000 goals to reduce the prevalence of birth defects (for details about these objectives, see the State Use of Birth Defects Surveillance chapter).

REFERENCES

1. Edmonds LD, Layde PM, James LM, Flynt JW Jr, Erickson JD, Oakley GP Jr. Congenital malformation surveillance: two American systems. Int J Epidemiol 1981;10:247–52.

2. Public Health Service. International classification of diseases, ninth revision, clinical modification. US Department of Health and Human Services, Health Care Financing Administration, 1991. DHHS publication no. (DHS)91-1260.

3. CDC. Use of folic acid for prevention of spina bifida and other neural tube defects—1983–1991. MMWR 1991;40:513–5.

4. Milunksy A, Jick H, Jick SS, et al. Multivitamins/folic acid supplementation in early pregnancy reduces the prevalence of neural tube defects. JAMA 1989; 262:2847–52.

5. Wald N, Sneddon J, Densem J, Frost C, Stone R. Prevention of neural tube defects: results of the Medical Research Council Vitamin Study. Lancet 1991; 338:131–7.

6. Mulinare J, Cordero JF, Erickson JD, Berry RJ. Periconceptional use of multivitamins and the occurrence of neural tube defects. JAMA 1988;260:3141–5.

7. Hewitt D. Geographical variations in the mortality attributed to spina bifida and other congenital malformations. Br J Prev Soc Med 1963;17:13–22.

State Use of Birth Defects Surveillance

Michele C. Lynberg, Ph.D., M.P.H.,[1] and Larry D. Edmonds, M.S.P.H.[1]

PUBLIC HEALTH IMPORTANCE

Birth defects are the leading cause of infant mortality in the United States, accounting for >21% of all infant deaths in 1991 (Figure 1) (1). In addition, birth defects are the fifth leading cause of years of potential life lost (2), and they contribute substantially to childhood morbidity and long-term disability. Major birth defects are diagnosed for 3%–4% of infants in their first year of life. Of the 100,000–150,000 infants born with a major birth defect each year (3), approximately 6,000 die during their first 28 days of life, and another 2,000 die before reaching their first birthday. The remaining 92,000–142,000 children who survived beyond the age of 1 year are affected by birth defects to various degrees.

Each year about 1.2 million infants, children, and adults are hospitalized for treatment of birth defects; children with birth defects account for approximately 25%–30% of pediatric admissions (4). Total costs for the care of children with birth defects exceed $1.4 billion annually (5). The continuum of care includes diagnostic and treatment services, education, vocational training, and custodial care. The cost for this care pales in comparison to the loss of creativity and earning power of individuals with handicapping conditions.

Much remains to be learned about the etiology of birth defects. Although several human teratogens have been identified, two thirds of birth defects are of unknown causes (6). One area where substantial progress may be made is the use of folic acid consumption to reduce the number of cases of spina bifida and other neural tube defects (NTDs). The Public Health Service estimates that as many as 50% of cases of spina bifida and other NTDs could be reduced if women

of childbearing age would consume 0.4 mg of folic acid daily (7). This is an important prevention opportunity in public health. Other types of birth defects that are entirely preventable include fetal alcohol syndrome, congenital rubella, and isotretinoin embryopathy.

Much work is being done to classify infants with birth defects according to biologically meaningful categories that would be useful in identifying etiologic and pathogenetic mechanisms. This improved classification is critical to our continued progress in understanding and preventing birth defects.

The basic definition of a birth defect is a structural abnormality present at birth; most but not all such defects are included within codes 740.0–759.9 of the *International Classification of Diseases, Ninth Revision, Clinical Modification* (8). These conditions include a heterogenous group of outcomes, each with a different morphogenesis: 1) malformations such as clefts and congenital heart defects, which involve poor tissue formation; 2) deformations such as clubfeet and congenital hip dislocations, which involve unusual forces on normal tissue; and 3) disruptions such as amniotic bands and gastroschisis, which involve the breakdown of normal tissue.

Birth defects are also classified by underlying etiologic or pathogenetic mechanisms including chromosomal aberrations, single-gene (Mendelian) disorders, and sequences (multiple defects that are related to a single problem in morphogenesis).

[1] Division of Birth Defects and Developmental Disabilities
National Center for Environmental Health
Centers for Disease Control and Prevention
Atlanta, Georgia

FIGURE 1. Leading causes of infant mortality — United States, 1991

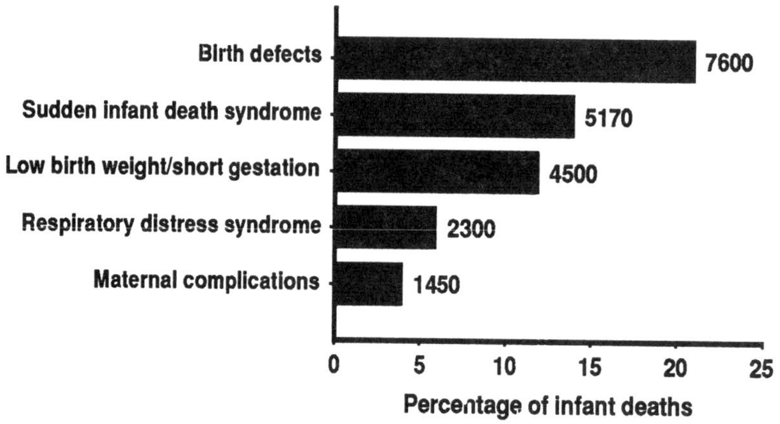

Additionally, birth defects can be classified as major or minor. Major birth defects are those that affect survival, require substantial medical care, or result in marked physiologic or psychologic impairment.

Most birth defects occur as isolated defects. In about 20%–30% of affected infants, however, multiple defects are involved. If two or more defects affect an infant, they are considered to be multiple if they occur in different organ systems or body sites, are not part of a known embryological sequence, and do not have a common primary defect.

Surveillance is a critical component in the effort to further reduce the impact of birth defects on public health. Surveillance is necessary to detect the occurrence of birth defects, to investigate potential etiologic agents, to plan and evaluate the effects of interventions, and to ensure appropriate care for persons in need of services (for additional information about related topics and surveillance activities, see the Prevalence of Birth Defects, Infant Mortality, and Neonatal and Postneonatal Mortality chapters).

HISTORY OF DATA COLLECTION

The earliest legislation requiring the reporting of birth defects in the United States was passed in New Jersey in 1926. Widespread interest in birth defects surveillance, however, was not generated until the early 1960s, where an epidemic of limb reduction deformities was associated with the prenatal use of thalidomide. Few specific causes of birth defects were known, and the epidemiologic patterns of several malformations suggested that unidentified teratogens were important in the etiology of major congenital malformations. Initially, birth defects surveillance systems were designed to monitor secular trends, especially patterns that might suggest environmental causes of birth defects. More recently, innovative, multipurpose systems have integrated traditional monitoring functions with new epidemiologic approaches and service-oriented objectives. Interest in birth defects surveillance has continued to grow, with programs currently monitoring outcomes at the state, national, and international levels.

CDC SURVEILLANCE ACTIVITIES

Twenty-eight states have established a plan to establish birth defects surveillance systems (Table 1). In 1992, seven states had surveillance systems that used active case ascertainment, providing information on approximately 700,000 births—19% of the U.S. births that year. Many of these state surveillance programs are modeled after the prototype surveillance system, CDC's Metropolitan Atlanta Congenital Defects Program (MACDP) (see the Prevalence of Birth Defects chapter for details about MACDP).

An additional 16 states had passive case-ascertainment surveillance systems, which provided information on 1,090,000 births (29% of

TABLE 1. State birth defects surveillance systems

State	Coverage	Legislation	Type of ascertainment
Alabama	None		None
Alaska	None		None
Arizona	Statewide	Yes	Active
Arkansas	Covers about one third of births	Yes	Active
California	Selected areas of state	Yes	Active
Colorado	Statewide	Yes	Passive
Connecticut	Statewide—inactive due to lack of funds	Planned	Passive—inactive due to lack of funds
Delaware	None		None
District of Columbia	None		None
Florida	None		None
Georgia	Five-county metropolitan Atlanta area		Active
Hawaii	Statewide	Yes	Active
Idaho	None		None
Illinois	Statewide	Yes	Passive
Indiana	Statewide	Yes	Passive
Iowa	Statewide	Yes	Active
Kansas	Statewide	Yes	Passive
Kentucky	Statewide—developing	Yes	Passive
Louisiana	None		None
Maine	Statewide—inactive due to lack of funds		Passive—inactive due to lack of funds
Maryland	Statewide	Yes	Passive
Massachusetts	Statewide—developing	Planned	Passive
Michigan	Statewide	Yes	Passive
Minnesota	None		None
Mississippi	None		None
Missouri	Statewide (up to 1988)		Passive
Montana	None		None
Nebraska	Statewide	Yes	Passive
Nevada	None		None
New Hampshire	None		None
New Jersey	Statewide	Yes	Passive
New Mexico	None		None
New York	Statewide	Yes	Passive
North Carolina	Statewide		Passive

TABLE 1. State birth defects surveillance systems — continued

State	Coverage	Legislation	Type of ascertainment
North Dakota	None		None
Ohio	None		None
Oklahoma	Pilot in part of state	Yes	Active
Oregon	None		None
Pennsylvania	None	Planned	None
Rhode Island	None		None
South Carolina	None		None
South Dakota	None		None
Tennessee	None		None
Texas	Developing in part of state	Yes	Active
Utah	Statewide	Planned	Passive
Vermont	None		None
Virginia	Statewide	Yes	Passive
Washington	Statewide	Yes	Passive
West Virginia	Statewide	Yes	Passive
Wisconsin	Statewide	Yes	Passive
Wyoming	None		None

the births in the United States), and one state had a system that was based on a supplement to vital records and provided information on 45,000 births. Examples of these passive case-ascertainment systems include systems created by legislative mandates for hospitals or physicians to report the occurrence of birth defects (such systems are now required in New York, New Jersey, and Nebraska); systems created by linkage of multiple data sources (such systems are used in Missouri and North Carolina); and systems that are based on vital statistics data (the Indiana Birth Problems Registry is one such system). Another five states are developing or planning to reactivate birth defects surveillance systems.

GENERAL FINDINGS

Because individual birth defects are rare, researchers have had difficulty obtaining enough cases for etiologic studies. The Birth Defects Monitoring Program (BDMP) provides some limited national data on the occurrence of birth defects.

Because the number of hospitals participating in BDMP continues to decline each year, CDC researchers are investigating new avenues for national birth defects surveillance, including collaboration among state birth defects monitoring programs. Such collaboration substantially increases researchers' power to study relatively rare birth defects, greatly enhancing our understanding of the occurrence and etiology of birth defects. Data from population-based state systems are an important source of information on the prevalence of birth defects, providing a more representative view than the nonrandom sample provided by BDMP (see the Prevalence of Birth Defects chapter).

For example, in a recent study of the incidence and descriptive epidemiology of spina bifida, CDC fostered the collaboration of 16 states (representing 23.5% of the U.S. population) with population-based birth defects surveillance systems (9). Through this cooperative effort, we were able to determine that spina bifida incidence declined from 5.9 per 10,000 births in 1993 to 3.2 cases per 10,000 births in 1990. State-specific rates varied substantially (range: 3.0 [Washington] to 7.8 [Arkansas]). Spina bifida rates also varied among racial and ethnic groups, being lowest among Asians and Pacific Islanders (2.3) and highest among Hispanics (6.0). The rate among Hispanics, however, declined substantially from 1983 to 1990, and the rate among blacks has remained stable since 1984. Consequently, spina bifida rates among whites, blacks, and Hispanics were nearly identical in 1990.

This collaboration—the first effort among multiple state systems to characterize the incidence of a major preventable birth defect—represents a new direction in birth defects surveillance and epidemiology. More state birth defects surveillance programs are needed in the continued effort to improve knowledge and understanding of birth defects and to further the ability to intervene and prevent this important public health problem.

INTERPRETATION ISSUES

The objective of collecting birth defects surveillance data is to characterize, as well as possible, the birth defects prevalence in a population, using available resources. In the ideal birth defects surveillance system, population-based information is reported in a timely manner. The timely recognition of a birth defect **epidemic**, such as that resulting from the introduction of a new teratogen, depends on rapid reporting of accurate data on the occurrence of birth defects. Timeliness is also important in the identification of children for early intervention programs to prevent secondary disabilities.

Case Ascertainment

To minimize underreporting, case ascertainment should be comprehensive and should usually require a review of data from multiple sources. The inclusion of personal identifiers facilitates follow-up studies and allows investigators to link infant, maternal, and paternal records. To be effective, a birth defects surveillance system should include these characteristics:

- Accurate and precise diagnostic criteria.

- Etiologically and pathogenetically meaningful classification schemes.

- A large database, permitting rate comparison and analysis of trends in the birth prevalence of a relatively rare birth defect.

- The capability to analyze the occurrence of multiple malformations.

- The ability to conduct meaningful and timely analysis.

- A system to disseminate data in a timely manner.

- A mechanism to ensure confidentiality of patient records.

Capacity to Analyze Multiple Malformations

The ability to analyze the occurrence of multiple malformations is also important. Most known teratogens are associated with a spectrum of birth defect combinations. Many birth defects monitoring systems, however, examine trends in rates of single defects, not combinations of anomalies. In some instances, an increase in the rate of birth defects caused by a teratogen may be detected more rapidly by monitoring rates of defect combinations rather than rates of individual defects. The monitoring of multiple birth defects is most effective in instances in which infants exposed to a given teratogen tend to have specific combinations of defects.

Components of a Birth Defects Surveillance System

The components of a birth defects surveillance system include case definition and case ascertainment (including case sources and the method of surveillance used to ascertain cases) as well as data collection, analysis, follow-up, and dissemination.

Cases to be included in the birth defects surveillance system must be clearly defined. Is any birth in which the infant has even a minor birth defect considered a case, or are cases limited to births in which the infants have at least one major malformation? CDC and a number of state systems maintain a well-developed list of birth defects that are considered normal variants or minor malformations, which are excluded from the case definition.

Age ranges of infants and children who are eligible for inclusion must also be specified (e.g., the newborn period, birth to 1 year, birth to 6 years). In determining which cases may be included, researchers must consider available resources for data collection and management.

Multiple-source case ascertainment provides the best potential for complete case finding. Usual data sources for birth defects surveillance systems include vital records (birth and death certificates), newborn or other hospital discharge summaries, hospital records, and data from cytogenetic laboratories. Each of these sources has strengths and weaknesses.

The advantages of using vital records are that they provide complete coverage of the population as well as some medical and parental data. Vital records also are a relatively inexpensive resource, and they provide data from previous years as well as the potential for follow-up of birth defects cases. The weaknesses of using vital records include the lack of timeliness in reporting data, the underreporting of birth defects (information is often limited to that obtained during the newborn period), and the lack of specific data on most birth defects.

Hospital discharge summary data on newborns are extremely useful in surveillance because they provide a more complete record of birth defects than birth certificates do; they are usually available with 6 months of discharge; they are already computerized and in digital form in many hospitals; and they allow potential follow-up of birth defects cases. Weaknesses of using hospital discharge summary data include the lack of maternal data; the lack of access to personal identifiers, which makes follow-up difficult; frequent difficulty in defining the population base, and frequent difficulty in establishing the representativeness of data. In addition, birth defects information may be incompletely recorded, or the data may reflect an incomplete diagnosis in the newborn period.

The strengths of multiple-source case ascertainment are that the system can be quite rapid, it allows a relatively complete recording, and diagnoses are more precise and accurate. In addition, researchers can more readily conduct follow-up studies of cases, and maternal and infant information is available.

Weaknesses of multiple-source case ascertainment include the expense which often limits use of this method to small populations and the time needed to establish baseline data.

Depending on the methods and sources of case ascertainment used, surveillance systems produce substantially varying birth defects rates (Table 2), ranging as high as 830 per 10,000 births (10).

Determining what data to collect is an important aspect of birth defects surveillance. Optimally, data should include precise descriptions of all birth defects, including syndrome identification by geneticists or dysmorphologists, demographic data, pregnancy history and other birth-related data, cytogenetic and laboratory data, family history, and etiologic information. These data provide the basis for initiating further follow-up studies. CDC currently recommends that workers in state birth defects surveillance programs collect a set of core data items (see the Appendix, p. 226 [11]).

Monitoring and Dissemination

By monitoring birth defects surveillance data, researchers can detect differing birth defects rates in different areas as well as rate changes over time. They can monitor the data by statistically evaluating the difference between observed and expected numbers of specific defects or defect combinations for a specified time in a specified area. Expected numbers are obtained from baseline prevalence data. Such comparisons may lead to the identification of clusters of birth defects; subsequent investigation of such clusters may yield useful etiologic information.

Researchers often conduct monitoring quarterly so they can determine whether flagged defects are increasing or decreasing. Such reviews may lead to investigations about the nature of the changes.

TABLE 2. Birth defects rates* determined by various surveillance approaches

Method and Source	Rate
Birth certificates[†]	88.9
Newborn hospital discharge data[§]	282.5
Mandatory hospital reporting data[•]	248.0
Linked data sources[**]	336.0
Active hospital surveillance data[††]	415.0
Physical exam of infant[§§]	830.0

* Per 10.000 births.
[†] National Center for Health Statistics. CDC. 1982–1983.
[§] Birth Defects Monitoring Program. 1982–1985.
[•] Nebraska Birth Defects Registry. 1982–1985.
[**] Missouri Birth Defects Registry. 1980–1984.
[††] Metropolitan Atlanta Congenital Defects Program. 1982–1987.
[§§] Collaborative Perinatal Project. 1959–1966 (10).

Dissemination of data is another important component of a birth defects surveillance system. Routine compilation of rates, changing trends, and other findings are useful to health care providers and to state and local officials. Feedback is also helpful to physicians and hospital officials who support surveillance efforts by providing medical information.

EXAMPLES OF USING DATA

Surveillance systems have numerous functions that extend beyond searching for increases in the incidence of specific malformations to detect the introduction of new teratogens or increased exposure to old ones. They can be used to develop baseline data, provide timely rates, and identify geographic areas of concern for cluster investigations. Surveillance systems also provide the basis for both ecologic investigations and follow-up studies. By monitoring national and local birth defects rates, investigators can correlate changing trends with changes in cultural, social, or environmental factors.

Moreover, state birth defects surveillance systems are useful in identifying infants and children with birth defects. These case registries can be used for etiologic investigations, studies of economic impact, and follow-up studies to assess survival rates and the long-term effects of birth defects,

including the development of cancer. Registries developed from birth defects surveillance systems are also useful in testing hypotheses and in conducting descriptive epidemiologic studies of various malformations. Another possible role of birth defects surveillance is in the identification of children who need special education, social services, and other programs. The use of surveillance systems can also assist in the evaluation of programs and services, including those that use new prevention and intervention strategies, such as prenatal diagnosis and improved genetics counseling. Additionally, data from surveillance systems can be used to educate health professionals and community members about the extent of a particular problem and to respond to the public's health concerns about environmental agents.

The collaborative effort on spina bifida surveillance is one good example of how state-specific surveillance data can be used. Another example is BDMP, which has been useful in evaluating potential environmental teratogens in specific geographic areas. For example, a 1975 investigation of the association between vinyl chloride monomer and an increased incidence of central nervous system defects in West Virginia showed no relationship between exposure and outcome (12). In a 1978 evaluation of the effect of the massive swine-influenza vaccination, no association between vaccination and birth defects was found. In several descriptive studies, researchers have

223

used BDMP data to characterize cases according to geographic location, seasonal pattern, and race to identify populations and areas with high or low rates of particular defects. In addition, BDMP has been used as a source for both case and control subjects in various case-control studies. Researchers have also used the data to evaluate the effectiveness of surveillance in the National Congenital Rubella Syndrome Registry.

CDC's Birth Defects Risk Factor Surveillance Project is another example of how birth defects data can be used. This project, an additional component to the ongoing MACDP program, involves about 300 selected case subjects and 100 control subjects each year. Parental interviews are conducted to identify possible risk factors, and additional clinical and laboratory studies are performed to identify markers of exposure and susceptibility. In addition to implementing this program within MACDP, CDC has funded two cooperative agreements with state birth defects surveillance systems to begin establishing a population-based network of collaborative institutions that can conduct birth defects risk factor surveillance in addition to their ongoing surveillance activities. Collaboration between increasing numbers of state surveillance systems is critical to the success of birth defects epidemiology as well as intervention and prevention strategies.

FUTURE ISSUES

Organizing a System

The single most important activity in the planning process is to define the purposes of the program. The primary question is, "How will the data be used?" In the past, most monitoring efforts focused on the epidemiologic uses of the data. More recently developed programs have begun to apply surveillance data to service planning and evaluation, professional and community education, and advocacy. Ideally, both epidemiologic and service objectives can be met by a newly established system.

A key step in designing a birth defects surveillance system is to develop a coordinated and unified approach to mobilizing resources within a state. Such a plan, tied to documented local and state needs, will help garner support for the program. A number of state agencies—in the areas of maternal and child health, genetics, developmental disabilities, epidemiology, vital statistics, and environmental health—have an interest in surveillance. Other organizations that may have an interest include university medical schools, voluntary agencies, advocacy groups, and the state legislature. Identifying potentially interested agencies and participants will facilitate the coordination of their efforts and also help establish a broad base of political and financial support. An advisory group can be helpful in obtaining community support and cooperation and in providing technical consultation.

Funding is a major determinant of the size and scope of a surveillance system. In most cases, creative funding approaches will be needed. States cannot count on obtaining funds from federal programs but must instead develop a base within the state for long-term support. In some cases, funding for systems can be underwritten by other programs in the health department that have peripheral interests in birth defects. A few states have obtained support from foundations, pharmaceutical companies, and universities, whereas others have obtained funding by linking the program to environmental issues. Other potential sources of funds within a state might come from the department of education, department of maternal and child health, department of environmental health, or developmental disabilities councils. In addition to state appropriations, other potential funding sources include Maternal and Child Health block grants and federal grants such as Special Projects of Regional and National Significance grants and grants from the National Institute of Child Health and Human Development and CDC.

Legislation

Before 1981, only Nebraska and New Jersey had legislation that required the reporting of birth defects to the state health department. Since 1981, 19 additional states have passed laws requiring the reporting of birth defects (Table 1). Four states have either pending or proposed legislation. Both the comprehensiveness and specificity of legislation in the various states differ substantially.

State planners should explore potential benefits and limitations of legislation early in the program development phase. Although legislation is not essential to the development and operation of a surveillance system, it can facilitate surveillance by providing 1) the authority and language to enforce rules and regulations regarding surveillance; 2) the authority to collect data for epidemiologic purposes or for case tracking, service provision, or follow-up; 3) a mandate for hospitals, physicians, and other providers to report birth defects; 4) specification of conditions and ages to be covered; 5) a means to access data on an individual patient while ensuring confidentiality; 6) designation of an organization to operate the surveillance activities; and 7) provisions for initial and continued funding. Each of these factors should be considered in drafting and introducing the legislation, because the mere omission or understatement of any single component may impede the full development of the surveillance system. For example, four states found their laws to be barriers because they were not specific enough in defining outcomes to be surveyed, and they did not provide the surveillance programs with enough authority to access data.

Researchers should draft birth defects surveillance legislation with a specific intent in mind and ensure that this intent is incorporated into the legislation. The legislation should define the purposes for which surveillance activities are undertaken such as epidemiologic surveillance, service provision, or both. This will also help states define outcomes and ages to be covered and the most important sources of data to be included.

For case-finding sources other than vital records, the legislation must provide surveillance systems with authority to require reporting, make available hospital discharge data, or allow a review of medical records. Legislation that allows access to hospital records provides surveillance systems with an opportunity to obtain more complete and reliable reporting of birth defects. Mandating reporting from various types of service providers ensures that the health community participates in the surveillance and that available malformation data sets are large enough to be useful.

Legislation that provides explicit authority and designates specific surveillance system functions decreases the need for continual interpretation of some broad authority to justify actions. The responsibility for enacting rules and regulations for reporting, determining reportable conditions, and developing and implementing reporting procedures must belong to the state health department and not be detailed in the legislation.

Surveillance systems often have a mandate to conduct various activities, including etiologic research, planning, evaluation, education, and service provision. Each of these activities requires the use of data on individual patients. Although confidentiality of patient data must be assured within the context of the program purposes and should be addressed in the legislation, confidentiality provisions should not be written in such a way as to inhibit the program from carrying out its lawful functions.

Year 2000 Objectives

Objective 22 of the year 2000 objectives outlines the necessity for conducting and coordinating birth defects surveillance *(13)*. Such programs can play an important role in defining problems and evaluating prevention programs. Adverse reproductive outcomes in general can be reduced through combined efforts—at the international, federal, state, and local levels—involving voluntary organizations, businesses, industries, and health professionals.

Developing a uniform approach that various programs can use to collect and analyze data is a major challenge. By responding to that challenge, we can further improve our knowledge of the causes of birth defects, develop preventive strategies, and assist in the evaluation and delivery of services to children with birth defects.

REFERENCES

1. CDC. National Center for Health Statistics. Annual summary of births, marriages, divorces, and deaths: United States, 1991. Hyattsville, Maryland: US Department of Health and Human Services, Public Health Service, CDC, 1992. (Monthly vital statistics report; vol. 40, no. 13.)

2. CDC. Years of potential life lost before age 65—United States, 1990 and 1991. MMWR 1993; 42:251–3.

3. Edmonds LD, Layde PM, James LM, Flynt JW, Erickson JD, Oakley GP Jr. Congenital malformations surveillance: two American systems. Int J Epidemiol 1981:10:247–52.

4. Flynt JW, Norris CK, Zaro S, Kitchen SB, Kotler M, Ziegler A. State surveillance of birth defects and other adverse reproductive outcomes: April 1987. Washington, DC: US Department of Health and Human Services, Office of the Assistant Secretary For Planning and Evaluation, 1987.

5. Hall JG, Powers EK, McIlvaine RT, Ean VH. The frequency and financial burden of genetic disease in a pediatric hospital. Am J Med Genet 1978;1:417–36.

6. Nelson K, Holmes LB. Malformations due to presumed spontaneous mutations in newborn infants. N Engl J Med 1989;320:19–23.

7. CDC. Recommendations for the use of folic acid to reduce the number of cases of spina bifida and other neural tube defects. MMWR 1992;41(no. RR-14):1–7.

8. Public Health Service. International classification of diseases, ninth revision, clinical modification. US Department of Health and Human Services, Health Care Financing Administration, 1991; DHHS publication no. (PHS)91-1260.

9. CDC. Spina bifida incidence at birth—United States, 1983–1990. MMWR 1993;41:497–500.

10. Chung CS, Myrianthopoulos NC. Congenital anomalies: mortality and morbidity, burden and classification. Am J Med Genet 1987;27:505–23.

11. Lynberg MC, Edmonds LD. Surveillance of birth defects. In: Halperin W, Baker E, eds. Public health surveillance. New York: Van Nostrand Reinhold, 1992.

12. Edmonds LD, Anderson CE, Flynt JW Jr, James LM. Congenital central nervous system malformations and vinyl chloride monomer exposure: a community study. Teratology 1978;17:137–42.

13. Public Health Service. Healthy people 2000: national health promotion and disease prevention objectives—full report, with commentary. Washington, DC: US Department of Health and Human Services, Public Health Service, 1991; DHHS publication no. (PHS)91-50212.

APPENDIX. Core data items for collection by state birth defects surveillance programs, as recommended by CDC's National Center for Health Statistics*

Data Item	Recommended Level of Inclusion	Recommended Use of Data	Recommended by NCHS
I. Infant			
A. Date of birth (month/day/year)	Recommended	National	Yes
B. Sex (male, female, ambiguous, unknown)	Recommended	National	Yes
C. Race (generated from parents)	Optional	National	Yes
D. Ethnicity (collected separately from race)	Optional	National	Yes
E. Name (including any alias)	Recommended	State	Yes
F. Unique health identifier	Optional	State	No
G. Date of report (month/day/year)	Recommended	National	Yes
H. Source of report (name, phone)	Recommended	National	Yes
I. Residence			
1. Mother at infant's birth			
City/county/state	Recommended	National	Yes
ZIP code	Recommended	National	Yes
Census tract (derived from address)	Optional	State	No
2. Mother at conception	Optional	National	No

APPENDIX. Core data items for collection by state birth defects surveillance programs, as recommended by CDC's National Center for Health Statistics* — continued

Data Item	Recommended Level of Inclusion	Recommended Use of Data	Recommended by NCHS
J. Place of birth	Recommended	National	Yes
1. Country	Recommended	National	Yes
2. City	Recommended	National	Yes
3. State	Recommended	National	Yes
4. County	Recommended	National	Yes
5. ZIP code	Recommended	National	No
6. Name of hospital/code	Recommended	State	Yes
K. Pregnancy outcome			
1. Live birth	Recommended	National	Yes
2. Still birth at >20 weeks	Recommended	National	Yes
3. Induced abortion	Optional	National	Yes
4. Spontaneous abortion	Optional	National	Yes
5. Unknown abortion	Optional	National	Yes
L. Birth weight in grams	Recommended	National	Yes
M. Apgar score	Optional	National	Yes
N. Plurality	Recommended	National	Yes
O. Gestational age			
1. By last menstrual period	Recommended	National	Yes
2. By newborn examination	Optional	National	Yes
3. By ultrasound	Optional	National	No
P. Diagnosis (description of all defects)	Recommended	National	No
Q. Source and place of diagnosis	Optional	National	No
R. Date of each diagnosis	Recommended	National	No
S. Date of death (month/day/year)	Recommended	National	Yes
T. Place of death			
1. Country	Recommended	National	Yes
2. City/state/county	Recommended	National	Yes
3. ZIP code	Recommended	National	Yes
4. Name of hospital/code	Optional	State	Yes
U. Cytogenetic studies			
1. Performed (yes, no, unknown)	Recommended	National	No
2. Results	Optional	National	No
V. Autopsy			
1. Performed (yes, no, unknown)	Recommended	National	Yes
2. Results	Optional	National	No

APPENDIX. Core data items for collection by state birth defects surveillance programs, as recommended by CDC's National Center for Health Statistics* — continued

Data Item			Recommended Level of Inclusion	Recommended Use of Data	Recommended by NCHS
	W.	Physicians of record			
		1. Pediatrician/obstetrician/family physician (name, phone)	Recommended	State	No
II.	**Mother**				
	A.	Date of birth (month/day/year)	Recommended	National	Yes
	B.	Race	Recommended	National	Yes
	C.	Ethnicity (collected separately from race)	Optional	National	Yes
	D.	Name (including maiden surname for matching)	Recommended	State	Yes
	E.	Unique health identifier	Optional	State	No
	F.	Occupation			
		1. Usual	Optional	National	No
		2. At time of conception or during first trimester	Optional	National	No
	G.	Education	Recommended	National	Yes
	H.	Method of payment	Optional	National	No
	I.	Summary totals of mother's previous pregnancies			
		1. Total of previous pregnancies	Recommended	National	Yes
		2. Live births	Recommended	National	Yes
		3. Still births at >20 weeks	Recommended	National	No
		4. Spontaneous abortions	Recommended	National	No
		5. Induced abortions	Recommended	National	No
		6. Neonatal deaths	Recommended	National	No
		7. Postneonatal deaths	Recommended	National	No
		8. Total number of pregnancies	Optional	National	No
	J.	Risk factors for the current pregnancy			
		1. Complications during pregnancy	Recommended	National	Yes
		2. Illnesses or conditions during pregnancy	Recommended	National	Yes
		3. Complications of labor and delivery	Optional	National	Yes
		4. Method of delivery	Optional	National	Yes
		5. Month prenatal care began	Optional	National	Yes
		6. Number of prenatal visits	Optional	National	Yes
		7. Parentally identified teratogenic exposures	Optional	National	No
		8. Use of tobacco	Optional	National	Yes
		9. Use of alcohol	Optional	National	Yes

APPENDIX. Core data items for collection by state birth defects surveillance programs, as recommended by CDC's National Center for Health Statistics* — continued

Data Item		Recommended Level of Inclusion	Recommended Use of Data	Recommended by NCHS
10.	Use of nonprescription drugs	Optional	National	No
11.	Prenatal diagnostic procedures	Optional	National	Yes
12.	Family history of malformations	Optional	National	No
III. Father				
A.	Date of birth (month/day/year)	Recommended	National	Yes
B.	Race	Recommended	National	Yes
C.	Ethnicity (collected separately from race)	Optional	National	Yes
D.	Name	Optional	State	Yes
E.	Unique health identifier	Optional	State	No
F.	Occupation			
1.	Usual	Optional	National	No
2.	At time of conception or during first trimester	Optional	National	No
G.	Education	Optional	National	Yes

* Adapted from Lynberg and Edmonds *(11)*.

Infant Mortality

Marian F. MacDorman, Ph.D.,[1] Diane L. Rowley, M.D., M.P.H.,[2]
Solomon Iyasu, M.B.B.S., M.P.H.,[2] John L. Kiely, Ph.D.,[3]
Paula G. Gardner, M.P.H.,[1] and Michelle S. Davis, M.S.P.H.[1]

PUBLIC HEALTH IMPORTANCE

Infant mortality is an important indicator of the health of a nation or community because it is associated with a variety of factors such as maternal health, quality and access to medical care, socioeconomic conditions, and public health practices (1–4) (National Center for Health Statistics [NCHS], unpublished data for 1987, 1992). The U.S. infant mortality rate has declined approximately tenfold since the beginning of this century, from an estimated 97.3 deaths per 1,000 live births in 1900 (5,6) to 9.2 deaths per 1,000 live births in 1990 (7).

Infant mortality declined rapidly for most of this period; however, rates of decline were slower from 1950 to 1964 and again from 1981 to 1990 (Figure 1). Despite this large decline, the problem of infant mortality remains substantial. In 1990, 38,351 infants died before their first birthday. Each of these deaths represents a tragedy for parents, siblings, and other family members.

Recent declines in infant mortality in the United States have not kept pace with declines in other countries. As a result, the United States' international ranking in infant mortality has fallen from 12th lowest in 1960 to 23rd lowest in 1988 (NCHS, unpublished data, 1993). In 1988, the U.S. infant mortality rate of 10 was about twice that of number one-ranked Japan. In addition, large disparities in the risk of infant death between various race and ethnic groups have persisted and even increased in recent years. For example, in 1990, the mortality rate for black infants was 18.0—2.4 times the rate of 7.6 for white infants (7) (see the General Findings section of this chapter).

Infant mortality is defined as the death of an infant before his or her first birthday. The infant mortality rate per 1,000 live births is computed by dividing the number of infant deaths for a given period by the number of live births for the same period and then multiplying by 1,000. Infant mortality rates may be computed either on a period or cohort basis (for additional information about related topics and surveillance activities, see the Behavioral Risk Factors Before and During Pregnancy, Prenatal Care, Preterm Birth, Low Birth Weight and Intrauterine Growth Retardation, Prevalence of Birth Defects, and Neonatal and Postneonatal Mortality chapters).

HISTORY OF DATA COLLECTION

The primary source of infant mortality statistics for the United States is the National Vital Statistics System. Through this system, virtually all vital events (births, deaths, and other events) occurring in the United States each year are registered; the data are then processed and made available to the public. Infant deaths comprise a subset of the approximately 2.2 million deaths registered on death certificates each year.

[1] Division of Vital Statistics
National Center for Health Statistics
Centers for Disease Control and Prevention
Hyattsville, Maryland

[2] Division of Reproductive Health
National Center for Chronic Disease Prevention
   and Health Promotion
Centers for Disease Control and Prevention
Atlanta, Georgia

[3] Division of Health and Utilization Analysis
National Center for Health Statistics
Centers for Disease Control and Prevention
Hyattsville, Maryland

FIGURE 1. Infant mortality rates, by race of mother —
United States, 1970–1990

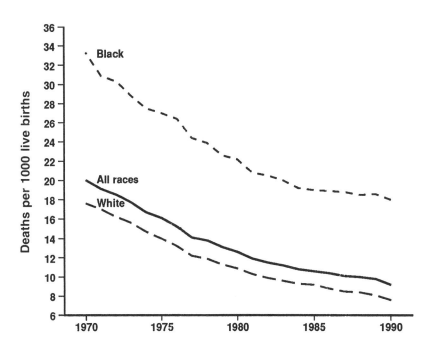

Periodic estimates of deaths and death rates have long been available, but in 1900, the U.S. Bureau of the Census began collecting mortality statistics annually for a death registration area of 10 states, the District of Columbia, and a number of cities. The death registration area gradually expanded and by 1933 included the entire United States. In 1946, the responsibility for providing vital statistics was given to the Public Health Service (8). This task now rests with CDC's National Center for Health Statistics (NCHS). *Vital Statistics of The United States*, which contains data on general and infant mortality and other vital events, has been published annually since 1937. From 1900 to 1936, the volume was entitled *Mortality Statistics*.

CDC SURVEILLANCE ACTIVITIES

National Vital Statistics System

MORTALITY DATA

Mortality data from the National Vital Statistics System provide information on the number of infant deaths by various characteristics of the decedent including age, sex, race and ethnic origin, and cause of death. These data also form the numerator when computing infant mortality rates. Data on the number of live births, used as the denominator for infant mortality rates, are also provided through the National Vital Statistics Program in a manner similar to that described for mortality data (live-birth data are described in more detail in the Prenatal Care and Low Birth Weight and Intrauterine Growth Retardation chapters).

Mortality data from the National Vital Statistics System are cooperatively produced by NCHS and state vital statistics offices under the Vital Statistics Cooperative Program. The basic source of mortality information is the death certificate. U.S. death registration is a state function; death certificates are filed and maintained in state vital statistics offices according to state legal requirements.

The U.S. Standard Certificate of Death, recommended by NCHS for use by states, is revised approximately once every 10 years in collaboration with the states, NCHS, other federal agencies, and subject-matter experts (9). The current certificate, revised in 1989, has been adopted with minor variations by the states (Figure 2). The information on the death certificate is provided by two groups of persons: 1) the certifying physician, medical examiner, or coroner, and 2) the funeral director. The certifying physician, medical examiner, or coroner certifies the causes of death *(10,11)*. The funeral director provides the demographic information (e.g., age, race, sex) and files the certificate with the state vital statistics office *(12)*. Coverage is universal because state laws require death certificates for disposition of bodies and because the certificates are often needed for legal purposes, including estate settlement.

In addition to making periodic revisions to the U.S. Standard Certificate of Death, NCHS promotes uniformity in the collection and processing of mortality data in a number of ways. NCHS also periodically updates the *Model State Vital Statistics Act and Model State Vital Statistics Regulations (13)* to help states develop and revise their vital statistics laws. In addition, NCHS offers training and technical assistance to state vital statistics offices to enhance their capabilities and provides states with annually updated instruction manuals containing information on standard coding and data processing procedures *(14)*. Most of the mortality data are coded in the state vital statistics offices according to standard NCHS procedures. In 1990, the demographic information for all states and the cause-of-death information for about half of the states were coded by the state vital statistics offices *(7)*. Information not coded in the state offices is coded by NCHS from microfilm copies of the original records.

Mortality data are subject to NCHS quality-control procedures at several processing stages to check for completeness, individual item code validity, and consistency between data items. First, NCHS checks problems or inconsistencies against the original source and corrects them, if possible. When corrections are not possible, lists of coding inconsistencies are returned to the states for information and corrective action. Second, NCHS codes a quality control sample of records and compares the sample with state-coded data to assess the accuracy of state coding. Third, numbers of deaths are compared between the current and the previous year's data for each county in the United States and for 282 cause-of-death

categories. States are contacted when large changes are noted, and any data problems are investigated. Counts and percentages of records with impossible or out-of-range codes are also reviewed and compared with the previous year's performance. Finally, according to written procedures, invalid or inconsistent values may be modified or assigned as unknowns. Selected missing items may be imputed.

FINAL AND PROVISIONAL DATA

Final infant mortality data from the National Vital Statistics System are generally available about 18–24 months after the close of a data year. These data are published annually in the *Advance Report of Final Mortality Statistics (7)* and in *Vital Statistics of the United States (15)*, as well as in periodic NCHS reports *(16,17)*. NCHS also produces a number of unpublished worktables each year and public-use data tapes containing individual-record information on all registered deaths occurring since 1968. The tape contents, file characteristics, and cost are described in the *Catalog of Electronic Data Products*, available from NCHS *(18)*.

Each month, NCHS also produces provisional infant mortality data. These data are published 3–4 months after the death certificates are filed in state vital statistics offices and are limited to estimates of the number of infant deaths and infant mortality rates, by state and selected causes of death *(19,20)*. Estimates are derived from 1) counts of the number of deaths and infant deaths registered during the month in state offices and 2) a 10% systematic sample (called the Current Mortality Sample) of death certificates filed in state offices and coded by NCHS. Although not considered as reliable as the final mortality data, provisional data are widely used for surveillance purposes because of their timeliness.

Role of the World Health Organization

The World Health Organization (WHO) plays a major role in collecting, classifying, and tabulating mortality statistics for the United States and other countries through its publication of the *Manual of the International Statistical Classification of Diseases, Injuries, and Causes of Death*

FIGURE 2.

U.S. STANDARD
CERTIFICATE OF DEATH

TYPE/PRINT IN PERMANENT BLACK INK
FOR INSTRUCTIONS SEE OTHER SIDE AND HANDBOOK

LOCAL FILE NUMBER

STATE FILE NUMBER

DECEDENT

1. DECEDENT'S NAME (First, Middle, Last)

2. SEX

3. DATE OF DEATH (Month, Day, Year)

4. SOCIAL SECURITY NUMBER

5a. AGE—Last Birthday (Years)

5b. UNDER 1 YEAR — Months | Days

5c. UNDER 1 DAY — Hours | Minutes

6. DATE OF BIRTH (Month, Day, Year)

7. BIRTHPLACE (City and State or Foreign Country)

8. WAS DECEDENT EVER IN U.S. ARMED FORCES? (Yes or no)

9a. PLACE OF DEATH (Check only one; see instructions on other side)
HOSPITAL: ☐ Inpatient ☐ ER/Outpatient ☐ DOA
OTHER: ☐ Nursing Home ☐ Residence ☐ Other (Specify)

9b. FACILITY NAME (If not institution, give street and number)

9c. CITY, TOWN, OR LOCATION OF DEATH

9d. COUNTY OF DEATH

10. MARITAL STATUS—Married, Never Married, Widowed, Divorced (Specify)

11. SURVIVING SPOUSE (If wife, give maiden name)

12a. DECEDENT'S USUAL OCCUPATION (Give kind of work done during most of working life. Do not use retired.)

12b. KIND OF BUSINESS/INDUSTRY

13a. RESIDENCE—STATE

13b. COUNTY

13c. CITY, TOWN, OR LOCATION

13d. STREET AND NUMBER

13e. INSIDE CITY LIMITS? (Yes or no)

13f. ZIP CODE

14. WAS DECEDENT OF HISPANIC ORIGIN? (Specify No or Yes—If yes, specify Cuban, Mexican, Puerto Rican, etc.) ☐ No ☐ Yes Specify:

15. RACE—American Indian, Black, White, etc. (Specify)

16. DECEDENT'S EDUCATION (Specify only highest grade completed)
Elementary/Secondary (0-12) | College (1-4 or 5+)

PARENTS

17. FATHER'S NAME (First, Middle, Last)

18. MOTHER'S NAME (First, Middle, Maiden Surname)

INFORMANT

19a. INFORMANT'S NAME (Type/Print)

19b. MAILING ADDRESS (Street and Number or Rural Route Number, City or Town, State, Zip Code)

DISPOSITION

20a. METHOD OF DISPOSITION
☐ Burial ☐ Cremation ☐ Removal from State
☐ Donation ☐ Other (Specify) _____

20b. PLACE OF DISPOSITION (Name of cemetery, crematory, or other place)

20c. LOCATION—City or Town, State

21a. SIGNATURE OF FUNERAL SERVICE LICENSEE OR PERSON ACTING AS SUCH ▶

21b. LICENSE NUMBER (of Licensee)

22. NAME AND ADDRESS OF FACILITY

PRONOUNCING PHYSICIAN ONLY

Complete items 23a-c only when certifying physician is not available at time of death to certify cause of death.

23a. To the best of my knowledge, death occurred at the time, date, and place stated.
Signature and Title ▶

23b. LICENSE NUMBER

23c. DATE SIGNED (Month, Day, Year)

ITEMS 24-26 MUST BE COMPLETED BY PERSON WHO PRONOUNCES DEATH

24. TIME OF DEATH ___ M

25. DATE PRONOUNCED DEAD (Month, Day, Year)

26. WAS CASE REFERRED TO MEDICAL EXAMINER/CORONER? (Yes or no)

CAUSE OF DEATH

27. PART I. Enter the diseases, injuries, or complications that caused the death. Do not enter the mode of dying, such as cardiac or respiratory arrest, shock, or heart failure. List only one cause on each line.

Approximate Interval Between Onset and Death

IMMEDIATE CAUSE (Final disease or condition resulting in death) → a. _____
DUE TO (OR AS A CONSEQUENCE OF):

Sequentially list conditions, if any, leading to immediate cause. Enter UNDERLYING CAUSE (Disease or injury that initiated events resulting in death) LAST

b. _____
DUE TO (OR AS A CONSEQUENCE OF):

c. _____
DUE TO (OR AS A CONSEQUENCE OF):

d. _____

PART II. Other significant conditions contributing to death but not resulting in the underlying cause given in Part I.

28a. WAS AN AUTOPSY PERFORMED? (Yes or no)

28b. WERE AUTOPSY FINDINGS AVAILABLE PRIOR TO COMPLETION OF CAUSE OF DEATH? (Yes or no)

29. MANNER OF DEATH
☐ Natural ☐ Pending Investigation
☐ Accident
☐ Suicide ☐ Could not be Determined
☐ Homicide

30a. DATE OF INJURY (Month, Day, Year)

30b. TIME OF INJURY ___ M

30c. INJURY AT WORK? (Yes or no)

30d. DESCRIBE HOW INJURY OCCURRED

30e. PLACE OF INJURY—At home, farm, street, factory, office building, etc. (Specify)

30f. LOCATION (Street and Number or Rural Route Number, City or Town, State)

CERTIFIER

31a. CERTIFIER (Check only one)

☐ CERTIFYING PHYSICIAN (Physician certifying cause of death when another physician has pronounced death and completed Item 23)
To the best of my knowledge, death occurred due to the cause(s) and manner as stated.

☐ PRONOUNCING AND CERTIFYING PHYSICIAN (Physician both pronouncing death and certifying to cause of death)
To the best of my knowledge, death occurred at the time, date, and place, and due to the cause(s) and manner as stated.

☐ MEDICAL EXAMINER/CORONER
On the basis of examination and/or investigation, in my opinion, death occurred at the time, date, and place, and due to the cause(s) and manner as stated.

31b. SIGNATURE AND TITLE OF CERTIFIER ▶

31c. LICENSE NUMBER

31d. DATE SIGNED (Month, Day, Year)

32. NAME AND ADDRESS OF PERSON WHO COMPLETED CAUSE OF DEATH (ITEM 27) (Type/Print)

REGISTRAR

33. REGISTRAR'S SIGNATURE ▶

34. DATE FILED (Month, Day, Year)

NAME OF DECEDENT: For use by physician or institution
SEE INSTRUCTIONS ON OTHER SIDE
SEE DEFINITION ON OTHER SIDE
SEE INSTRUCTIONS ON OTHER SIDE
SEE DEFINITION ON OTHER SIDE

DEPARTMENT OF HEALTH AND HUMAN SERVICES — PUBLIC HEALTH SERVICE — NATIONAL CENTER FOR HEALTH STATISTICS — 1989 REVISION

PHS-T-003
REV. 1/89

FIGURE 2. — continued

INSTRUCTIONS FOR SELECTED ITEMS

Item 9. – Place of Death
If the death was pronounced in a hospital, check the box indicating the decedent's status at the institution (inpatient, emergency room/outpatient, or dead on arrival (DOA)). If death was pronounced elsewhere, check the box indicating whether pronouncement occurred at a nursing home, residence, or other location. If other is checked, specify where death was legally pronounced, such as a physician's office, the place where the accident occurred, or at work.

Items 13-a-f. – Residence of Decedent
Residence of the decedent is the place where he or she actually resided. This is not necessarily the same as "home State," or "legal residence." Never enter a temporary residence such as one used during a visit, business trip, or a vacation. Place of residence during a tour of military duty or during attendance at college is not considered as temporary and should be considered as the place of residence.

If a decedent had been living in a facility where an individual usually resides for a long period of time, such as a group home, mental institution, nursing home, penitentiary, or hospital for the chronically ill, report the location of that facility in items 13a through 13f.

If the decedent was an infant who never resided at home, the place of residence is that of the parent(s) or legal guardian. Do not use an acute care hospital's location as the place of residence for any infant.

Items 23 and 31 – Medical Certification
The PRONOUNCING PHYSICIAN is the person who determines that the decedent is legally dead but who was not in charge of the patient's care for the illness or condition which resulted in death. Items 23a through 23c are to be completed only when the physician responsible for completing the medical certification of cause of death (Item 27) is not available at time of death to certify cause of death. The pronouncing physician is responsible for completing only items 23 through 26.

The CERTIFYING PHYSICIAN is the person who determines the cause of death (Item 27). This box should be checked only in those cases when the person who is completing the medical certification of cause of death is not the person who pronounced death (Item 23). The certifying physician is responsible for completing items 27 through 32.

The PRONOUNCING AND CERTIFYING PHYSICIAN box should be checked when the same person is responsible for completing Items 24 through 32, that is, when the same physician has both pronounced death and certified the cause of death. If this box is checked, items 23a through 23c should be left blank.

The MEDICAL EXAMINER/CORONER box should be checked when investigation is required by the Post Mortem Examination Act and the cause of death is completed by a medical examiner or coroner. The Medical Examiner/Coroner is responsible for completing items 24 through 32.

Item 27. – Cause of Death
The cause of death means the disease, abnormality, injury, or poisoning that caused the death, not the mode of dying, such as cardiac or respiratory arrest, shock, or heart failure.

In Part I, the immediate cause of death is reported on line (a). Antecedent conditions, if any, which gave rise to the cause are reported on lines (b), (c), and (d). The underlying cause, should be reported on the last line used in Part I. No entry is necessary on lines (b), (c), and (d) if the immediate cause of death on line (a) describes completely the train of events. ONLY ONE CAUSE SHOULD BE ENTERED ON A LINE. Additional lines may be added if necessary. Provide the best estimate of the interval between the onset of each condition and death. Do not leave the interval blank; if unknown, so specify.

In Part II, enter other important diseases or conditions that may have contributed to death but did not result in the underlying cause of death given in Part I.

See examples below.

235

(ICD) (21). The *ICD* specifies the detailed title for >5,000 categories to which medical entities and circumstances of death may be assigned. The *ICD* also recommends broad categories to be used for tabulating and ranking mortality data and provides information on standard definitions and reporting requirements. The *ICD* has been revised about once each decade since the beginning of this century to take into account advances in medical knowledge. The ninth revision of the *ICD (ICD-9)* was implemented in 1979 and is currently used in the United States *(21)*. The 10th revision should be implemented in the United States in the mid- to late-1990s.

Cause of death in the United States and other countries is traditionally presented in terms of the underlying cause of death, defined as "(a) the disease or injury which initiated the train of morbid events leading directly to death, or (b) the circumstances of the accident or violence which produced the fatal injury" *(21)*. The underlying cause of death is selected from the several possible morbid conditions listed on the death certificate, according to rules specified in the *ICD*. However, underlying-cause data can be augmented with additional information on other conditions reported as contributing to death on the death certificate *(22)*. For this reason, NCHS also produces reports and a public-use data tape on multiple causes of death *(18,23)*.

The National Linked Birth and Infant Death Data Set

Another important source of data on infant mortality is NCHS's linked birth and infant death data set. In this data set, the death certificate is linked with the corresponding birth certificate for each infant who dies in the United States. The purpose of this linkage is to use the many additional variables available from the birth certificate in infant mortality analysis and to use the more accurate race data from the birth certificate in calculating race-specific infant mortality rates (see the Interpretation Issues section of this chapter). Information on all of the approximately 4 million live births in the United States each year is also included in the data set to enable researchers to compare deaths with survivors and to facilitate the computation of rates. The most recent of an

annual series of national linked files is the 1987 birth cohort file, which includes infants born in 1987 who died in 1987 or 1988 before their first birthday *(24)*.

The linked birth and infant death data set (linked file) is constructed as a cohort file, with a one-to-one match of birth and death records from the NCHS's annual Natality and Mortality Vital Statistics Files. The linked file itself consists of two separate files. The first, the numerator file, is made up of the matched birth and death records of all deceased infants from a given cohort; the second, the denominator file, consists of the natality file for a given year plus any birth records from that cohort filed after the closing date of that year's natality file. Approximately 2% of each cohort's certificates cannot be linked, resulting in an underestimate of infant mortality of about 2% compared with the annual files.

The national linked file is processed in two stages. In the first stage, NCHS creates an initial file. NCHS takes advantage of the fact that most states routinely link infant death certificates to their corresponding birth certificates for their own linked files to obtain a list of birth and death certificate numbers from state vital statistics offices. Using these identifiers, NCHS selects birth and death records from the final, edited NCHS natality and mortality statistical files and creates a single record containing information from both.

In the second stage, NCHS works with states to correct problems identified during the processing of the initial file; unlinked death certificates are identified and records with inconsistent data are reviewed. To link unlinked death certificates, NCHS provides a list of unlinked certificates to the states in which the infant deaths occurred. If the state of death is different from the state of birth, the state of death is responsible for contacting the state of birth identified on the death certificate to obtain the original birth certificate number. If a third state is identified as the state of residence at the time of birth or death, that state is also sent a copy of the appropriate certificate.

If the birth certificate had been filed after the close of the NCHS statistical files, the state provides NCHS with a copy of the late-filed birth certificate. Because the linked file includes late filed certificates, it differs slightly from the natality file, and rates may differ from those that have been computed by using data from the mortality and natality files.

Four items common to the birth and death certificates are used to link the files and assess the validity of the match: date of birth, sex, state of birth, and race. A link is rejected if two or more items are inconsistent, if the date of birth is inconsistent by >1 day, if the date of death is earlier than the date of birth, or if the infant's sex is inconsistent between the birth and death records. NCHS provides states with certificate numbers of records in need of review to confirm that both the data and the link are correct.

The follow-up process confirms that questionable matches are correct and improves the overall match rate. For 1987, the overall match rate increased from 94.5% in the initial file to 97.8% in the final file. For infants whose births and deaths occurred in the same state, matching increased from 95.7% to 98.3%; for infants whose births and deaths occurred in different states, matching increased from 66.5% to 87.3%.

Both its construction as a cohort and the processing procedure add to the linked file's processing time. Two years of mortality data are necessary if all infant deaths to a cohort are to be included. The multiple steps taken to ensure correct matching also add to the processing time. As a result, linked files are available later than annual mortality data from the vital statistics system. The linked birth and infant death data sets for the 1983–1987 birth cohorts are available for public use in magnetic tape format.

National Maternal and Infant Health Survey

In addition to the data sources mentioned above, periodic sample surveys can provide a wealth of more detailed data on infant mortality in the United States. The most recent of these is the 1988 National Maternal and Infant Health Survey (NMIHS) (25). The NMIHS is a vital records follow-back survey (the sample is drawn by using vital records, and then supplementary information is collected through mail or telephone

surveys). NCHS conducted the 1988 NMIHS in collaboration with state vital records offices and 17 additional federal or state organizations. The objective of the NMIHS was to collect data needed by the research community to study factors related to pregnancy and the health of infants up to 6 months of age. Black infants and low-birth-weight infants were oversampled because of their higher risk of adverse outcomes.

Questionnaires were sent out for a sample of 9,953 live births, 5,332 infant deaths, and 3,309 fetal deaths. A stratified random probability sample design was used. Surveys were sent to the sampled mother, hospitals where she and her infant received care, and her prenatal-care providers. The mother's questionnaire included questions on sociodemographic characteristics, barriers to prenatal care, smoking, alcohol and drug use, infant immunizations, and participation in the Special Supplemental Food Program for Women, Infants, and Children. The hospital questionnaire included questions on diagnoses and procedures, maternal and infant hospitalization, fetal monitoring, and charges for care. The prenatal-care provider questionnaire included questions on patient education, advice and referral, sonograms, x-rays, medications, and vitamins. In addition, information on weight, blood pressure, hematocrit, urine glucose, urine protein, and hemoglobin was collected for each prenatal visit.

The data collected from the mother, her prenatal-care providers, the hospital, and vital records are linked to produce a single data tape that can be linked to other sources of information for additional analyses on other topic areas.

GENERAL FINDINGS

Trends

The infant mortality rate in the United States has declined rapidly during much of this century. In 1900, about 1 in 10 infants died within the first year of life (5,6), whereas in 1990, <1 in 100 infants died within their first year (26). The infant mortality rate declined rapidly from 1900 to 1950; by 1950, the rate of 29.2 infant deaths per 1,000 live births was less than one third the rate in

1900. However, from 1950 to 1964, the decline in the infant mortality rate slowed markedly to average only 1% per year. From 1965 to 1981, the infant mortality rate again declined rapidly, by an average of 4.5% per year from 24.7 to 11.9. However, from 1981 to 1989, the rate of decline again slowed markedly to average 2.5% per year. Between 1989 and 1990, the infant mortality rate decreased 6% to 9.2 per 1,000. A 24% decline in deaths caused by respiratory distress syndrome was a major contributor to the rapid reduction in the infant mortality rate from 1989 to 1990 *(26)*.

Leading Causes of Infant Death

In 1990, the four leading causes of infant death were congenital anomalies, sudden infant death syndrome, disorders relating to short gestation and unspecified low birth weight, and respiratory distress syndrome (Table 1). Together, these four causes accounted for about half (48.8%) of all

TABLE 1. Number of infant deaths, mortality rate,* and percentage of deaths for each cause of death, by race of mother — United States, 1990

Race/rank order	Cause of death (ICD-9 codes)	No.	Rate	Distribution (%)
Total[†] All Causes		38,351	922.3	100.0
1	Congenital anomalies (740–759)	8,239	198.1	21.5
2	Sudden infant death syndrome (798.0)	5,417	130.3	14.1
3	Disorders relating to short gestation and unspecified low birth weight (765)	4,013	96.5	10.5
4	Respiratory distress syndrome (769)	2,850	68.5	7.4
5	Newborn affected by maternal complications of pregnancy (761)	1,655	39.8	4.3
6	Newborn affected by complications of placenta, cord, and membranes (762)	975	23.4	2.5
7	Accidents and adverse effects (E800–E949)	930	22.4	2.4
8	Infections specific to the perinatal period (771)	875	21.0	2.3
9	Intrauterine hypoxia and birth asphyxia (768)	762	18.3	2.0
10	Pneumonia and influenza (480–487)	634	15.2	1.7
All other causes (residual)		12,001	288.6	31.3
White All Causes		24,883	756.3	100.0
1	Congenital anomalies (740–759)	6,418	195.1	25.8
2	Sudden infant death syndrome (798.0)	3,643	110.7	14.6
3	Disorders relating to short gestation and unspecified low birth weight (765)	2,004	60.9	8.1
4	Respiratory distress syndrome (769)	1,798	54.6	7.2
5	Newborn affected by maternal complications of pregnancy (761)	1,044	31.7	4.2
6	Newborn affected by complications of placenta, cord, and membranes (762)	657	20.0	2.6
7	Accidents and adverse effects (E800–E949)	609	18.5	2.4
8	Infections specific to the perinatal period (771)	569	17.3	2.3
9	Intrauterine hypoxia and birth asphyxia (768)	505	15.3	2.0
10	Pneumonia and influenza (480–487)	375	11.4	1.5
All other causes (residual)		7,261	220.7	29.2

TABLE 1. Number of infant deaths, mortality rate,* and percentage of deaths for each cause of death, by race of mother — United States, 1990 — continued

Race/rank order	Cause of death (ICD-9 codes)	No.	Rate	Distribution (%)
Black **All Causes**		**12,290**	**1,795.9**	**100.0**
1	Disorders relating to short gestation and unspecified low birth weight (765)	1,912	279.4	15.6
2	Sudden infant death syndrome (798.0)	1,578	230.6	12.8
3	Congenital anomalies (740–759)	1,530	223.6	12.4
4	Respiratory distress syndrome (769)	984	143.8	8.0
5	Newborn affected by maternal complications of pregnancy (761)	571	83.4	4.6
6	Infections specific to the perinatal period (771)	291	42.5	2.4
7	Newborn affected by complications of placenta, cord, and membranes (762)	291	42.5	2.4
8	Accidents and adverse effects (E800–E949)	289	42.2	2.4
9	Pneumonia and influenza (480–487)	235	34.3	1.9
10	Intrauterine hypoxia and birth asphyxia (768)	231	33.8	1.9
	All other causes (residual)	4,378	639.7	35.6

* Rate per 100,000 live births in specified group.
† Includes infants of races other than black or white.

infant deaths. The first four leading causes of death were the same for black and white infants, although their rank order differed. The leading cause of death for black infants was disorders relating to short gestation and unspecified low birth weight.

Low Birth Weight

Overall, the percentage of infants with low birth weight has declined by only 8% since 1950, whereas the 1990 infant mortality rate of 9.2 is less than one third the rate of 29.2 in 1950. So, the vast majority of the decline in the infant mortality rate since 1950 has been the result of declines in birth-weight-specific infant mortality rates, rather than a decline in the percentage of infants with low birth weight. Linked infant death and birth certificate data can be used to make a more accurate estimate of how improvements in birth-weight-specific mortality and in birth-weight distribution have contributed to the decline in infant mortality (27,28). The statistical methods that have been used in such analyses of time

trends are a straightforward extension of direct standardization of rates and are discussed in detail elsewhere (29).

In the most recently published analysis of national time trends that used this statistical approach, infant mortality rates in 1983 were compared with those in 1960 (28). Among white infants, 90% of the decline in mortality for single delivery infants was attributed to lower birth-weight-specific mortality and 10% was attributed to an improved birth-weight distribution. Among black infants, all of the decrease in mortality was attributed to lower birth-weight-specific rates because the incidence of low birth weight actually **increased** among blacks during this 23-year period.

These results clearly show that birth-weight-specific mortality rates have declined drastically but birth-weight distributions have improved very little. Thus, most of the progress in improving infant survival has resulted from improved obstetric and neonatal care, and very little has resulted from the prevention of low birth weight (27,28).

When we review national data on birth-weight-specific infant mortality for the 1987 birth cohort, comparing infant death rates in three weight categories for the 1960 and 1987 birth cohorts, we see that the declines are quite striking (Table 2). Because very little change occurred in the weight distributions of U.S. births between 1983 and 1987 (the percentage of infants with low birth weight was 6.8% in 1983 and 6.9% in 1987 [30]), the conclusions of the Kleinman et al. study (28) remain valid: improvement in perinatal medical care is the major contributor to the infant mortality decline, whereas efforts to prevent low birth weight have had little impact on infant mortality.

Racial and Ethnic Differences

Infant mortality rates vary substantially by race and ethnicity (Table 3). Mortality rates are highest for the infants of black, Native American, and Puerto Rican mothers, and they are lowest for the infants of Asian mothers. We must use caution, however, when interpreting race and ethnic data from different data sources. Some data sources have measurement problems, whereas others do not have sufficient socioeconomic covariates available in the data set to allow researchers to control for confounding factors (see the Interpretation Issues of this chapter).

Although Puerto Rican and Native American infants also experience elevated mortality rates, the highest mortality rates are for black infants. In 1990, the mortality rate for black infants was 18.0—2.4 times the rate of 7.6 for white infants. A number of interrelated factors may help to explain the high mortality rates for black infants. In 1990, nearly three times as many black infants (56%) as white infants (20%) were members of families with incomes below the poverty level (U.S. Bureau of the Census, unpublished data for 1990, 1993). Infants of families of low-socioeconomic status are at an increased risk of death (1,31). In addition, largely because of income differentials, black women are less likely to have health insurance that covers the cost of care for pregnancy and childbirth (32) and therefore are less likely to obtain adequate prenatal care (30).

Table 2. Infant mortality rates, by birth weight and race of mother — United States, 1960 and 1987 birth cohorts

Birth weight and race of mother	Birth cohort		
	1960	1987	% change
All birth weights, all races	25.1	9.8	−61.0
White	22.2	8.2	−63.1
Black	42.1	17.8	−57.7
<1,500 g	752.6	351.4	−53.3
White	769.4	354.8	−53.9
Black	706.4	346.5	−51.0
1,500–2,499 g	91.9	25.5	−72.3
White	93.9	26.2	−72.1
Black	85.1	23.6	−72.3
≥2,500 g	11.2	4.0	−64.3
White	9.7	3.6	−62.9
Black	20.2	5.9	−70.8

Risk Factors

Although all infants born in the United States are at some risk of death, the probability of death varies markedly according to the risk factors of the mother, the baby, and the pregnancy. Maternal and family characteristics that influence infant mortality include age, education, marital status, family income, access to medical care, and the use of cigarettes, alcohol, and other drugs during pregnancy. Infant and pregnancy-related variables include birth order, previous history of infant or fetal loss, adequacy of prenatal care, period of gestation, birth weight, Apgar scores, sex, and plurality.

As we discuss the relationships between some of the most important of these variables and infant mortality, please keep in mind that these results show differentials in infant mortality rates for each variable **unadjusted for the possible effects of other variables**. In the real world, women

TABLE 3. Infant mortality rates, by race and Hispanic origin of mother — United States, 1987 birth cohort

Race and Hispanic origin of mother	Birth cohort 1987
All mothers	9.8
White	8.2
Black	17.8
American Indian or Alaska Native	13.0
Asian or Pacific Islander	7.3
Chinese	6.2
Japanese	6.6
Filipino	6.6
Other Asian or Pacific Islander	7.9
Hispanic origin*	8.2
Mexican American	8.0
Puerto Rican	9.9
Cuban	7.1
Central and South American	7.8
Other and unknown Hispanic	8.7
Non-Hispanic White	8.1
Non-Hispanic Black	17.4

* Includes mothers of all races. Data are shown only for states with a Hispanic origin item on their birth certificates. In 1987, 23 states and the District of Columbia included this item.

with one risk factor often have other risk factors as well. Thus, teenaged mothers are more likely to also be unmarried and of a low-income status. Mothers who do not receive prenatal care are more likely to be of a low-income status and uninsured. The preferred method for disentangling the multiple interrelationships between risk factors is multivariate analysis; however, an understanding of the basic relationships between risk factors and infant mortality is a necessary precursor to more sophisticated types of analysis.

Infant mortality rates exhibit a curvilinear relationship with the age of the mother, with infants of teenaged mothers and mothers ≥40 years of age having a substantially higher risk of death than mothers aged 20–39 years. For the 1987 birth cohort, the infant mortality rate was 14.5 for teenaged mothers, compared with 8.4 for mothers

aged 25–29 years and 8.1 for mothers aged 30–34 years. For mothers aged ≥40 years, the rate was 12.6 (*NCHS, unpublished data for 1987, 1992*). Both biological and sociological factors may contribute to the elevated mortality risks for infants born to teenaged and older mothers (*33–35*).

Infant mortality rates were also higher for mothers with fewer years of education. For the 1987 birth cohort, the infant mortality rate was 14.6 for infants whose mothers did not complete high school compared with 6.3 for infants whose mothers were college graduates. These differentials may reflect actual differences in knowledge as well as socioeconomic differences because women with more education tend to have higher family income levels (*35*).

Infants born to unmarried mothers are also at an elevated risk of death. For the 1987 birth cohort, mortality rates for the infants of unmarried white mothers (12.5) were 1.7 times those for the infants of married white mothers (7.3); rates for the infants of unmarried black mothers (19.6) were 1.3 times those for the infants of married black mothers (14.8). Altogether, 17% of white infants and 63% of black infants were born to unmarried mothers.

Infants born from multiple pregnancies are also at an elevated risk of death. For the 1987 birth cohort, the infant mortality rate was 8.9 for single births compared with 50.0 for multiple births. Multiple pregnancies can lead to an accentuation of maternal risks and complications associated with pregnancy (*36*). Infants from multiple pregnancies are also much more likely to be born with low birth weights or at preterm gestational ages. Other specific biological risks associated with multiple births are described in detail elsewhere (*28,36,37*).

The timing and quality of prenatal care received by the mother during pregnancy are also important to the infant's subsequent health and survival (see the Prenatal Care chapter) (*38*). For the 1987 birth cohort, the mortality rate for infants whose mothers began prenatal care during the first trimester of pregnancy was 8.4 compared with 41.5 for infants whose mothers received no prenatal care.

One preventable maternal behavior that consistently has been associated with an increased risk of infant mortality is cigarette smoking. Several studies have used linked birth and infant death files from states that include maternal smoking as an item on the birth certificate *(39–41)*. In the 1988 NMIHS, the estimated risk of mortality was 46% higher among infants of mothers who smoked during pregnancy (13.1 per 1,000 live births) than among infants of mothers who did not smoke (9.9 per 1,000 live births) *(NCHS, unpublished data, 1993)*.

Geographic Variations

Substantial geographic variation in infant mortality has been observed in the United States. A twofold to threefold difference exists between the highest and the lowest state-specific infant mortality rates *(15,42,43)*. Similarly, data for 1985–1989 for cities with a population of >100,000 (1980 census) showed that the highest city-specific infant mortality rate was three times that of the lowest rate *(44)*. Some of these differences relate to differences in race and ethnic composition and income distribution between geographic areas. However significant geographic variations persist even after race differences and birth weight are taken into account. When the comparison is limited to normal-birth-weight infants born to low-risk women (those with ≥13 years of education who are ≥20 years of age and who initiated prenatal care in the first trimester), substantial differences still exist between states *(45)*. These findings suggest that differences in access to high-quality prenatal and perinatal care may be important contributors to the geographic variation in infant mortality.

INTERPRETATION ISSUES

Period versus Cohort Rates of Infant Mortality

In the conventional definition used in most reports of vital statistics, the **period infant mortality rate** (per 1,000 live births) is calculated as follows:

$$\frac{\text{Number of infant deaths during a year}}{\text{Number of live births during the same year}} \times 1,000^{*}$$

Because this rate is calculated by comparing infant deaths with live births during the same period instead of following the birth cohort[†] to determine its mortality experience, the numerator and denominator may relate to different populations. For example, an urban renewal project may result in a rapid, sudden change in the characteristics of an area's population. In this case, the infant deaths during the year would be compared with a very different population of births for that year, and the rate would be misleading. Keep in mind these types of population shifts when analyzing mortality rates for small areas.

This problem does not occur, however, in analyses of linked birth and infant death files because these files allow us to analyze the infant mortality experience of birth cohorts. A **cohort infant mortality rate** is calculated as follows:

$$\frac{\text{Number of infant deaths that occurred among live births during a year}}{\text{Number of live births during a year}} \times 1,000$$

An important difference exists between this rate and the **period infant mortality rate** defined previously. Two years of data on infant deaths are needed to calculate the cohort rate for a given year. For example, the numerator of the cohort infant mortality rate for 1987 would include deaths in both 1987 and 1988 among infants born in 1987.

---

[*] Cause-specific infant mortality rates are generally calculated per 100,000.

[†] A cohort consists of "a group of individuals who experienced the same significant demographic event during a specified brief period of time, usually a year, and who may be identified as a group at successive later dates on the basis of this common demographic experience. Examples are a birth cohort, persons born during the same year or years. . ." *(46)*.

An additional problem with analyses using period infant mortality rates is that the source of information for the numerator is the death certificate whereas the source for the denominator is the birth certificate. Lack of comparability in certain items has been noted by researchers who have compared birth and death certificates for the same infant (47). The problem does not occur in analyses of linked birth and infant death files because these files use the more accurate data on race and other socioeconomic characteristics from the birth certificate, regardless of whether the infant died.

Data on Race and Ethnicity

Surveillance of infant mortality outcome by race and ethnicity is useful in monitoring the success of the national year 2000 goal of reducing the disparity in health outcomes (48). We must recognize, however, that surveillance reports have some limitations, including potential problems in the classification of race and ethnicity in vital records. In addition, potential socioeconomic and cultural factors that may underlie differences in health status by race and ethnicity are often not available in surveillance data. Also, misinterpretation of racial and ethnic information can lead to stigmatization and racism.

Inconsistencies in the classification of race and ethnicity on birth and death certificates can lead to problems in the accurate estimation of race-specific infant mortality rates. A study comparing the race assigned on the birth certificate to the race assigned on the death certificate for the same infant found that 3.7% of infant deaths in the 1983–1985 birth cohorts were classified to different races on birth and death certificates (47). Discrepancies in race classification were greatest for infants of races other than black or white, with 43.2% assigned to different races on birth and death certificates. Substantial differences were also found for Hispanic origin subgroups (47). In part to address these problems, NCHS created the linked birth and infant death data set that allows researchers to use more accurate race data from birth certificates in tabulating infant mortality statistics.

In 1989, to further improve the quality of race data on vital records, NCHS changed the method of tabulating race for live births to the race of the mother as reported directly on the birth certificate. Before 1989, birth tabulations were by race of child as determined by an algorithm based on information reported for the mother and father. Briefly, children of mixed-race parentage with one white parent were assigned the other parent's race. When neither parent was white, the child was assigned the father's race (30). The change to tabulating live births by race of the mother affects infant mortality data because live births comprise the denominator of infant mortality rates. The method of tabulating mortality data by race has not changed; race is that of the decedent as reported on the death certificate. The change to tabulating live births by race of the mother provides a more consistent indicator of race and helps to reduce the magnitude of differences between race-specific infant mortality rates from vital statistics data and the linked file (49). Unless otherwise specified, all infant mortality rates shown in this chapter are based on live births tabulated by race of the mother.

Surveillance program staff who include information on race and ethnicity should exercise caution when using race as a substitute for socioeconomic status (if the race is black, it is usually interpreted to mean low-socioeconomic status). The validity of routinely adjusting for race as a method for controlling for missing socioeconomic data has been questioned (50).

Race and ethnicity should not be used as an etiologic risk factor for infant mortality. Race sometimes has been used as a genetic marker, and therefore, assumed to be a risk factor. Race has not been demonstrated to directly increase physiologic risk for disease, except for a few genetic diseases. Specific racial or ethnic populations may be socially, culturally, environmentally, or economically exposed to risk factors that put them at a higher or lower risk for death (51,52). Ideally, potential intervening variables such as socioeconomic status and environmental exposures should be collected and analyzed in relation to race and ethnicity data because misinterpretation of the meaning of reporting of race or ethnicity may sometimes impede prevention research activities (53).

Birth-Weight-Specific Rates

In nonexperimental evaluations of medical care, the need to adjust for differences in disease severity between groups receiving different therapies has long been recognized. For example, in comparisons of postoperative mortality in different hospitals, elaborate statistical techniques have been developed for case-mix adjustment.

In the surveillance and monitoring of infant mortality rates, the need for some sort of case-mix adjustment has also been acknowledged, but the situation is simplified by the overwhelming importance of birth weight as a predictor of infant death. Therefore, when comparing infant mortality rates between geographic areas, time periods, or hospitals, the common practice is to look separately at two components of these rates: 1) the **birth-weight distribution** and 2) the mortality within each birth-weight category or **birth-weight-specific mortality**. The first component is generally considered to be strongly affected by the socioeconomic and demographic circumstances of the mother. The second component is often used as a measure of the quality of perinatal care *(54)*.

In analyses of birth-weight-specific mortality, the use of 500-g categories has been commonly used. However, in small areas, the number of infants falling into many of the 500-g categories are quite small. Therefore, a more practical option may be to use the following categories: <1,500 g, 1,500–2,499 g, and ≥2,500 g.

For each birth-weight category, the **birth-weight-specific mortality rate** is calculated by using the following formula:

$$\frac{\text{Number of deaths in the birth-weight category}}{\text{Number of births in the birth-weight category}} \times 1,000$$

Because birth-weight-specific infant mortality rates may not always be a direct measure of the effect of perinatal medical care, factors such as these must be considered: 1) female infants usually have lower birth-weight-specific mortality rates than males; 2) black infants usually have lower

mortality rates at low birth weights and higher rates at normal and high birth weights; and 3) postneonatal mortality has several causes—such as intestinal infections, pneumonia, influenza, sudden infant death syndrome, and unintentional injuries—that have little association with obstetric or neonatal care. For this reason, postneonatal deaths are often excluded from evaluations of perinatal care, and birth-weight-specific **neonatal** mortality rates are compared.

Quality of Cause-of-Death Data

Identifying the cause of death among infants presents particular challenges to the physician, medical examiner, or coroner certifying the death. More than half of all infant deaths occur during the first 7 days of life *(15)*. For these deaths, the certifier does not have access to a medical history of illness that would help him or her in identifying the underlying cause of death. Therefore, he or she is much more likely to rely on postmortem examination in determining the cause of death. In 1989, 44.1% of infant deaths resulted in autopsies, compared with 11.5% of deaths at all ages *(55)*. Few studies focus on the validity of cause-of-death information for infants. However, because of the high autopsy rate, the quality of cause-of-death certification for infants is believed to be at least as good as that for persons at all ages. The validity of cause-of-death data for deaths at all ages has been discussed extensively elsewhere *(56,57)*.

Stability of Rates

An area's observed infant mortality rate should be considered an estimate of the true underlying mortality rate.§ As is the case with any estimate, the infant mortality rate is subject to chance variation. If the area has very few births, the observed infant mortality rate may be very different from the true rate. Thus, if rates for two areas are compared in a given year and one (or both) of the area's rates is based on a small number of

---

§ The number of infant deaths in an area varies by chance, depending on the number of births and the probability of infant death (the *true* infant mortality rate). As the number of births increases, the chance component becomes less important, and the observed infant mortality rate becomes a better estimate of the true rate.

births, it would not be unusual for the findings to be reversed the following year.

Therefore, a method is needed to assess the adequacy of the observed infant mortality rate as an estimate of its true value. The most common method is the use of confidence intervals. Calculation of confidence intervals is explained in detail elsewhere (58–60). Basically, a **95% confidence interval** is defined so that the probability is 95% that the true rate is included in the interval. If the interval is very wide, the true rate is not estimated with much precision. The interval generally becomes narrower as the number of births on which the rate is based increases. Two common methods of increasing the numbers of births are to combine years and to combine smaller areas into larger ones.

Although aggregation over years and areas permits us to compute stable rates, loss of information occurs. Combining heterogeneous areas to obtain a stable rate may be more misleading than helpful. Combining years involves the assumption that in each of the years, the ranking of the areas is the same—that is, annual changes in the rates are the same for all areas.

The stability issue is especially important when comparing areas or determining whether real changes have occurred over time within an area. In these situations, confidence limits should be used to assess the magnitude of the differences. Two areas (or two time periods for one area) can be compared by using the absolute difference in their rates or by using the ratio of their rates. The ratio of rates (or relative risk as it is sometimes called) is usually preferred because it allows for comparison of areas or time over a wide range of rates.

Multivariate Analysis

When investigating factors that may affect infant mortality, researchers must always consider the possibility of confounding variables. An apparent association between a factor and infant mortality may be related to the effect of other variables. This is especially true in studies of social and demographic factors because the effects of such variables are often relatively small, and the addition of a confounding variable into the analysis

could easily reduce relative risks to 1. By social and demographic factors, we mean such variables as the parents' income, occupation, race, ethnicity, and education as well as the mother's age, parity, and gravidity. This is in contrast to biological variables such as very low birth weight, abruptio placentae, and prolapsed umbilical cord, whose associations with mortality are so strong that it is unlikely that the control of any confounder could reduce their effects to the null.

In investigations of infant mortality, one of the most common solutions to the problem of confounders has been to perform **multivariate analyses**. Detailed discussions of dealing with confounding, and of the problems of carrying out a careful multivariate analysis, can be found elsewhere (61–63). Several examples of multivariate analyses of infant mortality have been published in the epidemiologic (64–66), sociological (67), and demographic (68) literature.

EXAMPLES OF DATA USE

Vital statistics data on infant mortality are used extensively by state and local health departments to track numbers of infant deaths and infant mortality rates for states, cities, counties, and other geographic areas. Major changes in numbers of deaths, in rates, or in the cause-of-death profile of a region can provide a strong indication of improvements in medical care, or conversely, problems that the health department needs to address. Some causes of death, such as whooping cough, serve as red flags to health departments for follow-up activities.

One example of state use of linked birth and infant death data is Mississippi's program for high-risk infant follow-up (69). The purpose of this program is to prevent postneonatal deaths of infants born at high risk of death. In the original system, birth certificates were marked if they contained one or more risk factors and were sent to county nurses for follow-up. The problem with the initial system was that it identified about one fourth of all births as high risk—too many births for the county nurses to effectively follow.

Mississippi's goal was to design a new system that would reduce the number of infants identified without running the risk of missing infants who needed follow-up. To redesign the system, the state used logistic regression on its linked files to calculate relative risk scores for a variety of risk factors relating to maternal age and education, race, prenatal care, pregnancy history, birth weight, Apgar score, and the presence of congenital anomalies. Because the risk scores were multiplicative, a total risk score could then be generated for each infant on the basis of its unique risk profile. Currently, risk scores are generated monthly, and information on high-risk infants is sent to county health nurses. The nurses follow up through letters, telephone calls, and/or home visits to provide information on the need for and availability of well-baby care and immunizations and to address parents' concerns. By using this system, the state reduced the number of infants identified for follow-up by almost two thirds, allowing county health nurses to concentrate their follow-up activities on the infants most in need of their help *(69)*.

FUTURE ISSUES

The national health objectives for the year 2000 relating to infant mortality are to reduce the infant mortality rate to 7 for the total population, 11 for black infants, 8.5 for Native American infants, and 8 for Puerto Rican infants *(48)*. The objective for the total population is the rate that we can expect to achieve if the average annual decline in infant mortality rates observed from 1981–1986 (2.8%) persists through the 1990s. To achieve the goal for black infants, we must accelerate the average annual decline in infant mortality from 2.2% per year from 1981–1986 to 3.5% *(48)*.

As previously stated, most of the decline in infant mortality over the past three decades can be attributed to improvements in perinatal medical care rather than improvements in prevention. In 1990, as in 1980, only 76% of mothers began prenatal care in the first trimester *(70)*. Even for those women who did get prenatal care, serious questions persist about the quality of that care, particularly for socioeconomically disadvantaged groups *(71)*. Similarly, the percentage of infants born with low birth weights has not declined during the 1980s and has actually increased for black infants *(70)*.

Future research must focus on some of the fundamental issues, such as low birth weight, that affect infant mortality. To address this need, the linked birth and infant death data set is being expanded to provide more detailed information on specific risk factors for infant death. Beginning with the 1989 birth cohort, the linked file contains the many additional variables available from the 1989 revision of the birth certificate. Included are items on smoking, alcohol use, and weight gain during pregnancy as well as check-box items on specific medical risk factors of the pregnancy, complications of labor and delivery, method of delivery, obstetric procedures, abnormal conditions of the newborn, and congenital anomalies of the child.

Although these research issues are important, we have an even greater need to apply what we already know to solve the fundamental problems surrounding infant mortality in the United States. For example, much of what is already known about preventing low birth weight—such as the need for universal access to quality prenatal care and substance abuse counseling—is not being applied in this country. Although improvements in perinatal medicine have lowered the mortality rate for low-birth-weight infants, these infants are at a substantially increased risk of morbidity, mental retardation, and neurological disorders that require increased levels of medical and parental care *(72–74)*. If our goal is not merely to reduce the infant mortality rate but to improve the quality of life for infants and children, we must prevent preterm and low-birth-weight births and increase prenatal care use. Future efforts should focus on making basic prevention and public health services available to all pregnant women.

REFERENCES

1. Gould JB, Davey B, LeRoy S. Socioeconomic differentials and neonatal mortality: racial comparison of California singletons. Pediatrics 1989;83:181–6.

2. Rosenbaum S, Layton C, Liu J. The health of America's children. Washington, DC: Children's Defense Fund, 1991.

3. Berkov B, Cheung M, Tashiro M. Trends in births and birth outcomes for unmarried and married women, California, 1966–1985. Sacramento, California: California Department of Health Services, 1988.

4. Babson SG, Clarke NG. Relationship between infant death and maternal age. J Pediatr 1983;103:391–3.

5. Department of the Interior. Census Reports, vol. IV, twelfth census of the United States, 1900. Vital statistics, part II. Washington, DC: US Census Office, 1902.

6. Department of the Interior. Census Reports, vol. III, twelfth census of the United States, 1900. Vital statistics, part I. Washington, DC: US Census Office, 1902.

7. NCHS. Advance report of final mortality statistics, 1990. Hyattsville, Maryland: US Department of Health and Human Services, Public Health Service, CDC, 1993. (Monthly vital statistics report; vol. 41, no. 7, suppl.)

8. Public Health Service. History and organization of the vital statistics system. In: Vital statistics of the United States, vol. I, 1950. Hyattsville, Maryland: US Department of Health, Education, and Welfare, Public Health Service, National Vital Statistics Division, 1978:2–19.

9. Freedman MA, Gay GA, Brockert JE, Potrzebowski PW, Rothwell CJ. The 1989 revisions of the U.S. standard certificates of live birth and death and the U.S. standard report of fetal death. Am J Public Health 1988;78:168–72.

10. NCHS. Physicians' handbook on medical certification of death. Hyattsville, Maryland: US Department of Health and Human Services, Public Health Service, 1987; DHHS publication no. (PHS)87-1108.

11. NCHS. Medical examiners' and coroners' handbook on death registration and fetal death reporting. Hyattsville, Maryland: US Department of Health and Human Services, Public Health Service, 1987; DHHS publication no. (PHS)87-1110.

12. NCHS. Funeral director's handbook on death registration and fetal death reporting. Hyattsville, Maryland: US Department of Health and Human Services, Public Health Service, 1987; DHHS publication no. (PHS)87-1109.

13. NCHS. Model state vital statistics act and model state vital statistics regulations, 1977 revision. Hyattsville, Maryland: US Department of Health, Education, and Welfare, Public Health Service, 1978; DHEW publication no. (PHS)78-1115.

14. NCHS. Instruction manual. Parts 1–20. Hyattsville, Maryland: US Department of Health and Human Services, Public Health Service, CDC, 1992.

15. NCHS. Vital statistics of the United States, 1988. Vol. II, mortality, part A. Hyattsville, Maryland: US Department of Health and Human Services, Public Health Service, CDC, 1991.

16. MacDorman MF, Rosenberg HM. Trends in infant mortality by cause of death and other characteristics, 1960–88. Hyattsville, Maryland: US Department of

Health and Human Services, Public Health Service, CDC, NCHS, 1993. (Vital and health statistics; series 20, no. 20.)

17. Maurer JD, Rosenberg HM, Keemer JB. Deaths of Hispanic origin, 15 reporting states, 1979–81. Hyattsville, Maryland: US Department of Health and Human Services, Public Health Service, CDC, NCHS, 1990. (Vital and health statistics; series 20, no. 18.)

18. NCHS. Catalog of electronic data products. Hyattsville, Maryland: US Department of Health and Human Services, Public Health Service, CDC, 1992; DHHS publication no. (PHS)92-1213.

19. NCHS. Births, marriages, divorces, and deaths for October 1992. Hyattsville, Maryland: US Department of Health and Human Services, Public Health Service, CDC, 1993. (Monthly vital statistics report; vol. 41, no. 10.)

20. NCHS. Annual summary of births, marriages, divorces, and deaths: United States, 1991. Hyattsville, Maryland: US Department of Health and Human Services, Public Health Service, CDC, 1992. (Monthly vital statistics report; vol. 40, no. 13.)

21. World Health Organization. Manual of the international statistical classification of diseases, injuries, and causes of death, based on the recommendations of the Ninth Revision Conference, 1975, and adopted by the Twenty-ninth World Health Assembly. Geneva: World Health Organization, 1977.

22. Israel RA, Rosenberg HM, Curtin LR. Analytical potential for multiple cause-of-death data. Am J Epidemiol 1986;124:161–79.

23. NCHS. Multiple causes of death in the United States. Hyattsville, Maryland: US Department of Health and Human Services, Public Health Service, 1984. (Monthly vital statistics report; vol. 32, no. 10, suppl. 2.)

24. NCHS. Public use data tape documentation. Linked birth/infant death data set: 1987 birth cohort. Hyattsville, Maryland: US Department of Health and Human Services, Public Health Service, CDC, 1992.

25. Sanderson M, Placek PJ, Keppel KG. The 1988 national maternal and infant health survey: design, content, and data availability. BIRTH 1991;18: 1:26–32.

26. CDC. Infant Mortality—United States, 1990. MMWR 1993;42:161–5.

27. Buehler JW, Kleinman JC, Hogue CJR, Strauss LT, Smith JC. Birth weight-specific infant mortality, United States, 1960 and 1980. Public Health Rep 1987;102: 151–61.

28. Kleinman JC, Fowler MG, Kessel SS. Comparison of infant mortality among twins and singletons: United States, 1960 and 1983. Am J Epidemiol 1991;133: 133–43.

29. Fleiss JL. Statistical methods for rates and proportions. 2nd ed. New York: John Wiley and Sons Inc., 1981:238.

30. NCHS. Vital statistics of the United States, 1988. Vol. I, natality. Hyattsville, Maryland: US Department of Health and Human Services, CDC, 1990.

31. Stockwell EG, Swanson DA, Wicks JW. Economic status differences in infant mortality by cause of death. Public Health Rep 1988;103:135–42.

32. Alan Guttmacher Institute. Blessed events and the bottom line: financing maternity care in the United States. New York: Alan Guttmacher Institute, 1987.

33. Friede A, Baldwin W, Rhodes PH, Buehler JW, Strauss LT. Older maternal age and infant mortality in the United States. Obstet Gynecol 1988;72:152–7.

34. Lawrence RA, Merritt TA. Infants of adolescent mothers: perinatal, neonatal, and infancy outcome. In: McArarney ER, ed. Premature adolescent pregnancy and parenthood. New York: Grove and Stratton, 1983:149–68.

35. US Bureau of the Census. 1980 census of population, detailed population characteristics, United States summary. Washington, DC: US Department of Commerce, US Bureau of the Census, 1984.

36. Fowler MG, Kleinman JC, Kiely JL, Kessel SS. Double jeopardy: twin infant mortality in the United States, 1983 and 1984. Am J Obstet Gynecol 1991;165: 15–22.

37. Kiely JL, Kleinman JC, Kiely M. Triplets and higher-order multiple births—time trends and infant mortality. Am J Dis Child 1992;146:862–8.

38. Institute of Medicine, National Academy of Sciences. Prenatal care: reaching mothers, reaching infants. Washington, DC: National Academy Press, 1988.

39. Kleinman JC, Pierre MB, Madans JH, Land GH, Schramm WF. The effects of maternal smoking on fetal and infant mortality. Am J Epidemiol 1988; 127:274–82.

40. Malloy MH, Kleinman JC, Land GH, Schramm WF. The association of maternal smoking with age and cause of infant death. Am J Epidemiol 1988;128: 46–55.

41. Weiss J, Cowan L. The burden of smoking on mothers and infants in Massachusetts: supplement to advance data: births and smoking: death, disease, and dollars. Boston: Massachusetts Department of Public Health, Bureau of Family and Community Health, April 1993.

42. Marks JS, Buehler JW, Strauss LT, Hogue CJR, Smith JC. Variation in state-specific infant mortality risks. Public Health Rep 1987;102:146–50.

43. Kleinman JC. State trends in infant mortality, 1968–83. Am J Public Health 1986;76:681–7.

44. CityMatCH. Urban infant mortality data 1985–1989. CityLights 1993;2:4–6.

45. Aoyama MC, Iyasu S, Marks J, McCarthy B. Variation in state-specific infant mortality rates, 1983–1987: the potential for reducing the U.S. infant mortality rate. Presented at the Epidemic Intelligence Service Conference, Atlanta, Georgia, April 19–23, 1993.

46. Shryock HS, Siegel JS, and Associates. The methods and materials of demography, condensed edition by EG Stockwell. Orlando, Florida: Academic Press Inc., 1976.

47. Hahn RA, Mulinare J, Teutsch SM. Inconsistencies in coding of race and ethnicity between birth and death in US infants: a new look at infant mortality, 1983 through 1985. JAMA 1992;267:259–63.

48. Public Health Service. Healthy people 2000: national health promotion and disease prevention objectives—full report, with commentary. Washington, DC: US Department of Health and Human Services, Public Health Service, 1991; DHHS publication no. (PHS)91-50212.

49. Gardner P, Hoyert D, MacDorman M. Classification and interpretation of race and ethnicity in infant mortality research. Presented at the annual meeting of the American Public Health Association, Washington, DC, November 8–12, 1992.

50. Mason JO. Understanding the disparities in morbidity and mortality among racial and ethnic groups in the United States. Ann Epidemiol 1993;3:120–4.

51. Blackmore CA, Ferré CD, Rowley DL, Hogue CJR, Gaiter J, Atrash H. Is race a risk factor or a risk marker for preterm delivery? Ethn Dis 1994 (in press).

52. Warren RC. The morbidity/mortality gap: What is the problem? Ann Epidemiol 1993;3:127–9.

53. David RJ, Collins JW Jr. Bad outcomes in black babies: race or racism? Ethn Dis 1991;1:236–44.

54. Paneth N. Infant mortality reexamined. JAMA 1982; 247:1027–8.

55. NCHS. Vital statistics of the United States, 1989. Vol. II, mortality, part A. Hyattsville, Maryland: US Department of Health and Human Services, Public Health Service, CDC, 1994.

56. Rosenberg, HM. The nature and accuracy of cause-of-death data. In: Report of the Workshop on Improving Cause-of-Death Statistics. Hyattsville, Maryland: US Department of Health and Human Services, Public Health Service, CDC, NCHS, 1989.

57. Gittelsohn AM, Royston PN. Annotated bibliography of cause-of-death validation studies, 1958–1980. Washington, DC: US Department of Health and Human Services, Public Health Service, NCHS, 1982. (Vital and health statistics; series 2, no. 89.)

58. Kleinman JC, Kiely JL. Infant mortality. Hyattsville, Maryland: US Department of Health and Human Services, Public Health Service, CDC, NCHS, 1991. (Healthy people 2000 statistical notes; vol. 1, no. 2.)

59. Gardner MJ, Altman DG, eds. Statistics with confidence: confidence intervals and statistical guidelines. London: British Medical Journal, 1989.

60. Armitage P, Berry G. Statistical methods in medical research. 2nd ed. Boston: Blackwell Scientific Publications, 1987.

61. Susser M. Causal thinking in the health sciences: concepts and strategies in epidemiology. New York: Oxford University Press, 1973.

62. Greenland S, Neutra R. Control of confounding in the assessment of medical technology. Int J Epidemiol 1980;9:361–7.

63. Kiely JL. Some conceptual problems in multivariable analyses of perinatal mortality. Paediatr Perinat Epidemiol 1991;5:243–57.

64. Bross DS, Shapiro S. Direct and indirect associations of five factors with infant mortality. Am J Epidemiol 1982;115:78–91.

65. Shoham-Yakubovich I, Barell V. Maternal education as a modifier of the association between low birthweight and infant mortality. Int J Epidemiol 1988;17:370–7.

66. Kiely JL. Mode of delivery and neonatal death in 17,587 infants presenting by the breech. Br J Obstet Gynaecol 1991;98:898–904.

67. Gortmaker SL. Poverty and infant mortality in the United States. American Sociological Review 1979;44:280–297.

68. Eberstein IW, Nam CB, Hummer RA. Infant mortality by cause of death: main and interaction effects. Demography 1990;27:413–30.

69. Gunter N. Using matched certificates for high risk infant followup in Mississippi. Proceedings of the Linked Birth and Infant Death Record Project, second evaluation meeting. Hyattsville, Maryland: US Department of Health and Human Services, Public Health Service, CDC, NCHS, 1990.

70. NCHS. Advance report of final natality statistics, 1990. Hyattsville, Maryland: US Department of Health and Human Services, Public Health Service, CDC 1993. (Monthly vital statistics report; vol. 41, no. 9, suppl.)

71. Hansell MJ. Sociodemographic factors and the quality of prenatal care. Am J Public Health 1991;81:1023–8.

72. Hunt JV, Cooper BAB, Tooley WH. Very low birthweight infants at 8 and 11 years of age: role of neonatal illness and family status. Pediatrics 1988;82:596–603.

73. Stanley FJ. Survival and cerebral palsy in low birthweight infants: implications for perinatal care. Paediatr Perinat Epidemiol 1992;6:298–310.

74. Overpeck MD, Moss AJ, Hoffman HJ, Hendershot GE. A comparison of the childhood health status of normal birth-weight and low birth-weight infants. Public Health Rep 1989;104:58–70.

249

Neonatal and Postneonatal Mortality

Diane L. Rowley, M.D., M.P.H.,[1] Solomon Iyasu, M.B.B.S., M.P.H.,[1]
Marian F. MacDorman, Ph.D.,[2] and Hani K. Atrash, M.D., M.P.H.[1]

PUBLIC HEALTH IMPORTANCE

By convention, infant mortality analysis is subdivided into two stages—the neonatal and postneonatal periods.* More than a century ago, William Farr recognized that factors affecting the death rate vary at different stages of infancy and wrote about the need to subdivide the first year of life into months or even days (1). He also noted that the effect of environmental factors on mortality varied by age of the infant, with those who are older experiencing substantially higher mortality rates than younger infants. Today, neonatal and postneonatal mortality are examined separately because most deaths during the neonatal period are associated with events surrounding the prenatal period and the delivery, whereas postneonatal deaths are more likely to be associated with conditions or events that arise after the delivery and, thus, reflect environmental factors. This division into neonatal and postneonatal periods is not completely satisfactory, however. For example, deaths from birth defects are common during both the neonatal and postneonatal periods, but the causes of birth defects are related to events that occur from conception to birth. Likewise, delivery of preterm infants (born <37 completed gestational weeks) is caused by conditions arising during the antepartum and intrapartum periods, but deaths related to prematurity may be postponed to the postneonatal period (2,3).

The proportionate contribution of neonatal and postneonatal mortality to the infant mortality rate has varied over the past century. In general, infant mortality declined throughout the 20th century. Rates of decline were rapid for the first four decades but were slower from 1950 to 1964 and again from 1981 to 1989. In the first two decades of this century, two thirds of infant deaths occurred during the postneonatal period, and until the late 1960s, improvement in infant mortality was primarily the result of declines in postneonatal mortality (1,4). Environmental changes that resulted in fewer infections, the use of antibiotics, and improved nutrition are thought to have contributed to the decline in postneonatal mortality from the 1900s to the 1950s (5). As a result, deaths in the postneonatal period contributed a progressively smaller proportion of total infant deaths in the United States: 50% in the 1920s, 35% in the 1940s, and 25% in the mid-1960s (4).

As early as the late 1920s, neonatal mortality began to command relatively greater attention as a health concern than postneonatal mortality. In the ensuing decades, while postneonatal mortality continued to fall, neonatal mortality rates also

---

[1] Division of Reproductive Health
National Center for Chronic Disease Prevention
 and Health Promotion
Centers for Disease Control and Prevention
Atlanta, Georgia

[2] Division of Vital Statistics
National Center for Health Statistics
Centers for Disease Control and Prevention
Hyattsville, Maryland

Acknowledgments

For providing advice and assistance, we thank Krista A. Kugaraj, B.S., National Center for Chronic Disease Prevention and Health Promotion, Centers for Disease Control and Prevention; William M. Sappenfield, M.D., M.P.H., South Carolina Department of Health and Environmental Control, assigned from the National Center for Chronic Disease Prevention and Health Promotion; and Qiduan Liu, M.Ed., South Carolina Department of Health and Environmental Control.

---

* **Neonatal mortality** — defined as the death of a live-born infant in <28 days of life — can be further subdivided into **early neonatal mortality**, an infant death that occurs in <7 days of birth, and **late neonatal mortality**, a death from 7 to <28 days of age. **Postneonatal mortality** is defined as the death of a live-born infant from 28 through 364 days of life.

declined, though less rapidly than postneonatal mortality. From 1950 to 1964, very little decline occurred in either neonatal or postneonatal mortality. From 1965 to 1970, a sharp drop in postneonatal mortality coincided with the implementation of Medicaid and other federal programs targeted at the poor (1,6). With the introduction of neonatal intensive care units that improved survival of low-birth-weight infants, neonatal mortality declined rapidly from 1970 through 1980. Beginning in 1970, the rate of decline in neonatal mortality exceeded that of postneonatal mortality for the first time. Although the rate of decline was slower, regionalization of perinatal intensive care services contributed to further improvements in the survival of low-birth-weight babies in the 1980s. In the late 1980s, therapeutic advances in the treatment of respiratory distress syndrome probably contributed substantially to the 6% decline in infant mortality reported between 1989 and 1990 (7).

Neonatal mortality continues to account for the largest proportion (63.5%) of infant deaths. However, since 1970, because postneonatal mortality has declined at a slower rate than neonatal mortality (8), the proportion of infant deaths occurring in the postneonatal period has increased steadily from 24.7% in 1970 (1) to 36.6% in 1990 (9). In recent years, postneonatal mortality has declined only slightly (10), and the United States continues to have higher postneonatal rates than many industrialized countries (6).

These trends since 1970, combined with the relative lack of improvement in postneonatal mortality rates in the 1980s, suggest that postneonatal deaths should receive more attention than they have in the past few decades. The reasons for the relatively low importance given to postneonatal mortality in the United States may include the false perception that postneonatal mortality is a disappearing problem, the possibility that infants dying in the postneonatal period are less likely to be seen by clinicians or hospital professionals before death and therefore tend to not attract their attention, and the possibility that factors related to postneonatal mortality deaths are social rather than medical and are less studied in a research environment dominated by the medical model of disease causation. For additional information about related topics and surveillance activities, see the Preterm Birth, Low Birth Weight and Intrauterine Growth Retardation, Prevalence of Birth Defects, Infant Mortality, and Injury and Child Abuse chapters.

HISTORY OF DATA COLLECTION

The concept of neonatal and postneonatal mortality surveillance is not new, but until recently, the purpose for tracking these rates was limited to the collection, analysis, and dissemination of data (11). Surveillance focused on reporting declines in rates of neonatal and postneonatal deaths by cause of death. In the late 1960s, public health surveillance for infectious disease incorporated the idea that surveillance should have an action component that results in disease prevention and control (12); however, action steps related to prevention, planning, and evaluation did not become a priority for neonatal and postneonatal surveillance until the 1980s, coinciding with the availability of linked birth certificates and infant death certificates (13). Surveillance is now used to describe families at risk for neonatal or postneonatal death so that they can be targeted for prevention services; to set priorities for directing scarce resources to programs that will do the most to improve neonatal and postneonatal survival; to evaluate the effectiveness of those programs; and to determine whether preventive public health services are reaching populations in need of those services. Neonatal surveillance has focused on planning and evaluating efforts to improve birth-weight-specific mortality and birth-weight distribution, such as early prenatal care and appropriate referrals to tertiary care facilities for women who have severe maternal risk factors or who are likely to deliver a very-low-birth-weight or preterm infant. Postneonatal surveillance has focused on planning and evaluating preventable causes of death such as infections and injuries.

Although vital records form the basis of surveillance, many state programs are beginning to link other health systems records such as Medicaid, the Special Supplemental Food Program for Women, Infants, and Children (WIC), and hospital discharge data to the birth and infant death certificate linked file. Linkage to information on sources and details of care allow for more extensive risk factor identification, assessment of the extent to which programs reach targeted populations, and a more complete evaluation of the effectiveness of programs. However, these additional linkages require a large commitment of resources for computer time and data management. Some program files may not contain an adequate set of variables to allow for individual linkage.

CDC SURVEILLANCE ACTIVITIES

Routine reports of mortality statistics remain an important source of information for surveillance. Mortality reports are available sooner than linked vital records data. Therefore, the cause of death can be examined within 2 years after the event.

The first national linkage of birth and infant death certificates was generated for the 1960 birth cohort by NCHS *(14)*. The 1980 birth cohort was linked by the National Infant Mortality Surveillance project *(15)*. This cohort provided information from 50 states, New York City, the District of Columbia, and Puerto Rico; the data were presented in tabular form rather than in individually linked birth and infant death certificate records. Beginning with the 1983 birth cohort, NCHS has generated individually linked birth and infant death certificates for each cohort. This method represents a change in the population used to estimate yearly neonatal mortality rates. The neonatal mortality rate estimated by using the linked file reflects the mortality experience of all infants born to a specific birth cohort based on the calendar year of birth. The major advantages of using the linked file is that it provides more information about the mothers and infants who died. The major disadvantage is the lack of timeliness in producing the files. State files are usually produced within 2–3 years of the last infant death. (See the Infant Mortality chapter.) National files lag 4–5 years behind the year of death.

Neonatal and postneonatal mortality rates are generally reported by race, with the most striking differences reported between white and black infants (neonatal and postneonatal rates) and between white and Native American infants (postneonatal rates). Before 1989, infant race, which served as the denominator for neonatal

and postneonatal mortality rates, was tabulated on the basis of the race of the child, as generated by an algorithm developed by NCHS. Since 1989, NCHS has tabulated infant race based on the race of the mother, as reported directly on the birth certificate. Race-specific rates of neonatal and postneonatal mortality may vary in the same year depending on whether the denominator of live births is based on the race of the child or of the mother. When reporting mortality by race, one must indicate whether rates are based on use of the race of the child or of the mother. Unless otherwise noted, rates reported in the General Findings section of this chapter are based on the mother's race. Variations in these rates may be related to socioeconomic factors rather than to race or ethnicity per se.

Ethnicity is classified as Hispanic or non-Hispanic. Reporting of ethnicity varies by state. For example, during 1983–1987, only 23 states and Washington, D.C., reported Hispanic ethnicity on the birth certificate. For these states, the Hispanic origin of the mother and father was reported; persons of Hispanic origin were further identified as being of Mexican, Puerto Rican, Cuban, Central or South American, or other Hispanic culture of origin, regardless of race. When reporting mortality by ethnicity, methods used to determine ethnicity should be cited in reports. In this chapter, and in most published reports, rates generated from the linked birth and infant death certificates are based on the mother's ethnicity.

GENERAL FINDINGS

Geographic, Race-Specific Time Trends

From 1978–1980 to 1988–1990, the U.S. neonatal mortality rate declined by 31%, from 8.9 per 1,000 live births to 6.1 per 1,000 live births (*see* Table 22 in NCHS [*16*]). Neonatal mortality rates varied by race and region of the country (time trends are based on unlinked files). Black infants experienced a twofold higher rate of neonatal deaths (15.1 for 1978–1980 and 11.8 for 1988–1990) than white infants (7.8 for 1978–1980 and 5.1 for 1987–1989).

In 1990, the black-to-white infant mortality rate ratio (based on race of the child) was 2.2—an increase of 22% over the lowest ratio of 1.77 attained in 1971. This overall trend was a product of two diverging trends: one for neonatal mortality and one for postneonatal mortality. From 1960 to 1973, neonatal mortality for black and white infants declined at similar rates so that the rate ratio remained relatively stable (1.62 in 1960 and 1.64 in 1973). Since 1973, however, neonatal mortality declined much more rapidly for white than for black infants, leading to an increase in the ratio from 1.64 in 1973 to 2.21 in 1990 (16–17).

In contrast to the trend in neonatal mortality, the black-to-white ratio in postneonatal mortality based on race of child declined rapidly between 1966 and 1975 (from 2.86 in 1966 to 2.08 in 1975), reflecting a more rapid rate of decline for black than white infants (17). From 1975 to 1988, black and white postneonatal mortality declined at about the same rate so that the rate ratio changed little. The rate ratio for postneonatal mortality in 1990 was 2.18 (see Table 20 in NCHS [16]).

From 1987 to 1990, neonatal mortality among white infants was lowest in the Pacific States (Washington, Oregon, California, Alaska, and Hawaii) and the West North Central States (Minnesota, Iowa, Missouri, North Dakota, South Dakota, Iowa, Nebraska, and Kansas); for that same period, neonatal mortality for black infants was lowest in the West South Central States (Arkansas, Louisiana, Oklahoma, and Texas). Between 1978–1980 and 1988–1990, the greatest percentage declines in neonatal mortality for both black and white infants occurred in the West North Central and the West South Central States.

From 1987 to 1990, postneonatal mortality among white infants was lowest in the New England States (Maine, New Hampshire, Vermont, Massachusetts, Rhode Island, and Connecticut). Black postneonatal mortality was also low in the New England States, but rates were based on only three of the six states because the small number of black live births in the other three states resulted in highly unreliable estimates of postneonatal mortality (see Table 22 in NCHS [16]). Among regions that had reliable estimates, postneonatal mortality was lowest in the South

Atlantic States (Delaware, Maryland, District of Columbia, Virginia, West Virginia, North Carolina, South Carolina, Georgia, and Florida).

For both races, the largest percentage declines in postneonatal rates occurred in the South Atlantic States (Delaware, Maryland, District of Columbia, Virginia, West Virginia, North Carolina, South Carolina, Georgia, and Florida) and the West South Central States (Arkansas, Louisiana, Oklahoma, and Texas).

Birth-Weight-Specific Mortality Rates

Birth weight is a major predictor of neonatal mortality. Neonatal mortality may improve because of a decline in the proportion of births that are low birth weight (LBW, <2,500 g) or because of improvements in the survival of LBW infants. Therefore, when evaluating neonatal mortality, we must examine both the proportion of births in each birth-weight category and the mortality experience in each category.

Compared with the 1960 U.S. birth cohort, the 1980 U.S. birth cohort experienced a substantially lower neonatal mortality rate (based on linked files)—16.7 vs. 7.3 per 1,000 live births—reflecting a decline of 56%. However, 91% of this decline can be attributed to reductions in the birth-weight-specific neonatal mortality risk and the remainder to improvements in birth-weight distribution. Although birth-weight-specific neonatal mortality risk decreased among all birth-weight groups, the greatest percentage decline occurred among infants weighing 1,500–1,999 g. A small shift from a lighter to a heavier range of birth weight accounted for the small contribution to the overall decline between 1960 and 1980. Similarly, virtually all of the change in postneonatal mortality risk between 1960 and 1980 resulted from declines in birth-weight-specific mortality. Postneonatal mortality risks decreased among all birth-weight groups except for neonatal survivors weighing 500–999 g (18).

In the United States, rate of very low birth weight (VLBW, <1,500 g) is the principal predictor of neonatal mortality (19). In the 1980s, <1.5% of all live-born infants were VLBW, but these infants account for >50% of all neonatal deaths (15).

Racial and Ethnic Differences in Neonatal and Postneonatal Mortality

The neonatal mortality rate is a crude weighted average of race and ethnicity, birth-weight distribution and birth-weight-specific experience, and many other factors. As noted previously, linked infant birth certificates and death certificates provide more accurate information on neonatal mortality by race and ethnicity (Table 1). Data for the 1985–1987 birth cohorts show that neonatal and postneonatal mortality risks varied widely by race and ethnicity. Infants born to black mothers had the highest neonatal mortality risks followed by those born to Puerto Rican mothers. Overall, Asians had the lowest neonatal mortality risks whereas the risks among whites, Native Americans, and Hispanics (except Puerto Ricans) were somewhat similar.

Postneonatal mortality risks were highest among Native Americans and blacks. Rates among Native Americans were 2.4 times the rates among non-Hispanic whites, and rates among blacks were 2.2 times the rates among non-Hispanic whites. Mortality risks among the other racial and ethnic groups were relatively low and showed little variation. Postneonatal deaths accounted for over half of the total infant deaths among Native Americans compared with approximately a third among other groups [20].

The variation in mortality risks among race/ethnic groups may be related to differences in birth-weight distribution or from differences in

TABLE 1. Infant, neonatal, and postneonatal mortality rates, by race and Hispanic origin of mother — United States, 1985–1987 birth cohorts

Race and Hispanic origin of mother	Deaths per 1,000 live births		
	Infant	Neonatal	Postneonatal
All mothers	10.1	6.6	3.6
Race			
White	8.5	5.5	3.0
Black	18.2	12.0	6.2
Native American or Alaska Native	13.3	6.1	7.2
Asian or Pacific Islander	7.6	4.7	2.9
Chinese	6.0	3.4	2.6
Japanese	6.6	3.9	2.7
Filipino	7.2	4.7	2.5
Other Asian or Pacific Islander*	8.3	5.2	3.2
Hispanic origin†	8.5	5.5	3.0
Mexican American	8.1	5.2	2.9
Puerto Rican	10.9	7.3	3.6
Cuban	7.7	5.5	2.2
Central and South American	7.8	5.2	2.6
Other and unknown Hispanic	9.1	5.7	3.4
Non-Hispanic white†	8.4	5.4	3.0
Non-Hispanic black†	17.9	11.6	6.3

* Includes Hawaiians and part Hawaiians.
† Includes mothers of all races. Data shown only for states with a Hispanic-origin item on their birth certificates. In 1986–1987, 23 states and the District of Columbia included this item.

Source: NCHS, linked birth/infant death data set.

255

birth-weight-specific mortality. Analysis of data from the 1983–1984 U.S. birth cohorts revealed that blacks had nearly three times (2.60%) and Puerto Ricans 1.6 times (1.48%) the incidence of VLBW as did non-Hispanic whites (0.93%) (21). Little or no excess in VLBW incidence was observed among other groups. Blacks and Puerto Ricans also had an elevated rate of moderate-low-birth-weight (MLBW, 1,499–2,499 g) births. The relatively high VLBW and MLBW incidence among blacks and Puerto Ricans is reflected in their high neonatal mortality risks. Mortality risks for VLBW did not vary substantially by race/ethnic groups, although Japanese and Filipino mothers had particularly low rates. However, elevated mortality risks among normal-birth-weight (NBW, 2,500–4,500 g) black and Puerto Rican infants contributed to their high neonatal mortality risks.

An examination of the mortality risk difference between non-Hispanic white and black infants for the 1983 birth cohort showed that black infants weighing <3,000 g had a lower neonatal mortality risk than whites. However, this survival advantage was outweighed by the far greater incidence of LBW in general and VLBW in particular among black infants than among white infants. In the postneonatal period, mortality risks for black infants were generally higher than risks for white infants in all birth-weight groups. After considering the relative contribution of differences in birth-weight distribution and birth-weight-specific neonatal mortality risks, investigators found that deaths among VLBW babies accounted for about 84% of the black-to-white gap in the neonatal mortality risks. In the postneonatal period, higher mortality risk among babies weighing >1,500 g—including those of MLBW (23.4%) and NBW (48%)—accounted for 72.3% of the black to white risk difference in postneonatal mortality (22).

In evaluating neonatal mortality surveillance among Hispanic populations, using the 1983 and 1984 linked birth and infant death data set, Becerra and colleagues identified infants born to Hispanic mothers in 24 reporting areas that included a Hispanic identifier on the birth certificate if the mother was reported as Hispanic (20). By also including infants born in any of the 50

states and Washington, D.C., whose mothers were born in Mexico, Puerto Rico, or Cuba, the investigators identified 3% more Mexican Americans, 27% more Puerto Rican Americans, and 17% more Cuban Americans than originally indicated on the linked data set. To compare outcomes by geographic location, the investigators included infants born to residents of the Commonwealth of Puerto Rico. The VLBW rate was higher among Puerto Ricans born in the continental United States (but not Puerto Rican islanders) than among other Hispanics. Compared with neonatal mortality rates among non-Hispanic whites, neonatal mortality rates were higher among Puerto Rican islanders and Puerto Ricans living in the continental United States. Puerto Rican islanders had the highest birth-weight-specific mortality for all groups except infants weighing >4,000 g.

Causes of Death

The leading cause of neonatal deaths for all infants (based on unlinked files) was birth defects, followed by disorders related to short gestation and unspecified low birth weight, and respiratory distress syndrome (Table 2) (23). However, among black infants, the ranking of leading causes of neonatal deaths was disorders related to short gestation and unspecified low birth weight, followed by respiratory distress syndrome and birth defects. In the postneonatal period, the leading cause of death was sudden infant death syndrome, followed by birth defects and injuries (Table 2). Native Americans and blacks had postneonatal mortality rates of sudden infant death syndrome, infections, and injuries that were two to three times the rates among whites. The least variation in cause-specific mortality among racial and ethnic groups occurred for deaths caused by birth defects.

INTERPRETATION ISSUES

Many of the methodologic and interpretation issues associated with the surveillance of neonatal and postneonatal mortality are similar to those cited for the surveillance of chronic diseases (24). Surveillance involves multiple diseases, rather than a single disease, as well as a complicated

TABLE 2. Mortality from 10 leading causes of neonatal and postneonatal death — United States, 1989

Rank order	Cause of death and rank (ICD codes)*	Number	Rate	Percentage of total deaths
Neonatal				
All causes		**25,168**	**622.8**	**100.0**
1	Congenital anomalies (740–759)	5,902	146.1	23.5
2	Disorders relating to short gestation and unspecified low birth weight (765)	3,878	96.0	15.4
3	Respiratory distress syndrome (769)	3,386	83.8	13.5
4	Newborn affected by maternal complications of pregnancy (761)	1,520	37.6	6.0
5	Newborn affected by complications of placenta, cord, and membranes (762)	973	24.1	3.9
6	Infections specific to the perinatal period (771)	833	20.6	3.3
7	Intrauterine hypoxia and birth asphyxia (768)	653	16.2	2.6
8	Sudden infant death syndrome (798.0)	398	9.8	1.6
9	Neonatal hemorrhage (772)	262	6.5	1.0
10	Birth trauma (767)	215	5.3	0.9
	All other causes (residual)	7,148	176.9	28.5
Postneonatal				
All causes		**14,487**	**358.5**	**100.0**
1	Sudden infant death syndrome (798.0)	5,236	129.6	36.1
2	Congenital anomalies (740–759)	2,218	54.9	15.3
3	Accidents and adverse effects (E800–E949)	900	22.3	6.2
4	Pneumonia and influenza (480–487)	536	13.3	3.7
5	Septicemia (038)	290	7.2	2.0
6	Homicide (E960–E969)	266	6.6	1.8
7	Respiratory distress syndrome (769)	245	6.1	1.7
8	Meningitis (320–322)	193	4.8	1.3
9	Human immunodeficiency virus infection (*042–*044)†	119	2.9	0.8
10	Viral diseases (045–079)	107	2.6	0.7
	All other causes (residual)	4,377	108.4	30.2

* ICD, International Classification of Diseases.
† Asterisks in HIV code indicate category numbers introduced in the United States in 1987.

Source: NCHS (23).

array of risk factors that vary with the disease. Surveillance staffers frequently use existing databases not designed or established for disease surveillance purposes. Furthermore, although mortality reduction will always be the surveillance goal, program managers need a system flexible enough to allow them to make modifications and track a variety of indicators that influence survival.

Another issue to consider is that the surveillance of nonbirth defects-related neonatal mortality has not focused on the individual causes of death but, rather, on the contribution of low birth weight to all-cause mortality. Although low birth weight is a very important determinant of neonatal mortality, this single-minded focus on low birth weight may lead to missed opportunities to conduct routine surveillance and to plan prevention activities for other causes of death (such as maternal medical complications or birth asphyxia) that have high case-fatality rates and that are amenable to medical intervention (25). Although some efforts have been made to address postneonatal mortality among normal-birth-weight infants, more attention needs to be directed to planning prevention strategies for this highly preventable subset of infant deaths (26,27).

EXAMPLES OF USING DATA

South Carolina

Public health surveillance data are useful when associated with action. In the area of neonatal and postneonatal mortality, these actions are usually related to policy development and resource allocation at the state and local levels. For example, neonatal surveillance data can be used to evaluate health service delivery issues related to regionalization. The South Carolina Department of Health and Environmental Control has a perinatal regionalization surveillance system that helps providers of maternofetal and neonatal intensive care services to evaluate risk-appropriate referral patterns and mortality experience and to identify areas for further improvement (28).

In an assessment of neonatal mortality experience, South Carolina analyzed birth-weight-specific neonatal mortality rates for VLBW

infants (500–1,499 g) by level of hospital care for selected years during 1983–1991 (Table 3) (28). Delivery and infant care in a tertiary care hospital (level III) that provides fetal medicine and neonatal intensive care improves the survival of this vulnerable group of infants. The 3-year neonatal mortality rate for white and black VLBW infants is given to smooth the variability associated with small annual numbers. For each period, infants who were born in a level III facility tended to have lower neonatal mortality. Those infants weighing 500–999 g who were born in level III facilities consistently had lower neonatal mortality rates than those treated in level I hospitals.

South Carolina's 3-year direct-adjusted neonatal mortality rate varied by perinatal region for infants weighing 500–1,400 g (Figures 1 and 2). The adjusted mortality rate was estimated by multiplying the birth-weight-specific neonatal mortality rate by the proportion of live births in each weight group of a standard population. This adjustment allowed the comparison of mortality between different regions and periods and removed the effect of differences in birth-weight distribution (28). Investigators observed a decline in neonatal mortality among white infants residing in three of the four regions (Figure 1). Similar declines were found for black and other minority infants, but not in the same regions (Figure 2).

Puerto Rico

Puerto Rico evaluated its regionalized perinatal health-care system after an initial study showed that from 1980 through 1984, the system was deficient and that the survival of newborns in Puerto Rico was much worse than for Puerto Ricans in the continental United States (29). Nevertheless, the neonatal mortality rate declined by an annual average of 5% from 1980 through 1988. Data for the 1981–1988 linked birth and infant death certificates were used to measure any contributions of the regionalized perinatal health-care system to the declining neonatal mortality rate in Puerto Rico. These data include approximately 265,000 singleton infants whose mothers were residents of Puerto Rico in 1981–1984 and 252,000 infants whose mothers were residents in 1985–1988. Analysts found that from 1981 to 1988, Puerto Rico experienced

FIGURE 1. Three-year, direct-adjusted neonatal mortality risk for white
live-born infants weighing 500–1499 g at birth, by perinatal
region — South Carolina, 1983–1992

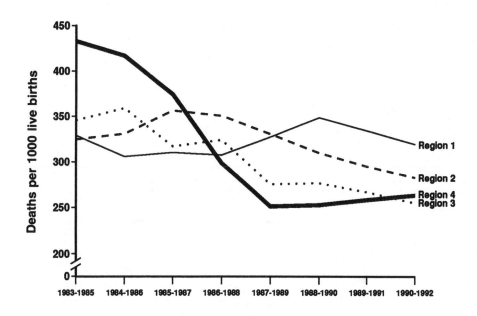

FIGURE 2. Three-year, direct-adjusted neonatal mortality risk for black and
other minority live-born infants weighing 500–1499 g at birth, by
perinatal region — South Carolina, 1983–1992

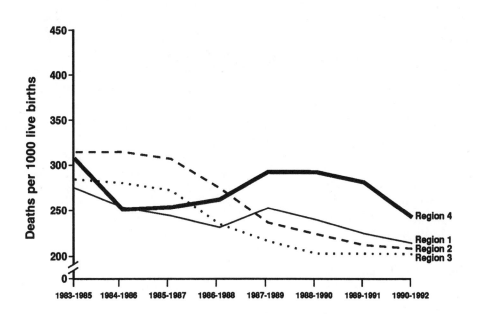

259

TABLE 3. Three-year low-birth-weight-specific neonatal mortality rate, by level of hospital care for white infants — South Carolina, 1983–1991

Birth weight (g)	Deaths per 1,000 live births								
	1983–1985			1986–1988			1989–1991		
	Level I	Level II	Level III	Level I	Level II	Level III	Level I	Level II	Level III
500–749	936	952	750	840	958	712	809	1,000	638
750–999	515	476	404	583	538	344	429	440	223
1,000–1,249	256	133	101	273	179	163	100	205	146
1,250–1,499	98	103	114	62	100	65	158	93	52
% of all births*	17	9	62	10	10	72	5	15	71
Total number of births		928			962			1,036	

* Percentages may not add to 100 because percentage distribution of all births is shown only for hospital births.

Source: Liu Q et al. *(28)*.

significant improvement in the regionalization of the perinatal health-care system. Improvement was reflected in the increased proportion of VLBW newborns delivered in hospitals with neonatal intensive care units and in the survival advantage provided by these hospitals to premature babies. In addition, from 1981 to 1988, Puerto Rico experienced significant reductions in the neonatal mortality rate because of better newborn survival—a reflection of better access to and quality of hospital care. Neonatal survival varied by perinatal region.

Florida

Surveillance also has been used to evaluate the effects of expanded services on neonatal mortality. The evaluation of Florida's statewide Improved Pregnancy Outcome (IPO) program examined how 1985–1988 neonatal mortality rates were affected by IPO comprehensive services (prenatal care, health and nutritional counseling, education, assistance with delivery arrangements, postpartum and well-baby care, family planning, and WIC and Medicaid enrollment) *(30)*. Birth certificate data, infant death certificate data, and program records of participating women were linked. Linked birth certificate and infant death records were used to identify nonparticipants matched for race, age,

education, marital status, and number of prenatal-care visits (<7 or ≥7). Neonatal mortality was 33% lower among black IPO enrollees than among black nonparticipants. Neonatal mortality declined faster among white enrollees than among white nonparticipants.

West Virginia

In West Virginia, health officials developed a birth scoring system to identify newborns at risk for postneonatal mortality. They used vital records data from 1980–1983 births to develop the risk score *(Myerberg and Myerberg, West Virginia University, unpublished data, 1992)*. Infants born in 1985–1987 were assigned a birth score. In an evaluation of the program, using birth scores linked to birth and infant death certificates, they demonstrated that the rate of postneonatal death was six times higher among infants with high birth scores than among those with lower scores.

United States

National surveillance for neonatal and postneonatal mortality can be useful for identifying areas in need of prevention activities. In a national study of 1986–1987 case-fatality rates associated with conditions arising in the perinatal period, the results indicated that maternal medical conditions were associated with high case-fatality rates *(25)*. Since then, national linked birth certificate and infant death certificate files for 1983–1987 are being used to describe infant deaths caused by maternal medical conditions. Preliminary results indicate that infants born to multiparous (parity of 2) women <20 years of age have the highest rates of neonatal death from medical conditions associated with the pregnancy.

FUTURE ISSUES

During the 1980s, the surveillance of neonatal and postneonatal mortality moved beyond monitoring to include public health action. In the future, state and local health officials will need to 1) clarify priority issues that should be addressed by surveillance; 2) determine whether the efficient linkage of additional health databases (such as Medicaid data, hospital discharge records, or WIC records) to vital records data at the state and local levels will be useful in addressing priority areas related to neonatal and postneonatal deaths; and 3) determine how surveillance can be used as a risk assessment tool.

Because so many causes of death and potential risk factors exist for neonatal and postneonatal death, the traditional surveillance loop of data collection, analysis, reporting, and action must include the establishment of priorities to determine which types of analyses must be done. Furthermore, because of the multifactorial etiologies and the difficulty in linking exposures, risk factors, interventions, and outcomes *(12)*, public health officials will continue to be in constant pursuit of more detailed data sets that provide more information on risk factors. Surveillance is usually based on the preventability of the outcome of interest. To prevent infant deaths, program directors expect surveillance data to help them identify infants at the highest risk of neonatal and postneonatal deaths. Like West Virginia and other states that use linked vital records data to develop risk assessment measures, more states need to begin using these data to determine which infants are at the highest risk of postneonatal mortality.

REFERENCES

1. Pharoah POD, Morris JN. Postneonatal mortality. Epidemiol Rev 1979;1:170–83.

2. Buehler JW, Hogue CJR, Zaro SM. Postponing or preventing deaths? Trends in infant survival, Georgia, 1974 through 1981. JAMA 1985;253:3564–7.

3. Friede A, Rhodes PH, Guyer B, Binkin NJ, Hannan MT, Hogue CJR. The postponement of neonatal deaths into the postneonatal period: evidence from Massachusetts. Am J Epidemiol 1988;127:161–70.

4. Starfield B. Postneonatal mortality. Annu Rev Public Health 1985;6:21–40.

5. McCormick MC. The contribution of low birth weight to infant mortality and childhood morbidity. N Engl J Med 1985;312:82–90.

6. Kleinman JC, Kiely JL. Postneonatal mortality in the United States: an international perspective. Pediatrics 1990;86:1091–7.

7. CDC. Infant mortality—United States, 1990. MMWR 1993;42:161–5.

8. Khoury MJ, Erickson JD, Adams MJ Jr. Trends in postneonatal mortality in the United States, 1962 through 1978. JAMA 1984;252:367–72.

9. NCHS. Advance report of final mortality statistics, 1990. Hyattsville, Maryland: US Department of Health and Human Services, Public Health Service, CDC, 1993. (Monthly vital statistics report; vol. 41, no. 7, suppl.)

10. Iyasu S, Lynberg MC, Rowley D, Saftlas AF, Atrash HK. Surveillance of postneonatal mortality, United States, 1980–1987. MMWR 1991;40(No. SS-1):43–55.

11. Langmuir AD. The surveillance of communicable diseases of national importance. N Engl J Med 1963;268:182–92.

12. Thacker SB, Berkelman RL. Public health surveillance in the United States. Epidemiol Rev 1988;10:164–90.

13. Zahniser C, Halpin G, Hollinshead W, Kessel S, Koontz A. Using linked birth and infant death files for program planning and evaluation: NIMS workshop lessons. Public Health Rep 1987;102:211–6.

14. NCHS. A study of infant mortality from linked records: method of study and registration aspects, United States, 1960 live birth cohort. Washington, DC: US Department of Health, Education, and Welfare, Public Health Service, Health Services and Mental Health Administration, 1970. (Vital and health statistics; series 20, no. 7.)

15. Hogue CJR, Buehler JW, Strauss LT, Smith JC. Overview of the National Infant Mortality Surveillance (NIMS) Project—design, methods, results. Public Health Rep 1987;102:126–38.

16. NCHS. Health, United States, 1992, and healthy people 2000 review. Hyattsville, Maryland: US Department of Health and Human Services, Public Health Service, CDC, 1993; DHHS publication no. (PHS) 93-1232.

17. MacDorman MF, Rosenberg HM. Trends in infant mortality by cause of death and other characteristics, 1960–88. Hyattsville, Maryland: US Department of Health and Human Services, Public Health Service, CDC, NCHS, 1993. (Vital and health statistics; series 20, no. 20.)

18. Buehler JW, Kleinman JC, Hogue CJR, Strauss LT, Smith JC. Birth weight-specific infant mortality, United States, 1960 and 1980. Public Health Rep 1987;102: 151–61.

19. Lee K, Paneth N, Garner LM, Pearlman M. The very low-birth-weight rate: principal predictor of neonatal mortality in industrialized populations. J Pediatr 1980;97:759–64.

20. Becerra JE, Hogue CJR, Atrash HK, Pérez N. Infant mortality among Hispanics: a portrait of heterogeneity. JAMA 1991; 265:217–21.

21. Kleinman JC. Infant mortality among racial/ethnic minority groups, 1983–1984. MMWR 1990;39(No. SS-3):31–9.

22. Iyasu S, Becerra JE, Rowley DL, Hogue CJR. Impact of very low birthweight on the black-white infant mortality gap. Am J Prev Med 1992;8:271–7.

23. NCHS. Vital statistics of the United States, 1989, Vol. II, mortality part A. Washington, DC: US Department of Health and Human Services, Public Health Service, CDC, 1992; DHHS publication no. (PHS)92-1102.

24. Garbe PL, Blount SB. Chronic disease surveillance. In: Halpin W, Baker EL Jr, Monson RR, eds. Public health surveillance. New York: Van Nostrand Reinhold, 1992:130–9.

25. Becerra JE, Rowley DL, Atrash HK. Case fatality rates associated with conditions originating in the perinatal period: United States, 1986 through 1987. Pediatrics 1992;89:1256–8.

26. Druschel CM, Hale CB. Postneonatal mortality among normal birth weight infants in Alabama, 1980 to 1983. Pediatrics 1987;80:869–72.

27. Schoendorf KC, Hogue CJR, Kleinman JC, Rowley D. Mortality among infants of black as compared with white college-educated parents. N Engl J Med 1992; 326:1522–6.

28. Liu Q, Sappenfield WM, Moniz KS, Kemick B, Holgren E. South Carolina perinatal regionalization surveillance system: report of perinatal indicators for 1983–1991. Vol. 1. Columbia, South Carolina: South Carolina Department of Health and Environmental Control, 1992.

29. Becerra JE, Pérez de Saliceti N, Smith JC. Evaluation of a regionalized perinatal care system through linked infant birth and death certificates: Puerto Rico, 1980–84. P R Health Sci J 1989;8:305–11.

30. Clarke LL, Miller MK, Vogel WB, Davis KE, Mahan CS. The effectiveness of Florida's "improved pregnancy outcome" program. J Health Care Poor Underserved 1993;4:117–32.

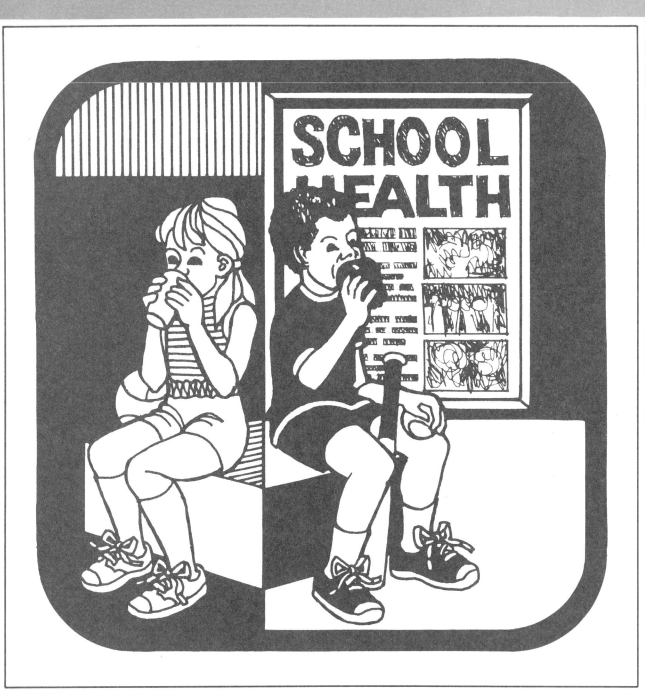

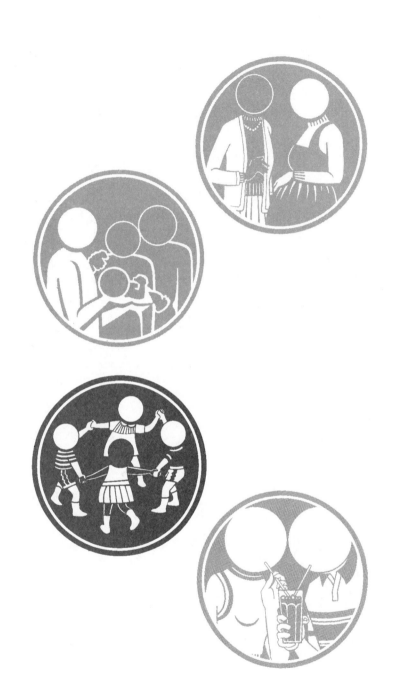

Commentary

on Child Health
from the University of Nebraska Medical Center and CityMatCH

A 5-year-old girl is about to start kindergarten. As she enters the classroom for the first time, information about her immunization status is captured for reporting to a surveillance system. If she contracts measles or another vaccine-preventable disease before that, her case probably would be reported to CDC through the National Electronic Telecommunications System for Surveillance. If this same child is struck by a car while riding her bike home, information about her injuries may be captured by hospital discharge data systems or reported to a trauma registry. If her younger sister becomes ill with an invasive bacterial disease like meningitis and her family lives in an active surveillance area, her case likely would be reported to CDC. If her sister develops significant hearing impairment or mental retardation as a sequela of meningitis and the family resides in the Atlanta metropolitan area, her case would have been captured by the Metropolitan Atlanta Developmental Disabilities Surveillance Program. And should any of the children in this family die, the death certificate would capture data for population-based surveillance.

From all of this surveillance activity, what can be learned? How do existing public health surveillance systems help us plan for the health of this child and her family? The Child Health section of this monograph is intended to serve as a road map to guide public health practitioners in the acquisition, use, and translation of the kinds of data illustrated above. Before proceeding, be forewarned—unlike data systems capturing risks and outcomes of the perinatal period, child health surveillance is far less straightforward. Existing health data for the surveillance of growing children are like the materials of an elementary art class—pieces of paper, bits, glitter, and glue. As the child creates unique images from these pieces, so must the skilled public health professional create a **collage** of information that illustrates the compelling story of the health and well-being of children. Public health practitioners at the local, state, and national levels must learn not only about the value of each piece of information but also about how best to apply the glue to link the pieces together.

CHILD HEALTH SURVEILLANCE AND CDC

The inventory of CDC's existing and forthcoming child health surveillance systems, as described in this section of the monograph, provides an excellent cornerstone in compiling a knowledge base of national surveillance activities. CDC surveillance systems address a wide range of problems, including infectious diseases, vaccine-preventable diseases, injuries, child abuse, lead poisoning, poor nutrition, developmental disabilities, and fetal alcohol syndrome. Readers are given a succinct overview of the public health importance and history of surveillance, a description of the current surveillance systems at CDC, and general findings from these systems. System-specific methodological and interpretational issues are reviewed, and forthcoming surveillance activities are described. In these chapters, the authors give specific examples of how the surveillance data have been used for program planning and policy development.

Despite CDC's efforts, few truly national, population-based systems are available for child health surveillance. Moreover, no single, overarching national surveillance system is in place to monitor children's health in the United States. Each of the individual surveillance systems with relevance to children addresses selected components of health risks, health services, and health outcomes of childhood. Each system seemingly was designed independent of most all others, driven by the data collection, analysis, and utilization needs related to the disease or condition of focus. Furthermore, when no data collection system exists—as is the case with injuries—surveillance relies on the acquisition, interpretation, and linkage of fragmented secondary data sources that commonly have been developed for other purposes. The key is for public health practitioners to have a firm understanding of the existence, content, and utility of the major separate surveillance systems. CDC scientists, like public health practitioners at the state and local levels, often must derive estimates from partial systems and extrapolate those findings to specific populations of children defined by geographic residence, age, race or ethnicity, sex, or other characteristics. The lack of national surveillance systems for the growing years of childhood is disappointing but not surprising. As a result of increased childhood survival, the epidemiology of children's health has shifted in recent decades from mortality to morbidity; death is a rare event in childhood. Moreover, the etiology of disease has moved from acute biologic causes (infectious pathogens) to more chronic environmental and socioeconomic factors (risk-related behavior, poverty, and access to care). CDC's current and developing surveillance systems for children reflect this pattern: death certificate vital statistics and infectious disease reporting are long-standing and population-based, whereas the surveillance of injury and fetal alcohol syndrome must rely on the linkage of multiple secondary data sources usually not designed for health monitoring. The number of emerging surveillance systems in child health at CDC reflects an impressive recognition of the need for change; indeed, the landscape of child health surveillance should look remarkably different in the next century. In the interim, we must develop effective approaches to using existing data resources.

COLLAGE STRATEGIES FOR LINKING CDC CHILD HEALTH DATA

Now let us move on to the craft of child health surveillance, using CDC data that are described in the following chapters. Let us examine the basic materials for the ensuing collage—paper, bits, glitter, and glue—and identify basic strategies for putting the pieces together.

- **The paper**. Just as the creation of a collage starts with a single piece of paper to support the various bits and glitter, so must users of CDC data at the state and local levels develop up front a clear vision of the primary purpose for which acquired data will be used. CDC's child health surveillance data are used in several primary ways: 1) as estimates of the national prevalence of selected conditions or events; 2) as baselines for the generation of synthetic estimates through extrapolation to the state and local levels;

and 3) as benchmarks for well-developed, robust methods and standardized definitions that can be used at the state and local levels to develop primary data collection activities. Clarifying how surveillance data are to be used before acquisition and analysis will secure the right piece of paper as a firm foundation for the resulting collage.

- **The bits**. Too often, the availability of data alone drives its use. When presented with an assortment of data fragments—ranging from reportable cases of Haemophilus influenzae and other vaccine-preventable childhood diseases to anthropometric and hemoglobin measurements of low-income children and malformations—public health planners may feel compelled to use all of the pieces to create the most comprehensive profile of children's health status. An alternate strategy is to first develop a keen understanding of all possible data of interest and to then select judiciously the elements that will influence the intended purpose of the data. One approach is to establish a brief profile of each potential data set that documents its strengths and caveats and use these profiles to influence both the selection process and subsequent use of the data.

- **The glitter**. Better data can make the collage glisten. Being aware of existing surveillance activities at CDC should stimulate communities to contribute more fully to state and national surveillance systems, thus improving the overall quality and use of the data. The providers of data need incentives to ensure greater participation in surveillance activities. One powerful incentive can be timely and substantive feedback to state and local health departments so that the benefits and products of data generation can be felt closer to home.

- **The glue**. How can we hold all of these pieces together? The first critical step is to fully realize the limitations of using existing data from various sources and systems. In the collection of fragmented data from multiple sources, having standard definitions of selected indicators across data sets is unlikely. Linking data from multiple sources may be hampered further by varying units of analysis (i.e., population-based [children] vs. program-based [encounters]). Valid and appropriate concerns regarding the protection of confidentiality may limit the use of data when numbers are small or outcomes are rare. Amid inconsistent legal bases for child health surveillance across jurisdictions, the incentives for reporting selected conditions or events will differ, yielding varying levels of data completeness. Measurement thresholds and case definitions for some conditions have changed over time, making trend analysis problematic. Extrapolations of prevalence estimates from national surveys to the state and local levels may be unadvisable when sociodemographic population characteristics are widely dissimilar. Being aware of such data caveats, although critical, may dissuade some state and local public health planners from using the substantial array of CDC surveillance data on growing children. In areas with no community-based data collection efforts, CDC data may be the only alternative to no surveillance at all. The best strategy in the short term is to remain cognizant of all potential limitations without becoming paralyzed by them. The long-term challenge is to identify unmet state and local data needs that CDC will be unlikely to address and to develop a plan for strengthening surveillance closer to home.

This monograph should yield many creative collages for child health surveillance at the state and local levels. Yet communities' surveillance activities should not be driven by the current array of fragmented child health information systems. Indeed, the art of child health surveillance is the creation of a shared vision for comprehensive surveillance at the national, state, and local levels. Ideally, in future decades the current collage will become transformed into a systematic, meaningful portrait of children's health in the United States.

Magda G. Peck, Sc.D.
Chief
Section on Child Health Policy
Assistant Professor, Pediatrics
University of Nebraska Medical Center
Executive Director/Chief Executive Officer, CityMatCH
Omaha, Nebraska

Bacterial and Other Infectious Diseases

Anne Schuchat, M.D.,[1] and Jacquelyn A. Polder, B.S.N., M.P.H.[2]

PUBLIC HEALTH IMPORTANCE

Despite important twentieth century advances such as improved sanitation and the availability of several safe and effective vaccines for infants, infectious diseases remain the most common cause of illness in children in the United States. In developing countries, infectious agents are still the predominant cause of mortality during childhood.

Infectious diseases among children range in severity from the self-limited common cold to potentially fatal infections like bacterial meningitis and hemolytic uremic syndrome associated with Escherichia coli O157:H7. Otitis media, usually a relatively minor infection, has the potential to permanently impair hearing and thus contribute to learning disability. Other childhood infectious diseases have substantial case-fatality ratios; for example, even when antibiotics are appropriately administered, 12% of meningococcal disease cases result in death.

The public health effects of childhood infections extend beyond the direct disability and death caused by these agents. For example, chronic antibiotic therapy for otitis media can lead to the emergence of antimicrobial resistance and can complicate the management of subsequent infections in the community. Other childhood infections may cause serious outcomes for contacts of the infected children, such as the complications that may occur when pregnant women are exposed to children with rubella or cytomegalovirus infection (1,2).

From a public health perspective, the most alarming manifestation of childhood infections is the potential for propagation of disease, particularly when transmission leads to widespread community involvement with disease. Infectious disease outbreaks can lead to the closing of schools or child day-care centers and may require emergency vaccination campaigns. The closing of restaurants, recall of contaminated foods, and litigation related to implicated vehicles in common-source outbreaks can have an important effect on a community's economy. Also important are the costs associated with loss of work for parents who must stay home to care for an ill child or one excluded from child day care until he or she is no longer considered contagious. Tourism has even been threatened when travelers fear their children might contract a serious infection in a proposed destination. Good surveillance data can prove invaluable in the management of public concerns.

Recent public health history provides several instances in which illness among children was a sentinel for a problem in the general community. Cases of acquired immunodeficiency syndrome (AIDS) among children with hemophilia were early alerts to the transmissibility of human immunodeficiency virus (HIV) through blood products. A community outbreak of foodborne listeriosis in 1981 was only recognized when >1% of newborns in a Halifax maternity hospital suffered from perinatal listeriosis (3). In

---

[1] Division of Bacterial and Mycotic Diseases
National Center for Infectious Diseases
Centers for Disease Control and Prevention
Atlanta, Georgia

[2] Hospital Infections Program
National Center for Infectious Diseases
Centers for Disease Control and Prevention
Atlanta, Georgia

1978, James Todd first described toxic-shock syndrome (TSS) in seven children with severe multisystem disease *(4)*. Investigation of epidemic TSS associated with tampon use in 1980 revealed that many TSS cases had occurred in earlier years *(5)*.

Many infectious diseases of childhood are preventable through relatively simple measures such as routine vaccination, good hygiene, and careful food preparation. Surveillance for infectious diseases permits us to identify high-risk populations in which improved access to preventive services and health education efforts might produce the greatest benefits. Surveillance for diseases that are not currently preventable provides a baseline to measure the effectiveness of interventions subsequently introduced, as was recently illustrated by surveillance data on *Haemophilus influenzae* type b (Hib) disease in the prevaccine and vaccine eras *(6)* (for additional information about related topics and surveillance activities, see the Vaccination Coverage and Vaccine-Preventable Diseases chapters).

HISTORY OF DATA COLLECTION

Surveillance for infectious diseases has one of the longest histories of all public health issues. The collection of U.S. data on plague, smallpox, and yellow fever began in 1878 *(7)*. By 1925, all states were reporting the occurrence of selected diseases to the U.S. Public Health Service. Public health surveillance originally referred to the quarantine of contacts of persons with communicable diseases to observe for early symptoms. Langmuir expanded the term's scope to include the surveillance of populations rather than individuals and used the term to refer to the collection, analysis, and dissemination of data *(7)*. Subsequent definitions incorporated certain disease control responsibilities. This action-oriented sense of surveillance for infectious diseases in children is the primary focus of this chapter.

In addition to CDC's well-established systems for the surveillance of nationally notifiable diseases *(8)*, several systems for the surveillance of specific infectious diseases are coordinated through programs at CDC. These surveillance systems monitor diseases of particular importance in childhood, such as viral hepatitis, AIDS, Reye's syndrome, TSS, outbreaks of foodborne and waterborne diseases, and vaccine-preventable diseases such as measles, rubella, and influenza. Infections associated with child day care have been included in recently established pilot projects for the surveillance of infectious diseases in child day-care settings. For several years, however, information regarding child care attendance has been a part of routine surveillance for specific infections, such as viral hepatitis, Hib disease, and giardiasis.

CDC SURVEILLANCE ACTIVITIES

Throughout this chapter, various general surveillance activities at CDC are mentioned, but the primary focus is on the Multistate Active Surveillance System to illustrate the use of surveillance data in directing and evaluating public health interventions. The multistate system, initiated in 1986, involves collaborative surveillance for invasive bacterial diseases of substantial importance in childhood. In recent years, diseases under active surveillance have included meningitis and other invasive diseases caused by *H. influenzae, Neisseria meningitidis*, group B streptococcus (GBS), *Listeria monocytogenes*, and *Streptococcus pneumoniae*. CDC defines a case as isolation of one of these pathogens from a usually sterile site (e.g., blood or cerebrospinal fluid) in a resident of the active surveillance area.

Standardized case report forms are completed for all cases. For a number of the pathogens, bacterial isolates are sent to CDC laboratories for further tests such as serotyping and molecular subtyping. Information routinely collected on case report forms includes demographic data, the outcome of infection, the clinical syndrome, the anatomic site from which the organism was isolated, and whether the child attended a child-care facility, was hospitalized, and required hospital transfer. For particular pathogens, information is collected on serogroup and antibiotic susceptibility. This population-based surveillance system has been used to detect cases for additional studies, including case-control studies of the efficacy of vaccines against Hib disease. In those studies, surveillance officers help to enroll control subjects and CDC personnel collect additional information on manufacturer, lot numbers, and number of vaccine doses administered. The surveillance system also has identified cases for studies of dietary risk factors for sporadic listeriosis; the results of these studies led to the development of dietary guidelines on how pregnant women can reduce their risk of foodborne listeriosis (9).

Surveillance areas have included entire states (e.g., Maryland, Missouri, New Jersey, Oklahoma, and Washington), metropolitan areas (e.g., San Francisco Bay and metropolitan Atlanta areas), several counties within a state (e.g., four counties in Tennessee), or a large geographic unit (e.g., Los Angeles County). Currently, the aggregate population under surveillance includes >20 million people and represents cases detected at 570 hospitals.

Surveillance is indeed **active**; surveillance personnel based at local and state health departments and academic institutions make biweekly calls to contacts in microbiology laboratories serving all acute care hospitals in the surveillance areas. Surveillance officers verify case eligibility (e.g., residence) and enter the data from case report forms into an Epi Info database. Computer diskettes are mailed monthly to CDC, where a surveillance coordinator reviews the data for accuracy and completeness. The central surveillance database is thus updated monthly, with corrections being made at the local levels. The results of additional laboratory tests performed at CDC are sent to the surveillance sites periodically. In addition, some surveillance officers provide local hospitals with periodic summaries of disease reports by coded hospital number. Hospital personnel know the code only for their own hospital and can thus compare disease occurrence in their institution with reported cases in the other area institutions.

Periodically, surveillance officers perform laboratory audits to assess the completeness of active surveillance and to identify additional cases. In some instances, microbiology records for a specified period are reviewed for all hospitals in the surveillance areas. In other audits, records are reviewed in a stratified sample of hospitals (e.g.,

auditing 100% of institutions with at least 200 beds and 20% of those with fewer beds).

Census data are used for denominators. Surveillance reports use age- and race-specific rates because age is strongly related to risk of disease, and rates of several of these infections are higher for certain racial and ethnic populations than they are for whites. These racial differences are not likely related to race per se but instead to behavioral and socioeconomic factors such as day care attendance, breast-feeding, household crowding, and access to health care.

Surveillance reports vary in frequency, depending on the subject or focus. Recent reports have summarized the entire active surveillance for bacterial meningitis (10) as well as several components of the system (6,9,11,12). Surveillance personnel meet every 1–2 years, offering additional forums for problem-solving, feedback, and the introduction of new components into the surveillance system. Periodically, the surveillance system has been adapted to exclude a disease for which surveillance is no longer considered feasible or of a high priority. Diseases also may be added to the system, when resources permit, in response to emerging public health needs; for example, in 1992, the active surveillance system was expanded to include the reporting of multidrug-resistant tuberculosis in certain surveillance areas.

A passive surveillance system, the National Bacterial Meningitis Reporting System (NBMRS), has provided information on culture-confirmed cases of bacterial meningitis since 1979. Reporting is less complete and not as timely as surveillance in the active system; however, the NBMRS does allow the evaluation of longitudinal trends, which would not be possible using surveillance systems that were only introduced recently (see the Interpretation Issues section of this chapter).

Another surveillance system that collects information on infectious diseases important in childhood is the National Notifiable Diseases Surveillance System (NNDSS) (8). To help state epidemiologists and health department staff establish a database for the surveillance of numerous diseases and to increase the ease and timeliness of reporting, CDC in 1984 introduced the National

Electronic Telecommunications System for Surveillance (NETSS) *(13)*. Six states initially used NETSS, and by 1989, all 50 states and 3 U.S. territories were using the system for the weekly reporting to CDC of 44 of the 49 nationally notifiable diseases *(8)*. This computer-based telecommunications system encompasses the collection, transmission, and analysis of the data and the publishing of weekly reports on notifiable diseases from all states as well as New York City, the District of Columbia, and U.S. territories. To enter data states use a variety of computer systems that are programmed to create data files in standard NETSS format for transmission to CDC. Tables of the number of cases reported by state and region appear each week in the *Morbidity and Mortality Weekly Report*. Although some of the reported conditions have little relevance for children, the reporting of conditions such as measles, mumps, pertussis, and rubella in this system underscores the important role that the NNDSS and NETSS can play in the surveillance of childhood infections (further details on surveillance for vaccine-preventable diseases appear in the Vaccine-Preventable Diseases and Vaccination Coverage chapters).

The Public Health Laboratory Information System (PHLIS) is yet another resource for the surveillance of infectious diseases. The system is based in state health department laboratories. Selected results are reported electronically from these laboratories to appropriate programs within CDC. Examples of data transmitted via PHLIS are the results of serotyping *Salmonella* isolates and, more recently, antimicrobial resistance of *Mycobacterium* tuberculosis isolates. The system is flexible, and new modules for reporting additional diseases can be introduced relatively quickly.

GENERAL FINDINGS

CDC's Multistate Active Surveillance System has consistently demonstrated a strong relationship between age and risk for invasive bacterial diseases *(10)*. The highest rates of disease caused by *N. meningitidis*, Hib, *S. pneumoniae*, GBS, and *L. monocytogenes* are among children <5 years old. GBS and *L. monocytogenes* primarily affect children during the first month of life, whereas the highest rates of disease caused by

the other three pathogens occur after the first few months, presumably once maternally acquired antibodies are no longer circulating.

In general, rates of invasive bacterial disease are higher for blacks than for whites. For example, the relative risk of meningococcal disease in 1989–1991 for blacks of all ages was 1.41 (95% confidence interval = 1.10, 1.80) the relative risk for persons of other races (Figure 1) *(14)*. Active surveillance in 1990 revealed that blacks had twice the rate of neonatal GBS disease as did whites (p <0.001) *(12)*. Although blacks have had higher rates of invasive disease caused by Hib than whites, a case-control study nested into a predecessor to the bacterial disease surveillance system in metropolitan Atlanta revealed that after controlling for child day-care attendance and breast-feeding, black race was no longer a risk factor for Hib disease *(15)*.

In general, rates of bacterial meningitis have been similar in different surveillance areas, with some regional variations in the incidence of Hib disease *(10)*. When New Jersey was stratified into counties with high vs. low prevalence of AIDS, important differences were identified in the rates of invasive pneumococcal disease. Among children of races other than white, those in areas with a high prevalence of AIDS had more than twice the rate of pneumococcal disease as did those living in the low-AIDS areas (p <0.05) *(16)*. This finding was consistent with the observation that persons with AIDS have a nearly 300-fold risk of invasive pneumococcal disease *(16)*.

Seasonal trends in the occurrence of disease caused by Hib and meningococcus also have been observed. Hib disease peaks in the fall and winter, whereas meningococcal disease peaks in late winter and early spring *(10)*. No consistent seasonal patterns have been detected for disease caused by *L. monocytogenes* or GBS.

Important trends in certain diseases have been evident over the last several years. The most striking example is the decline of childhood Hib disease in the Hib vaccine era. Active surveillance data for 1989–1991 were recently reported along with NBMRS data for 1980–1991, permitting us to compare disease incidence before and after any Hib vaccines were introduced and after the introduction of conjugate vaccines for disease pre-

FIGURE 1. Incidence of meningococcal disease by race — selected U.S. areas, 1989–1991

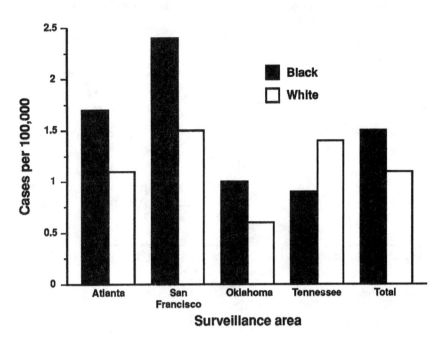

vention *(6)*. Because the passive system consistently reported only on cases of meningitis (not all cases of invasive disease) and could not distinguish disease caused by type b from disease caused by other *H. influenzae*, the active surveillance system was important in confirming trends in disease occurrence. In addition, the very high sensitivity of the active system assured that the reduction in disease occurrence was not an artifact of decreased reporting. Active surveillance revealed a 71% decrease in the incidence of Hib disease among children <5 years old, from 37 per 100,000 persons in 1989 to 11 per 100,000 persons in 1991 (Figure 2) *(6)*. Increases in doses of Hib vaccine distributed in the United States coincided with declines in Hib disease *(6)*.

Active surveillance for neonatal GBS disease has revealed both a lower incidence and case-fatality ratio than data from hospital-based series reported in the medical literature *(12)*. However, rates of GBS disease among preterm infants are much higher than rates among term deliveries, and many hospital-based series are conducted in tertiary centers or hospitals serving indigent populations, where rates of prematurity and other risk factors may be elevated. The distribution of preterm deliveries in the active surveillance population is similar to national estimates. Therefore,

incidence determined through active surveillance is probably a better reflection of disease occurrence nationally than estimates from a few hospitals. The reduced case-fatality ratio for neonatal GBS disease, identified in the active surveillance population (<6% compared with 15%–50% in previous series), probably reflects recent improvements in the management of neonatal sepsis as well as the fact that recent studies reporting higher mortality rates were conducted in relatively high-risk patient populations.

INTERPRETATION ISSUES

The reduced incidence of Hib disease documented by CDC's active surveillance system has raised numerous questions *(6)*. Although the striking decrease in disease occurrence coincided with the vaccine era, disease in infants <18 months of age declined dramatically before vaccines were licensed for use in that age-group. Was the decline an artifact of decreased reporting, a reflection of natural variation in disease activity, or a biologically explicable phenomenon?

Laboratory audits confirmed that the active surveillance system was quite sensitive in detecting cases of invasive disease caused by Hib. In 1990,

275

FIGURE 2. *Haemophilus influenzae* type 6 vaccine doses distributed and *H. influenzae* meningitis cases among children <5 years old — 20 states participating in the National Bacterial Meningitis Reporting System — 1980–1991

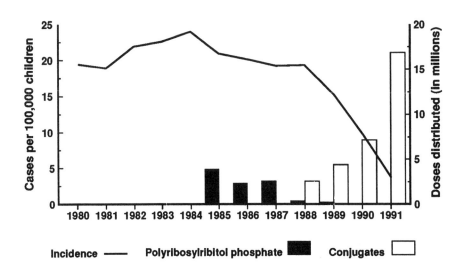

surveillance officers audited 81 hospital laboratories to identify case patients <5 years old who were missed by routine surveillance in 1989. This audit demonstrated that active surveillance had identified 95.6% of all Hib cases among children <5 years old. An artifact of decreased reporting in a system this sensitive could not account for the >70% reduction in disease occurrence. Laboratory audits for all hospitals participating in surveillance throughout 1991 suggested that the sensitivity of active surveillance for Hib disease remained high (6).

Although data from the passive NBMRS are available for a longer period than data from the active system, case reports do not distinguish disease caused by Hib from disease caused by other *H. influenzae*. Some investigators have postulated that a vaccine-related decrease in Hib disease might be accompanied by an increase in disease caused by nontypeable and other serotypes of *H. influenzae* (17). The very specific case definition used in active surveillance permits an ongoing assessment of the possible emergence of other types of *H. influenzae* disease.

Another strength of the active surveillance system for Hib disease is that the system is quite sensitive for both meningitis and nonmeningitic disease. In previous studies, researchers have

suggested that Hib vaccines might have higher efficacy for meningitic disease than other forms of Hib disease (18). Because the NBMRS tracks meningitis cases only, stable or increasing rates of nonmeningitic Hib disease during the vaccine era would go undetected. The active surveillance system confirmed that both meningitis and nonmeningitic disease caused by Hib have declined during the conjugate vaccine era.

The best explanation to date for the decline in Hib disease among infants before the vaccine was licensed for use in that age-group is that vaccine use among older children interrupted transmission of the organism to younger children. In support of this hypothesis, a recently published study suggested that conjugate vaccines may decrease pharyngeal carriage of Hib (19). The possibility that vaccine recipients are protected from disease directly (through vaccine-induced antibody) and are less likely to transmit the disease (by elimination of nasopharyngeal carriage) suggests that Hib disease could be practically eliminated with adequate vaccine coverage. Continued sensitive surveillance is therefore critical to our efforts to follow trends in disease occurrence and to identify populations needing enhanced vaccination coverage.

Recently, NETSS reporting of disease caused by *H. influenzae* was expanded to collect information about the subject's vaccination history. The sensitivity of the NETSS system for Hib reporting needs to be determined. However, the apparent decline in Hib disease during the vaccine era must be monitored. A resurgence of disease among young children because of inadequate vaccination or emergence of disease in older children or adults because of a waning of immunity could herald the need to revise vaccination efforts. Because NETSS provides national data on the occurrence of Hib disease, maintaining this system will be an important means of monitoring this disease throughout the country.

To appropriately interpret surveillance data for **any** disease, we must be aware of the dynamics of clinical practice. Although the case definition used in CDC's active surveillance system requires the isolation of specific bacteria by culture, advances in biotechnology have led to the development of methods for the rapid detection of bacterial antigen, potentially obviating the perceived need for culture methods. The cost, timeliness, and convenience of such methods may lead clinicians to favor rapid methods over classical culture methods. Surveillance systems will need to adapt to such changes in diagnostic practices to assure that case reporting correlates with disease occurrence. Of even more concern is that the replacement of bacterial isolation methods with antigen-based rapid diagnostic methods could severely threaten our ability to evaluate trends in the antimicrobial resistance of various pathogens—an important goal of many infectious disease surveillance systems.

EXAMPLES OF USING DATA

Health authorities can use accurate estimates of the incidence and characteristics of childhood infectious diseases for a variety of purposes. In this section, I present examples of how surveillance data are being used to 1) compare the cost-effectiveness of various strategies for preventing neonatal GBS disease, and 2) determine the need for alternative vaccination strategies for preventing hepatitis B.

Prenatal Screening for Group B Streptococcus

Substantial controversy has surrounded the issue of prenatal screening for GBS carriage. A randomized clinical trial demonstrated that intrapartum antibiotics prevented neonatal GBS disease when given to pregnant women who were identified as GBS carriers and who developed prolonged rupture of membranes (PROM) or preterm labor (20). However, maternal carriage of GBS is relatively common (10%–40%), and neonatal GBS disease occurs in only 1%–2% of infants born to carrier mothers. Clinicians and professional organizations questioned whether screening all women for the bacteria during pregnancy would be cost-effective in identifying a high-risk population for intrapartum antibiotics.

Active surveillance data were incorporated into a cost-effectiveness model regarding strategies for the prevention of neonatal GBS disease. Using current population-based rates of neonatal disease, investigators estimated that prenatal screening and the use of intrapartum antibiotics in GBS carriers with PROM or premature delivery would prevent about 3,300 cases annually in the United States and save approximately $16 million in direct medical costs (21).

Despite this demonstration that GBS disease prevention using routine prenatal screening and selective intrapartum antibiotics is cost-effective, the practice has not been widely accepted. The Georgia Department of Human Resources is surveying obstetrical providers in Georgia about their knowledge, attitudes, and practices regarding the prevention of neonatal GBS disease to identify barriers to the use of prevention strategies. This survey may be followed by a targeted educational campaign to improve the implementation of prevention strategies. Because metropolitan Atlanta is an area in the active surveillance system, the state health department can use trends in the incidence of neonatal GBS disease in Atlanta to estimate the effect of educational campaigns on disease occurrence.

Alternative Vaccination Strategies for Hepatitis B

Intensive surveillance for viral hepatitis was conducted in four sentinel U.S. counties during 1981–1988; the findings suggest that the strategy of targeting high-risk groups for hepatitis B immunization did not significantly affect disease incidence and that <1% of hepatitis B cases occurred among persons <15 years old *(22)*. However, the rise in cases of hepatitis B despite the introduction of hepatitis B vaccine in 1982 suggests that the vaccination strategy was not working. At least 30% of patients with hepatitis B could not be associated with an identifiable risk factor, indicating they would not be identified for a selective immunization strategy. Another problem with the selective strategy was the difficulty in reaching the **high-risk** population to deliver vaccine before infection could occur. After reviewing the surveillance data and considering the obstacles to selective immunization, policymakers concluded that a policy of universal immunization of infants would be preferable. Although the surveillance data did not suggest that hepatitis B was a disease of childhood, the data led to the introduction of another vaccine for universal use in infancy. Long-term surveillance will be needed to determine how the current policy of universal hepatitis B vaccination of infants affects disease occurrence.

FUTURE ISSUES

The future holds tremendous potential for enhancing surveillance for infectious diseases in children. Efforts to link vaccination registries with databases for disease occurrence are a natural goal of efforts to improve the level of childhood vaccination in this country. Streamlining communication among health departments, health-care providers, and federal agencies can enhance the level of compliance with surveillance efforts. One obvious need is to eliminate unnecessary redundance in reporting. Moreover, future surveillance activities will need to target the major public health issues that threaten the health of children, particularly infectious diseases in child day-care settings and the emergence of new pathogens.

Child Day-Care Settings

By the year 2000, an estimated 80% of women with children aged <6 years will be in the workforce; most of their children will be cared for in settings outside their homes. Studies conducted by CDC and others have shown that children who receive outside-the-home child care have an overall risk of acquiring certain infections that is two to three times the risk among children who are cared for exclusively at home *(23)*. The health of children in child day-care settings also will have significant economic consequences. Some investigators have attributed more than $1.8 billion in annual excess costs to these illnesses *(23)*. Others have suggested that >60% of employee absenteeism in the United States may be directly related to unmet child care needs *(24)*.

Fortunately, child day-care settings provide ideal opportunities for disease surveillance, but such efforts will require close networking among health departments, other health professionals, and the facilities that provide the majority of care to U.S. children. Over the coming years, infectious diseases surveillance in child day-care settings will continue to have three critical functions: 1) the early detection of outbreaks of illness in child care settings, many of which have significant potential for spread to the community (for example, a citywide outbreak of shigellosis in Lexington, Kentucky, was perpetuated through transmission at multiple child day-care centers); 2) the identification of facilities with unusually high incidences of infectious diseases requiring public health intervention; and 3) ongoing data collection to monitor the effectiveness of public health and regulatory interventions.

In the future, CDC will continue to conduct epidemiologic studies to identify risk factors for infectious disease and to develop targeted prevention and intervention strategies. CDC also is developing surveillance methodologies that can serve as models to help public health agencies determine the content and extent of infectious disease problems in child day-care settings. To begin evaluating such surveillance methodologies, CDC has cooperative agreements with several local health departments. Various other research, intervention, and evaluation projects are in progress and are planned for the future.

New Pathogens

The emergence of new pathogens has been a continual threat to children's health (25). A recent illustration of this phenomenon was a multistate outbreak of bloody diarrhea and hemolytic uremic syndrome caused by *E. coli* O157:H7, traced to contaminated hamburger patties. During the outbreak investigation in the winter of 1993, investigators promptly conducted multistate surveillance for disease caused by *E. coli* O157:H7 by adapting computer software that was already in place in public health laboratories for the surveillance of other diseases. *E. coli* has recently been added to the list of nationally notifiable diseases. The emergence of penicillin-resistant pneumococci in the United States is another important threat to children's health, and multidrug-resistant tuberculosis has introduced critical concerns regarding treatment and prevention of tuberculosis in all age-groups. Effective surveillance to monitor antimicrobial resistance for numerous pathogens is needed. As the identification of an apparently new hantavirus associated with an outbreak of acute respiratory failure among young people in the Southwestern states dramatically illustrated (26), emerging infectious diseases continue to challenge the public health system at the local, state, and federal levels.

As we approach the turn of the century, we need to go beyond merely responding to public health emergencies by improving our capacity to anticipate and control their occurrence.

REFERENCES

1. Pass RF, Little EA, Stagno S, Britt WJ, Alford CA. Young children as a probable source of maternal and congenital cytomegalovirus infection. N Engl J Med 1987;316:1366–70.

2. Lindegren ML, Fehrs LJ, Hadler SC, Hinman AR. Update: rubella and congenital rubella syndrome, 1980–1990. Epidemiol Rev 1991;13:341–8.

3. Schlech WF, Lavigne PM, Bortolussi RA, et al. Epidemic listeriosis—evidence for transmission by food. N Engl J Med 1983;308:203–6.

4. Todd J, Fishaut M, Kapral F, Welch T. Toxic-shock syndrome associated with phage-group-I staphylococci. Lancet 1978;2:1116–8.

5. CDC. Toxic-shock syndrome—United States. MMWR 1980;29:229–30.

6. Adams WG, Deaver KA, Cochi SL, et al. Decline of childhood *Haemophilus influenzae* type b (Hib) disease in the Hib vaccine era. JAMA 1993;269:221–6.

7. Langmuir AD. The surveillance of communicable diseases of national importance. N Engl J Med 1963; 268:182–92.

8. Chorba TL, Berkelman RL, Safford SK, Gibbs NP, Hull HF. Mandatory reporting of infectious diseases by clinicians. In: CDC Recommendations and Reports, June 22, 1990. MMWR 1990;39:(No. RR-9):1–17.

9. Schuchat A, Deaver K, Wenger JD, et al. Role of foods in sporadic listeriosis, I: case-control study of dietary risk factors. JAMA 1992;267:2041–5.

10. Wenger JD, Hightower AW, Facklam RR, Gaventa S, Broome CV. Bacterial meningitis in the United States, 1986: report of a multistate surveillance study. J Infect Dis 1990;162:1316–23.

11. Pinner RW, Gellin BG, Bibb WF, et al. Meningococcal disease in the United States—1986. J Infect Dis 1991;164:368–74.

12. Zangwill KM, Schuchat A, Wenger JD. Group B streptococcal disease in the United States, 1990: report from a multistate active surveillance system. In: CDC Surveillance Summaries, November 20, 1992. MMWR 1992;41:(No. SS-6):25–32.

13. CDC. National Electronic Telecommunication System for Surveillance—United States, 1990–1991. MMWR 1991;40:502–3.

14. Jackson LA, Wenger JD. Laboratory-based surveillance for meningococcal disease in selected areas, United States, 1989–1991. In: CDC Surveillance Summaries, June 4, 1993. MMWR 1993;42(No. SS-2):21–30.

15. Cochi SL, Fleming DW, Hightower AW, et al. Primary invasive *Haemophilus influenzae* type b disease: a population-based assessment of risk factors. J Pediatr 1986;108:887–96.

16. Schuchat A, Broome CV, Hightower A, Costa SJ, Parkin W. Use of surveillance for invasive pneumococcal disease to estimate the size of the immunosuppressed HIV-infected population. JAMA 1991;265:3275–9.

17. Wenger JD, Pierre R, Deaver K, et al. Invasive *Haemophilus influenzae* disease: a population-based evaluation of the role of capsular polysaccharide serotype. J Infect Dis 1992;165(Suppl.1):S34–5.

18. Wenger JD, Pierre R, Deaver KA, et al. Efficacy of *Haemophilus influenzae* type b polysaccharide-diphtheria toxoid conjugate vaccine in US children aged 18-59 months. Lancet 1991;338:395–8.

19. Takala AK, Eskola J, Leinonen M, et al. Reduction of oropharyngeal carriage of *Haemophilus influenzae* type b (Hib) in children immunized with an Hib conjugate vaccine. J Infect Dis 1991;164:982–6.

20. Boyer KM, Gotoff SP. Prevention of early-onset neonatal group B streptococcal disease with selective intrapartum chemoprophylaxis. N Engl J Med 1986; 314:1665–9.

21. Mohle-Boetani J, Schuchat A, Plikaytis BD, Smith D, Broome CV. Comparison of prevention strategies for neonatal group B streptococcal disease: a population-based economic analysis. JAMA 1993;270:1442–8.

22. Alter MJ, Hadler SC, Margolis HS, et al. The changing epidemiology of hepatitis b in the United States: need for alternative vaccination strategies. JAMA 1990;263:1218–22.

23. Thacker SB, Adiss DG, Goodman RA, Holloway BR, Spencer HC. Infectious diseases and injuries in child day care: opportunities for healthier children. JAMA 1992;268:1720–6.

24. NCHS. Disability days: United States, 1980. Hyattsville, Maryland: US Department of Health and Human Services, Public Health Service, 1983. (Vital and health statistics; series 10, no. 143.)

25. Lederberg J, Shope RE, Oaks SC Jr, eds. Emerging infections: microbial threats to health in the United States. Washington, DC: National Academy Press, 1992.

26. CDC Update: outbreak of hantavirus infection—southwestern United States, 1993. MMWR 1993;42: 441–3.

Vaccine-Preventable Diseases

Melinda Wharton, M.D., M.P.H.,[1] and Peter M. Strebel, M.B.Ch.B., M.P.H.[1]

PUBLIC HEALTH IMPORTANCE

Vaccination is one of the most important interventions available for preventing serious diseases among infants, children, and adults. Vaccination programs have resulted in the elimination of smallpox worldwide and the virtual elimination of indigenous poliomyelitis in the Western Hemisphere. In the United States, vaccine-preventable diseases predominately affecting children have been greatly reduced since the introduction of vaccination programs (Table 1). Vaccination programs are also highly cost-effective. For example, the benefit-cost ratio for the U.S. measles-mumps-rubella immunization program has been estimated at approximately 14:1 (1). Similar positive benefit-cost ratios have been reported for pertussis (2), poliomyelitis (3), and other vaccine-preventable diseases (4) (for additional information about related topics and surveillance activities, see the Bacterial and Other Infectious Diseases and Vaccination Coverage chapters).

HISTORY OF DATA COLLECTION

The reporting system for infectious diseases, including most of the vaccine-preventable diseases of childhood, was developed during the first half of the twentieth century primarily as an archival system of long-term documentary importance rather than a means of providing epidemiologically significant indicators of current problems (5). As national immunization programs developed, so did surveillance for vaccine-preventable diseases, as was illustrated by the rapid development of the Poliomyelitis Surveillance Unit in 1955 (5–8). During the 2 weeks following the announcement of the re-

sults of the successful field trial of formaldehyde-inactivated poliomyelitis vaccine, approximately 4 million doses of vaccine were administered, mostly to elementary schoolchildren. On April 25, 1955, an infant with paralytic poliomyelitis was admitted to a Chicago hospital, 9 days following vaccination with formaldehyde-inactivated poliomyelitis vaccine. The next day, five additional cases of paralytic poliomyelitis were reported from California among children who had received vaccine produced by the same manufacturer of the vaccine administered to the child in Chicago. In each case, paralysis first developed in the limb in which vaccine had been given. On April 27, the Surgeon General asked the manufacturer to recall all remaining lots of vaccine. The following day, the Poliomyelitis Surveillance Unit was established.

State health officers were asked to designate a polio reporting officer responsible for reporting cases of poliomyelitis among vaccinated individuals; later, cases among their family members and other contacts were included. Case reports were transmitted by telephone or telegraph to the Poliomyelitis Surveillance Unit, where the data were collated, analyzed, and disseminated via poliomyelitis surveillance reports, the first of which was mailed out on May 1, 1955—only 3 days after the surveillance activity was initiated. The report was prepared and distributed daily for 5 weeks, weekly for the remainder of the summer and fall, and once every 3–4 weeks during the winter.

[1] National Immunization Program
Centers for Disease Control and Prevention
Atlanta, Georgia

TABLE 1. Comparison of maximum and current reported morbidity of vaccine-preventable diseases and current preschool morbidity — United States, 1921–1992

Disease	Maximum cases		1992 reported cases		
	No.	(Year)	Total cases	% change	Cases among children 0–4 years of age (% of total)*
Diphtheria	206,939	(1921)	4	− 99.998	1 (33)
Measles	894,134	(1941)	2,237	− 99.7	1,116 (50)
Mumps[†]	152,209	(1968)	2,572	− 98.3	364 (17)
Pertussis	265,269	(1934)	4,083	− 98.5	2,261 (158)
Poliomyelitis (paralytic, wild virus)	21,269	(1952)	0	−100.0	0 (0)
Rubella[§]	57,686	(1969)	160	− 99.7	24 (24)
Congenital rubella syndrome	20,000[¶]	(1964–1965)	3	− 99.98	3 (100)
Tetanus**	601	(1948)	45	− 92.5	0 (0)
Haemophilus influenzae[††]	20,000[¶]	(1984)	1,412	− 92.9	592 (45)

* Among those with known ages.
[†] First reportable in 1968.
[§] First reportable in 1966.
[¶] Estimated.
** First reportable in 1947.
[††] First reportable in 1991.

During the first days of the surveillance program, as more cases were reported, the data demonstrated with increasing certainty that the problem was confined to vaccine produced by a single manufacturer. Production procedures were reviewed, and other manufacturers were encouraged to continue vaccine production. Without the surveillance program and the rapid clarification of the scope of the problem that was provided by analysis of surveillance data, the manufacture of poliomyelitis vaccine might have been halted in the United States.

This episode highlights several important aspects of modern public health surveillance. Data were collected, analyzed, and disseminated rapidly to allow policymakers to base their decisions on the best information available. Morbidity data were not collected for publication in archival tables but rather to characterize important public health problems and to facilitate effective public health action.

CDC SURVEILLANCE ACTIVITIES

In cooperation with state health departments and CDC's Epidemiology Program Office (EPO), the National Immunization Program (NIP) at CDC performs national surveillance for measles, mumps, rubella, congenital rubella syndrome, diphtheria, tetanus, pertussis, poliomyelitis, and varicella (Table 2). In this chapter, we focus primarily on the surveillance of those diseases monitored by NIP. Responsibility for the surveillance of other vaccine-preventable diseases (hepatitis B, *Haemophilus influenzae* type b, influenza, and pneumococcal disease) rests with CDC's National Center for Infectious Diseases.

State communicable disease reporting requirements mandate physicians and other health-care providers to report specified diseases (in most states, this includes all vaccine-preventable diseases of childhood) *(9)*. In some states, data from providers are supplemented by laboratory data; however, laboratory-based reporting is much less uniformly available *(10)*. State health departments have established various mechanisms for reporting; many use morbidity cards that are sent through the mail whereas others report data by telephone, facsimile machine, modem, and other systems.

After receiving the report, state and local health departments initiate a case investigation and disease control efforts. Therefore, at the local and state levels, timeliness is extremely important.

Cases reported to state health departments are reported to the National Notifiable Disease Surveillance System (NNDSS), overseen by EPO. In general, CDC encourages health departments to report provisional data to the NNDSS before completing case investigations, but there are exceptions; since 1983, only confirmed cases of measles have been reported to the NNDSS. For other vaccine-preventable diseases, cases that are classified as suspect, probable, or under investigation may be reported provisionally. (The data reported in the *Morbidity and Mortality Weekly Report* [*MMWR*], however, include only confirmed cases of paralytic poliomyelitis; suspect cases are enumerated in a footnote.)

All state health departments now have their surveillance data computerized, and development of these systems during the 1980s allowed electronic reporting to supplant the previous system of reporting aggregate data to the NNDSS by telephone. Since 1989, all state health departments have reported data electronically to the NNDSS via the National Electronic Telecommunications System for Surveillance (NETSS) *(11)*. With the introduction of computerized data management, additional demographic information on age, sex, race, and ethnicity for each case patient has been collected and reported to the NNDSS, along with county of residence and date of onset of illness.

The data collected by the NNDSS are supplemented by other surveillance systems operated by NIP (Table 2). Supplemental surveillance systems provide data on vaccination status,

TABLE 2. Surveillance for vaccine-preventable diseases — National Immunization Program, 1994

Diseases	Surveillance systems
Diphtheria	National Notifiable Diseases Surveillance System (NNDSS) Requests for diphtheria antitoxin
Measles	NNDSS Rapid Surveillance Helper (RASH)
Mumps	NNDSS
Pertussis	NNDSS Supplementary Pertussis Surveillance System
Poliomyelitis	Paralytic Poliomyelitis Surveillance System
Rubella	NNDSS* National Congenital Rubella Syndrome Registry
Tetanus	NNDSS Supplemental Tetanus Surveillance System
Varicella	NNDSS

* Although no supplemental system for collecting detailed, disease-specific information exists, limited additional information is collected by some state health departments and is reported electronically via the National Electronic Telecommunications System for Surveillance.

laboratory confirmation, complications, and epidemiologic linkage to other cases; these data provide important information for disease control activities and policy making. Most of the supplemental systems continue to be paper-based, but efforts are under way to develop integrated electronic data management and reporting systems that will make surveillance data more useful for state health departments. Electronic reporting will also facilitate more rapid analysis and dissemination of results at the national level.

CDC publishes NNDSS data weekly in *MMWR* and yearly in the *Annual Summary of Notifiable Diseases*. NNDSS data and data reported to supplemental surveillance systems are analyzed by NIP staff and disseminated through articles in *MMWR*, *CDC Surveillance Summaries*, and other published articles.

Descriptions of supplemental and related data collection systems follow.

Diphtheria

Reports of diphtheria cases from state health departments to the NNDSS are supplemented by additional cases identified through requests received by NIP for diphtheria antitoxin. Clinical data on the severity of illness, vaccination status, outcome, and final diagnosis are obtained for all suspected diphtheria cases identified through diphtheria antitoxin requests. No supplemental surveillance system for diphtheria exists at present, but a supplemental system is being developed.

Measles

Since 1978, substantial effort has been invested in measles surveillance at the state and local levels. In 1979, a standard clinical case definition for measles was adopted, and cases were further classified as suspected, probable, or confirmed. Since 1983, only confirmed cases have been reported *(12)*.

NIP developed the Rapid Surveillance Helper (RASH) system to electronically.collect supplemental data on measles cases. The software was first introduced in 1985 and has since undergone several modifications, most recently in 1990–1991 to allow the entry of data on multiple doses of measles vaccine. The software is now used in all state health departments by state immunization program personnel. Data on vaccination status, complications, setting of transmission, and serologic confirmation of cases are collected. Cases identified with particular outbreaks can also be linked in the RASH database. Although local and state program personnel can enter data on suspected and probable measles cases into the program, only data on confirmed cases are sent to CDC. Files are transmitted to an electronic bulletin board operated by NIP. The RASH system is currently being integrated into the NETSS system; this integration will eliminate the need for duplicate data entry and separate reporting to the NNDSS and RASH.

Mumps

No supplemental surveillance system for mumps exists, although CDC has future plans to collect data on mumps vaccination status and other characteristics via NETSS.

Pertussis

Since 1979, health departments have reported detailed clinical, demographic, and laboratory information on each case of pertussis through the Supplementary Pertussis Surveillance System (SPSS). Information is collected on age, diphtheria-tetanus-pertussis vaccination history, and selected clinical characteristics, including duration of cough and the occurrence of complications such as pneumonia, seizures, encephalopathy, hospitalization, and death. Results of laboratory tests, including cultures and direct fluorescent antibody tests for *Bordetella pertussis*, and information on antimicrobial therapy are also collected. Reports of encephalopathy and death are confirmed by telephone.

During 1989–1991, case reports of pertussis were sent to SPSS on 9,480 (83%) of the 11,446 patients reported to the NNDSS *(13)*. The SPSS report forms (CDC Form 71.14A. Rev. 8/85) are currently mailed to CDC, but in the future, SPSS will be integrated into the NETSS system.

Poliomyelitis

Detailed demographic, clinical, and epidemiologic data are collected on all suspected cases of paralytic poliomyelitis reported to CDC. Experts who are not affiliated with CDC review suspected cases and determine whether they meet the case definition for paralytic poliomyelitis. Since the adoption of a new case classification system in the 1980s, cases have been classified as sporadic, epidemic, imported, or occurring in immunologically abnormal persons, and as being related to wild virus or vaccine virus *(14)*.

Rubella and Congenital Rubella Syndrome

No supplemental surveillance system for rubella exists, although some states include vaccination status and pregnancy status in the data they report to the NNDSS via NETSS. The expansion of reporting of these supplemental data to all states and the addition of laboratory confirmation status are anticipated.

The National Congenital Rubella Syndrome Registry (NCRSR) collects additional clinical and laboratory information on cases of suspected congenital rubella syndrome in the United States (CDC Form 71.17, Rev. 1/83). The registry, established in 1969, includes data on only cases classified as confirmed or compatible. Cases are also classified as indigenous (exposure within the United States) or imported (exposure outside the United States) and are tabulated by year of birth. In contrast, cases reported to the NNDSS are tabulated by year of report.

Tetanus

Since 1965, state health departments have reported supplemental clinical and epidemiologic information on reported cases of tetanus to the Supplemental Tetanus Surveillance System. They collect information on the clinical history, presence, and nature of associated risk factors, vaccination status, wound care, and clinical management. Data are reported on tetanus surveillance case report forms (CDC Form 71.15, Rev. 9/86).

GENERAL FINDINGS

Diphtheria

During 1980–1992, 40 cases of diphtheria and three diphtheria-related deaths were reported in the United States. Although the risk of acquiring diphtheria in the United States is very low, importation of the organism from developing countries where the infection is endemic continues to be a threat (15).

Measles

The measles resurgence of 1989–1991 followed almost a decade of greatly diminished measles activity. Between 1981 and 1988, an average of approximately 3,000 cases were reported each year. During 1989–1991, approximately 55,000 cases of measles and 132 measles-associated deaths were reported. The resurgence was characterized by the occurrence of urban outbreaks affecting large numbers of unvaccinated preschool children; compared to 1981–1988, an increasing proportion of cases were among preschool children and, to a less striking degree, among adults, with a corresponding decrease in the proportion of reported cases among children of school age (16).

In 1992, only 2,237 cases of measles were reported. Through July 3, 1993, CDC recorded a provisional total of 167 measles cases—the lowest total ever reported for the first 6 months of any year in the history of measles surveillance. This reduction in measles activity in 1992 and the first half of 1993 likely reflects improvement in measles vaccine coverage among preschool children (17).

Mumps

Reported cases of mumps decreased in the United States from 8,576 cases in 1980 to 2,982 cases in 1985. A relative resurgence occurred in 1986–1987, when outbreaks occurred among high school and college students as well as other adults. The increase in reported disease incidence was concentrated among those states lacking comprehensive school immunization requirements for mumps vaccination (18). Since 1987, reported cases have continued to decline, and in 1992, an all-time low of 2,572 cases was reported. Of the cases in which age was known, 364 cases (17%) were reported among children <5 years of age, and 980 cases (47%) were reported among children 5–14 years of age.

Pertussis

With the number of measles cases currently at an all-time low in the United States and

Haemophilus influenzae type B (Hib) disease declining rapidly because of the widespread use of Hib conjugate vaccines, pertussis has emerged as the most frequently reported vaccine-preventable disease among children <5 years of age (Table 1). In 1992, 4,083 cases of pertussis were reported to CDC, with all states except Wyoming reporting cases.

Analysis of pertussis surveillance data for 1980–1989 reveals a moderate seasonal pattern that peaked in July and August. The interepidemic interval for pertussis was 3–4 years, a pattern seen in both the prevaccine era and now (19). During 1989–1991, age-specific incidence for reported pertussis was highest among infants (especially infants <6 months of age) and decreased with increasing age. Infants <6 months of age also had the highest rates of pertussis-associated hospitalization (69%), pneumonia (16%), seizure (2%), encephalopathy (0.2%), and death (0.4%). Failure to vaccinate children on time was a major factor contributing to pertussis morbidity; 65% of children 3 months to 4 years of age who had reported cases of pertussis had not been vaccinated appropriately for their age (13).

Poliomyelitis

Since 1980, no cases of paralytic poliomyelitis caused by indigenously acquired wild poliovirus infection have been reported in the United States. The last reported outbreak of poliomyelitis (10 paralytic cases) in the United States occurred in 1979 among religious communities opposed to vaccination (20). Thorough surveillance for paralytic poliomyelitis has also documented the exceedingly low but stable risk of vaccine-associated paralytic poliomyelitis (VAPP) in the United States. This problem was first reported in September 1962, approximately 6 months after the licensure of type 3 monovalent poliovirus vaccine in the United States. During the 1980s, 80 cases of VAPP were reported in the United States, reflecting a risk of one case of VAPP per 2.5 million doses of trivalent oral poliomyelitis vaccine (OPV) distributed. Among immunologically normal persons, the risk of VAPP is higher following the first dose than following subsequent doses

(1 recipient case per 1.4 million first doses of OPV and 1 contact case per 1.9 million first doses). Among immunologically abnormal persons, an overall risk of 1 case of VAPP per 14.5 million doses distributed has been observed, or 1 case of VAPP per 6.2 million first doses of OPV distributed (21).

Rubella and Congenital Rubella Syndrome

Reported cases of rubella decreased in the United States from 3,904 in 1980 to only 225 cases in 1988. A relative resurgence of rubella occurred in 1990–1991, when >1,000 cases were reported each year. California alone accounted for almost half of the 1,125 cases reported nationally in 1990. A large outbreak in southern California in early 1990 resulted in a cluster of cases of congenital rubella syndrome in late 1990 (22), and other outbreaks occurred throughout the state in prisons and colleges (23). In 1990–1991, outbreaks occurred in several states among the Amish and other groups that objected to immunization (24,25). Reported cases of congenital rubella syndrome to the NCRSR have generally paralleled rubella incidence, with 25 cases born in 1990 and 31 cases born in 1991. In 1992, only 160 cases of rubella were reported—a new all-time low— and as of September 1, 1993, three cases of congenital rubella syndrome among babies born in 1992 were reported to NCRSR.

Tetanus

During 1976–1985, an average of 83 cases of tetanus were reported each year (range = 72 to 95) in the United States. Since 1986, fewer than 65 cases were reported each year; in 1992, only 45 cases were reported, representing an all-time low. Of 109 patients of known age whose tetanus cases were reported during 1989–1990, 63 (58%) were ≥60 years of age and only 3 (1%) were <5 years of age (26). In 1989, one case of neonatal tetanus was reported in an infant born to an unimmunized woman who delivered at home, and the umbilical cord was cut with unsterilized scissors; this represented the first case of neonatal tetanus reported in the United States since 1984 (27).

INTERPRETATION ISSUES

We know that the reporting of vaccine-preventable disease by physicians and other providers to passive surveillance systems is incomplete. Periodic community canvasses in Hagerstown, Maryland, in 1922–1923 identified 560 cases of measles among the 7,424 residents. Sixty-four percent of these patients were seen by physicians, and only 40% of these cases were reported to the health department; overall, only 26% of cases were reported to local health authorities (28). We have little evidence that reporting by physicians has improved dramatically in the years since the Hagerstown study. Only an estimated 11.6% of pertussis cases in the United States are reported (29). Although the reporting of sporadic cases of measles is thought to be more complete than that estimated for pertussis, a recent investigation of reporting during an urban outbreak suggested that only 45% of measles patients treated in hospitals were reported (30).

The completeness of reporting to supplemental surveillance systems has been evaluated by using capture-recapture methods (31,32). After comparing congenital rubella syndrome cases reported to the NCRSR with those identified by the Birth Defects Monitoring Program during 1970–1985, Cochi and colleagues determined that only 22% of these cases were reported to the NCRSR (33). By comparing the number of deaths reported to CDC surveillance systems with the number reported on death certificates to CDC's National Center for Health Statistics, Sutter and colleagues estimated that 40% of tetanus-related deaths during 1979–1984 and 33% of pertussis-related deaths during 1985–1988 were reported to CDC supplemental surveillance systems (29,34). Likewise, during 1985–1988, an estimated 32% of pertussis-related hospitalizations were reported to SPSS (29), and during 1985–1991, 41% of measles-related hospitalizations were reported to RASH (CDC, unpublished data, 1993).

Those cases reported to a surveillance system may not be representative of all cases. A comparison of hospitalized pertussis case patients reported to SPSS with hospital data collected by the Commission on Professional and Hospital Activities Professional Activities Survey (CPHA) revealed that the case patients reported to CDC were more likely to have pneumonia, seizures, and encephalitis than those identified in the CPHA sample. The average hospitalization was longer for those case patients reported to SPSS than for those in the CPHA sample, suggesting that more severe cases were more likely to be reported to CDC (29).

To improve specificity and enhance comparability of state-reported cases of vaccine-preventable diseases, case definitions for surveillance have been developed. A standard case definition of paralytic poliomyelitis was introduced in 1958, and a clinical case definition of measles was adopted in 1979. Standard case definitions for the surveillance of all vaccine-preventable diseases have recently been published (35). However, implementation of uniform case definitions for reporting by state health departments has been incomplete.

Because of the relative insensitivity of bacterial culture for *Bordetella pertussis*, the development and evaluation of clinical case definitions are particularly important in the surveillance of pertussis. A surveillance case definition of cough illness lasting for ≥14 days was found to be 84% sensitive and 63% specific for detecting culture-positive pertussis cases in outbreaks in 1985 and 1986 (36). In a more recent outbreak, a case definition of cough illness with whoop lasting ≥14 days was found to have a sensitivity of 81% and a specificity of 58% (37).

We have observed increasing interest in alternative approaches to traditional morbidity surveillance systems. Hospital discharge data sets may be useful for some purposes, although they are of limited usefulness in providing timely data for disease control purposes. Ultimately, computerized medical records in physicians' offices and clinics may provide data that are timely, accurate, and complete. The development of such systems is perhaps most advanced in large health maintenance organizations and other large group practices, but it lies in the future for smaller practices. Aside from the other technological barriers, maintaining patient confidentiality remains a primary concern.

EXAMPLES OF USING DATA

State and local health departments promptly investigate reports of suspected cases of vaccine-preventable diseases to institute appropriate measures to limit the spread of disease. Analysis of disease reports also provides important information on groups at highest risk for disease. Such data are important for allocating resources, targeting interventions, and making policies.

Even in the absence of wild virus transmission, surveillance for paralytic poliomyelitis continues to be crucial in determining the optimal poliomyelitis vaccination policy for the United States. The continued occurrence of vaccine-associated paralytic poliomyelitis—together with the licensure of an enhanced-potency inactivated poliovirus vaccine (eIPV) in 1987—led the Institute of Medicine to reassess poliomyelitis vaccination options (38). National surveillance data clearly demonstrate that most cases of VAPP among immunologically normal persons follow administration of the first dose of OPV. A proportion of these cases, especially the recipient cases, can be prevented by initially administering eIPV, followed by doses of OPV. In contrast, cases among immunologically abnormal persons who received OPV show no such association with the dose number (21). How a sequential schedule would affect the occurrence of VAPP among contacts of recipients is uncertain, but it probably would not reduce such cases dramatically.

Surveillance data have also influenced measles vaccination policy in the United States. In 1985–1986, 101 outbreaks of measles were reported among school-age children. In these outbreaks, the majority of cases occurred among vaccinated children (39). In response to the occurrence of measles among vaccinated children of school age, the Advisory Committee on

Immunization Practices in 1989 recommended a routine two-dose schedule for measles vaccine, with the first dose at 15 months (12 months in areas with recurrent measles transmission), followed by a second dose at school entry (40). Such a strategy had already been adopted by New York State, following the occurrence of 91 outbreaks in college, high school, and middle school during the spring semester of 1989 (41).

FUTURE ISSUES

To maximize the usefulness of vaccine-preventable disease surveillance data at the state level, the existing supplemental surveillance systems need to be fully integrated with state notifiable disease data systems. This process is already under way, with the development of a combined RASH-NETSS system. Electronic reporting of supplemental data for pertussis and other vaccine-preventable diseases is anticipated in the near future. Eliminating missed opportunities for vaccination is an important component of the national objective to achieve 90% vaccination coverage among 2-year-old children by the year 2000 (42). Missed opportunities occur when children eligible for vaccination are seen by health-care providers but are not vaccinated, or when only some of the recommended vaccines are given at a visit. NIP, in consultation with state health departments, is currently developing a surveillance system to monitor missed opportunities among children with vaccine-preventable diseases. The occurrence of vaccine-preventable diseases in a community is a sentinel event that should alert health authorities to possible failures in the vaccine delivery system. This type of surveillance information will help state and local health departments develop programs to improve vaccination coverage in both the private and public sectors by further characterizing the type of missed opportunities in the community.

The use of both current and new data sources needs to be improved. Laboratory-based reporting is a valuable adjunct to traditional provider reports. It is essential for the surveillance of some conditions for which the case definition is based on results of laboratory testing (e.g.,

Hib) and for certain conditions where clinical diagnosis is unreliable (e.g., rubella); laboratory-based reports may be the only source of accurate information. Improved links between laboratories and communicable disease surveillance activities within state health departments are needed. The Public Health Laboratory Information System, the electronic reporting system developed by the Association of State and Territorial Public Health Laboratory Directors and the National Center for Infectious Diseases, may provide an important electronic link within state health departments *(43)*. In the future, electronic links with commercial laboratories, and ultimately large group practices and clinics, may provide more complete and timely data than are now available.

As the Institute of Medicine noted in its 1988 report, *The Future of Public Health*, in recent years essential surveillance activities have had difficulty competing for scarce resources at the state and local levels with more visible public health activities *(44)*. At the same time, increasingly complex data needs have resulted in increasing personnel demands, as state and local support has diminished. Support for surveillance is a crucial problem as we approach the public health challenges of the 1990s.

REFERENCES

1. White CC, Koplan JP, Orenstein WA. Benefits, risks and costs of immunization for measles, mumps and rubella. Am J Public Health 1985;75:739–44.

2. Hinman AR, Koplan JP. Pertussis and pertussis vaccine: reanalysis of benefits, risks, and costs. JAMA 1984;251:3109–13.

3. Weisbrod BA. Costs and benefits of medical research: a case study of poliomyelitis. J Polit Econ 1971;79:527–44.

4. Willems JS, Sanders CR. Cost-effectiveness and cost-benefit analyses of vaccines. J Infect Dis 1981;144:486–93.

5. Langmuir AD. The surveillance of communicable diseases of national importance. N Engl J Med 1963;268:182–92.

6. Nathanson N, Langmuir AD. The Cutter incident: poliomyelitis following formaldehyde-inactivated poliovirus vaccination in the United States during the spring of 1955. I. Background. Am J Hyg 1963;78:16–28.

7. Etheridge EW. Sentinel for health: a history of the Centers for Disease Control. Berkeley, California: University of California Press, 1992.

8. Langmuir AD, Nathanson N, Hall WJ. Surveillance of poliomyelitis in the United States in 1955. Am J Public Health 1956;46:75–88.

9. CDC. Mandatory reporting of infectious diseases by clinicians. MMWR 1990;39(No. RR-9):1–17.

10. Sacks JJ. Utilization of case definitions and laboratory reporting in the surveillance of notifiable communicable diseases in the United States. Am J Public Health 1985;75:1420–2.

11. CDC. National Electronic Telecommunications System for Surveillance—United States, 1990–1991. MMWR 1991;40:502–3.

12. CDC. Classification of measles cases and categorization of measles elimination programs. MMWR 1983;31:707–11.

13. Davis SF, Strebel PM, Cochi SL, Zell ER, Hadler SC. Pertussis surveillance—United States, 1989–1991. In: CDC Surveillance Summaries, December 1992. MMWR 1992;41(No. SS-8):11–9.

14. Sutter RW, Brink EW, Cochi SL, et al. A new epidemiologic and laboratory classification system for paralytic poliomyelitis cases. Am J Public Health 1989;79:495–8.

15. Farizo KM, Strebel PM, Chen RT, Kimbler A, Cleary TJ, Cochi SL. Fatal respiratory disease due to *Corynebacterium diphtheriae*: case report and review of guidelines for management, investigation, and control. Clin Infect Dis 1993;16:59–68.

16. Gindler JS, Atkinson WL, Markowitz LE, Hutchins SS. Epidemiology of measles in the United States in 1989 and 1990. Pediatr Infect Dis J 1992;11:841–6.

17. CDC. Measles—United States, 1992. MMWR 1993;42:378–81.

18. Cochi SL, Preblud SR, Orenstein WA. Perspectives on the relative resurgence of mumps in the United States. Am J Dis Child 1988;142:499–507.

19. Farizo KM, Cochi SL, Zell ER, Brink EW, Wassilak SG, Patriarca PA. Epidemiological features of pertussis in the United States, 1980–1989. Clin Infect Dis 1992;14:708–19.

20. CDC. Poliomyelitis—Pennsylvania, Maryland. MMWR 1979;28:49–50.

21. Strebel PM, Sutter RW, Cochi SL, et al. Epidemiology of poliomyelitis in the United States one decade after the last reported case of indigenous wild virus-associated disease. Clin Infect Dis 1992;14:568–79.

22. Lee SH, Ewert DP, Frederick PD, Mascola L. Resurgence of congenital rubella syndrome in the 1990s: report on missed opportunities and failed prevention policies among women of childbearing age. JAMA 1992;267:2616–20.

23. CDC. Increase in rubella and congenital rubella syndrome—United States, 1988–1990. MMWR 1991; 40:93–9.

24. CDC. Outbreaks of rubella among the Amish—United States, 1991. MMWR 1991;40:264–5.

25. Briss PA, Fehrs LJ, Hutcheson RH, Schaffner W. Rubella among the Amish: resurgent disease in a highly susceptible community. Pediatr Infect Dis J 1992;11:955–9.

26. Prevots R, Sutter RW, Strebel PM, Cochi SL, Hadler S. Tetanus surveillance—United States, 1989–1990. In: CDC Surveillance Summaries, December 1992. MMWR 1992;41(No. SS-8):1–9.

27. Kumar S, Malecki JM. A case of neonatal tetanus. South Med J 1991;84:396–8.

28. Sydenstricker E, Hedrich AW. Completeness of reporting of measles, whooping cough, and chicken pox at different ages. Public Health Rep 1929;44: 1537–48.

29. Sutter RW, Cochi SL. Pertussis hospitalizations and mortality in the United States, 1985–1988: evaluation of the completeness of national reporting. JAMA 1992;267:386–91.

30. Davis SF, Strebel PM, Atkinson WL, et al. Reporting efficiency during a measles outbreak in New York City, 1991. Am J Public Health 1993;83: 1011–5.

31. Sekar CC, Deming WE. On a method of estimating birth and death rates and the extent of registration. J Am Stat Assoc 1949;44:101–15.

32. Cormack RM. The statistics of capture-recapture methods. Oceanogr Mar Biol Annu Rev 1968;6: 455–506.

33. Cochi SL, Edmonds LE, Dyer K, et al. Congenital rubella syndrome in the United States, 1970–1985: on the verge of elimination. Am J Epidemiol 1989; 129:349–61.

34. Sutter RW, Cochi SL, Brink EW, Sirotkin BI. Assessment of vital statistics and surveillance data for monitoring tetanus mortality, United States, 1979–1984. Am J Epidemiol 1990;131:132–42.

35. CDC. Case definitions for public health surveillance. MMWR 1990;39(No. RR-13):1–43.

36. Patriarca PA, Biellik RJ, Sanden G, et al. Sensitivity and specificity of clinical case definitions for pertussis. Am J Public Health 1988;78:833–6.

37. Strebel PM, Cochi SL, Farizo KM, Payne BJ, Hanauer SD, Baughman AL. Pertussis in Missouri: evaluation of nasopharyngeal culture, direct fluorescent antibody testing, and clinical case definitions in the diagnosis of pertussis. Clin Infect Dis 1993;16: 276–85.

38. Institute of Medicine. An evaluation of poliomyelitis vaccine policy options. Washington, DC: National Academy of Science, 1988.

39. Markowitz LE, Preblud SR, Orenstein WA, et al. Patterns of transmission in measles outbreaks in the United States, 1985–1986. N Engl J Med 1989;320: 75–81.

40. CDC. Measles prevention: recommendations of the Immunization Practices Advisory Committee (ACIP). MMWR 1989;38(No. S-9):1–18.

41. Birkhead GS, Morse DL, Mills IJ, Novick LF. New York State's two-dose schedule for measles immunization. Public Health Rep 1991;106:338–44.

42. Public Health Service. Healthy people 2000: national health promotion and disease prevention objectives—full report, with commentary. Washington, DC: US Department of Health and Human Services, Public Health Service, 1991; DHHS publication no. (PHS) 91-50212.

43. Bean NH, Martin SM, Bradford H. PHLIS: an electronic system for reporting public health data from remote sites. Am J Public Health 1992;82:1273–6.

44. Institute of Medicine. The future of public health. Washington, DC: National Academy Press, 1988.

Vaccination Coverage

Paul A. Stehr-Green, Dr.P.H., M.P.H.[1]

PUBLIC HEALTH IMPORTANCE

One of the U.S. health objectives for the year 2000 is to ensure that at least 90% of children complete the basic vaccination series by 2 years of age *(1)*. We are still far from achieving this goal, however, as is evident by the resurgence of measles in 1989–1991, particularly among preschool children *(2)*, and results of national, state, and city vaccination coverage surveys conducted during and immediately after this epidemic *(3–6) (CDC, unpublished data, 1992 and 1993)*.

A comprehensive strategy for controlling vaccine-preventable diseases by raising vaccination coverage levels should include research into the nature of causal problems and effective solutions for low-coverage levels, activities to improve vaccination service delivery, information and education programs for consumers and providers, policy development, and ongoing assessments of overall program effectiveness. Arguably, the last of these activities is critical in that it provides the data necessary to stimulate and guide all these other actions.

Although such information per se is not the solution to any problem, it can lead to solutions. The power of measurement data is illustrated by the organization theorist Mason Haire *(7)*. Quite simply, Haire said, "What gets measured, gets done." The basic insights embodied in his remark are that measurement data display exactly where one is relative to where one wants or needs to be, and when this distance is greater than one can accept, the desire and commitment to close the gap is aroused (for additional information about related topics and surveillance activities, see the Bacterial and Other Infectious Diseases and Vaccine-Preventable Diseases chapters).

HISTORY OF DATA COLLECTION

A combination of various assessment methods has been used to monitor the successes and failures of immunization programs since the late 1950s. Among the oldest of these assessment efforts, the United States Immunization Survey (USIS) comprised annual population-based surveys of children of all ages throughout the United States; these surveys were discontinued in 1985 but were recommenced as part of the National Health Interview Survey (NHIS) in 1991. In recent years, a few state and local health departments have begun to conduct similar population-based coverage surveys among preschool children. Audits of clinic records have also recently been used more widely to assess coverage levels and evaluate program performance at the service-provision level.

The assessment approach used most widely by state and local immunization programs over the past 30 years has been the collection of data on children's vaccination status at school entry. In the last few years, as a result of changing epidemiologic patterns of vaccine-preventable diseases (especially measles), we have witnessed an increased use of data collected at school entry to retrospectively estimate children's coverage levels at the age of 2 years. Data routinely collected for management purposes (e.g., for vaccine inventory control and billing) have also

---

[1] National Immunization Program
  Centers for Disease Control and Prevention
  Atlanta, Georgia

been used throughout this period to monitor vaccine use patterns and general trends in vaccination coverage at the local, state, and national levels.

In the future, to improve program effectiveness and to raise vaccination coverage to desired levels, we will need quality information to stimulate and guide the management of our programs as well as to track individual children's vaccination histories and needs. To meet these needs, efforts are now under way to develop viable, comprehensive vaccination registries.

SURVEILLANCE ACTIVITIES

Immunization Surveillance

To maximize the effectiveness of immunization programs, health officials should thoroughly evaluate the effects of their programs, using measurement data from a variety of sources (5):

- Assessments of vaccination coverage.

- Surveillance of vaccine-preventable diseases.

- Outbreak investigations.

- Serologic surveys.

- Postlicensure field studies of vaccine efficacy.

- Monitoring of the vaccine **cold-chain** (i.e., ensuring that vaccines are shipped, stored, and handled under prescribed temperatures and physical conditions so that they retain their optimal effectiveness).

- Surveys of knowledge, attitudes, and behaviors among health-care consumers and providers.

- Monitoring of vaccine-associated adverse events.

Assessment of vaccination coverage and the surveillance of disease incidence and vaccine-associated adverse events should be regular, ongoing activities; the remainder of these

immunization surveillance activities should be conducted periodically or as specific needs arise. Each source of information offers a different perspective and is valuable in managing disease control programs and developing policies.

This chapter focuses on options for monitoring the vaccination status of children through vaccination coverage assessments and includes examples of the historical use of several assessment approaches, what has been learned from their application, and what is planned for the future (current surveillance programs for vaccine-preventable diseases and vaccine-associated adverse events are described in the Vaccine-Preventable Diseases chapter).

Vaccination Coverage Assessment

Four general methods are used to estimate vaccination coverage: coverage surveys, the use of management data on vaccines, registries, and retrospective assessments.

COVERAGE SURVEYS

Coverage surveys use sampling techniques to derive estimates for targeted populations. These surveys are conducted by collecting relevant data for a representative sample of a targeted population (e.g., at a national, state, local, or clinic level) to estimate vaccination coverage rates and determine reasons for nonvaccination.

The principal advantages of conducting surveys on vaccination coverage are that they do not require the establishment or maintenance of a permanent infrastructure (and, therefore, can be conducted relatively quickly and inexpensively in most local settings); we have a wealth of experience with sampling survey approaches for evaluating vaccination coverage; and these surveys can be used simultaneously to collect information on other health issues. Generally, estimates of key population attributes (e.g., vaccination coverage levels among 2-year-old children) derived from such surveys provide a valid assessment of the effects of public health programs.

The principal disadvantage of using sampling approaches is the lack of information that would facilitate identification of at-risk individuals and that could allow the sending of timely reminders to children who are due for vaccinations or the sending of recall notices to children who are behind schedule for their vaccinations (i.e., as a basis for reminder and recall systems). Further, unless parent- or provider-held vaccination records are readily available to verify the data collected, the validity of coverage estimates derived from these sources will be questionable. And because the data are historical, estimates can reflect only the situation at some time in the past. Finally, to assess changes over time in a given population or simultaneously characterize the situation in different targeted populations, we must conduct separate surveys; the cost of conducting regular national surveys or multiple simultaneous surveys in all local jurisdictions can be very high.

USE OF MANAGEMENT DATA

Management data—which include data that are collected for monitoring vaccine inventories and health-care services billing, for example—can also be used to roughly estimate vaccination coverage in selected jurisdictions. The principal means of estimating vaccination coverage with management information has been through the use of data routinely collected on the number of doses of publicly purchased vaccine that are administered (commonly referred to as **doses administered** data). In addition, some local immunization programs and individual vaccination providers regularly use billing information to estimate coverage levels in their service areas and practices and to monitor individual children's vaccination status.

The principal advantage of using such data to estimate vaccination coverage is that they are already routinely collected (e.g., doses administered data are collected quarterly by all public immunization programs) and are, therefore, readily available at a minimal cost. In addition, these data can provide useful information on the access to and use of immunization and other health-care services, program performance (e.g., drop-out rates), and trends in public sector vaccine delivery.

The principal disadvantages of using these data are that they reflect vaccinations administered

to a nonrepresentative subgroup of children (e.g., doses administered data reflect only publicly purchased doses and, thus, include only about half the number of vaccine doses administered nationwide), represent only **numerator** information (i.e., information on the targeted population, the denominator, can only be inferred from census data or client lists), and may not always distinguish multiple-dose vaccines (e.g., first diphtheria-tetanus-pertussis vaccine dose [DTP1] vs. the second dose [DTP2] vs. the third dose [DTP3]). Therefore, at best, these data can only be used to derive crude estimates of vaccination coverage. Like survey sampling approaches, management data lack information on individuals that would facilitate the identification, reminder, and recall of individual children who are due or overdue for vaccinations.

REGISTRIES

Registries monitor the vaccination status of all children in a given area. National, state, health district, or primary provider-based registries collect real-time coverage data by enrolling all children in their area into a tracking system and continuously recording and monitoring their use of immunization services (and, possibly, other health care and social services).

The principal advantage of enrolling all children into registries—whether at a national, state, health district, or primary provider level—and monitoring their vaccination status is that such registries can provide current information on coverage levels in the general population and in selected subpopulations. In addition, if locating information is kept current, registries provide a basis for tracking individual children's needs and special conditions and for operating effective reminder and recall systems. This approach has achieved success in parts of the United Kingdom, where individuals are given unique identification numbers, they are required to receive immunization services from specific assigned providers, and a system is in place to facilitate the routine exchange of relevant patient information among primary vaccination providers.

Expense is the principal disadvantage of registries. The cost to establish and maintain

293

registries at a national, state, or health district level is likely to be high because the supporting infrastructure has to be built anew in most cases. Depending on local circumstances, building on to existing systems might be possible, although, even in these instances, additional personnel and data processing costs will be incurred to reconfigure hardware, rewrite software, and hire additional data management staff. On a smaller scale, establishing primary provider-based registries, complemented by the promotion and more extensive use of parent-held records, would not require the development and maintenance of a centralized infrastructure for data collection and handling, but it would require expenditures for initial development, promotion, and training for primary providers. Another limitation to consider is that identifying and tracking individuals from place to place and over time—especially persons who may not have regular access to health-care services—requires careful attention to not only the associated logistics and costs, but also the ethics and likely societal acceptance of doing so. Finally, because of the long period of development required, registries are not likely to provide representative vaccination coverage data for at least the first 2–5 years. Therefore, health departments must incur the costs associated with conducting other types of assessments (e.g., vaccination coverage surveys) in the interim.

RETROSPECTIVE ASSESSMENTS

In retrospective assessments, vaccination coverage data are collected for all children in a targeted population at key milestones of their lives when they are expected to have contact with the health-care system (e.g., at school entry). These data are used to calculate measures of current vaccination coverage levels (or levels at some point in the past, such as at the child's second birthday). Unlike sampling surveys, retrospective assessments usually collect relevant data for **all** children, although valid estimates of vaccination coverage can be, and often are, derived from representative samples of children entering school.

Retrospective assessments combine some of the best elements of both survey sampling methods

and registries. Collecting data in this way relies on existing points of contact with each individual. As a result, establishing a separate infrastructure for data collection is not necessary, and initial costs are relatively low. Because children are required by law to show vaccination records at the time of school registration and entry, the validity of vaccination coverage measurements derived from these sources is assured. Moreover, if a complete census is conducted, the vaccination status of each child can be evaluated, and necessary catch-up vaccinations can be administered (albeit, behind schedule).

As with all of the options for assessing vaccination coverage, costs are incurred for maintaining and analyzing the data that are collected through such assessments of children entering school. The biggest drawback of using retrospective assessments to estimate vaccination coverage among preschool children, however, is that the data collected at school entry (on children's vaccination status at their second birthday) are 3–5 years out-of-date. This drawback can seriously hinder efforts to monitor the overall effects of current immunization programs and focused interventions; it also limits the ability to keep children on schedule for receiving vaccinations.

GENERAL FINDINGS

Nationwide data from unverified parental reports, collected as part of the USIS and the NHIS between 1962 and 1991, revealed that among 2-year-old children, coverage with three or more doses of DTP gradually but consistently dropped from a peak of 77.9% in 1967 to 66.6% in 1991 (Figure 1). A similar trend was seen for coverage with three or more doses of polio vaccine, which dropped from a peak of 63.6% in 1975 to 52.2% in 1991. In contrast, coverage with measles-containing vaccines among 2-year-old children rose from the mid-60% range, where it remained for most of the 1970s and early 1980s, to an all-time high of 80.4% in 1991. This increase probably resulted, in large part, from the emphasis on measles vaccination following the 1989–1991 nationwide measles epidemic (8).

FIGURE 1. Series-complete vaccination status of U.S. children at their second birthday, by state — retrospective surveys of children entering school* — 1991–1992

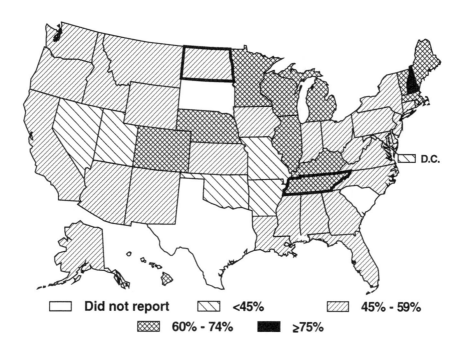

| Did not report | ☒ <45% | ▨ 45% - 59% |
| 60% - 74% | ■ ≥75% |

* Tennessee and North Dakota conducted surveys of 2-year-old children rather than children entering school.

In recent years, a few states and local jurisdictions (e.g., Tennessee, Mississippi, North Dakota, and Oklahoma) have also conducted similar population-based coverage surveys of 2-year-old children, with results generally being comparable to findings obtained at the national level. For example, results from a 1991 survey in North Dakota revealed coverage levels of 61.0% for four doses of DTP, 65.8% for three doses of polio vaccine, and 74.8% for one dose of measles-containing vaccine by the second birthday. In 1991, **series-complete** coverage levels (i.e., four DTP doses, three polio doses, and one measles-containing dose received by the second birthday) were reported to be 58.3% in North Dakota and 69.5% in Tennessee.

As mentioned previously, the assessment approach used most widely by state and local immunization programs has been the collection of data on children's vaccination status at school entry. Among these children entering school, vaccination coverage levels of ≥95% are now routinely achieved in all states; in large

part, these high levels of vaccination coverage at school entry are responsible for the ≥90% reductions in the incidence of all vaccine-preventable diseases in the United States. However, because of the changing epidemiologic patterns of these diseases, especially the large nationwide epidemic of measles that occurred in 1989–1991, vaccination coverage data collected at school entry have been used increasingly to retrospectively estimate coverage levels among children at age 2 years.

In 1991, 45 states and the District of Columbia estimated preschool coverage levels by examining the vaccination histories of a representative sample of children who entered school in the 1991–1992 school year. These combined assessments showed that median coverage levels at 2 years of age were 59.8% for four doses of DTP (range = 37.9%–78.1%), 75.0% for three doses of polio vaccine (range = 58.3%–88.9%), and 78.3% for one dose of measles-containing vaccine (range = 57.5%–90.8%); overall, series-complete coverage levels among children at 2 years of age

295

were even lower (median = 56.3%; range = 35.8%–78.9%) (Figure 2) *(CDC, unpublished data, 1993)*. Results from similar assessments conducted in >20 urban areas during the same time showed that series-complete coverage levels were 10%–15% lower, on average, than the respective state estimates *(3–6). (CDC unpublished data, 1992)*.

INTERPRETATION ISSUES

All of these data sources have inherent inaccuracies and, in some cases biases, which limit their usefulness. The most egregious of these problems are as follows:

- The data are often old (e.g., estimates of preschool coverage levels from retrospective assessments of children entering school may be as much as 3–5 years old) and, therefore, may not yield estimates that are representative of current population levels.

- The data often do not reflect the vaccination experience of a representative sample of all children (e.g., doses administered data reflect the vaccination experience of only the estimated 50% of children who receive publicly purchased vaccines).

- The data are based on unverified parental reports (e.g., historically, the USIS, NHIS, and most state and locally conducted population-based surveys have relied predominantly on parental recall of their children's vaccination histories), thereby introducing inaccurate information.

Because of these limitations, we need to establish an ongoing system of data collection that will provide up-to-date, complete, verified information that is necessary to stimulate and guide the management of our programs and to assess individual children's vaccination histories and needs. A potential solution—viable, comprehensive vaccine registries—will be discussed later in this chapter.

EXAMPLES OF USING DATA

Numerous general approaches for assessing vaccination coverage have been used to varying degrees and with varying effectiveness at the national, state, local, and clinic levels. The collection of vaccination coverage data at all of these levels is necessary because of the different uses for the information generated at each level. National assessment data are useful in guiding federal planning efforts and evaluating

FIGURE 2. Vaccine-specific coverage rates among 2-year-old children — United States, 1962–1991*

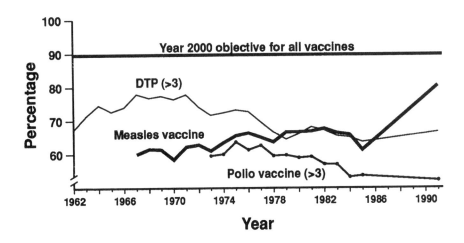

*Surveys were discontinued in 1985 but were recommenced in 1991.

Source: United States Immunization Survey and National Health Interview Survey.

funding needs. Data from smaller geographic areas or populations, such as states or cities, are also valuable for planning purposes and for allocating both financial and professional resources; in addition, these data can be used to compare various programs' performances, thereby stimulating poorly performing programs to improve and good programs to get even closer to their goals. Finally, assessment data at the clinic or private practice level are essential to bringing about necessary changes in clinic policies and procedures and to better managing staff, time, and financial resources.

Since 1978, state and local immunization programs have relied primarily on data collected through assessments of children entering school to measure progress and guide programs. In the earlier years of the immunization programs, these data were used primarily to stimulate increases in vaccination levels among children entering school. For example, CDC previously published vaccination rates according to whether states had laws requiring vaccination for school entry. In addition, these data were important in guiding efforts to control vaccine-preventable diseases because, at that time, the highest incidence for these diseases were observed among children 5–9 years of age, the group in which most outbreaks occurred. However, since the late 1970s and early 1980s, the age-specific incidence of these diseases has shifted, largely as a result of the ≥95% vaccination levels now routinely achieved among children entering school. Therefore, as previously mentioned, we have observed an increased use of vaccination coverage data collected at school entry to retrospectively estimate coverage levels among 2-year-old children and thus guide efforts to raise coverage levels among preschoolers.

Doses administered data have also been used throughout this period as a decision-making aid for managing programs at the local, state, and national levels. These data, which are routinely collected by all state and local immunization programs and are reported quarterly to CDC, have been used predominantly to track the distribution of publicly purchased vaccines. More recently, they also have been used to monitor trends in vaccination coverage as a decision-making aid for directing intervention efforts to

raise vaccination coverage levels among preschoolers.

Potentially, the most effective use of vaccination assessment information is in the clinics and practices where vaccination services are actually delivered. In these settings, information on clinic-specific coverage levels and performance indicators—such as rates of children who start their vaccination series later than 3 months of age or who drop out of the vaccination system before completing their full series—can be used to modify clinic policies and procedures and to optimize the use of professional and financial resources. In recognition of the importance of this powerful management tool, the *Standards for Pediatric Immunization Practices (9)*, which has been developed and endorsed by numerous professional medical organizations in the United States, recommends regular clinic audits of vaccination coverage as a part of good clinic practice, in both the public and private sectors. To facilitate the widespread use of clinic-based assessments, CDC has prepared a manual on how to conduct, analyze, and interpret clinic audits *(10)*.

FUTURE ISSUES

The results from retrospective assessments, management information systems, and sampling surveys have highlighted the successes and deficiencies in our immunization programs and have guided our decisions on how to distribute resources to address these problems. However, as mentioned above, we have had to rely on data that are old, that do not reflect the vaccination experience of all children, or that are based on unverified reports. By establishing and using comprehensive registries, we have the potential to mitigate these deficiencies and, further, to provide the basis for facilitating the development and use of quality vaccination service programs.

Registries to track children's vaccination status in the United States and elsewhere around the world have been used by vaccination providers—both public clinics and by private practices. In these settings, provider-based registries have successfully facilitated the reminder and recall of patients for vaccinations, resulting in significant improvements in vaccination coverage levels. Furthermore, such provider-based registries can be used as a basis for monitoring vaccination coverage levels in the overall population through periodic surveys of vaccination providers or direct data sharing and electronic links.

So far, only a few states—most notably Arkansas and South Dakota—have piloted computerized registries for tracking children's vaccination status. However, the development of a comprehensive vaccination tracking system for the United States is a principal component of the *Comprehensive Child Immunization Initiative*—a blueprint for the future immunization program in the United States *(11)*. Under this blueprint, each state will be encouraged to develop a fully operational tracking system and to assure that vaccination providers report all necessary information for each dose of vaccine administered.

The potential benefits of a nationwide system of state-based vaccination registries are many and varied. If each state provides CDC with aggregate vaccination data, we will be able to monitor vaccination coverage at the local, state, and national levels and identify areas where additional technical assistance may be needed. This proposed system would also enable public health officials to monitor the safety and efficacy of vaccines by linking vaccine administration information with adverse events reporting and disease outbreak patterns. In addition, such tracking systems would enable us to identify children who need vaccination and notify parents and providers to ensure that children are age-appropriately immunized. Finally, monitoring distribution patterns and the uptake of vaccines would provide a basis for guiding management decisions at all levels regarding the purchase and distribution of vaccines.

The immunization initiative calls for the initiation of a nationwide system of state-based vaccination registries. Until such comprehensive systems of registries are fully in place, however, population-based surveys will be conducted quarterly to continue to monitor progress toward meeting the nation's goal of fully vaccinating at least 90% of our preschool children by the year 2000 *(1)*.

The challenge is clear as we continue the initiative to reach 90% age-appropriate vaccination coverage. Of the objectives outlined in our national strategy for increasing coverage, the assessment of vaccination coverage at all population levels has been given one of the highest priorities. Having high-quality, timely assessment data can generate both the will **and** the way to solve our vaccination coverage problems.

REFERENCES

1. Public Health Service. Healthy people 2000: national health promotion and disease prevention objectives—full report, with commentary. Washington, DC: US Department of Health and Human Services, Public Health Service, 1991; DHHS publication no. (PHS)91-50212.

2. CDC. Measles—United States, 1990. MMWR 1991; 40:369–72.

3. CDC. Update: measles outbreak—Chicago, 1989. MMWR 1990;39:317–9, 325–6.

4. CDC. Measles vaccination levels among selected groups of preschool-aged children—United States. MMWR 1991;40:36–9.

5. Orenstein WA, Bernier RH. Surveillance: information for action. Pediatr Clin North Am 1990;37:709–34.

6. CDC. Retrospective assessment of vaccination coverage among school-aged children—selected U.S. cities, 1991. MMWR 1992;41:103–7.

7. Peters TJ, Waterman RH Jr. In search of excellence: lessons from America's best-run companies. New York: Harper and Row Publishers, 1984.

8. Stehr-Green PA, Zell ER, Eddins DL. Childhood vaccinations: are rates really declining? [Letter]. JAMA 1993;270:1932.

9. CDC. Standards for pediatric immunization practices. MMWR 1993;42(no. RR-5):1–13.

10. National Center for Prevention Services. Guidelines for assessing vaccination levels of the 2-year-old population in a clinic setting. Atlanta: US Department of Health and Human Services, Public Health Service, CDC, 1992.

11. Robinson CA, Sepe SJ, Lin KFY. The president's child immunization initiative—a summary of the problem and the response. Public Health Rep 1993;108:419–25.

Injury and Child Abuse

Suzanne M. Smith, M.D., M.P.H.,[1] Joseph E. Sniezek, M.D., M.P.H.,[2]
Jennifer J. Luallen, M.D.,[1,3] Philip W. McClain, M.S.,[2]
Robert G. Froehlke, M.D.,[4] Philip L. Graitcer, D.M.D., M.P.H.,[5]
and Juan G. Rodriguez, M.D., M.P.H.[1,6]

PUBLIC HEALTH IMPORTANCE

Injuries to children require special consideration. Because of their vulnerability, children are particularly dependent on society for protection from injuries. Over the last century in the United States, injury has surpassed disease as the leading cause of childhood mortality. Among children aged 1–19 years, injuries cause more deaths than all diseases combined and are a leading cause of disability (1). In the last 60 years, rates of death caused by infectious diseases have declined 90%, but rates of death caused by injuries have declined only 40% (2). Thus, the relative importance of injuries has increased substantially. To reduce childhood injuries, we need to launch a coordinated, committed effort similar to that given to lower the rate of death from infectious diseases.

In the past two decades, injuries have begun to gain widespread recognition as a problem amenable through public health measures (3). However, intervention programs have been hampered because injuries have been perceived as **accidents** that are unpredictable and uncontrollable. Parents may believe **accidents** won't happen to their own children because they are confident in the level of supervision they provide for their children. Injuries, like diseases, actually occur in predictable patterns and are therefore preventable and controllable. **Accidents** are more accurately described as **unintentional events that produce injuries**. Children and adolescents sustain injuries from both unintentional events and events in which harm is purposeful (e.g., interpersonal and self-directed violence).

Injury Mortality

Injury causes almost 40% of deaths among children aged 1–4 years and more than half of all deaths among children aged 5–14 years (1,4,5). In 1990, injuries caused >6,000 deaths among U.S. children under the age of 10 years (Table 1). Among children in their first year, injuries rank third after perinatal complications and congenital anomalies as a cause of death. After the first year of life, unintentional injuries are the most frequent cause of death for children of all ages (and persons up to 35 years of age). Violent injuries among children increase with age; for example, homicide as a

[1] Division of Unintentional Injury Prevention
National Center for Injury Prevention and Control
Centers for Disease Control and Prevention
Atlanta, Georgia

[2] Division of Acute Care, Rehabilitation Research,
and Disability Prevention
National Center for Injury Prevention and Control
Centers for Disease Control and Prevention
Atlanta, Georgia

[3] Epidemic Intelligence Service
Epidemiology Program Office
Centers for Disease Control and Prevention
Atlanta, Georgia

[4] Department of Pediatrics
Michigan State University
East Lansing, Michigan

[5] Office of the Director
National Center for Injury Prevention and Control
Centers for Disease Control and Prevention
Atlanta, Georgia

[6] Deceased

Acknowledgments

For their contributions, we thank Sue N. Mallonee, R.N., M.P.H., Injury Prevention Service, Oklahoma State Department of Health; Roger W. Rochat, M.D., Georgia Department of Human Resources; Daniel A. Pollock, M.D., Division of Acute Care, Rehabilitation Research, and Disability Prevention, National Center for Injury Prevention and Control, Centers for Disease Control and Prevention (CDC); and Stephen P. James, B.A., and Joann M. O'Neil, B.S., Office of Statistics, Programming, and Graphics, National Center for Injury Prevention and Control, CDC.

TABLE 1. Ten leading causes of death* among children, by age-group — United States, 1990

	Age-groups (years)		
Rank	<1	1–4	5–9
1	Perinatal complications 17,482	Unintentional injuries 2,566	Unintentional injuries 1,771
2	Congenital anomalies 8,239	Congenital anomalies 896	Malignant neoplasms 569
3	Unintentional injuries 930	Malignant neoplasms 513	Congenital anomalies 286
4	Heart disease 794	Homicide 378	Homicide 156
5	Pneumonia and influenza 634	Heart disease 282	Heart disease 124
6	Homicide 332	Pneumonia 171	Pneumonia 76
7	Septicemia 267	Perinatal complications 134	HIV infection 64
8	Meningitis 197	HIV infection 123	Benign neoplasms 53
9	Nephritis 151	Septicemia 100	Bronchitis, emphysema, and asthma 34
10	Cerebrovascular disease 148	Meningitis 81	Cerebrovascular disease 33

* Causes and numbers of deaths are represented in each cell. To promote comparability between infant and child causes of death, leading causes of infant death shown in this table are ranked on the basis of 72 cause-of-death tabulation list, rather than on the 61 infant cause-of-death list as is more commonly used for ranking infant deaths. Because of this difference, rankings for leading causes of infant death are not identical to those shown in Table 1 of the Infant Mortality chapter.

Source: National Center for Health Statistics, CDC, mortality tapes.

cause of death increases in rank from sixth for children <1 year of age to fourth among those 1–9 years old.

Injury Morbidity

Injuries lead to 20% of all hospitalizations among children, closely following respiratory illnesses (23%), the leading cause of hospitali-zations among children (1). Each year an estimated 600,000 children are hospitalized be-cause of injuries, and almost 16 million more are seen in emergency departments. Injuries result in more hospital days of care than any disease, cause the highest proportion of dis-charges to long-term care facilities, and result in the highest proportion of children requiring home health care after discharge. Although estimates of injury costs are difficult to develop, one 1986 study found that for the 22,000 injury fatalities among persons ≥19 years old, the cost of future lost productivity amounted to nearly $8.3 billion (in 1985 dollars) (6).

Children are exposed to injury hazards both within and outside the home. A recent study estimated that 60% of children <5 years of age regularly received child care outside the home (7). Although an increased risk from infectious diseases in child-care settings is apparent (see the Bacterial and Other Infectious Diseases chapter), increasing evidence suggests that injury rates in child care centers are relatively low and that the injuries are predominantly minor. Most severe injuries in child care centers occur on playgrounds where lowering the height of equipment and providing more resilient surfaces could reduce children's risk of injury.

Cross-National Comparisons

The United States leads the industrialized world in childhood death rates (1). Virtually all of the excess mortality among children in the United States is attributed to unintentional injuries and violence. Factors that contribute to cross-national variations in injury rates include socioeconomic and cultural patterns as well as differences in agents of unintentional injury and violence (such as motor-vehicle use patterns, the level of safety-belt use, the prevalence of swimming hazards, and access to firearms). For additional information about related topics and surveillance activities, see the Pregnancy-Related Morbidity, Infant Mortality, and Unintentional Injuries and Violence chapters.

HISTORY OF DATA COLLECTION

Because injury has only recently been recognized as a problem requiring the attention of the public health community, adequate public health surveillance systems for injury have only begun to be developed. The limited injury-related data now available are often found among disparate data systems, many of which are maintained outside of the public health community—for example, police and fire reports. Coordinated and standardized data systems are critical for injury

surveillance. Linking existing data systems may prove to be an effective way to address these limitations.

Injury prevention and control programs depend on having access to information that describes the injury-producing event (i.e., the external cause of injury). Fortunately, because of the uniform death certificate coding standards in the United States, these data are available for fatalities. Unfortunately, standardized cause-of-injury data are not widely available in most nonfatal injury data systems such as hospital discharge data systems. Often only data on the injury outcomes, (e.g., cerebral concussion or fractured femur), are available without reference to the causative event. Therefore, the available nonfatal injury data are useful only for estimating the burden of injuries. The injury burden may be useful for setting priorities, but if the data lack details about the underlying cause, they are not useful in designing effective injury-control measures.

Mortality Data

A number of existing data systems are used for the surveillance of fatal injuries (Table 2) (8). Currently, vital records provide the only virtually complete reporting source for fatalities. The other systems provide more detailed information but are limited in other ways. With few exceptions, these data systems are not readily linked to other data sources that might help to reduce some data limitations. Eleven states* currently have computerized, statewide medical examiner data, although these systems are not standardized; in North Carolina the data are regularly linked to vital records (Parrish RG, unpublished data, 1993).

In a study of deaths related to three-wheeled all-terrain vehicles (ATVs), Alaska used identifying information from existing mortality databases to link records such as vital statistics; medical examiner, coroner, and magistrate records; state department of transportation police reports; deaths recorded by the Consumer Product Safety

---

* Connecticut, Delaware, Iowa, North Carolina, New Jersey, New Mexico, Oklahoma, Rhode Island, Tennessee, Utah, and Vermont.

TABLE 2. Major sources of data on fatal injuries among children — United States, 1993

Data Source	Usefulness	Injury types	Comments
Vital records	High	All injuries	Underlying cause of death is cause of injury.
Medical examiner— coroner systems	Moderate	Various types— usually most traumatic deaths	Contain detailed information about circumstances surrounding death; not uniform across jurisdictions; rarely computerized.
Child fatality reviews	Undetermined*	Childhood deaths	Not uniform across jurisdictions; few states have mature activities.
Fatal Accident Reporting System	High	Fatal injuries from motor vehicle crashes on public roads	Limited to deaths occurring on public roadways and within 30 days of crash; contain little medical information.
Drug Abuse Warning Network	Moderate	Fatal injuries in which drug abuse was causal or contributory	More timely than vital statistics with more detailed drug data; may not be uniform across jurisdictions; limited to persons aged >6 years.
Uniform crime report— supplementary homicide report	High	Homicides	Complete for 90%–95% of murder and nonnegligent manslaughter cases.

* Child fatality reviews are newly established. The text summarizes an evaluation of the Georgia system.

Commission; emergency medical services records; and information from the Indian Health Service and the U.S. Armed Forces. Although no single data system identified all deaths related to ATVs, vital statistics and medical examiner data each captured 85% of all deaths; together they provided an adequate mechanism for monitoring ATV-related fatalities (9).

A specialized data set is available to monitor fatal motor vehicle crashes. The National Highway Traffic Safety Administration (NHTSA) maintains the Fatal Accident Reporting System (FARS), which contains data on all motor vehicle crashes occurring on public roadways that resulted in a fatality within 30 days of the incident (excluding crashes resulting from natural disasters). FARS analysts in all 50 states, the District of Columbia, and Puerto Rico use available data sources to collect information on crash, vehicle, and occupant characteristics (10). The FARS is particularly valuable for monitoring risk factors associated with fatal crashes. A major limitation of FARS is the absence of medical information.

Morbidity Data

Data systems to adequately measure the impact of nonfatal U.S. injuries are currently not well developed, and the data are much less available than injury fatality data. Because these data sources usually do not include external-cause-of-injury information, they have limited use in designing injury control programs. However, some existing data, such as hospital discharge data, have the benefit of being widely available, and some data sources, such as the National Electronic Injury Surveillance System and trauma registries provide detailed information, albeit for a specialized subset of injuries (Table 3) (8).

The Behavioral Risk Factor Surveillance System (BRFSS), sponsored by CDC's National Center for Chronic Disease Prevention and Health Promotion, collects limited injury risk factor information in participating states. The BRFSS permits analyses of risk factors. For example, researchers with CDC's National Center for Injury

TABLE 3. Major sources of data on nonfatal injuries among children — United States, 1993

Data source	Usefulness	Injury types	Comments
Hospital discharge data	Moderate	Injuries requiring hospitalization	Rarely contain external-cause-of-injury information; capture of less severe injuries is sensitive to treatment patterns; often not timely.
National Electronic Injury Surveillance System	High	Injuries associated with consumer products	Have been used for special projects (e.g., firearm-related injuries); utility limited to national estimates.
Trauma registry data	Moderate	Injuries treated at trauma registry hospitals	Inclusion criteria may vary; often difficult to define population at risk; mix of injuries referred for tertiary care and for those in hospital catchment area.
NCHS* surveys such as the National Health Interview Survey	Moderate	Injuries in past 14 days resulting in restricted activity or requiring medical attention	Contain little cause of injury information; provide national and regional estimates only; have little utility for injury control programs.
National Hospital Discharge Survey	Low	Injuries requiring hospitalization	No external-cause-of-injury information; capture of less severe injuries is sensitive to treatment patterns; provide national and regional estimates only; have little utility for injury control programs.

* National Center for Health Statistics, CDC.

Prevention and Control (NCIPC) used BRFSS data to characterize the association between reduced adult safety-belt use and reduced adult-reported use of occupant restraints for children <11 years old (11).

CDC SURVEILLANCE ACTIVITIES

To monitor the magnitude of fatal and nonfatal injuries in the United States, NCIPC primarily uses existing data systems such as vital statistics databases, the National Hospital Discharge Survey, and the National Health Interview Survey, which are maintained by CDC's National Center for Health Statistics. In addition, NCIPC provides national coordination for injury surveillance activities, standard definitions and methodologies in certain areas, and support to help states build their injury surveillance capacity. Several prototype surveillance systems are also under development (see the Future Issues section of this chapter).

GENERAL FINDINGS

Unintentional Injuries

Injury risks vary considerably with the child's age and developmental level. Across age-groups, marked differences in injury rates, by cause, reflect changes in cognitive, perceptual, motor/language abilities, and associated behaviors as well as changes in the environment and exposure to hazards. For example, toddlers exploring their homes are at risk for different injuries than older children who are frequently outside the home.

Injuries related to motor vehicle crashes are the leading cause of childhood injury death, accounting for 33.5% of all injury deaths among children <10 years old (Table 4). CDC and NHTSA researchers used FARS data to assess trends in fatalities among motor vehicle occupants <5 years old. They found that despite overall increases in the use of restraint devices, fatalities among children <5 years old increased overall between 1982 and 1989 *(10)*. Of motor vehicle occupants <5 years old killed in crashes in 1990, an estimated 70% were not restrained.

Among children aged 5–9 years, pedestrian injuries cause more deaths than do any other injury cause (Table 4). Pedestrian fatality rates are nearly twice as high for males as for females *(12)*. The risk of pedestrian injury is inversely related to socioeconomic status, with poor children having two to three times the risk of other children. **Dart-out** incidents, in which the child darts out into the street in front of a moving vehicle, account for 50%–70% of pedestrian injuries among children <10 years of age. Incidents in which a vehicle backs up over a child account for about 5%–7% of pedestrian deaths; these fatal events occur primarily among children <5 years of age.

Among all children, falls are the leading cause of hospitalizations, whereas sports injuries are the leading cause of emergency department visits *(13)*. According to national estimates based on data from a Massachusetts surveillance system *(13)*, falls and sports injuries were by far the most frequent cause for emergency department visits among all persons <20 years of age. Emergency department visits for the next most frequent cause—motor vehicle occupant injuries—were outnumbered by more than fivefold by visits for

falls and by almost fourfold by visits for sports injuries.

More than half of burn deaths occurring before the age of 20 are among children <5 years of age, and almost 75% are among those <10 years of age *(1)*. Residential fire deaths are most common among children <5 years of age. Although black children make up only about 15% of the pediatric population, they accounted for 40% of all pediatric fire and burn deaths in 1990. Historically, race categories have been collected in surveillance data for convenience. Race itself is certainly not a risk factor for burn death, but future research may help discern whether race is a proxy measure for a variety of socioeconomic factors that put children at greater risk: poor housing, improper heating, and greater exposure to homes with smokers *(1)*. Children living in the South, especially the Southeast, have the greatest risk of dying in a house fire.

Although they make up only 26% of the pediatric population, children <5 years of age account for 37% of all pediatric drowning deaths *(1)*. In California, Arizona, and Florida, drowning is the leading cause of injury death among children under the age of 5 years *(14)*. Children aged 1–3 years are at greatest risk of drowning death. Up to 90% of drownings in this age-group occur in residential swimming pools.

TABLE 4. Leading causes of injury-related deaths among children aged 9 years or less, by age and sex — United States, 1990

Age and sex	All injuries*		Motor vehicle crash		Homicide		Drowning		Pedestrian incident	
	Number	Rate	Number	Rate	Number	Rate	Number	Rate	Number	Rate
<5 years										
Boys	2,519	26.24	623	6.49	386	4.02	420	4.38	287	2.99
Girls	1,771	19.34	500	5.46	324	3.54	220	2.40	169	1.85
Total	4,290	22.87	1,123	5.99	710	3.79	640	3.41	456	2.43
5–9 years										
Boys	1,216	13.17	595	6.49	70	0.76	176	1.91	278	3.01
Girls	735	8.35	375	4.26	86	0.98	72	0.82	128	1.45
Total	1,951	10.82	970	5.38	156	0.86	248	1.38	406	2.25

*Rates per 100,000 population; categories may not be mutually exclusive.

Source: National Center for Health Statistics mortality tapes.

Injuries Caused by Violence

Over the past 25 years, homicide rates among children have at least doubled for each age-group *(15)*. Homicide is now the third leading cause of injury death among children <10 years of age (Table 4). Most child homicides are among boys (68%), and 46% are among blacks *(1)*. Race is not a causal factor but may be a marker for other yet-to-be-understood risk factors. Homicide rates are quite high during the first 3 years of life but are relatively low among children aged 5–10 years. For homicides among children <5 years of age, about half are the result of blows, and about 10% are the result of shootings. The proportion of homicides that are inflicted with firearms increases with age, regardless of the child's sex or race. In 1990, firearms accounted for 1.3% of deaths among children aged 1–4 years and 3% of deaths among those aged 5–9 years *(16)*.

Surveillance of child abuse, both fatal and non-fatal, is severely hampered by inconsistent definitions and legal requirements and by varying record-keeping practices. No valid national estimates for the magnitude of child abuse cases are available. In two surveys, investigators found that reported cases of child maltreatment increased 66% from 1980 to 1986 *(17)*, primarily because of an increase in reported child abuse. Reported cases of physical abuse increased 68%, and reported cases of sexual abuse rose >300% during the same period. Whether these trends represent a true increase in incidence or reflect increased reporting (or both) is not known.

INTERPRETATION ISSUES

Establishing effective public health systems for the surveillance of childhood injuries is especially challenging because of the enormous effect of injuries and the wide variety of injury-producing events and outcomes. Data needs are diverse and include the characteristics of injured children and causative events, etiologies, injury diagnoses, contributing factors, and long-term outcomes. Current data collection systems are fragmented and have critical gaps in information.

Injury surveillance systems may use data from many sources. Because these systems have been developed for other purposes, they frequently lack essential information needed to plan, carry out, and evaluate injury control programs *(8)*. Therefore, existing data sources frequently need to be modified or linked to other data sources to be useful for public health and prevention activities.

Medical sources such as hospital discharge databases often provide rich information about the magnitude and types of injuries that occur. Without cause-of-injury information, these sources' usefulness is limited to measuring the injury burden. Changing patterns of medical care, access, and reimbursement may influence the nature of injury data captured by these sources, complicating the capability to monitor the injury burden over time.

Trauma registries—specialized medical data systems developed primarily to assess quality of care—are another potential source of childhood injury data. Although trauma registries typically include critical external-cause-of-injury information, they are not population-based. Defining the population at risk is difficult because the catchment areas are often poorly defined. The main impediment to calculating population-based rates is that generally not all acute care hospitals in a population-defined geographic area participate in multihospital registries. As trauma registries mature and all acute care hospitals become participants (as has happened throughout Alaska and in San Diego, California), trauma registries will become population-based. Trauma registries generally include information on trauma patients who are admitted to the hospital, who die in the emergency department, or who are transferred to other facilities—patients whose records generally do not become part of hospital discharge databases.

Many states maintain specialized registries of persons sustaining selected injuries such as severe burns, traumatic brain injuries, and spinal cord injuries. Although these registries may be valuable sources of surveillance data on childhood injury, their primary purpose is to monitor service delivery to the injured persons. See the Unintentional Injuries and Violence chapter for more detailed information on state-based registries.

Nontraditional (from a public health perspective) sources of data used in injury surveillance systems include police, fire, and motor vehicle crash reports. We can greatly increase the usefulness of these data sources by linking them to other data systems containing information on injury outcomes and cost.

We also must consider limitations related to data on child abuse and neglect. Our most notable concern is that no consensus definitions exist for either child abuse or neglect. Definitions, legal reporting requirements, and record-keeping practices often vary by jurisdiction. Increasing evidence suggests that child neglect, physical abuse, and sexual abuse are epidemiologically distinct entities requiring different prevention strategies (17). Available data are often based on a combination of voluntary and mandated reporting. Although the surveillance of many adverse health events is based on such reporting systems, data on child abuse and neglect are particularly vulnerable to reporting bias. Differences in clinical judgments, variability in recognition of cases, reluctance to report, and campaigns to increase awareness all may influence the reporting of child abuse and neglect. To address these limitations, CDC is involved in various activities to assess and improve mechanisms for the surveillance of child abuse and neglect.

Graitcer has suggested that we apply the following principles when addressing injury surveillance (18):

1. The design of any surveillance system needs to take into consideration the purposes of surveillance. The means of data collection will vary by the purposes of surveillance.

2. Various data sources are available for injury surveillance. Existing data systems may be most useful—obviating the need to develop new data systems. The accessibility of computerized data, the availability of cause-of-injury information, and the representativeness of the data must be considered.

3. A minimal amount of data should be collected in a surveillance system. Existing data systems may provide basic information—allowing investigators to study risk factors in more focused studies.

4. Injury surveillance is not the same as case investigation. Although surveillance may identify cases, more focused epidemiologic studies are the most effective way to define risk factors.

5. Local data should be used for local programs. This may limit available data to vital records and hospital discharge data.

EXAMPLES OF USING DATA

Oklahoma Residential Fire Injury Prevention Project

Burn injuries that require hospitalization or that result in death have been reportable conditions in Oklahoma since November 1986. The state established an active surveillance system using data from the three burn centers in the state and the state medical examiner. Data from the first 32 months of surveillance revealed that residential fires caused 313 (18%) of the 1,720 burn injuries reported and 201 (63%) of the 320 burn fatalities reported.

Using surveillance and fire department data, the Oklahoma injury prevention staff calculated injury rates per 100 residential fires to identify a high-risk area in need of a smoke detector give-away program. The targeted area had the highest rate of residential fire-related burn injuries in Oklahoma City. It also had low median household incomes and a high prevalence of Hispanic, Asian, and Native American minorities. The annual burn injury rate was nearly three times higher in the targeted area (4.8 per 100 residential fires) than in the rest of the city (1.7 per 100 residential fires). Thirty-six months after the intervention, the injury rate in the targeted area had declined 83% (p <0.001, Fisher's exact test) while the injury rate for the rest of the city increased by 33%, although the citywide increase was not statistically significant (p = 0.2, Fisher's exact test). Surveillance data played a critical role in targeting and ameliorating the high rate of residential fire injuries in this high-risk population.

Georgia Child Fatality Review System

Georgia is one of only 22 states currently conducting statewide multidisciplinary child fatality reviews (CFRs) aimed primarily at preventing fatal child abuse and neglect *(19,20)*. Georgia conducted one third of all CFRs reported to the National Center for Child Abuse Prevention and Research in 1991. Reviews are mandated in Georgia for childhood deaths that are sudden, unexpected, or unexplained. Cases are referred to county CFR teams at the discretion of the county coroner or medical examiner. The results of county CFR reports are reviewed by a state-level panel.

In an analysis of this review system, the Georgia Department of Human Resources and CDC found that the CFR system reviewed 13.5% of all childhood deaths during 1991, the first full year of operation. Deaths among older children, boys, children from minority populations, and those whose deaths were attributed to injury were more likely to be reviewed than other childhood deaths in the state. Injury was the underlying cause in 24.4% of all deaths and in 49.4% of the deaths investigated by CFRs. The highest proportion of deaths reviewed were those caused by violence (40.5%). CFR reviews judged 71% of firearm-related deaths to be preventable. CFR reviews also identified a cause of death different from the cause listed on the death certificate in 21 cases; in five of these cases, this difference was found to be related to evidence of fatal abuse or neglect.

The Georgia CFR system has had an immediate public health impact. As a result of cases reviewed, the following actions have taken place:

- In a case originally attributed to sudden infant death syndrome, an autopsy required by the CFR led to a different determination for the external cause of death and a subsequent homicide prosecution.

- A traffic light was installed at an intersection where several adolescents had been killed in motor vehicle crashes.

- A court order was issued to prevent deliveries by a lay midwife.

- State rules regarding the certification of midwives have been revised to require all midwives to be licensed nurses.

- CFR data on failure to use child restraints convinced legislators to pass tougher motor vehicle child restraint laws in 1993.

FUTURE ISSUES

External-Cause-of-Injury and Poisoning Codes

Although 99% of all injuries in the United States are nonfatal, mechanisms to collect national nonfatal injury surveillance are severely limited. The current standard for coding external causes of nonfatal injury is the *International Classification of Diseases, Ninth Revision, Clinical Modification (ICD-9-CM), Supplementary Classification of External Causes of Injury and Poisoning*, also known as E codes[†] *(21)*. Modifying existing hospital discharge data systems by requiring the use of E codes would be a practical and cost-effective way to collect information about severe nonfatal injuries *(22)*. The Indian Health Service, U.S. Public Health Service, which for more than a decade has required the use of E codes in hospital records, has successfully used its computerized medical records system to target and monitor injury prevention efforts *(23)*. Fourteen states[§] currently or will soon require the use of E codes in their hospital discharge data systems. The revised national uniform billing format, also known as UB92, used for third-party reimbursement now provides a separate, labeled space for E codes where none was previously available. The usefulness of E codes can be improved. E-code users and potential users would benefit from standardized coding guidelines and definitions and from increased availability of training.

[†] Two types of codes are used to describe injuries under the ICD-9-CM systems. The injury and poisoning codes (N codes) specify the anatomical nature of the injury (i.e., the injury diagnosis). The external-cause-of-injury and poisoning codes (E codes) are a supplementary system that classifies the environmental events, circumstances, intentionality, and conditions that cause injury, poisoning, and other adverse effects.

[§] California, Delaware, Maryland, Massachusetts, Missouri, Nebraska, New Jersey, New York, Pennsylvania, Rhode Island, South Carolina, Vermont, Washington, and Wisconsin.

Physicians and coroners who complete death certificates should also be trained in the nature and limitations of the system so that their diagnoses and comments about external causes of childhood injuries and contributing conditions can be accurately translated into *ICD-9-CM* codes. Although a more rigorous evaluation of the E-code scheme is currently under way, certain limitations still exist. Because the number of E codes for certain injury agents or events is restricted or absent (e.g., all-terrain vehicles, drowning in swimming pools vs. open bodies of water), the detail needed to conduct surveillance on certain injury problems is not available through E-coded data, regardless of coding accuracy. Also, important data on contributing factors, such as the role of alcohol and other drugs, are not captured in the current coding scheme. Some of these limitations are expected to be addressed in the 10th revision of the *International Classification of Diseases*, expected to be released in 1999.

Injury Control and Risk Factor Surveillance System

NCIPC is currently developing the Injury Control and Risk Factor Surveillance System (ICARIS), a prototype national computer-assisted telephone interview survey. The ICARIS is intended to be a flexible and rapid mechanism to collect injury risk factor information. The ICARIS follows the paradigm of other CDC computerized, telephone survey models such as the BRFSS and the Youth Risk Behavior Surveillance System. A national pilot survey is being conducted to determine the feasibility of this mechanism as a tool for evaluating injury control programs. The ICARIS also is intended to be useful for conducting state and local surveys.

National Electronic Injury Surveillance System

The National Electronic Injury Surveillance System (NEISS) is an ongoing surveillance system maintained by the U.S. Consumer Product Safety Commission. The NEISS tracks product-related injuries treated in hospital emergency departments across the United States. The NEISS is the only national system that collects data on injuries that are severe enough to require medical atten-

tion but not necessarily hospitalization. CDC has conducted special analyses to determine the system's usefulness in identifying certain injuries (e.g., product-related head injuries) *(Greenspan AI, personal communication, 1993)*. In addition, CDC has supported expansion of the NEISS for special studies, such as a recent national survey of boating- and boat propeller-related injuries *(24)*. One important special effort involving the NEISS and CDC has been the Firearm Injury Surveillance Study, which is intended to evaluate the feasibility and cost of using the NEISS to provide national data on nonfatal firearm injuries. This study will provide useful information on the feasibility of using the NEISS to obtain data on other injuries. For more details, see the Unintentional Injuries and Violence chapter.

Head and Spinal Cord Injury Surveillance

Working with government agencies, professional organizations, and consumer groups, NCIPC has developed standard guidelines (case definitions and a minimal data set) for the surveillance of head and spinal cord injuries. These guidelines, which use the CDC National Electronic Telecommunications Surveillance System format, are currently being field-tested. NCIPC currently receives spinal cord injury data from five states (see the Unintentional Injuries and Violence chapter for more details).

Data Linkage

CDC is collaborating with the National Highway Traffic Administration on a project to improve data on nonfatal motor vehicle-related injuries by linking police crash reports with hospital discharge records. The project will include 1) an inventory of linkages that have already been made in some states; 2) descriptions of the methodologies employed to make these linkages; 3) descriptions of the data elements in existing linked data sets, including the elements used for linkage; 4) descriptions of data sets that other states use to form linkages; and 5) an inventory of agencies in other states with interests in achieving data linkages.

When completed, the data linkage project will provide us with improved epidemiologic data, especially on the injuries sustained, the vehicles involved, and the circumstances of each crash. Linked data can be used to 1) measure the impact and cost of failure to use safety belts, child restraints, and motorcycle helmets; 2) measure the impact and cost of alcohol use in motor vehicle crashes; and 3) provide data of value to legislators drafting prevention legislation.

Child Abuse and Neglect

The NCIPC is involved in a number of activities intended to foster a better understanding of child abuse and neglect. In recent years, reports of child abuse and neglect have increased, but we have reason to believe that this increase may be related largely to increased awareness and reporting rather than to increased incidence. The NCIPC has developed a methodology to estimate confirmed, probable, and possible child abuse and neglect fatalities using vital records supplemented with Federal Bureau of Investigation crime data (25). In addition, NCIPC is assessing the adequacy of existing state records systems for identifying child abuse and neglect and is supporting the development of a model system for child fatality review.

Long-Term Goals

As more resources become available for NCIPC, CDC's newest center, our long-term surveillance goals will include the development of a comprehensive surveillance system that can provide data useful for state and local programs and for national estimates. Through the data linkage project, NCIPC and NHTSA also hope to refine data linkage methodology. Dissemination of this methodology will allow more states and local health agencies to improve the quality of injury surveillance data. In addition, NCIPC staff will use their findings from the national pilot test to make the ICARIS useful at the state and local levels.

Finally, we recognize the critical need for external-cause information on nonfatal injuries, and we will encourage all states to include external-cause-of-injury information in their hospital discharge data systems. We anticipate that the National Hospital Discharge Survey will be more useful for injury surveillance when E codes are routinely available. In the meantime, additional methods to capture information about injuries not requiring hospitalization need to be developed.

REFERENCES

1. Public Health Service. Childhood injuries in the United States. Atlanta: US Department of Health and Human Services, Public Health Service, CDC, 1989.

2. Baker SP, O'Neill B, Ginsburg MJ, Li G. The injury fact book. 2nd ed. New York: Oxford University Press, 1992.

3. Committee on Trauma Research, Commission on Life Sciences, National Research Council, Institute of Medicine. Injury in America: a continuing public health problem. Washington, DC: National Academy Press, 1985.

4. National Safety Council. Accident facts. 1992 ed. Itasca, Illinois: National Safety Council, 1992.

5. NCHS. Mortality tapes; 1968–1990. Hyattsville, Maryland: US Department of Health and Human Services, Public Health Service, CDC, 1968-1990.

6. Rice DP, MacKenzie EJ, Jones AS, et al. Cost of injury in the United States: a report to Congress—1989. San Francisco: Institute for Health and Aging, University of California, Injury Prevention Center, The Johns Hopkins University, 1989.

7. Briss PA, Sacks JJ. A nationwide study of the risk of injury associated with day care center attendance. Pediatrics 1994 (in press).

8. Graitcer PL. The development of state and local injury surveillance systems. J Safety Res 1987;18:191–8.

9. Smith SM, Middaugh JP. An assessment of potential injury surveillance data sources in Alaska using an emerging problem: all-terrain vehicle-associated injuries. Public Health Rep 1989;104:493–8.

10. Chorba TL, Klein TM. Increases in crash involvement and fatalities among motor vehicle occupants younger than 5 years old. Pediatrics 1993;91:897–901.

11. CDC. Impact of adult safety-belt use on restraint use among children <11 years of age—selected states, 1988 and 1989. MMWR 1993;42:275–8.

12. Rivara FP. Child pedestrian injuries in the United States: current status of the problem, potential interventions, and future research needs. Am J Dis Child 1990;144:692–6.

13. Guyer B, Ellers B. Childhood injuries in the United States: mortality, morbidity, and cost. Am J Dis Child 1990;144:649–52.

14. Wintemute GJ. Childhood drowning and near-drowning in the United States. Am J Dis Child 1990;144:663–9.

15. O'Carroll PW, Smith JC. Suicide and homicide. In: Wallace HM, Ryan G Jr, Oglesby AC, eds. Maternal and child health practices. 3rd ed. Oakland, California: Third Party Publishing, 1988:583–97.

16. Fingerhut LA. Firearm mortality among children, youth, and young adults 1–34 years of age, trends and current status: United States, 1985–90. Hyattsville, Maryland: US Department of Health and Human Services, Public Health Service, CDC, NCHS, 1993. Advance data from vital and health statistics; no. 231.

17. Study findings: study of the national incidence and prevalence of child abuse and neglect, 1988. Washington, DC: US Department of Health and Human Services, National Center on Child Abuse and Neglect, 1988.

18. Graitcer PL. Injury surveillance. In: Halperin W, Baker EL, Monson RR, eds. Public health surveillance. New York: Van Nostrand Reinhold, 1992:142–56.

19. Luallen JJ, O'Neil J. Protecting the future: the Georgia Child Fatality Review, 1991: a report to the statewide Child Fatality Review Panel. Atlanta: CDC, National Center for Injury Prevention and Control, 1993.

20. The Georgia Department of Human Resources. Communities learn to prevent deaths of children: child fatality reviews in Georgia—progress during the first year. GA Epi Rep 1992;8(9):1–3.

21. Public Health Service. International classification of diseases, ninth revision, clinical modification. Washington, DC: US Department of Health and Human Services, Public Health Service, Health Care Financing Administration, 1991;DHHS publication no. (PHS)91-1260.

22. Sniezek JE, Finklea JF, Graitcer PL. Injury coding and hospital discharge data. JAMA 1989;262:2270–2.

23. Smith SM, Colwell LS Jr, Sniezek JE. An evaluation of external cause-of-injury codes using hospital records from the Indian Health Service, 1985. Am J Public Health 1990;80:279–81.

24. Branche-Dorsey CM, Smith SM, Johnson D. A study of boat and boat-propeller-related injuries in the United States, 1991–1992. Atlanta: CDC, National Center for Injury Prevention and Control, 1993.

25. McClain PW, Sacks JJ, Froehlke RG, Ewigman BG. Estimates of fatal child abuse and neglect, United States, 1979 through 1988. Pediatrics 1993;91:338–43.

Lead Poisoning

Carol A. Pertowski, M.D.[1]

PUBLIC HEALTH IMPORTANCE

Lead poisoning is one of the most common environmental health problems affecting young children. The Environmental Protection Agency estimates that in 1990, 3 million children had blood-lead (PbB) levels high enough (≥10 μg/dL) to cause adverse health effects (1). Health effects from lead exposure vary with the PbB level. Severe neurologic problems, such as coma and seizures, and death have been associated with blood-lead levels of ≥80 μg/dL (2). Renal damage and decreased hematopoiesis have occurred among patients with PbB levels of 40–80 μg/dL (2). Adverse health effects can also occur at low levels, however. PbB levels at least as low as 10 μg/dL have been associated with decreased intelligence and impaired neurobehavioral development (3,4). Most children with elevated PbB levels are asymptomatic (5), and lead exposure is usually a diagnosis based on laboratory findings.

Childhood lead poisoning is a preventable disease. Most childhood lead exposure in the United States results from exposure to household lead-based paint or dust from this paint (6). In 1989–1990, the U.S. Department of Housing and Urban Development evaluated the extent of lead paint hazards in the nation's housing stock (7). The results of this survey suggest that 3.8 million housing units containing either lead-based paint in deteriorated condition or high levels of lead in dust are occupied by families with children <7 years of age. Also preventable are exposures to lead through drinking water, soil, traditional or folk medicines, fishing sinkers, bullets, materials used to make ceramics and stained glass, and **take-home** exposure from household members occupationally exposed to lead. All children are at risk for lead exposure; young children living in deteriorated housing in inner cities are at the highest risk (6).

In October 1991, CDC revised its policy statement on preventing lead exposure among young children (6). In this statement, CDC lowered the PbB level of concern from 25 to 10 μg/dL; recommended the phasing in of **virtually universal screening** (i.e., screening of all young children except in communities where large numbers or percentages of children were screened and did not have elevated PbB levels); emphasized the importance of primary prevention (i.e., identification and remediation of lead hazards before a child's PbB level is elevated); and identified PbB measurement as the screening test of choice. The lead statement also included an approach for investigating sources of lead, remediating lead hazards, and conducting medical follow-up based on an affected child's PbB level.

In February 1991, the Department of Health and Human Services announced its *Strategic Plan for the Elimination of Childhood Lead Poisoning* (8). Surveillance of lead exposure is one of the key program components of the *Strategic Plan*. Surveillance is needed to identify children at highest risk for lead exposure, target interventions, and track our progress in

[1] Division of Environmental Hazards and Health Effects
National Center for Environmental Health
Centers for Disease Control and Prevention
Atlanta, Georgia.

Acknowledgments

I thank Jennifer Flattery, M.P.H., California State Department of Health Services; Rita Gergely, Iowa Department of Public Health; and Mary Jean Brown, Massachusetts Department of Public Health, for their assistance with the Examples of Using Data section.

eliminating lead exposure. To develop surveillance systems at the state level, programs may need to integrate information from several sources: childhood lead poisoning prevention programs at the state and local levels, public and private laboratories, and health, environment, and housing agencies.

Lead exposure among children is a worldwide health issue, although the predominant sources of lead in other parts of the world may differ from those in the United States. Increased lead levels in air and soil have been measured in areas such as Eastern Europe where environmental controls of industrial sources have not been fully implemented. Lead contamination from cottage industries, such as battery repair shops, have also been associated with elevated PbB levels among children *(9)*. In countries where leaded gasoline is used, automobile emissions may contribute to elevated PbB levels among children *(10,11)*. Other sources of lead include improperly fired or unfired lead-glazed pottery *(12,13)* and lead in canned foods *(13)*. For additional information about related topics and surveillance activities, see the Pediatric Nutrition chapter.

HISTORY OF DATA COLLECTION

During the 1970s and early 1980s, CDC funded childhood lead poisoning prevention projects in state and local health departments, where program staff hand-tallied the number of children screened for lead exposure and the number of children with elevated PbB levels. During 1981, 62 childhood lead poisoning prevention programs reported screening >500,000 children, >18,000 of whom had PbB levels above 30 μg/dL, the CDC level of concern at the time *(14)*. The reporting process was difficult, however, and children tested several times a year may have been counted more than once.

In 1981, funding for childhood lead poisoning prevention programs was folded into CDC's Maternal and Child Health Services Block Grants. Each state was allowed to decide how it would allocate resources provided by these grants. The federal reporting requirements for

childhood lead levels were eliminated, and the surveillance system was discontinued.

Less than a decade later, the Lead Contamination Control Act of 1988 authorized money for CDC to administer a childhood lead poisoning prevention grant program. Most of the money is provided as grants to state and local agencies to screen children for elevated PbB levels, to assure medical and environmental follow-up, and to conduct educational programs about lead exposure in communities with children who have elevated PbB levels.

Recently, CDC collaborated with the Council of State and Territorial Epidemiologists (CSTE) to develop a national surveillance system for monitoring PbB levels among children. In 1990, CSTE approved a position statement recommending that states require that elevated PbB levels be reported to state health departments and establish surveillance for elevated PbB levels in all age-groups.

At the state or local level, the primary source of data for surveillance is usually the childhood lead poisoning prevention program. These programs are responsible for screening children, ensuring that children with elevated PbB levels receive appropriate medical follow-up and environmental management, and for collecting, managing, and reporting data. The collaboration and coordination of activities by staffs at the health department, housing authority, and environmental agencies are crucial for assuring complete medical and environmental management of children with elevated PbB levels and for carrying out primary prevention of lead exposure. Because young children are at an increased risk for lead exposure, screening programs focus on children <6 years of age.

Information from public health screening programs is a valuable resource for surveillance data; however, these data have limitations. First, data from these programs are restricted to populations targeted by the program. Because prevention programs usually target children thought to be at a high risk for elevated PbB levels, the population screened may not be representative of the entire population. Data from these programs are inadequate to assess population rates or to estimate a community's burden from lead exposure, and they are of limited use in monitoring trends. Second, although many state and local agencies gather data from environmental investigations and medical management of children with elevated PbB levels, in some states these data are not organized into a single database that can be used to track trends over time.

The National Health and Nutrition Examination Surveys serve as another source of national data for estimating the number of children with elevated PbB levels. Although these surveys provide national estimates of the prevalence of elevated PbB levels among children, they do not provide information at the state or local level. Also, these surveys do not directly measure incidence, and the data cannot be used to follow short-term trends.

Other sources of data that can provide supplemental information on childhood lead exposure are the National Health Interview Survey, Injury Control and Risk Survey, National Hospital Discharge Survey, and surveys conducted by state health departments.

The national surveillance system for PbB levels among children is based on systems developed and maintained at the state level. One key component for surveillance at the state level is a law mandating that laboratories report PbB levels to state health departments. A 1989 survey examining state and territorial laws for reporting childhood PbB levels indicated that a majority of jurisdictions required the reporting of elevated PbB levels among children but that the PbB concentrations that had to be reported varied (15). Of the 29 jurisdictions with mandatory reporting requirements, only 2 states mandated the reporting of all test results, regardless of the PbB value. The majority of the jurisdictions required the reporting of PbB values of ≥ 25 µg/dL—the level defining childhood lead poisoning at the time of the survey. Of the jurisdictions that specified age-groups, all required the reporting of elevated PbB levels among children ≥ 5 years old. The mechanism of reporting also varied among these 29 jurisdictions: 24 required private laboratories to report; 22 required public laboratories to report;

and 13 required both in-state and out-of-state laboratories to report. In addition, 23 jurisdictions required physicians to report, and 11 required screening programs to report. Since the survey was conducted, several states have modified their reporting requirements.

In September 1992, CDC awarded cooperative agreement funds to eight state health departments to help them in carrying out PbB surveillance activities. The goals of the national childhood PbB surveillance program are to increase the number of state health departments with surveillance systems for PbB levels among children; build the capacity of states and territories to conduct laboratory-based surveillance of PbB levels; use data from these systems to establish a national surveillance system; disseminate data on the extent of elevated PbB levels among children to government agencies, researchers, and medical care providers; and direct intervention efforts to reduce environmental lead exposure.

CDC SURVEILLANCE ACTIVITIES

CDC's National Center for Environmental Health is responsible for developing and maintaining the national surveillance system for childhood lead levels. This system is based on data collected by state health departments. For national surveillance, a child is considered to meet the case definition if any venous sample contains a lead level of ≥ 10 µg/dL or if two capillary samples taken within 12 weeks of each other both contain levels of ≥ 10 µg/dL. The system is based on laboratory reporting, which may simplify and help achieve completeness of reporting (16).

In conjunction with the eight states that received 1992 cooperative agreement funds to develop surveillance systems, CDC developed new data fields for the national surveillance system of children with PbB levels (Table 1) and an approach for data management and transfer. The surveillance data can be extracted from laboratory reports and from information collected by health departments as part of the medical and environmental management of a child with elevated PbB levels. To organize data from environmental and medical follow-up of a child

313

with elevated PbB levels, many state and local health departments use computer software such as the System for Tracking Elevated Lead Levels and Remediation (STELLAR), a public domain program developed by CDC *(17)*. CDC is developing computer programs that will allow health departments to directly import data from laboratories into STELLAR and to extract surveillance data from the STELLAR database.

The degree and use of technology, number of children with elevated PbB levels, and approaches to case-management vary from state to state; however, a state surveillance system for children <16 years of age who have elevated PbB levels should include several basic components (Table 2). This database will allow states to describe children aged <16 years with elevated PbB levels over time, by person, place, and likely source of exposure. Additional information on funding sources for screening, type of screening program, medical treatment, and environmental follow-up of children with elevated PbB levels will be available.

The database will also provide information to calculate case-rates among children aged <6 years who receive PbB tests. Data on all children aged <6 years who have been tested for lead exposure, regardless of the test result, may be maintained in the same database as that for children with elevated PbB levels. These data will provide denominator estimates for calculating rates of elevated PbB levels among children in this age-group who have been tested. Data on children aged <6 years without elevated PbB levels are limited to laboratory slip information, because these children do not receive medical or environmental follow-up. The number of children aged <6 years may be large, and limited resources may prevent states from collecting data for a full year. Therefore, data on these children may be collected for less than a full year and be extrapolated to yearly estimates. To maximize representativeness, states should include data from all quarters.

States transfer quarterly data by using CDC WONDER/PC, a public-domain software system developed by CDC for public health programs. This system also links sites together via an elec-

tronic mail system and will soon allow state surveillance programs to perform a set of basic analyses on their data.

GENERAL FINDINGS

The surveillance system is currently being developed, and no national data are available. When these data are available, they will have numerous useful applications. First, a descriptive picture of children with elevated PbB levels will be provided. The importance of paint and nonpaint sources can then be determined, and clusters of children with elevated PbB levels can be identified. Second, an estimate of children newly identified as having elevated PbB levels (prevalence of new cases at screening) and an estimate of all children with elevated levels (prevalence of all cases) among children tested can be calculated.

INTERPRETATION ISSUES

Advantages of the System

Advantages of the system include its usefulness and relative simplicity. The case definition is simple because it requires only the reporting of elevated PbB levels. The use of laboratory-based reporting will simplify the system. Automated data transfer will facilitate management of the large numbers of PbB reports. The surveillance system also does not require the collection of data beyond the information usually obtained during the investigation and treatment of a child with an elevated PbB level.

State and local health departments will be able to use information from this system for planning or modifying prevention programs. The data also will be useful for evaluating the cost-effectiveness of specific screening activities such as door-to-door screening. Collecting information on both the number of children with elevated PbB levels and the number tested will allow states to identify neighborhoods or towns with children **at high risk** or those **not at risk** for elevated PbB levels. Interventions or screening programs can then be directed to high-risk groups.

TABLE 1. Proposed data fields for the national surveillance of children with elevated blood-lead levels — Centers for Disease Control and Prevention, 1993

VARIABLES SUBMITTED ON LABORATORY SLIP*

Child ID Number	Date of birth
Sex	Race
Ethnicity	Address ID
City	County
State	ZIP code
Medicaid enrolled	
Type of sample (venous or capillary)	Results (μg/dL)
Date sample drawn	Date sample analyzed by lab
Laboratory type (public health or commercial)	

DATA FROM CASE INVESTIGATION†

Program data

Date sample received by state health department

Child previously with elevated blood-lead level

Type of provider ordering test (fixed site specific to lead, door-to-door program, other screening program such as WIC, private health-care provider)

Reason for test (screening an asymptomatic child, confirmatory test after an elevated value by finger-stick, follow-up of confirmed elevated level, clinical suspicion of lead poisoning.)

Funding source (public, including Medicaid, state or local programs; private insurance; self-pay)

Treatment data

Child received chelation therapy

Type of chelation therapy (inpatient, outpatient, both)

Source of funding for chelation therapy

Paint hazard data

Age of child's residence

Ownership of child's residence (private or public, owned or rented)

Residence with peeling, chipping, or flaking paint

Date child moved to present residence

Residence renovated

Date renovation started

Date renovation completed

Environmental investigation information (Highest value obtained)

Location (current or former residence, child care facility, residence of relative)

Dust samples in μg/ft^2 or ppm (floors, window sills, window wells)

X-ray fluorescence reading

Paint chip analysis

Soil sample analysis

Water sample analysis

Nonpaint hazards

Traditional medicines

Household member with occupation using lead (e.g., welder, battery repair shop operator)

Child with occupation involving lead exposure

Household member with hobby using lead (stained glass, pottery/ceramics, making bullets or fish sinkers, using firearms or artist paints)

Improperly fired or imported pottery used for eating, cooking, or food storage

Industrial facility near home

---

* Information collected on all blood tests, regardless of lead level.
† Information collected for children with lead levels above the action level for environmental and medical investigation defined by the state. The action levels vary from state to state.

Limitations of the System

One inherent limitation of the system results from reliance on information reported by laboratories because the data are often incomplete. Assuring the reporting of all PbB tests, especially those submitted to private or out-of-state laboratories, may be difficult. The data on laboratory reports are a vital component of the surveillance database; information on children with PbB levels of 10–19 μg/dL and <10 μg/dL may be limited to data provided on the laboratory

315

TABLE 2. Components of a state surveillance system for children aged <16 years with elevated blood-lead levels.

1. A law or regulation mandating the reporting of blood-lead (PbB) levels.

   Reports are submitted by both private and public laboratories.

   Reports contain sufficient demographic information to allow states to identify the child and assure appropriate follow-up.

2. Development of a state database of information, children with elevated PbB levels (≥10 µg/dL)

   Data on children are entered into the database with the first report of a PbB level of ≥10 µg/dL.

   Subsequent blood test results on children already in the database are added to the children's files.

   States add to the data set the type of laboratory (i.e., public or private) performing the test, the date the sample was received by the health department, and the data from the laboratory slip (Table 1).

   States coordinate the collection of information from environmental and medical case-management (Table 1) and add this information to the database.

3. An age-dependent approach to data management.*

   For children aged <6 years:

   A child remains in the database until the child's 6th birthday.

   For children aged 6–16 years:

   An indication of whether the child previously had a PbB level of ≥10 µg/dL is also added to the data set.

   A child remains in the database only for the calendar year in which the elevated PbB level was drawn.

4. Estimates of children tested.

   Data on all children aged <6 years who have been tested for lead, regardless of test result, may also be maintained in this database.

   These data will provide denominator estimates for calculating rates of elevated PbB levels among children aged <6 years who have been tested for lead exposure.

5. Data transmission and analysis.

   Identifying information is removed, and a unique number is assigned to each child.

   The surveillance database is transmitted quarterly to CDC.†

   The final database for a calendar year is compiled by CDC from data received by March 31 of the following year.

   States perform quarterly analyses and release annual reports of descriptive data; they generate yearly case-rates among tested populations.

6. Use of automated data transfer.

   To facilitate the management of large amounts of data, programs focus on the use of automated data transfer whenever possible.

---

* Because screening programs focus on children aged <6 years, the data for these children are obtained in a manner different from that for children aged ≥6 years.

† States with a large number of children may wish to transfer data more frequently than quarterly.

---

slip. To facilitate reporting, CDC is working with CSTE and the Association of State and Territorial Public Health Laboratory Directors to establish core variables for reporting from public and private laboratories.

Another potential limitation to initiating a state surveillance activity is the time needed to establish the system. To promote efficient use of time and resources, states should avoid duplicating efforts conducted during case-management activities and use computerized data management and transfer. However, organizing a state surveillance system may require pulling data together from several childhood lead poisoning prevention programs within the state and assuring complete reporting of data. Assuring complete data reporting may involve educational programs for physicians and for laboratory staff. Once the system is established, states must provide personnel to maintain the surveillance database and to analyze and disseminate the data.

In addition, we must consider the limitations related to the representativeness of the data. Currently, many children are tested in screening programs. Because screening programs usually focus on children at high risk, the population of children tested in the state and the population with elevated PbB levels may not be representative of all children in the age-group of interest. The number and demographic characteristics of children tested by private health-care providers and screening programs may also reflect awareness campaigns by state and local health departments. The amount and type of information on children with elevated PbB levels may not be comparable across sites because the approach to medical follow-up and environmental management at the state and local levels varies with the PbB value and the resources of the agency. When interpreting the data, we must take these limitations into account.

Another limitation is the potential for false negatives. Screening for elevated PbB levels can be conducted on samples obtained from either a venipuncture or a finger-stick (capillary sample). Although **one** elevated PbB level from a sample obtained by venipuncture defines a case, **two** finger-stick specimens taken within 12 weeks of each other with levels of >10 μg/dL are needed to define a case. Because sequential finger-stick samples with elevated PbB levels taken within 12 weeks of each other may not be available, some children with persistently elevated PbB levels may be incorrectly classified as not meeting the case definition.

EXAMPLES OF USING DATA

Although data collection for the national surveillance system has just begun, several states have already used their surveillance data to develop legislation supporting lead poisoning prevention activities, obtain funding, identify risk groups, and target screening and prevention activities.

California

In 1986, California established a Childhood Lead Poisoning Prevention Program (CLPPP) and reporting requirements for a laboratory-based surveillance system for all persons with PbB levels ≥ 25 μg/dL. The surveillance system documented an increasing number of children with elevated PbB levels in 1989 and 1990. In response to this increase, the legislature in 1991 passed additional laws supporting childhood lead poisoning prevention efforts. One law mandated that all children in California be screened according to standards set by regulations that are at least as stringent as the CDC guidelines and authorized the CLPPP to change the reporting requirements for PbB levels as necessary. In addition, under the Child Health and Disability Prevention Program, physicians providing health care to low-income children are required to provide PbB screening to all children who attend publicly funded well-child day-care facilities.

Data from the surveillance system have shown that children living outside metropolitan areas also have elevated PbB levels. The California CLPPP has used this information to educate health care providers about the need to screen children not usually thought to be at risk for lead exposure. In addition to paint sources of lead, the system has shown the importance of nonpaint sources such as traditional medicines (18) and ceramic ware. Because the system currently collects only reports of elevated PbB levels—rather than reports of all PbB levels measured—rates of elevated PbB levels among

317

children cannot be calculated. The California CLPPP is adapting its reporting requirement and surveillance system to collect reports of all PbB levels.

Iowa

Since September 1992, Iowa has used both laboratory-based and physician reporting for the surveillance of all PbB levels among children. Data from the surveillance system suggest that children in both rural and urban parts of the state have elevated PbB levels. Because the surveillance system collects reports of all PbB levels, the Iowa CLPPP has been able to calculate rates of elevated PbB levels among all children tested for lead exposure. The rates of children with elevated PbB levels in many small towns and rural areas are higher than rates in some urban regions of the state. These findings—and data suggesting that many children screened by private health-care providers have elevated PbB levels—are being used to educate physicians about the need to screen all children for lead.

The state and county health departments have used data from the surveillance system to build communitywide coalitions and to develop and fund local CLPPPs. The state CLPPP also used these data to inform legislators of the need for authority to inspect and require remediation of lead hazards in the residences of children with elevated PbB levels and to develop a contractor certification program to assure that lead hazards are remediated properly.

Massachusetts

In a study using 1988 data from the Massachusetts lead poisoning prevention program, researchers found that only 43% of children aged 13–24 months and 29% of children aged 25–36 months were screened for elevated PbB levels (19). They also found that 30% of children with elevated PbB levels lived in rural or suburban communities. The screening schedule subsequently adopted by Massachusetts requires that all children be assessed for the risk of exposure to lead and be screened for elevated

PbB levels periodically during early childhood. In 1990, Massachusetts established a laboratory-based surveillance system that requires reporting of PbB levels among children. Data from the surveillance system are used to evaluate state programs and to target screening activities.

FUTURE ISSUES

In 1990, an estimated 3 million children aged 6 months through 5 years had PbB levels exceeding 10 μg/dL (1). The U.S. Department of Health and Human Services has defined the year 2000 objective for childhood lead exposure as "reducing the prevalence of PbB levels exceeding 15 μg/dL and 25 μg/dL among children aged 6 months through 5 years to no more than 500,000 and zero, respectively" (20). For inner-city black children, special targets have been set at 75,000 children with levels of 15–25 μg/dL and no children with levels above 25 μg/dL.

During the next few years, a major challenge to surveillance will be to collect data from portable blood lead analyzers. Equipment that will allow us to analyze blood samples in the field may soon be available. Analysis in the field may facilitate the notification of parents about their child's PbB test results and allow us to collect more accurate demographic data. However, assuring that all test results are reported to state health departments will require innovative approaches.

We also can expect an increased use of automated data transfer and improvements in the scope and quality of data collected. Continued progress in the development and use of computerized systems will enhance surveillance systems at the local, state, and national levels. Automated data transfer is a crucial time-saving measure, especially in programs where different agencies maintain separate databases and are responsible for different components of case-management. For example, the use of electronic data transfer systems such as the Public Health Laboratory Information System will facilitate the reporting of PbB test results from laboratories to state or local health departments. Advancements in the CDC WONDER/PC system will simplify data analysis by expanding the number and type of data analyses available to state surveillance programs as menu-driven programs.

Over the next few years, more states will be submitting data to the national surveillance system, thus improving the representativeness of the data. At the state level, data quality will likely improve as reporting is standardized (e.g., as laboratories begin using a set of core variables). With time, state surveillance programs will be better able to obtain data from laboratories performing PbB analyses and to identify and complete missing risk factor and environmental information.

Achieving the year 2000 objective for reducing childhood lead exposure requires an increased use of primary prevention measures. Improvements in the scope and quality of the surveillance database will provide a clearer picture of the extent and determinants of childhood lead exposure in the United States and will help programs allocate resources and coordinate primary prevention efforts.

REFERENCES

1. US Environmental Protection Agency. U.S. Environmental Protection Agency strategy for reducing lead exposures. Washington, DC: US Environmental Protection Agency, 1991.

2. Agency for Toxic Substances and Disease Registry. The nature and extent of lead poisoning in children in the United States: a report to Congress. Atlanta: US Department of Health and Human Services, Public Health Service, 1988.

3. Bellinger DC, Stiles KM, Needleman HL. Low-level lead exposure, intelligence and academic achievement: a long-term follow-up study. Pediatrics 1992; 90:855–61.

4. Dietrich KN, Berger OG, Succop PA, Hammond PB, Bornschein RL. The developmental consequences of low to moderate prenatal and postnatal lead exposure: intellectual attainment in the Cincinnati Lead Study Cohort following school entry. Neurotoxicol Teratol 1993;15:37–44.

5. Piomelli S, Rosen JF, Chisolm JJ Jr, Graef JW. Management of childhood lead poisoning. J Pediatr 1984;105:523–32.

6. CDC. Preventing lead poisoning in young children: a statement by the Centers for Disease Control—October 1991. Atlanta: US Department of Health and Human Services, Public Health Service, 1991.

7. US Department of Housing and Urban Development. Comprehensive and workable plan for the abatement of lead-based paint in privately owned housing: report to Congress. Washington, DC: US Department of Housing and Urban Development, 1990.

8. CDC. Strategic plan for the elimination of childhood lead poisoning. Atlanta: US Department of Health and Human Services, Public Health Service, 1991.

9. Matte TD, Figueroa JP, Ostrowski S, et al. Lead poisoning among household members exposed to lead-acid battery repair shops in Kingston, Jamaica. Int J Epidemiol 1989;18:874–81.

10. Romieu I, Palazuelos E, Meneses F, Hernandez-Avila M. Vehicular traffic as a determinant of blood-lead levels in children: a pilot study in Mexico City. Arch Environ Health 1992;47:246–9.

11. Lyngbye T, Hansen ON, Grandjean P. Predictors of tooth-lead level with special reference to traffic: a study of lead exposure in children. Int Arch Occup Environ Health 1990;62:417–22.

12. Hernandez-Avila M, Romieu I, Rios C, Rivero A, Palazuelos E. Lead-glazed ceramics as major determinants of blood lead levels in Mexican women. Environ Health Perspect 1991;94:117–20.

13. Lara-Flores E, Alagon-Cano J, Bobadilla JL, Hernandez-Prado B, Ciscomani-Begona A. Factores asociados a los niveles de plomo en sangre en residentes de la ciudad de México [Risk factors for high blood-lead levels in residents of Mexico City]. Salud Publica Mex 1989;31:625–33.

14. CDC. Annual summary 1981: reported morbidity and mortality in the United States. MMWR 1982; 30:112–3.

15. CDC. Surveillance of children's blood lead levels—United States, 1991. MMWR 1992;41:620–2.

16. Istre GR. Disease surveillance at the state and local levels. In: Halperin W, Baker EL Jr, eds. Public health surveillance. New York: Van Nostrand Reinhold, 1992:42–55.

17. CDC. STELLAR user guide. Version 2.0a. Atlanta: US Department of Health and Human Services, Public Health Service, 1993.

18. CDC. Lead poisoning associated with use of traditional ethnic remedies—California, 1991–1992. MMWR 1993;42:521–4.

19. Brown MJ, DeGiacomo JM, Gallagher G, et al. Lead poisoning in children of different ages [Letter]. N Engl J Med 1990;323:135–6.

20. Public Health Service. Healthy people 2000: national health promotion and disease prevention objectives—full report, with commentary. Washington, DC: US Department of Health and Human Services, Public Health Service, 1991; DHHS publication no. (PHS) 91-50212.

FROM DATA TO ACTION · CDC'S PUBLIC HEALTH SURVEILLANCE FOR WOMEN, INFANTS, AND CHILDREN

Nutrition

Ibrahim Parvanta, M.S.,[1] Bettylou Sherry,[1] Ph.D., R.D.,[1]
and Ray Yip, M.D., M.P.H.[1]

PUBLIC HEALTH IMPORTANCE

Nutritional status is an integral component of the overall health of individuals and populations. Among children, nutritional status can affect growth, development, and resistance to disease. The main nutrition-related health problems among Americans result from overconsumption of calories, fats, cholesterol, and sodium (1). Although the U.S. food supply is adequate to prevent severe undernutrition and deficiency-related diseases, some subgroups of Americans have inadequate dietary intake and deficiencies in nutrients—especially iron, which continues to represent the most common nutrient deficiency (1). The risk of nutrition-related health problems is greatest among low-income populations, with young children being especially vulnerable (2).

We can assess the nutritional status of individuals and populations in a variety of ways, including dietary, anthropometric (growth), and hematologic evaluations. The CDC Pediatric Nutrition Surveillance System (PedNSS) is designed to monitor the nutritional status of low-income children served by various publicly funded health and nutrition programs. The PedNSS uses anthropometric and hematologic measurements to assess the three most common nutrition-related problems among U.S. children—linear growth retardation, overweight, and iron deficiency anemia (3)—as well as birth weight and breast-feeding practices.

One of the Public Health Service's year 2000 objectives for the nation is to reduce growth retardation among low-income children aged <5 years to <10% (4). Growth retardation or stunting is an indicator of the long-term health and nutritional history of a child or a population.

On an individual level, shortness can reflect the normal variation of growth within a population. Stunted growth, however, can result from poor nutrition, an increased number of infections, or both (2). A poor psychosocial environment can also retard growth. Among young infants, such growth failure is associated with a generalized failure to thrive as well as short stature, whereas among older children, it primarily affects stature (5). The PedNSS is not designed to identify specific causes of short stature for each child under surveillance. However, on a population level, an increased prevalence of stunting generally reflects poor socioeconomic and health conditions (6).

Overweight or obesity can adversely affect health and longevity and is associated with numerous chronic diseases among adults (1). Childhood obesity affects about 25% of children in the United States (7) and increases their likelihood of obesity during adulthood (8). Many factors—including inherited, environmental, cultural, and socioeconomic conditions—can result in excessive weight gain (4). The PedNSS is not designed to determine specific causes of overweight in the population being monitored; however, it does provide data on the prevalence of overweight so that high-risk population groups can be identified and targeted for intervention.

The PedNSS is also useful in identifying children at highest risk for anemia, which usually is caused by iron deficiency (9). Iron deficiency

[1] Division of Nutrition
National Center for Chronic Disease Prevention
    and Health Promotion
Centers for Disease Control and Prevention
Atlanta, Georgia

anemia is associated with impaired learning and increased susceptibility to lead poisoning (10). This deficiency can be prevented and treated through the consumption of adequate dietary iron, or supplementation, or both. A year 2000 objective for the nation is to reduce iron deficiency among low-income children aged 1 to 2 years to 10%, and among children aged 3–4 years to 5% (4).

Another national objective is to reduce the proportion of low-birth-weight births to 5% of live births (4). Although monitoring birth weight in the United States is not the main focus of the PedNSS, the system can provide information on low-income population groups at highest risk for low birth weight. Birth weight is an indicator of maternal pregnancy health status and a predictor of morbidity and mortality during infancy and childhood. It is also a strong predictor of later childhood growth (11).

The Public Health Service also recommends that 75% of newborns be breast-fed at hospital discharge and of those, 50% be breast-fed until 5–6 months of age (4). The benefits of breast-feeding have been emphasized by many health authorities and organizations in the United States. Human milk contains the ideal balance of nutrients, enzymes, hormones, and other substances to provide physiologic benefits for the newborn infant. Breast milk consumption and breast-feeding are effective in preventing and reducing the burden of infections in infants (12). Further, breast-feeding provides intense maternal-infant interaction (4). Therefore, breast-feeding promotion is an important component of publicly funded maternal and child health programs. For additional information about related topics and surveillance activities, see the Pregnancy-Related Nutrition chapter.

HISTORY OF DATA COLLECTION

Several national nutrition surveys have been conducted to document the health of the U.S. population: the National Health Examination Surveys (NHES I in 1960–1962, NHES II in 1963–1965, and NHES III in 1966–1970); the

National Health and Nutrition Examination Surveys (NHANES I in 1971–1974, NHANES II in 1976–1980, and NHANES III, now in progress); and the Hispanic Health and Nutrition Examination Survey (1982–1984) (13).

The growth curves developed by CDC's National Center for Health Statistics (NCHS) evolved from NHES and NHANES I data. Specifically, the current growth curves (NCHS growth reference) published in 1979 for 2- to 18-year-old children are based on cross-sectional data collected from 1963–1975 on >20,000 children selected on a weighted sample to be representative of all children in the United States (14). Growth curve data for children from birth to 2 years of age included in the NCHS curves for 1979 are based on longitudinal data collected on white children in Yellow Springs, Ohio, by the Fels Research Institute between 1929 and 1978. These sex-specific growth curves, which evolved as a result of the national nutrition surveys, serve as a tool integral to the interpretation of the surveillance system. The growth curves provide a way of comparing the growth of a child with the average growth of all children in the United States. They also can be used as a screening tool to target children in need of food program support and can serve as an indicator of a program's effects on a child.

In the late 1960s, the Ten-State Nutrition Survey characterized the nutritional status of U.S. children from low-income families as being less than satisfactory (15). As a result, CDC began in 1973 working with Arizona, Kentucky, Louisiana, Tennessee, and Washington to develop a system for continuously monitoring the nutritional status of specific high-risk population groups (3). By 1992, the PedNSS had expanded to include public health and nutrition programs from 41 states, the District of Columbia, Puerto Rico, the Intertribal Council of Arizona, the Navajo Nation, and the Mt. Plains Tribes; however, the pattern of participation has fluctuated. As PedNSS coverage has expanded, so has the number of records submitted to the system each year. In 1992, CDC processed >6 million PedNSS records.

CDC SURVEILLANCE ACTIVITIES

Objectives of the System

The PedNSS is operated by CDC's National Center for Chronic Disease Prevention and Health Promotion. It is a program-based nutrition surveillance system that uses information collected by publicly funded health and nutrition programs throughout the United States and its territories. These programs include the Special Supplemental Food Program for Women, Infants, and Children (WIC), the Early and Periodic Screening, Diagnosis and Treatment Program, Head Start, and other programs funded by Maternal and Child Health Block Grants. As of 1992, 4,500 publicly funded health and nutrition clinics participated in the PedNSS. Because most of these public health programs serve low-income families, the PedNSS could be regarded as a nutrition surveillance system for low-income U.S. infants and children.

The system has three primary objectives:

- To monitor trends in the prevalence of health and growth problems among children.

- To rapidly provide summary data to participating programs for their use in program planning and evaluation.

- To promote the development and use of standardized pediatric nutrition surveillance methods.

Data Items

The PedNSS collects four types of data:

- Demographic: clinic, county, date of birth, date of visit, race/ethnic group, sex, type of program, and type of visit (initial visit vs. follow-up visit).

- Anthropometric: birth weight, height, and weight.

- Hematologic: hemoglobin, hematocrit, and erythrocyte protoporphyrin levels.

- Method of feeding: whether the child has ever been breast-fed and whether the child is currently breast-fed.

The nutritional status indicators used in the PedNSS relate to the most prevalent nutritional problems and correspond to data inexpensively and routinely collected by local public health programs (3). For example, nearly all health-oriented programs require that children be weighed, measured, and tested to measure their hemoglobin or hematocrit levels. The WIC program specifically uses these indicators for eligibility screening.

Data Collection

In the majority of cases, local public health clinic staff collect all demographic, health, and nutrition-related information on children applying for services, using state- and program-specific protocols and forms (direct-entry computer screens are replacing paper forms). Some programs, however, rely partially on information collected by other health-care providers. For example, anthropometric and hematologic measurements are performed by private health-care providers, and the results are reported to public health clinic staff who incorporate the information into their records. A difference among WIC programs specifically is that some agencies report PedNSS data only for those children certified for WIC benefits, whereas others report data for all children applying for WIC services, regardless of their certification status. This factor should be considered when comparing data between programs.

Local clinics send completed client information to each respective state health department, which enters the information into computer databases or forwards it to private vendors that maintain state-specific databases. The PedNSS data are then downloaded onto computer magnetic tapes or diskettes for submission to CDC for analysis and inclusion in the national surveillance database, which is maintained on a mainframe computer in Atlanta, Georgia.

At CDC, a surveillance record is generated for each visit by a child to a participating program. Thus, a child with more than one visit to a clinic will have multiple records in the surveillance system. On average, 2.1 records per child are recorded in the PedNSS (2).

Data Quality

Each state and private vendor performs edit checks on all data submitted to the PedNSS. CDC staff then check the records for critical errors (missing key information needed by the PedNSS software) and for data with biologically implausible values (BIVs) (one chance in a thousand of being real). Records with critical errors are excluded from the database. Records containing data with BIVs are included in the PedNSS database, but the variables for these data are excluded from routine analyses.

Definitions

GROWTH INDEXES

With the NCHS growth reference (14), the height, weight, and age data for each child at each clinic visit are interpreted into the height-for-age, weight-for-age, and weight-for-height indexes. The growth indexes can be expressed as percentile values or standard deviation values, (Z-scores), which are more useful for statistical analysis (16). Because the Z-score scale is linear, summary statistics such as means, standard deviations, and standard errors can be computed from Z-score values. The expected mean Z-score for the reference population is zero, and the standard deviation value of the Z-score is 1.0. The Z-score of each growth index for each child is calculated as follows:

$$Z\text{-score} = \frac{\text{Observed value - Reference mean value}}{\text{Reference standard deviation value}}.$$

A corresponding relationship exists between the percentile scale and the Z-score scale.

For the PedNSS, the cutoff level of abnormal indexes is below the 5th percentile or above the 95th percentile, corresponding to Z-scores of below −1.65 and above 1.65. (Table 1). Public health programs involved in PedNSS use growth indexes for screening and evaluation. These cutoffs enable program personnel to identify children with borderline growth status. Because the defined cutoffs for the reference are the 5th and 95th percentiles, the expected baseline prevalence is 5% for either an abnormally low or high growth index. A prevalence above the baseline level of 5% would be cause for concern (2).

HEIGHT-FOR-AGE

Height-for-age allows us to compare a child's height with the reference height of children of the same age and sex. The NCHS growth reference curves for children <24 months of age were based on a sample of children who were taller than average U.S. children. This contributes to an observed negative Z-score, or a higher-than-expected prevalence of low height-for-age, for average children 1–2 years of age (17,18). For children ≥2 years of age, the NCHS growth reference curves were based on a representative sample of U.S. children. As a result, the expected rate of low height-for-age for children ≥2 years of age is 5%.

TABLE 1. Criteria for anthropometric indexes used in the Pediatric Nutrition Surveillance System

Indexes	Measurement parameter	Defining cutoff	
		NCHS* percentile	Z-score
Stunting, shortness, or linear growth retardation	Height-for-age	<5th	<− 1.65
Overweight	Weight-for-height	>95th	>1.65
Thinness	Weight-for-height	<5th	<− 1.65

* National Center for Health Statistics pediatric growth reference (14).

The difference in height characteristics between the Fels sample and the U.S. sample also causes an abrupt change in the prevalence of low height-for-age and mean Z-score when children reach 2 years of age *(18)*.

WEIGHT-FOR-HEIGHT

Weight-for-height is an expression of weight in relation to height, or an index of body mass. High weight-for-height indicates overweight as a proxy for obesity (increased fat mass).

Low weight-for-height, or thinness, is often associated with recent severe disease. In developing countries, thinness indicates acute malnutrition, which is commonly the result of insufficient food supply, infectious disease, especially diarrheal disease, or both *(2)*. The prevalence of thinness in a population is usually low except during disaster conditions, such as famine and war, that result in severe food shortages and disease outbreaks.

Although weight-for-age is summarized in the PedNSS data, this index is not as easy to interpret as height-for-age or weight-for-height. Low weight-for-age could result from either chronic or acute short-term problems. A high weight-for-age could indicate obesity or a proportionate but large child. Thus, weight-for-age is not an indicator of primary focus in the PedNSS.

IRON DEFICIENCY ANEMIA

Both hemoglobin and hematocrit measurements are used by public health programs to screen for iron deficiency anemia. The CDC criteria for anemia are based on NHANES II data *(19)*. For children <24 months of age, the cutoff is a hemoglobin measurement of <11.0 g/dL or a hematocrit of <33%. For children 2–5 years of age, the cutoff is a hemoglobin measurement of <11.2 g/dL or a hematocrit measurement of <34% *(19)*.

LOW BIRTH WEIGHT

Low birth weight is defined as a birth weight <2,500 g (5 lbs, 8 oz). Although the PedNSS birth-weight data are reported by parents, a study comparing birth weights recorded in the PedNSS with those on birth certificates found close agreement between the two data sources. No significant misclassification of low birth weight was found *(20)*.

BREAST-FEEDING

For the PedNSS, WIC programs are encouraged to collect breast-feeding information on children up to 2 years of age. WIC programs define a breast-fed child as one who receives breast milk at least once a day. Because the year 2000 breast-feeding objective refers to exclusive breast-feeding, rather than breast-feeding once a day, national breast-feeding prevalence and patterns reported through the PedNSS may be somewhat misleading. However, the PedNSS breast-feeding data are useful for states and local programs that conduct and evaluate breast-feeding promotion projects.

Data Reporting

A key component of any surveillance system is to promptly and routinely provide summary data to local program leaders so that they can use the information for program planning and evaluation. CDC sends monthly, semiannual, and annual PedNSS reports to participating states.

The two monthly reports provided to each clinic include lists of all children with one or more **high/low** nutritional status indicators and the **clinic error** reports. The **high/low** lists are designed primarily for use in the follow-up of children at nutritional risk. The **clinic error** lists are designed to identify and follow up records with critical errors or BIVs.

The semiannual and annual reports include data tables summarizing the distribution, prevalence, and trends of various demographic and nutritional status indicators, by clinic, county, and state and for all participating states and territories. In addition, annual reports to participating states include graphic illustrations of the PedNSS data.

GENERAL FINDINGS

Although the PedNSS has operated since the early 1970s, the major findings presented in this chapter are based on data for the years 1980–1991. Birth weight data are not reported.

Height-for-Age

In 1991, the overall prevalence of stunting for PedNSS children <24 months of age was 10%—twice the expected level of 5%. For children 2–5 years of age, the prevalence was 7.1% slightly higher than the expected 5% level. In general, a greater-than-expected prevalence of low height-for-age indicates that some of the children were stunted because of health reasons, nutritional reasons, or both *(2)*.

Only long-term and significant changes in environmental factors, nutritional status, and health status can affect the height distribution in a population *(2)*. Over the last decade, the prevalence of low height-for-age has been stable among the populations monitored by the PedNSS. However, among children of Asian descent, mostly Southeast Asian refugees, we observed a substantial decrease in the prevalence of low height-for-age. Among Asian children <2 years of age, the prevalence of

stunting declined from approximately 22% in 1982 to 10% in 1991—a relative reduction of 54%. A similar decrease in prevalence was observed for Asian children aged 2–5 years *(2)*.

The improvement in the height-for-age index for Asian children from 1980 to 1991 was associated with a general upward shift in the height distribution; for Asian children 2–5 years of age, the mean height-for-age Z-score in 1980 was −1.03; by 1991 it had increased to −0.33 (Figure 1) *(2)*. This improvement of 0.7 in Z-score over a 10-year period indicates a significant change in the nutritional, health, and socioeconomic status of Southeast Asian refugee families since their arrival in the United States in the late 1970s and early 1980s *(21)*. Thus, a genetic factor was not the main reason for the shorter stature observed among Southeast Asian refugee children soon after they arrived in the United States *(2)*. This observation supports the concept that one growth reference can be valid for children of different racial and ethnic origins *(22)*.

In our assessment of race- and ethnicity-specific patterns in height-for-age from birth to 5 years of age (Figure 2), we found that black children had the lowest mean height-for-age near birth when compared with other groups. However, by 2 years of age, they had the highest mean

FIGURE 1. Height-for-age Z-score distribution of Asian children >2 years old compared with NCHS growth reference — United States, 1980 and 1991

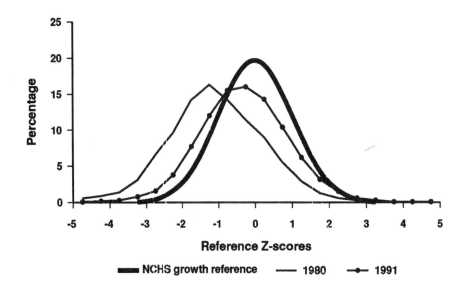

FIGURE 2. Age-specific mean height-for-age Z-scores for children ≤5 years of age — United States, 1991

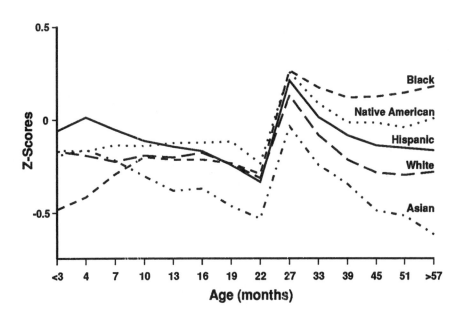

height-for-age, indicating possible minor variations in childhood growth patterns among different race and ethnic groups. However, for practical purposes these variations do not negate the use of one common growth reference (2).

The abrupt change of mean height-for-age Z-scores for all groups at the 24-month juncture (Figure 2) is an artifact related to the use of two different population samples to determine the NCHS growth reference.

The WIC program preferentially retains those children with the greatest health and nutritional risks; low height-for-age is one retention criterion for older children. Therefore, the progressively lower mean height-for-age Z-score among 2- to 5-year-old children monitored by PedNSS (Figure 2) is more likely related to public health program selection factors than to a general worsening of the nutritional status of PedNSS children as they age (2). Also, in the NHANES II data set, the inconsistency of measuring the supine and standing height of children 24–36 months of age may have affected the growth curves.

In an earlier study of PedNSS data, investigators evaluated the influence of altitude on child-

hood growth in the United States (23). When they analyzed data from eight mountain states and controlled for confounding factors, they found that the height of children was significantly shorter starting at an elevation of >1,500 meters. Therefore, when comparing nutritional survey or clinical assessment data obtained in areas of moderately high altitudes with data from lower altitudes, we must consider the effect of potential altitude-related growth retardation.

Weight-for-Height

OVERWEIGHT

Overall, the prevalence of high weight-for-height has remained stable among the children monitored by PedNSS. However, from 1980 to 1991, the prevalence of overweight increased by nearly 50% among Asian children and nearly 20% among Hispanic children (Figure 3) (2). The relative increase in overweight among Asian children was primarily related to a lower baseline prevalence of overweight during the early 1980s and a general improvement in the growth status of this group (2). Reasons for the increase among Hispanic children are not clear and need further study.

327

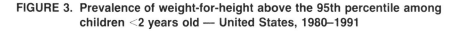

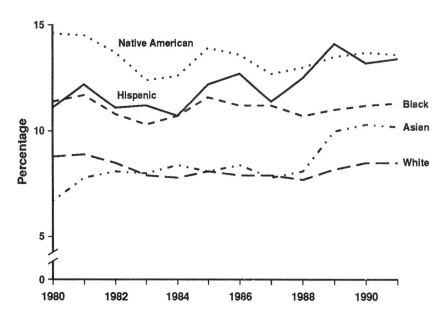

FIGURE 3. Prevalence of weight-for-height above the 95th percentile among children <2 years old — United States, 1980–1991

Although the prevalence of overweight was stable among Native American children monitored by the PedNSS, this population has consistently exhibited the highest weight-for-height Z-scores (Figure 3 and Table 2). Other studies have indicated a very high prevalence of obesity among Native Americans of all age-groups, and it appears to begin in early childhood or even in the intrauterine period *(24)*. Even though genetic predisposition is a significant factor in obesity among Native Americans, environmental factors such as inappropriate diet and physical inactivity have contributed substantially to the epidemic *(24)*. Culturally appropriate interventions are needed to prevent and treat obesity at a young age in this population.

THINNESS

Among children <2 years of age, the overall prevalence of weight-for-height below the 5th percentile has been <5% during 1980–1991, and the mean weight-for-height Z-score has remained near or slightly above the expected value of 0.0. This finding indicates that few children have suffered from acute or severe malnutrition *(2)*. However, the prevalence of low weight-for-height among Hispanic children increased during 1985–1988, primarily because

Puerto Rico was added to the surveillance system in 1984 (more Hispanic children in Puerto Rico are thin compared with those living in the contiguous United States). Because Puerto Rico added a significant number of thinner Hispanic

TABLE 2. Race- and ethnic-specific prevalence of underweight and overweight and mean weight-for-height Z-scores among children 2–5 years of age — Pediatric Nutrition Surveillance System, 1991.

	Prevalence (%)*		Weight-for-height Z-score	
	Underweight	Overweight	Mean†	SD§
White	2.5	5.7	0.11	0.95
Black	3.3	6.9	0.11	1.01
Hispanic	2.7	11.7	0.34	1.10
Native American	1.6	11.9	0.45	1.01
Asian	3.2	7.6	0.13	1.04

* The expected prevalence is 5%; values of <5% indicate a less-than-expected prevalence.
† A Z-score of zero would be equivalent to the 50th percentile. Values greater than zero indicate a mean weight-for-height above the 50th percentile. A Z-score of 1.00 would be equivalent to the 84th percentile.
§ SD, standard deviation.

children to the PedNSS database, the prevalence of low height-for-age among that ethnic group increased. With the addition of California to the PedNSS in 1988 and New York in 1989, the prevalence of low weight-for-height among Hispanics decreased because Hispanic children from those two large states have a higher weight-for-height status (2).

Iron Deficiency Anemia

A detailed study of six states consistently participating in the PedNSS from 1975 to 1984 revealed a significant decline in the prevalence of iron deficiency anemia (25). Among children <2 years of age monitored by the PedNSS, anemia declined from 23.3% in 1981 to 19.6% in 1991, reflecting a relative decrease of 16%. A similar trend was evident among children 2–5 years old (2). A decline in the prevalence of anemia also occurred among most race and ethnic groups. Black children monitored by PedNSS consistently had a higher prevalence of anemia than the other groups. They also had lower mean hemoglobin and hematocrit values (2). Recent studies indicate that black children and adults have a slightly lower hemoglobin level than their white counterparts, even when iron status is comparable. This indicates that the higher prevalence of anemia among blacks may be related to factors other than iron nutrition (26).

Although the current prevalence of anemia among PedNSS children is lower than in previous years, it is much higher than the expected prevalence of 5%, primarily because the PedNSS monitors a low-income, high-risk population and the WIC program preferentially enrolls and retains children with anemia. Despite these factors, we have a substantial need for appropriate and effective prevention and treatment programs to reduce the risk of iron deficiency among low-income children in the United States.

Breast-Feeding

The quality of breast-feeding data varies from state to state. Overall in 1991, about 28% of records for children 6–8 months old included breast-feeding information. This amounted to 133,741 records. Among those children, 34.5% were being breast-fed on the date of hospital discharge whereas 17% were consuming some breast milk at 6 months of age. Because a large number of records lacked breast-feeding information, these prevalence data do not likely represent the entire population being monitored. However, states that have more complete information (infant feeding data for >90% of records) can assess breast-feeding prevalence and duration among the low-income children monitored by the PedNSS. In any event, the available data indicate that the level of breast-feeding among low-income infants is significantly lower than the national average. Thus, greater effort must be made to promote breast milk as the preferred source of nutrition for young infants.

INTERPRETATION ISSUES

Public Health Implications

The purpose of the PedNSS is to efficiently and rapidly provide information on gross trends regarding the nutritional status of low-income children to allow for planning, implementing, and evaluating intervention programs. The PedNSS is not designed to provide specific details; rather, it provides a broad picture. If significant positive or negative changes in trends are noted, follow-up investigations are conducted.

After comparing PedNSS data with national survey findings, we have found that the nutritional status of low-income children monitored by the PedNSS is comparable with that of average U.S. children. However, these low-income children do have an increased prevalence of key nutritional status indicators such as stunting, overweight, and anemia.

The high prevalence of overweight among low-income Native American children and the increasing prevalence of overweight among low-income Hispanic children are of concern. At present, effective public health intervention strategies to prevent and treat overweight are not available. Because significant association exists between childhood and adult obesity, and because adult obesity is a risk factor for numerous chronic diseases, appropriate interventions should be developed to address weight control among low-income children. Among Native American populations specifically, we have witnessed a growing epidemic of diabetes mellitus type II that may be related to obesity *(24)*. Thus, programs must be developed to prevent and ameliorate obesity among Native Americans as a means to reduce morbidity and mortality associated with diabetes and other chronic diseases.

The high rate of anemia among the low-income children monitored by PedNSS suggests that they probably have poor iron nutrition, as has been shown in other research *(9)*. Because iron deficiency in childhood is associated with impaired learning and increased susceptibility to lead poisoning *(10)*, greater efforts toward effective prevention and interventions are needed. One important issue to be addressed at the state level is the standardization of screening procedures and cutoff values for anemia across public health programs and private health-care providers. Anecdotal reports from states indicate that private physicians rarely accept the results of anemia screening performed by public health clinics. Thus, patients are confused as to their health status, and appropriate follow-up of at-risk individuals is jeopardized.

Overall, the data indicate that nutritional status varies among different race and ethnic groups monitored by the PedNSS. Black children have the highest rates of low birth weight and anemia; Hispanic and Native American children have the highest rates of overweight; and Asian children have the highest rate of shortness.

Currently, the PedNSS is the only system in the United States that allows continuous monitoring of the overall nutrition-related health status of infants and children. Because the level of major nutritional status indicators in the system is similar to the level of indicators among U.S. children in general, PedNSS findings and trends may very well reflect the nutritional status of all children. In fact, the declining prevalence of anemia was first observed in the low-income PedNSS population and later confirmed in the general population.

Advantages and Disadvantages

To date, the PedNSS has been a very successful surveillance system, processing >6 million records annually. Data collection is simple, and reporting is rapid. Increasing automation and computer capabilities at the state and local levels will further enhance these features.

Because the PedNSS is designed to rapidly monitor the nutritional status of the target population and provide a broad picture, it lacks some of the detailed information that could be used to more fully interpret some of the findings. For example, the system does not discriminate among causes of low height-for-age such as genetic variations, inadequate diet, or certain medical conditions. Children with special needs, such as handicaps or developmental delays, may be included in the PedNSS and represent a subpopulation with indicators outside cutoff limits for reasons other than poor nutrition. Thus, local programs that serve significant numbers of this subpopulation need to interpret their PedNSS data accordingly and only compare their data with those of other similar programs.

Because the system is program-based, changes in an individual state program can affect the data for that state and, to a lesser degree, national data. Changes in technology, such as programs converting from one method of hemoglobin testing to another, could affect the data on prevalence of anemia. Therefore, a systematic process of maintaining up-to-date information for all programs participating in PedNSS is needed to overcome this limitation.

EXAMPLES OF USING DATA

State health departments have used PedNSS data in a variety of ways:

- To quantify nutritionally at-risk populations so as to obtain state funds for the WIC program.

- To assist with annual program planning required by the WIC program.

- To conduct program evaluations of factors such as population coverage and targeting.

- To identify the training needs of public health personnel.

- To present results in statewide public health-related conferences.

Alaska has made extensive use of the PedNSS data. The Nutrition Services Unit of the Alaska Department of Health and Social Services has used PedNSS data to determine the most effective way to direct health promotion resources and efforts through routine program planning channels. Unit staffers have used the surveillance information to evaluate the quality of anthropometric measurements and to identify specific nutrition-related problems among the children under surveillance. Using information derived from the PedNSS data, they targeted nutrition interventions to reach children with low hemoglobin concentrations and WIC mothers to increase breast-feeding incidence and duration. Alaska also uses the PedNSS data to monitor the accuracy of local WIC data and to evaluate outcomes of program interventions. The PedNSS results may also help state and local WIC advocates obtain program funding.

In addition, Alaska has used the PedNSS data in conjunction with data from the Pregnancy Nutrition Surveillance System and the Behavioral Risk Factor Surveillance System to provide a statewide nutrition prospective for baseline information to establish nutrition objectives for *Healthy Alaskans 2000 (27)*. A nutrition community work group has selected seven of the national year 2000 nutrition objectives to target in the state's comprehensive health plan, which is being finalized for public comment and acceptance.

At the national level, the PedNSS has been used in two ways:

- To monitor our progress toward meeting the year 2000 objectives for the nation.

- To demonstrate the WIC program's effectiveness in reducing the prevalence of anemia.

FUTURE ISSUES

CDC continuously strives to improve the PedNSS by improving the efficiency of data reporting, making reports more user-friendly, exporting PedNSS software to more states, and widely distributing graphic illustrations of the data. A number of future improvements are also planned:

- Adding dietary assessment variables to the PedNSS.

- Incorporating the PedNSS into lead screening programs.

- Screening to detect risk factors for chronic diseases, such as high cholesterol.

- Expanding the PedNSS to cover other pediatric populations such as school-children.

- Linking PedNSS data to vital statistics data at the state level for expanded use of surveillance data.

- Standardizing data collection techniques (e.g., direct measurement of all children).

- Standardizing the use of specific reference standards for hemoglobin and hematocrit measurements.

This surveillance system is flexible and allows states and local programs to monitor specific health and nutritional parameters that are not routinely included in the PedNSS. Data fields referred to as **state use fields** can be used to code such parameters. For example, if a state were interested in monitoring breast-feeding patterns, it might want to include the education level of the mother as a question to be asked in the **state use field**.

The national WIC program and Maternal and Child Health Block Grant requirements call for better data collection and monitoring by state public health programs. The PedNSS readily serves as a data source to assess current nutrition status profiles of low-income children at the state and local levels and to continuously and inexpensively monitor trends in the prevalence of various nutritional status indicators. In addition, CDC plans to help state health departments to better use the PedNSS in evaluating specific nutrition-related activities such as iron deficiency anemia intervention projects and breast-feeding promotion campaigns.

Overall, the size of the database makes the PedNSS a very robust surveillance system. Expanding it to school systems and more public health programs such as Head Start and the Early Periodic Screening, Diagnosis, and Treatment Program, which only require income eligibility, would provide data on a broader segment of children and permit the follow-up of cohorts to evaluate the long-term effectiveness of intervention programs.

REFERENCES

1. Life Sciences Research Office, Federation of American Societies for Experimental Biology. Nutrition monitoring in the United States: an updated report on nutrition monitoring. Hyattsville, Maryland: US Department of Health and Human Services, Public Health Service, and US Department of Agriculture, Food and Consumer Services, 1989; DHHS publication no. (PHS)89-1255.

2. CDC. Pediatric Nutrition Surveillance System—United States, 1980–1991. In: CDC Surveillance Summaries, November 27, 1992. MMWR 1992;41(no.SS-7): 1–24.

3. CDC. Nutrition surveillance: annual summary, 1983. Atlanta: US Department of Health and Human Services, Public Health Service CDC, 1985; DHHS publication no. (CDC)85-8295.

4. Public Health Service. Healthy people 2000: National health promotion and disease prevention objectives— full report, with commentary. Washington, DC: US Department of Health and Human Services, Public Health Service, 1991; DHHS publication no. (PHS)91-50212.

5. Johnson DE, Miller LC, Iverson S, et al. The health of children adopted from Romania. JAMA 1992; 268:3446–51.

6. Keller W. The epidemiology of stunting. In: Waterlow JC, ed. Linear growth retardation in less developed countries. New York: Vevey/Raven Press, 1988. (Nestlé Nutrition Workshop Series, vol. 14).

7. Rosenbaum M, Leibel RL. Obesity in childhood. Pediatr Rev 1989;11:43–55.

8. National Research Council. Obesity and eating disorders. In: Diet and health: implications for reducing chronic disease risk. Washington, DC: National Academy Press, 1989:563–92.

9. Dallman PR, Yip R, Johnson C. Prevalence and causes of anemia in the United States, 1976 to 1980. Am J Clin Nutr 1984;39:437–45.

10. Yip R. The interaction of lead and iron. In: Filer LJ Jr, ed. Dietary iron: birth to two years. New York: Raven Press, 1989:179–81.

11. Binkin NJ, Yip R, Fleshood L, Trowbridge FL. Birth weight and childhood growth. Pediatrics 1988; 82:828–34.

12. Oxtoby MJ. Human immunodeficiency virus and other viruses in human milk: placing the issues in broader perspective. Pediatr Infect Dis J 1988;7:824–35.

13. Interagency Board for Nutrition Monitoring and Related Research. Nutrition monitoring in the United States: the directory of federal and state nutrition monitoring activities. Hyattsville, Maryland: US Department of Health and Human Services, Public Health Service, 1992; DHHS publication no. (PHS)92-1255-1.

14. Hamill PVV, Drizd TA, Johnson CL, et al. Physical growth: National Center for Health Statistics percentiles. Am J Clin Nutr 1979;32:607–29.

15. CDC. Ten-State Nutrition Survey: 1968–1970. III: clinical, anthropometry, dental. Atlanta: US Department of Health, Education, and Welfare, Health Services and Mental Health Administration, CDC, 1972; DHEW publication no. (HSM)72-8131.

16. Dibley MJ, Staehling N, Neiburg P, Trowbridge FL. Interpretation of Z-score anthropometric indicators derived from the international growth reference. Am J Clin Nutr 1987;46:749–62.

17. Yip R, Trowbridge F, Wotaki C. International reference for child growth: current research and future plans. In: Kim WY, ed. Proceedings of the 14th International Congress of Nutrition. Vol. II. Seoul: Ewha Women's University 1989;150–1.

18. Dibley MJ, Goldsby JB, Staehling NW, Trowbridge FL. Development of normalized curves for the international growth reference: historical and technical considerations. Am J Clin Nutr 1987;46:736–48.

19. CDC. CDC criteria for anemia in children and childbearing-aged women. MMWR 1989;38:400–4.

20. Gayle HD, Yip R, Frank MJ, Nieburg P, Binkin NJ. Validation of maternally reported birth weights among 46,637 Tennessee WIC program participants. Public Health Rep 1988;103:143–7.

21. Yip R, Scanlon K, Trowbridge F. Improving growth status of Asian refugee children in the United States. JAMA 1992;267:937–40.

22. Graitcer PL, Gentry EM. Measuring children: one reference for all. Lancet 1981;2:297–9.

23. Yip R, Binkin NJ, Trowbridge F. Altitude and childhood growth. J Pediatr 1988;113:486–9.

24. Byers T. The epidemic of obesity in American Indians [Editorial]. Am J Dis Child 1992;146:285–6.

25. Yip R, Binkin NJ, Fleshood L, Trowbridge F. Declining prevalence of anemia among low-income children in the United States. JAMA 1987;258:1619–23.

26. Perry GS, Byers T, Yip R, Margen S. Iron nutrition does not account for the hemoglobin differences between blacks and whites. J Nutr 1992;122:1417–24.

27. Alaska Department of Health and Social Services. Healthy Alaskans 2000: health promotion and disease prevention objectives [Draft]. Juneau, Alaska: Alaska Department of Health and Social Services, 1993.

Developmental Disabilities

Pierre Decouflé, Sc.D.,[1] Marshalyn Yeargin-Allsopp, M.D.,[1]
Coleen A. Boyle, Ph.D.,[1] and Nancy S. Doernberg, B.A.[1]

PUBLIC HEALTH IMPORTANCE

Developmental disabilities are a group of heterogeneous conditions that are attributable to mental and/or physical impairments, manifested before the person attains the age of 22 years, and likely to continue indefinitely. Persons with developmental disabilities require specialized services and have substantial functional limitations in at least three of the following areas: self-care, receptive or expressive language, learning, mobility, self-direction, capacity for independent living, and economic self-sufficiency (1). Examples of developmental disabilities include mental retardation, neuromuscular disorders such as cerebral palsy, blindness and deafness, learning disabilities, epilepsy, and autism. As a group, these conditions may have similar etiologies because they often coexist.

Although precise prevalence rates for developmental disabilities in the United States are not available, an estimated 8%–16% of school-age children have difficulties that justify specialized educational services (1). These conditions are costly to the individual, affected families, and the country as a whole. In 1984, federal, state, and local governments spent about $16.5 billion for mental retardation and developmental disabilities services (2).

Surveillance of developmental disabilities is challenging, in general, and more so in the United States than in some European countries. Conducting surveillance is difficult because of a number of factors. The case definitions for developmental disabilities often rely on clinical examinations and clinical judgment rather than on results from laboratory reports or pathology findings. No standard national or state-specific case definitions or terminologies have been established for developmental disabilities, although

recent attempts to address this problem have been made (3). Also, because these conditions evolve over time and are related to the maturation of the nervous system, a child may be several years old before a definitive diagnosis of a developmental disability can be made. Despite these limitations that are inherent to the surveillance of developmental disabilities, ongoing mental retardation registries have been maintained in Great Britain since the 1940s (4).

Although various studies of developmental disabilities have been conducted in the United States, few meet the explicit criteria for surveillance, as defined by the CDC (5). In the absence of large, population-based centralized registries of individuals receiving services for developmental disabilities, as in Europe, an efficient developmental disabilities surveillance system in this country should attempt to identify cases from sources that see the most children with these conditions. Because we do not have a uniform system of health care in the United States, to obtain information on all preschool children with developmental disabilities it is necessary to access records from multiple community agencies. A recent mandate for preschool services through state departments of education may eventually help to overcome this problem, although not all children with developmental disabilities are served by public school systems (6). Identifying school-age children with developmental disabilities from school records alone yields more complete ascertainment of cases than any other single source because of the more than 15-year requirement that all school-age children with specific physical, emotional,

[1] Division of Birth Defects and Developmental Disabilities
National Center for Environmental Health
Centers for Disease Control and Prevention
Atlanta, Georgia

or cognitive impairments be identified and that educational services be provided (7).

U.S. surveys of children with developmental disabilities have usually yielded prevalence rates that are similar to those from other countries. For example, in population-based studies of school-age children in the United States and other countries' researchers have reported that the prevalence for cerebral palsy is around 1.5–2.5 per 1,000 children. However, rates as high as 5.0–5.8 per 1,000 children have also been reported from other studies conducted in the United States (8). These differences in rates are likely to be related to differences in case definitions, methods of ascertainment, characteristics of the populations studied such as age and sociodemographic factors, and the periods studied. For additional information about related topics and surveillance activities, see the Prevalence of Birth Defects chapter.

HISTORY OF DATA COLLECTION

Surveillance of developmental disabilities at CDC is a relatively recent activity. In 1992, we began our major effort in developmental disabilities surveillance, the Metropolitan Atlanta Developmental Disabilities Surveillance Program (MADDSP).

Before the inception of the MADDSP, CDC and the Georgia Department of Human Resources conducted the Metropolitan Atlanta Developmental Disabilities Study (MADDS), a population-based study of five developmental disabilities (mental retardation, cerebral palsy, hearing impairment, vision impairment, and epilepsy) in 10-year-old children living in five metropolitan Atlanta counties between 1985 and 1987 (9). MADDS was funded from 1984 to 1990 by the Agency for Toxic Substances and Disease Registry through a cooperative agreement involving CDC and the Georgia Department of Human Resources.

Because the MADDS was the first population-based study of multiple disabilities among U.S. school-age children, a major focus of the study was to develop methods for the surveillance of children with developmental disabilities. Many education, health, and social service agencies

in the Atlanta area were used as sources to ascertain cases for the study (9).

After the first year of MADDS surveillance, we calculated the prevalence rates of epilepsy and compared it with previously reported rates in the literature. Our rates were much lower than we had expected. We suspected that children with isolated epilepsy (i.e., without other disabilities) would be less likely than children with multiple disabilities to attend special education programs or require special services. We therefore added the 22 laboratories in Atlanta that regularly perform electroencephalograms as additional sources for identifying epilepsy cases. As a result, our estimated prevalence rate of epilepsy nearly doubled, increasing from 3.3 to 6.5 per 1,000 10-year-old children.

MADDS was unique in that we used individual school records to identify children with disabilities. By using these records, we were able to identify about 95% of the children with either mental retardation, cerebral palsy, vision impairment, or hearing impairment (Table 1).

CDC SURVEILLANCE ACTIVITIES

Metropolitan Atlanta Developmental Disabilities Surveillance Program

Surveillance of developmental disabilities at CDC is the responsibility of the National Center for Environmental Health. This center conducts the MADDSP, which is an active, population-based surveillance system for mental retardation, cerebral palsy, vision impairment, and hearing impairment among children aged 3–10 years whose parents are residents of the Atlanta metropolitan area.

MADDSP has two main purposes:

- To provide regular and systematic monitoring of prevalence rates of selected developmental disabilities according to various demographic, maternal, and child characteristics.

- To provide a framework and database for conducting studies of children with the selected conditions.

TABLE 1. Percentage of 10-year-old children identified as having selected developmental disabilities by three types of sources — Metropolitan Atlanta Developmental Disabilities Study, 1985–1987

Source	Mental retardation	Cerebral palsy	Hearing impairment	Vision impairment
Public schools and other Georgia Department of Education programs	97.8	85.0	97.0	93.5
Georgia Department of Human Resources, various programs	1.8	6.3	3.0	4.9
Selected hospitals	0.4	8.7	0.0	1.6

CASE DEFINITIONS

Under the MADDSP case definition, children must meet the following three criteria:

- They must be 3–10 years of age at any time during the calendar year of ascertainment.

- They must have one or more of the four conditions of interest.

- Their parents or legal guardians must reside in the surveillance area at some time during the calendar year of ascertainment.

The age range of 3–10 years was chosen because the lower bound corresponds with the beginning of the age span covered by Part B of the Education for All Handicapped Children Act (7), which mandates that public school systems provide services to children with special needs (public school systems being a major source of case ascertainment for our surveillance system), and because the vast majority of children served under that act enter the special education system by the age of 10 years (10).

The MADDSP defines the four developmental disabilities as follows:

- Mental retardation. Either 1) an intelligence quotient (IQ) of 70 or less on the most recent psychometric test performed by a psychometrist; or 2) a written statement by a psychometrist that a child's intellectual functioning falls within the mentally handicapped range.

- Cerebral palsy. Either 1) a diagnosis made by a qualified health professional and so noted on a medical record; or 2) physical findings in a medical record that are consistent with the condition. For the purposes of the MADDSP, cerebral palsy is defined as a group of nonprogressive disorders afflicting young children in which abnormalities of the brain cause paralysis, involuntary movement, or incoordination. The definition excludes motor disorders caused by spinal cord abnormalities.

- Vision impairment. A measured visual acuity of 20/70 or worse in the better eye with correction. In the absence of a measured visual acuity, a child is considered to meet the case definition if the medical record includes 1) a functional description, by an eye specialist, of visual acuity of 20/70 or worse (e.g., light perception only), or 2) a statement by an eye specialist that the child has low vision or blindness.

- Hearing impairment. A measured bilateral pure tone hearing loss averaging 40 decibels or worse, unaided, in the better ear at frequencies of 500, 1,000, and 2,000 hertz. In the absence of a measured bilateral hearing loss, a child is considered to meet the case definition if the medical record includes a description, by a licensed and/or certified audiologist or qualified physician, of a hearing level of 40 decibels or worse in the better ear.

POPULATION CHARACTERISTICS

The surveillance area for the MADDSP is the five-county Atlanta metropolitan area (Clayton, Cobb, DeKalb, Fulton, and Gwinnett counties) that includes the city of Atlanta. In 1990, the area had a population of about 2.2 million, which included about 250,000 children aged 3–10 years. Slightly >30,000 births a year are recorded in the area. A special feature of the area is the existence of an active birth defects surveillance program operated by CDC—the Metropolitan Atlanta Congenital Defects Program. (See the Prevalence of Birth Defects chapter.) Consequently, we can link children identified in the MADDSP to the birth defects registry to obtain additional medical data.

ASCERTAINMENT PROCEDURES

Cases are ascertained by reviewing existing educational, medical, and social service records at selected sources within the surveillance area. The ascertainment methodology of the MADDSP relies, in large part, on the experience of its predecessor, the MADDS. As was pointed out earlier, in the MADDS it was found that information needed to identify and describe most children with the four conditions of interest is available from the special education departments of local public school systems (Table 1).

The first step in identifying children with any of the chosen conditions is to acquire electronic data files from these selected primary sources:

- The nine public school systems serving the five-county area.

- Other Georgia Department of Education programs for children with developmental disabilities (e.g., the psychoeducational centers in the five-county area, state schools for the blind or deaf).

- Georgia Department of Human Resources programs for children with mental retardation and other special health care needs (e.g., county mental retardation service centers, state hospitals and residential care facilities. Children's Medical Services).

- The large public hospital (and selected associated clinics) offering specialized infant and pediatric care in Atlanta and the two major private pediatric care hospitals (and selected associated clinics) in the surveillance area.

DATA COLLECTED

In addition to identifying information and a standard array of demographic data on each case, the MADDSP collects the most recent and earliest evaluation data relevant to the specific type of developmental disability. For example, for a child with mental retardation, scores on tests of cognitive and adaptive functioning are recorded. The hearing level in each ear and the type of hearing loss are noted for children classified as hearing impaired. The best corrected vision (in each eye) or general description of visual acuity (e.g., light perception only) is recorded for children with vision impairment. For children with cerebral palsy, a medical diagnosis and/or functional description of the child's disability is recorded as well as a level of functioning determined by ambulation ability and the use of assistive devices. For all children identified, we record the presence of selected other medical conditions (e.g., major birth defects, autism, epilepsy) and information on etiology. For children identified through the public schools, we record information on all special education services the children receive through the public schools, the primary program for which they are eligible to receive special education services, the delivery model, and the servicing school.

DATA MANAGEMENT

Detailed data at each primary source are entered on laptop computers by MADDSP staff and are edited on-line at the point of entry to reduce the amount of batch editing done at CDC. Batch edit programs are run monthly to eliminate duplicate records for the same child and to check for errors not identified at the point of entry. Children born in Georgia are linked to Georgia birth certificates so that demographic and medical data from the birth certificates can be added to the case records. For children born outside Georgia, requests are made in writing to the appropriate state or city vital records office for copies of the birth certificates. The data are stored in a series of files on the CDC mainframe. Various types of analytical files are created, with personal identifiers removed.

REPORTING OF FINDINGS

Rates produced from the MADDSP may be of two types:

- **Point prevalence rates** of a specific developmental disability for a given age use the estimated number of children of that age living in the five-county area (from census data) as the denominator. Such rates permit the use of all case children, regardless of where they were born.

- **Birth cohort prevalence rates** of a specific condition use the number of live births in a given year in the five-county area (minus infant deaths) as the denominator and the number of case children aged 3–10 years who were born in that year in the surveillance area. Case children born outside the surveillance area are excluded from these rates.

Either of these two types of rates can be computed for children of a specific age, sex, or race to examine variations in the occurrence of the conditions. Further, we are able to examine the prevalence rate for multiple disabilities, for example, for the joint occurrence of mental retardation and cerebral palsy. Mental retardation can be analyzed according to four standard severity levels: mild (IQ, 50–70), moderate (IQ, 35–49), severe (IQ, 20–34), and profound (IQ, <20).

The first surveillance report from the MADDSP will be released in 1994. Subsequent reports will be released yearly.

Disability Prevention Programs

In addition to the intramural MADDSP, CDC supports developmental disabilities surveillance activities extramurally in 28 states through its Disability Prevention Program (11). The approaches used for developmental disabilities surveillance in those states range from a multitiered, active case-finding system in Rhode Island to a passive, data linkage system in Florida. Technical information about these state-based developmental disabilities surveillance programs are available from CDC (see the Additional Resources section of this chapter).

GENERAL FINDINGS

Because the MADDSP is a new surveillance system, data are not yet available. However, data collection in the MADDS, the prototype for MADDSP, ended in 1990, and some results have recently been published. In the MADDS, developmental disabilities were identified among 1,608 case children aged 10 years who resided in metropolitan Atlanta in 1985–1987. The prevalence rates for the five conditions studied in the MADDS were within the ranges described from previous population-based studies (Table 2) (8,9,12).

The overall surveillance methods and overall prevalence rates for each disability have been described elsewhere (9), and detailed data on children with vision impairment have been published, allowing an examination of variations in the prevalence, by race and by sex (13). Demographic differences in prevalence rates permit identification of subgroups that may be at an unusual risk for the conditions of interest. Sixty-one 10-year-old children in metropolitan Atlanta were identified as having vision impairment (defined as legal blindness). The prevalence of legal blindness was higher among whites than among blacks and was higher among boys than among girls. Of the four race-sex groups, black boys were found to have the highest prevalence of legal blindness, whereas black girls were found to have the lowest prevalence of legal blindness (Table 3). This low prevalence among black girls is noteworthy and warrants further investigation.

Plans are under way to publish data on other MADDS topics such as the sociodemographic characterization of children with mental retardation and children with cerebral palsy; biomedical conditions in children with mental retardation as well as children with cerebral palsy; the prevalence and methods used to identify children with epilepsy; the association between mothers' reported alcohol use during pregnancy and mental retardation; and links between maternal occupational exposures and mental retardation.

INTERPRETATION ISSUES

Because the MADDSP covers a well-defined population, its output is representative of that population. Moreover, the program has some inherent flexibility in that other developmental disabilities, such as autism and cystic fibrosis, could be added to its coverage with minimal effort. The MADDSP is relatively noninvasive in that only existing records are reviewed. No attempts are made to contact children, their families, or individual physicians, psychologists, or other health-care professionals to gather data. Further, the agencies and institutions that are the primary data sources for the MADDSP appear to accept and support the program.

TABLE 2. Prevalence* of five developmental disabilities among 10-year-old children in selected study areas

Disability	Prevalence MADDS† (1985–1987)	Estimates previous studies
Mental retardation	12.0	3.1–43.6§
Epilepsy	6.1	3.6–6.7¶
Cerebral palsy	2.3	2.0–3.0**
Hearing impairment	1.1	0.8–2.0§
Visual impairment	0.7	0.3–0.6§

* Per 1,000 children.
† Based on an estimated 89,534 children aged 10 years residing in the area, 1985–1987 (9).
§ See Yeargin-Allsopp et al. (9).
¶ See Hauser and Hesdorffer (12).
** See Paneth and Kiely (8) and Yeargin-Allsopp et al. (9).

Regarding coverage and representativeness, the MADDSP may have some limitations. Racially and ethnically, the MADDSP covers large numbers of black and white Americans, but Hispanics, Asians, and Native Americans probably are underrepresented. Even for black and white Americans, certain factors peculiar to residents of the Atlanta area may limit the generalizability of some MADDSP findings to other geographic areas (e.g., rural areas, other urban areas with different ethnic mixes, and areas with a very different socioeconomic makeup).

When interpreting findings from the MADDSP, we also must consider limitations in the surveillance methodology. Perhaps the most important point to keep in mind is that, for the sake

TABLE 3. Prevalence* of legal blindness among 10-year-old children by race and sex — Metropolitan Atlanta Developmental Disabilities Study, 1985–1987

Sex	White N	White Rate	Black N	Black Rate	Total N	Total Rate
Male	25	8.6	15	8.8	40	8.7
Female	18	6.7	3	1.8	21	4.9
Total	43	7.7	18	5.4	61	6.8

* Per 10,000 children.

of simplicity, the MADDSP uses only selected sources in the Atlanta area to identify case children. In general, the children identified at those sources receive medical, educational, or social services related to their conditions. Thus, only children in need of special services are ascertained by the MADDSP. Children with very mild forms of these conditions—presumably those who do not need special services—may not be included. Nevertheless, we believe that the MADDSP includes almost all children with moderate-to-severe forms of the four conditions of interest. One exception may be a child with a severe disability who is not served through any of the mechanisms we use as primary sources or who is in a residential program outside Georgia (for example, a child with severe mental retardation who has been placed in a residential facility outside Georgia without any contact with local agencies). On the other hand, any child included in the MADDSP almost surely has the condition, at least as we have defined the conditions for surveillance purposes (i.e., predictive value positive is virtually 100%).

Because the MADDSP is relatively new, it will most likely need time to mature into a surveillance system of known dimensions and scope. CDC analysts are engaged in an ongoing examination of the data to test the system's coverage of children at different ages for each of the selected conditions under surveillance. As new resources become available, special studies may be initiated to check the completeness of the system for a particular condition and to document characteristics of missing cases.

EXAMPLES OF USING DATA

Because the United States has no other ongoing population-based surveillance systems for multiple developmental disabilities, the MADDSP is expected to serve as an important resource for current data on developmental disabilities affecting U.S. children.

Potential uses of MADDSP data include 1) detecting the introduction of new and potent etiologic agents into the population, 2) correlating disability rates for smaller geographic areas with environmental exposure data to identify the presence of possible environmental exposures of concern, 3) identifying subgroups that have a higher-than-expected risk for developmental disabilities, 4) documenting the effects of new prevention activities, and 5) identifying overall services needs of the community and possibly projecting future needs.

FUTURE ISSUES

Year 2000 Objective for Serious Mental Retardation

The year 2000 national health objectives call for a reduction in the prevalence of serious mental retardation (IQ <50) in school-age children to no more than two cases per 1,000 children (14). The baseline rate—2.7 cases per 1,000 children aged 10 years in 1985–1987—was derived from data collected in MADDS. Using data collected in the MADDSP, we can track our progress toward meeting this objective during the 1990s.

Public Laws Affecting Services for Children With Special Needs

The MADDSP's efficiency in identifying children with developmental disabilities is greatly influenced by federal laws under which the vast majority of these children are identified at a single source (6,7). As the scope of such legislation changes, our ability to ascertain children with developmental disabilities could be facilitated or hindered. Recent legislation requires states to serve certain groups of children from birth to the age of 3 years (6,15). As this law is enacted locally, we may see increases in our counts of children above the age of 3 years, mainly because of a greater awareness and attention to those younger children who are at a high risk of developmental problems. These developments might enable us to extend our coverage to children under the age of 3 years. We also need to be aware of new trends in special education placement (e.g., mainstreaming) that may affect our case ascertainment method.

Data Needs

In the future, we will have numerous opportunities for enhancing our surveillance of developmental disabilities.

- Other developmental conditions such as autism need to be included in the system.

- We need to improve ascertainment of children with milder forms of cerebral palsy who do not require special services. Such an effort might necessitate canvassing additional sources in the area.

- We need to retrieve and review hospital birth records for children with developmental disabilities, thereby acquiring detailed data on medical risk factors.

- We must conduct clinical examinations and laboratory studies of selected children to gain more data on biomedical factors associated with their disabilities.

- We need to assess cognitive and adaptive functioning of groups of children to estimate the sensitivity of the MADDSP procedures for identifying children with mild mental retardation.

ADDITIONAL RESOURCES

For technical information about state-based developmental disabilities surveillance programs supported by CDC, contact Joseph G. Hollowell, M.D., Chief, Developmental Disabilities Branch, National Center for Environmental Health, Centers for Disease Control and Prevention, Mailstop F–15, 4770 Buford Highway, NE, Atlanta, GA 30341-3724, (404) 488-7360.

REFERENCES

1. Crocker AC. The spectrum of medical care for developmental disabilities. In: Rubin IL, Crocker AC, editors. Developmental disabilities: delivery of medical care for children and adults. Philadelphia, Pennsylvania: Lea and Febiger, 1989:10–1.

2. Braddock D, Hemp R. Governmental spending for mental retardation and developmental disabilities, 1977–1984. Hosp Community Psychiatry 1986;37:702–7.

3. American Association on Mental Retardation. Mental retardation: definition, classification, and systems of supports, 9th ed. Washington, DC: American Association on Mental Retardation, 1992.

4. Fryers T. The epidemiology of severe intellectual impairment. London, England: Academic Press, 1984:69–76.

5. Thacker SB, Parrish RG, Trowbridge FL, and Surveillance Coordination Group. A method for evaluating systems of epidemiological surveillance. World Health Stat Q 1988;41:11–6.

6. Education of the Handicapped Act Amendments of 1986. Public Law 99–457.

7. Education for All Handicapped Children Act of 1975. Public Law 94–142.

8. Paneth N, Kiely J. The frequency of cerebral palsy: a review of population studies in industrialized nations since 1950. In: Stanley F, Alberman E, eds. The epidemiology of the cerebral palsies. Oxford, England: Blackwell Scientific Publications Ltd., 1984:46–56.

9. Yeargin-Allsopp M, Murphy CC, Oakley GP, Sikes RK. A multiple-source method for studying the prevalence of developmental disabilities in children: the Metropolitan Atlanta Developmental Disabilities Study [published erratum appears in Pediatrics 1992;90:1001]. Pediatrics 1992;89:624–30.

10. US Office of Special Education and Rehabilitative Services. To assure the free and appropriate public education of all handicapped children. Eleventh annual report to Congress on the Implementation of the Education of the Handicapped Act. Washington, DC: US Department of Education, 1989.

11. Adams MJ Jr, Hollowell JG. Community-based projects for the prevention of developmental disabilities. Ment Retard 1992;30:331–6.

12. Hauser WA, Hesdorffer DC. Epilepsy: frequency, causes, and consequences. New York: Demos Publications, 1990:1–51.

13. Drews CD, Yeargin-Allsopp M, Murphy CC, Decouflé P. Legal blindness among 10-year-old children in metropolitan Atlanta: prevalence, 1985 to 1987. Am J Public Health 1992;82:1377–9.

14. Public Health Service. Healthy people 2000: national health promotion and disease prevention objectives—full report, with commentary. Washington, DC: US Department of Health and Human Services, Public Health Service, 1991; DHHS publication no. (PHS)91-50212.

15. Individuals With Disabilities Education Act Amendments of 1991. Public Law 102–119.

Fetal Alcohol Syndrome

R. Louise Floyd, R.N., D.S.N.,[1] Margarett K. Davis, M.D., M.P.H.,[1]
M. Louise Martin, D.V.M.,[1] Daniel Hungerford, Dr.P.H.,[1]
and Karen J. Hymbaugh, M.P.A.[1]

PUBLIC HEALTH IMPORTANCE

Fetal alcohol exposure is an important cause of birth defects and central nervous system impairment including mental retardation, developmental delay, and other cognitive and behavioral abnormalities. Fetal alcohol syndrome (FAS) can be prevented by discouraging alcohol consumption during pregnancy or preventing pregnancy during periods of alcohol consumption.

For centuries researchers have observed associations between the alcoholism of parents and the growth and development of their children. ·
Theories about etiology ranged from genetic causes to adverse environmental influences in the homes of alcoholic parents. The theory we now accept had its origins in France in the 1950s. In 1957, Heuyer et al. reported that children born to alcoholics had an excessive prevalence of neurological disorders as well as delayed growth and development (1). Christiaens et al. reported similar findings in 1960 (2). In 1968, Lemoine and colleagues described a pattern of abnormalities observed in the children of alcoholic mothers (3). In 1973, Jones and Smith observed the same pattern of abnormalities in Seattle, Washington, and coined the term fetal alcohol syndrome (4).

Published estimates of FAS prevalence range from 0.3 to 20 cases per 1,000 live births in various populations (5). Abel and Sokol reviewed studies of women in the United States, Canada, Australia, and several European countries during the 1970s and 1980s. Pooling the estimated cases in these various studies as well as the estimated total live births, they derived an overall rate of 1.9 cases of FAS per 1,000 live births. However, the studies used to generate

this estimate were biased in ascertainment for a number of reasons: 1) they were not population-based, 2) diagnosticians exhibited a degree of subjectivity in their diagnoses, and 3) varying methods of population selection and screening were used among the different racial and ethnic groups represented in the studies.

Abel and Sokol have recently reexamined the same literature and excluded studies that did not prospectively select consecutive pregnancies. As a result, they have lowered their revised estimate to 0.33 cases of FAS per 1,000 (6). Because this estimate was based on prospective studies only, does not include data on Native Americans, and is admittedly an underascertainment of the true prevalence of FAS, the commonly accepted estimate continues to be about 1 case per 1,000 births. Data comparing prevalence rates for this country and other countries are limited, but studies from European countries show rates of 1 to 2 cases per 1,000 live births (7).

Based on a birth prevalence estimate of 0.33 cases per 1,000, the annual financial burden of FAS in the United States is estimated to be $74.6 million (6). Approximately 78% of this amount is attributed to costs associated with mental retardation and low birth weight. Mental retardation is believed to be present in about 53% of FAS cases. The fact that these estimates were based on cases of FAS only is noteworthy. If we assessed all other documented

[1] Division of Birth Defects and Developmental Disabilities
National Center for Environmental Health
Centers for Disease Control and Prevention
Atlanta, Georgia

alcohol-related effects—low birth weight, specific birth defects, and other cognitive and behavioral disorders—the costs would be much higher.

The surveillance of FAS is the foundation for assessing trends in occurrence and in planning and evaluating prevention activities. Reducing FAS and increasing the number of women who abstain from drinking during pregnancy are among the maternal and infant health objectives for the year 2000 (8). To establish these objectives, the U.S. Department of Health and Human Services used baseline data for FAS rates from the Birth Defects Monitoring Program (BDMP) and baseline rates for alcohol use in pregnancy from the 1988 National Maternal and Infant Health Survey (NMIHS). In addition, state health departments were mandated to monitor and report annually the proportion of infants born with FAS. For additional information about related topics and surveillance activities, see the Behavioral Risk Factors Before and During Pregnancy, Pregnancy-Related Nutrition, Low Birth Weight and Intrauterine Growth Retardation, and Prevalence of Birth Defects chapters.

HISTORY OF DATA COLLECTION

Although FAS has been recognized as a clinical entity in the United States since 1973, no surveillance system has been designed expressly to monitor its occurrence. CDC has, however, conducted surveillance for birth defects for 25 years through the Metropolitan Atlanta Congenital Defects Program (MACDP) and the national BDMP. The MACDP, begun in 1967, is the oldest active birth defects surveillance system in the United States and is the prototype for many developing state systems. The BDMP, CDC's nationwide birth defects surveillance system, has been in operation since 1974. These two systems were designed primarily to monitor major congenital defects in infants; they were not designed to address some of the more specific problems encountered in tracking syndromes, such as FAS, that have less distinct anomalies associated with the syndrome.

Surveillance efforts have improved over the past 15 years because of the evolution of the case definition and designation of an *International Classification of Diseases, Ninth Revision, Clinical Modification (ICD-9-CM)* code that can be used for FAS (9). In 1980, an FAS case definition was accepted by the Fetal Alcohol Study Group of the Research Society on Alcoholism (10). With some modification, the definition was updated in 1989 to specify that a child must manifest signs of abnormality in each of the following categories to have a secure diagnosis (11):

- Prenatal and/or postnatal growth retardation (weight and/or length or height below the 10th percentile when corrected for gestational age).

- Central nervous system involvement including neurological abnormality, developmental delay, behavioral dysfunction or deficit, intellectual impairment, and/or structural abnormalities such as microcephaly (head circumference below the third percentile) or brain malformations found on imaging studies or autopsy.

- A characteristic face, currently qualitatively described as having short palpebral fissures, an elongated midface, a long and flattened philtrum, thin upper lip, and flattened maxilla.

Fetal alcohol effects (FAE) is frequently used to designate children with milder or less complete manifestations of fetal alcohol impairment not meeting a full FAS definition. This term is used when alcohol exposure during pregnancy has been documented. It is a controversial term with a less clear definition than the definition for FAS.

The complexity of the FAS case definition, the variability of physical expression at birth, and the enhancement of diagnosis with age are features of FAS that have posed serious challenges for complete case ascertainment in birth defects surveillance systems that focus case-finding in the neonatal and infancy periods. Nevertheless, birth defects surveillance systems can identify and track those infants for which manifestations of FAS are evident in the neonatal period.

CDC SURVEILLANCE ACTIVITIES

Birth Defects Monitoring Program

The BDMP collects data on births occurring in some 1,200 community hospitals throughout the country; hospital participation is voluntary. Because the birth data are obtained from a non-random sample of U.S. hospitals, BDMP birth data are not population-based and do not constitute a random sample of all U.S. births. For a detailed description of the BDMP, see the Prevalence of Birth Defects chapter.

The surveillance of FAS was influenced by the 1979 publication of the ICD-9-CM—the first revision of the coding scheme since the recognition of FAS as a clinical entity in the United States (9). In this newest revision, an ICD-9-CM code that includes FAS was first assigned. Because BDMP coding is based on this scheme, the program began in 1979 collecting information on infants assigned this code during the newborn period. Since then, the BDMP has accumulated almost 15 years of national data on infants diagnosed at birth as having FAS.

Metropolitan Atlanta Congenital Defects Program

The MACDP, CDC's population-based birth defects surveillance system, monitors all births occurring in the five-county metropolitan Atlanta area—approximately 38,000 births each year. In the 25 years that the MACDP has been in operation, it has monitored >700,000 births. The MACDP includes information on all live-born and stillborn infants with a diagnosis of at least one major birth defect within the first year of life; diagnoses continue to be ascertained on these infants up until the sixth birthday. For a detailed description of the MACDP, see the Prevalence of Birth Defects chapter.

For 20 years, CDC has tracked trends for infants affected with FAS. In 1974, 1 year after FAS was recognized in the United States as a

clinical entity, FAS was added to the list of defects monitored by the MACDP. Because the coding system for MACDP is a specific modification of the ICD-9-CM and the British Pediatric Association coding schemes for use with birth defects surveillance systems, coding for FAS was structured more definitively than coding used in the BDMP. In the MACDP, FAS has its own unique code (760.710), distinguishable from the code for **probable** FAS (760.718), which may also include FAS facies.

GENERAL FINDINGS

Even though the BDMP and MACDP have differed considerably in ascertainment methods, geographic focuses, and periods monitored, they have produced very similar crude FAS prevalence estimates for infants in the first year of life. Between 1979 and 1992, the BDMP generated an overall prevalence estimate of 0.2 cases per 1,000 births. Between 1974 and 1991, the MACDP generated a birth prevalence estimate of 0.2 cases per 1,000 live births for FAS (codes 760.710 and 760.718), an estimated prevalence of 0.1 cases per 1,000 live births for **definitive** FAS (code 760.710), and an estimated prevalence of 0.08 cases per 1,000 live births for **probable** FAS (code 760.718). We suspect that the estimates from both systems underestimate the true prevalence for FAS because they are based on the recognition and diagnosis of FAS in infancy. Many FAS researchers believe that the clinical features of this syndrome become more prominent as a child ages, suggesting that more cases would be identified beyond the birth and infancy periods and that recognition in the newborn period is difficult at best.

Even though the two systems give the same overall estimate of the prevalence of FAS, they give a different sense of trends over the period monitored (Figure 1). The estimated prevalence of FAS among newborns identified through the BDMP has increased from 0.1 cases per 1,000 births in 1979 to 0.4 cases per 1,000 in 1992 (chi-square test for linear trend = 346.4, p <0). Rates calculated from MACDP data are not stable from year to year and do not show a trend during the same period. This instability may be

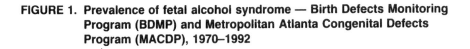

FIGURE 1. Prevalence of fetal alcohol syndrome — Birth Defects Monitoring Program (BDMP) and Metropolitan Atlanta Congenital Defects Program (MACDP), 1970–1992

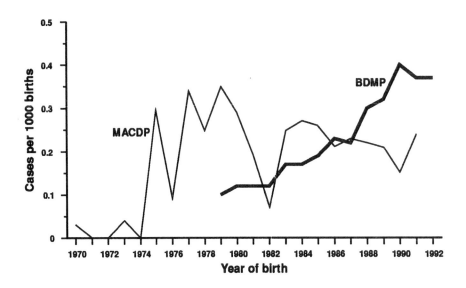

a function of the smaller number of births followed by the MACDP. Given the increased awareness of FAS among health-care providers during the last decade, we have difficulty determining whether the statistically significant increase in prevalence shown in BDMP data represents a true increase in prevalence or whether it reflects the role that increased awareness might play in identifying an increasing proportion of the cases in a population with an essentially stable attack rate.

Serdula et al. (12) report that between 1985 and 1988, the percentage of women who drank during pregnancy declined, but this decline was not evident for less educated and younger women. Moreover, for women who did drink during pregnancy, the median number of drinks remained the same during this 4-year period. Even though we have background information on alcohol exposure in the population of interest, we do not have comparable population-based data on FAS outcome. Therefore, it is difficult to predict whether the true prevalence of FAS might be stable, decreasing, or increasing over the period. Reports suggest that FAS prevalence is underascertained by a wide margin, particularly in the newborn period

(13). If this is true, increasing ascertainment could easily produce a spurious trend estimate. Analyzing trends by racial and ethnic groups might be instructive.

BDMP data show FAS to be a widespread problem in the U.S. population (Table 1); racial and ethnic differences may be related to economic, social, and additional factors other than race per se. In the BDMP and MACDP, the number of cases per group has been small enough each year to compromise the validity of stratified trend estimates. Even though rates vary considerably by race and ethnicity, the burden of the disease affects all groups. For example, whites exhibit a lower prevalence (0.11 cases per 1,000 births) than other racial and ethnic groups. However, because whites account for more than three fourths of all U.S. births, roughly a third of FAS births are white. Compared with rates for other groups, rates among both Native Americans and blacks are quite high; nevertheless, the overall public health burden is quite different for the two groups because Native American births represent about 1% of all U.S. births, and black births represent >15% of all U.S. births.

TABLE 1. Prevalence of fetal alcohol syndrome (FAS), by race/ethnicity — Birth Defects Monitoring Program (BDMP), 1981–1991

	FAS cases		BDMP births (in 1,000s)		Prevalence
	N	(%)	N	(%)	per 10,000
Black	710	(47.0)	873	(12.4)	8.1
White	537	(35.6)	4,887	(69.2)	1.1
Native American	77	(5.1)	25	(0.4)	31.0
Hispanic	45	(3.0)	382	(5.4)	1.2
Asian	3	(0.2)	101	(1.4)	0.3
Other	137	(9.1)	791	(11.2)	1.7
Overall	1,509	(100.0)	7,059	(100.0)	2.1

INTERPRETATION ISSUES

Problems in Identifying FAS

CDC's goal is to improve FAS surveillance methods in order to determine the scope of the problem and better serve prevention efforts. Successful, sound surveillance of FAS depends on accurate clinical diagnosis and more generally on a clearly understood and commonly accepted case definition that can be arrived at easily by clinicians. FAS does not conform to this requirement.

First, the diagnosis of FAS is difficult and subjective. Because we have no invariable core of specific features that designates a case patient, the diagnosis depends on FAS dysmorphology expertise to make the judgment, given some objective findings and a subjective impression.

Second, some FAS experts have said that ages 3–8 years are the best times for recognition because the distinct pattern of FAS facial abnormalities is fully expressed at these ages. Further, cognitive and behavioral delays manifest themselves at these ages when FAS children fail to perform developmental skills (e.g., kindergarten readiness at 4 years and reading and math skills at 7 years). However, no screening methods have been developed for this age-group, and identifying a single capture point for surveillance is difficult. Birth defects surveillance

systems capture diagnoses made during infancy, sometimes only during the early neonatal period, a time when the diagnosis is particularly difficult.

Finally, numerous sources of biases are inherent in the case ascertainment process. For example, practical diagnosis depends on knowledge of the mother's alcohol consumption during pregnancy. Many, if not most, clinicians are reluctant to make a diagnosis without this knowledge. Dependence on alcohol exposure information creates a tautological relationship between the exposure and the outcome, increasing the potential for biased judgments in a diagnostic setting already subject to bias.

Another possible source of bias in FAS diagnosis is reflected in the 1975—1992 MACDP data, which revealed 76 FAS diagnoses at Hospital A, a large inner-city public and teaching hospital serving poor women, most of whom are black, and only two FAS diagnoses at Hospital B, a large suburban hospital serving affluent women, most of whom are white. Interpreting this large discrepancy in rates between two different populations is difficult. Do women who deliver at Hospital B drink less than those at Hospital A? Do environmental factors such as nutrition and smoking influence outcome? Are clinicians at Hospital A more willing than those at Hospital B to elicit the history of alcohol consumption in pregnancy, to make the diagnosis, and to record it in the chart? Are clinicians at Hospital A more knowledgable about FAS and therefore more confident about making the diagnosis because they are in a teaching hospital and because there is an FAS research presence there? Perhaps children born at Hospital A are more likely to be followed at Hospital A outpatient departments if they have medical problems because they are less likely to have private pediatricians than children born at Hospital B. FAS may be overdiagnosed in some hospitals and underdiagnosed in others, but it is generally believed to be underascertained nationally. One report revealed that the MACDP failed to capture approximately 30% of cases of FAS that were diagnosed by other sources in infancy and early childhood *(Cordero J, Tosca M, unpublished data, 1993).*

FAS surveillance differs from the traditional surveillance approaches that have worked so well for infectious diseases and major congenital malformations. Even the best active birth defects surveillance systems such as the MACDP cannot be expected to capture FAS well without major modifications because of the subjectivity and the timing of the diagnosis, the lack of widespread FAS diagnostic expertise, and questionable tendencies toward social class and racial and ethnic biases in case ascertainment. Factors such as these are important to consider when interpreting FAS rates and designing methods for FAS ascertainment. To improve surveillance, we need to focus on four goals: 1) developing a more specific and objective case definition, 2) developing better age-specific screening and diagnostic methods, 3) training physicians and health-care providers to accurately screen and diagnose FAS, and 4) creating state and national systems for aggregating FAS data from a variety of sources.

Alternative Systems of Case Ascertainment

CDC provides both financial and technical support to state health departments and universities in an effort to establish affordable and efficient methods for estimating the prevalence of fetal alcohol syndrome. Cooperative agreements with these agencies and institutions support the

investigation of clinic-, school-, and social services-based approaches to FAS case ascertainment. The state of Washington is piloting a school-based program to screen all students in grade 1 by using a two-tier approach. Children are first screened on the basis of growth parameters and facial malformations; they are then referred to a special diagnostic clinic for examination by a dysmorphologist. Missouri is designing a case-finding system to refer all children removed from the home by protective services to a physician for a medical examination, which will include FAS assessment. In addition, the University of New Mexico is conducting population-based FAS diagnostic clinics patterned after a project that was conducted in the early 1980s among Native American communities.

A final methodology, which has been derived by CDC scientists working in Alaska, involves cross-linkage of existing data sets containing FAS diagnostic information. Data from birth certificates, death certificates, Medicaid, the Indian Health Service, and private physician practices were used to derive prevalence estimates for native populations *(14).* This approach provides a low-cost strategy for capturing cases that may be missed by surveillance systems that monitor rates among newborns only.

EXAMPLES OF USING DATA

In 1991, CDC entered into an agreement with the Indian Health Service and Alaska to provide epidemiologic assistance in determining the prevalence of FAS among all racial and ethnic groups in the state and to assist in the design of FAS prevention and evaluation activities. An FAS case file was developed to serve as the basis for a preliminary estimate of the prevalence rate of FAS among Alaska Native women. Earlier efforts at determining prevalence had been nonsystematic and biased in the ascertainment process. Relevant data from Indian Health Service data files and state files were cross-linked to produce an unduplicated number of FAS cases. Next, medical records were abstracted to confirm the presence of FAS. Using live births per year for the birth years of cases identified, researchers established a preliminary estimate of 2.1 cases of FAS per 1,000 live births *(14)*. This estimate was believed to be an underascertainment of the true prevalence because of the very stringent case definition used and because of certain inherent methodological constraints (underreporting in medical charts, unavailability of medical charts, and lack of access to all cases diagnosed by private physicians). Continued efforts are being made to increase ascertainment in order to generate more reliable estimates for all racial and ethnic groups in the state. These estimates will be used to justify the need to expend resources on prevention efforts and to explore the use of this methodology for tracking the effects of past and ongoing prevention efforts.

In 1983, May et al. published the results of an extensive effort to determine the prevalence of FAS among Southwestern Indians *(15)*. The method used for case finding in this study was to go into a community and organize diagnostic clinics aimed at identifying children with FAS. Community preparation and the education of providers were key elements of the success of this approach, which resulted in what remains to date the most reliable estimates of FAS among this population. In 1993, the University of New Mexico was funded by CDC to replicate this model statewide to determine the feasibility of using this approach on a population basis to determine prevalence rates of all racial and ethnic groups. This methodology could provide yet another alternative to determining prevalence rates for FAS.

In 1991, Oklahoma analyzed data from its Pregnancy Risk Assessment and Monitoring System and found that 12% of pregnant women in Oklahoma consumed a median of 8.2 alcoholic beverages per month during pregnancy. Using this and other information, the state developed an FAS Prevention Cooperative Agreement proposal, funded by CDC. Their project identified college-educated women as a targeted group for prevention activities. Further efforts are being developed to determine the level of drinking among this group, and early intervention approaches are being explored among college-aged men and women on one university campus in the state. The state is also exploring the surveillance of newborns and the

feasibility of a cross-linkage project similar to that done by Alaska.

FUTURE ISSUES

BDMP data will be used to monitor our progress in meeting the year 2000 national health objective for the reduction of FAS *(8)*. Current trends indicate an increase in FAS that relates in part to increased awareness and recognition of the syndrome *(13)*. Reaching a national rate of 0.12 cases per 1,000 live births over the next 6 years, given our current rate of 0.40 cases per 1,000 live births, will be a challenge. Further, we must consider the need to monitor the occurrence of other alcohol-related birth disorders. Facial malformations and central nervous system deficits that are characteristic of FAS have been noted among children whose symptoms do not meet the full case definition of FAS as defined by the Alcohol Working Group of the Society for Research on Alcoholism. The practice of assigning a diagnosis of fetal alcohol effects to these milder alcohol-related conditions has been discouraged by the working group *(11)*. The working group recommends the use of the term **alcohol-related birth defects** to "connote attribution of an observed anatomic or functional outcome to the impact of alcohol on the offspring," but it does not offer a case definition *(11)*. Thus, a fundamental measurement problem exists because we have no case definition for children affected by in utero exposure other than those who have full-blown FAS. Future progress in surveillance will require a more concise case definition of FAS as well as a case definition for alcohol-related birth disorders.

The lack of precision in definition relates to two other important concerns in FAS surveillance—biased ascertainment and misclassification. In the Alaska study, potential cases of FAS were identified from major health data sets and were confirmed by in-depth medical chart review by using a case definition developed for the study *(14)*. In that process, we discovered that only 14 of the 53 cases abstracted met the case definition for FAS. Documentation of alcohol exposure was present in 44 of the 53 potential cases given the *ICD-9-CM* code for FAS, which may be evidence of a lack of specificity of the code. The paucity of population-based prevalence data has contributed to biases among clinicians and health officials in recognizing the potential problems of FAS among persons of all socioeconomic statuses, races, and ethnicities. Therefore, in the future, we must expand surveillance systems to include population-based, systematic methods of identifying children with FAS at ages that optimize correct diagnoses.

REFERENCES

1. Heuyer H, Mises R, Dereux JF. La descendance des alcooliques [The offspring of alcoholics]. Nouvelle Presse Medicale 1957;29:657–8.

2. Christiaens L, Mizon JP, Delmarie G. Sur la descendance des alcooliques [On the offspring of alcoholics]. Annales de Pediatrie 1960;36:37–42.

3. Lemoine P, Harasseau H, Borteryu JP, Menuet JC. Les enfants de parents alcooliques: anomalies observées à propos de 127 cas [The children of alcoholic parents: anomalies observed in 127 cases]. Quest Medicale 1968;21:476–82.

4. Jones KL, Smith DW, Ulleland CN, Streissguth AP. Pattern of malformation in offspring of chronic alcoholic mothers. Lancet 1973;2:1267–71.

5. Abel EL, Sokol RJ. Incidence of fetal alcohol syndrome and economic impact of FAS-related anomalies. Drug Alcohol Depend 1987; 19:51–70.

6. Abel EL, Sokol RJ. A revised conservative estimate of the incidence of FAS and its economic impact. Alcohol Clin Exp Res 1991;15:514–24.

7. Abel EL. Fetal alcohol syndrome. Oradell, New Jersey: Medical Economics Books, 1990.

8. Public Health Service. Healthy people 2000: national health promotion and disease prevention objectives—full report, with commentary. Washington, DC: US Department of Health and Human Services, Public Health Service, 1991; DHHS publication no. (PHS)91-50212.

9. Public Health Service. International classification of diseases, ninth revision, clinical modification. Washington, DC: US Department of Health and Human Services, Public Health Service, Health Care Financing Administration, 1991; DHHS publication no. (PHS)91-1260.

10. Rosett HL. A clinical perspective of the fetal alcohol syndrome [Editorial]. Alcohol Clin Exp Res 1980;4:119–22.

11. Sokol RJ, Clarren SK. Guidelines for use of terminology describing the impact of prenatal alcohol on the offspring. Alcohol Clin Exp Res 1989;13: 597–8.

12. Serdula M, Williamson DF, Kendrick JS, Anda RF, Byers T. Trends in alcohol consumption by pregnant women: 1985 through 1988. JAMA 1991;265: 876–9.

13. CDC. Fetal alcohol syndrome—United States, 1979–1992. MMWR 1993;42:339–41.

14. CDC. Linking multiple data sources in fetal alcohol syndrome surveillance—Alaska. MMWR 1993;42: 312–4.

15. May PA, Hymbaugh KJ, Aase JM, Samet JM. Epidemiology of fetal alcohol syndrome among American Indians of the Southwest. Soc Biol 1983; 30:374–87.

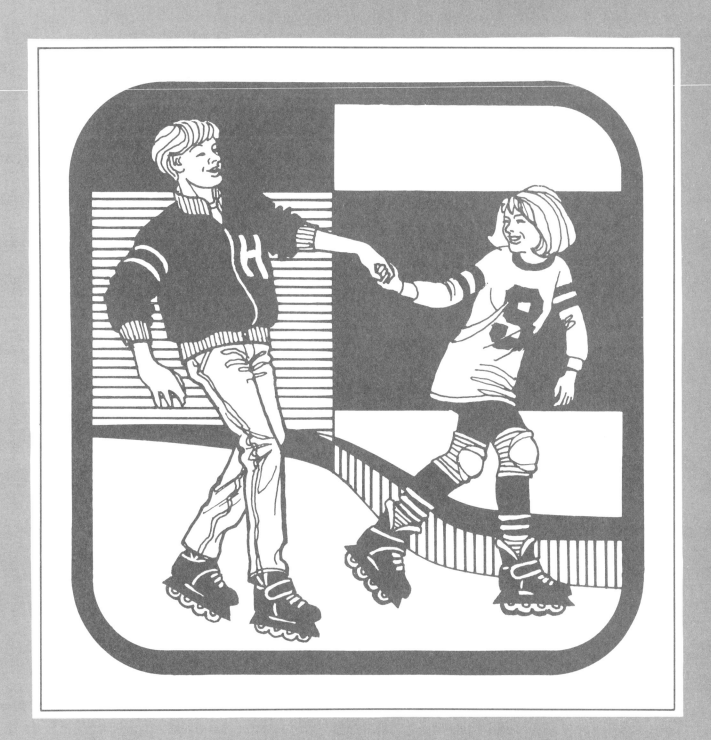

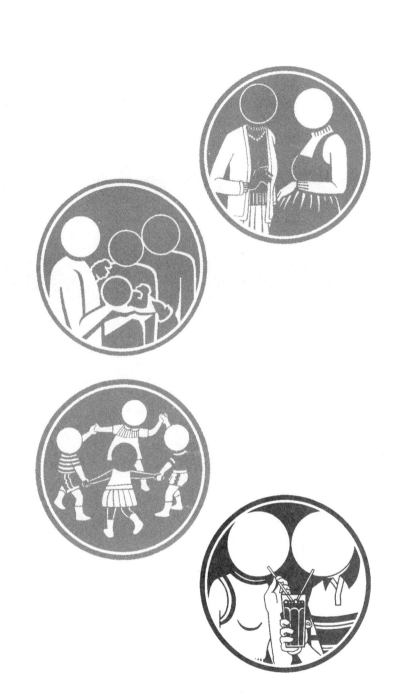

COMMENTARY

on Adolescent Health
from the Massachusetts Department of Public Health

Over the past decade, adolescent health issues have gradually begun to receive more attention. Today, we must recognize adolescence as an important developmental period between childhood and adulthood if we are to understand key health status indicators and to design appropriate health and related services to address these indicators. Although numerous commissioned papers and special reports have been published on the health and well-being of adolescents in our society, sufficient resources have not been allocated at any level of government to meet the needs of our nation's adolescents.

We need to develop an adequate surveillance system to monitor adolescent health and well-being and thus guide future planning and action. Unfortunately, the existing system for the surveillance of adolescents is not as comprehensive or focused as that available for the surveillance of pregnant women, infants, and children. Hence, in the next decade, we should place more attention on the development and implementation of an adolescent health surveillance system. This section of the monograph provides a good beginning for such an effort.

A system for the surveillance of adolescent health is needed to guide the planning and implementation of programs and policies as well as to assess the effects of existing community-based systems. Although state and local funding levels have not been adequate to focus on adolescent health and human services, all maternal and child health agencies at the state level embrace the goal of developing systems for the surveillance of adolescent health. All state maternal and child health agencies have adolescent specialists who assist in planning and advocacy for adolescent issues. Many of the existing state and local systems have been funded with Title V Maternal and Child Health Services Block Grant dollars. These community-based systems include a range of health and human services that address all domains of development (e.g., physical, cognitive, emotional, and social) in a culturally competent and youth-oriented manner. Although the specifics of the actual service delivery system vary by community—depending on the needs and the infrastructure available—most systems of adolescent services include primary care with appropriate links to tertiary care, school-linked and school-based services, and community-based and school-based prevention activities. The goal is to provide adolescents with services that meet their immediate needs, respect their individuality, and maintain their confidentiality.

A focused adolescent health surveillance system is crucial to our nation's ability to improve the health status and functioning of adolescents and adults in the future. To be most useful to state and local practitioners involved in program planning and evaluation, a surveillance system must have standardized definitions across data sets, be comprehensive in content and scope, and be able to generate community-based data. Although the data presented in this section represent an excellent beginning for an adolescent health surveillance system, all of these goals cannot be met through the adolescent health indicators currently available.

First, we need to agree on the definition of **adolescence** so that data can be collected and reported in at least standardized age increments. When defining adolescence, we must consider a wide range of issues. For example, is adolescence a developmental period that begins with the physiological markers of puberty or the transition from concrete operational to formal operational thinking? Or is it best characterized by cultural and societal rites of passage such as the age when one joins a religious group or the ages designated by society as the time when youths can assume adult roles such as driving a car, drinking, voting, or marrying without parental consent. Although age markers can never universally match biological, social, or cognitive transition markers of adolescence, they are the most convenient way to standardize a definition for a surveillance system. Currently, adolescence is defined by age categories ranging from 10 through 25 years. One of the most frequently used age categories in the existing data systems is 15–19 years. The age categories that are most useful for translation to action are those that correspond with existing markers such as the age when attendance in school is no longer compulsory (16 years), the age when voting is allowed and many youths graduate from high school (18 years), and the age when special education law ends coverage of services (21 years). Ideally, data should be available for each age and should be aggregated by state and local users in groupings that make sense for a specific planning or evaluation issue.

Second, an adolescent health surveillance system needs to be comprehensive in scope and include health status indicators, service utilization measures, sociodemographic and environmental measures, and behavioral risk indicators. The three chapters in this section highlight valuable contributions to a basic adolescent data system, but the actual data available to state and local planners cover a broader range of topics than those covered by these chapters alone. These data, combined with data from other major systems (education, welfare, mental health, substance abuse, nutrition, and employment), would provide local and state practitioners with valuable tools to use in guiding and evaluating policies and services.

Finally, data must be readily available at the state and local levels if they are to be maximally used on an ongoing basis. Much of the data reported in this volume are available at the state level with adequate technical characteristics but are not available for more local level analyses. Clearly, system planners need to consider resources and other variables to create such a flexible and comprehensive surveillance system. However, the availability of current technology and the pressure for community-based systems to meet local data needs may reinforce each other, thus creating an adolescent data system that is more responsive at the local level.

To evaluate the nation's progress in meeting the *Healthy People 2000* health objectives for adolescents, we need a responsive monitoring and surveillance system so that we can assess adolescent health status and well-being. This section of the monograph highlights the current CDC data systems that serve as a basis for a national system.

Deborah Klein Walker, Ed.D.
Assistant Commissioner
Bureau of Family and Community Health
Massachusetts Department of Public Health
Boston, Massachusetts

Youth Risk Behavior

Laura Kann, Ph.D.,[1] Charles W. Warren, Ph.D.,[1]
Janet L. Collins, Ph.D.,[1] and Lloyd J. Kolbe, Ph.D.[1]

PUBLIC HEALTH IMPORTANCE

In the United States, almost 70% of all deaths among persons 1–24 years of age are the result of only four causes. Motor vehicle crashes cause 31% of all deaths in this age-group, other unintentional injuries cause 14%, homicides cause 13%, and suicides cause 10% (1). A considerable amount of acute and chronic morbidity also results from these causes.

The use of alcohol and other drugs is associated with much of this mortality and morbidity among youths. Alcohol use is a factor in about half of all deaths from motor vehicle crashes, homicides, and suicides (2). The use of alcohol and other drugs also contributes to many important social problems—including dysfunctional families, crime, school dropout, and lost economic productivity—that are not reflected in vital statistics (3,4).

Substantial morbidity and social problems result from the >1 million pregnancies that occur among adolescents each year in the United States. The high rate of teenage pregnancy in the United States, in turn, contributes to the nation's high rate of infant mortality and morbidity (5).

Finally, significant morbidity results from the estimated 12 million cases of sexually transmitted diseases (STDs) that occur each year among persons 15–29 years of age (6). Relatedly, 20% of AIDS cases are diagnosed among persons 20–29 years of age (7). Because the median incubation period between infection with human immunodeficiency virus (HIV) and onset of AIDS is estimated to be 10 years, we suspect that many persons aged 20–29 years with AIDS were infected during adolescence (8). In 1989, AIDS ranked as the sixth leading cause of death among persons aged 15–24 years (1).

When we consider the leading causes of death among all age-groups combined, we find that >60% of all deaths in the United States, and an enormous amount of acute and chronic morbidity, are caused by only three conditions: heart disease (34%), cancer (23%), and stroke (7%) (1). A relatively small number of behaviors—including tobacco use, unhealthy dietary patterns, and physical inactivity—contribute greatly to mortality and morbidity from these three diseases.

In summary, many health problems among persons <24 years of age are caused by a relatively small number of preventable behaviors such as drinking and driving, failing to wear safety belts, and engaging in unprotected sexual intercourse. Also, other behavior often begun during adolescence, such as tobacco use, unhealthy dietary patterns, and physical inactivity, contributes to the leading causes of mortality and morbidity for persons >24 years of age. All of these behaviors often are established during youth, extend into adulthood, and are interrelated. For additional information about related topics and surveillance activities, see the Contraception, Sexually Transmitted Diseases, Human Immunodeficiency Virus, Legal Induced Abortion, Pregnancy in Adolescents, and Unintentional Injuries and Violence chapters.

[1] Division of Adolescent and School Health
National Center for Chronic Disease Prevention
   and Health Promotion
Centers for Disease Control and Prevention
Atlanta, Georgia

HISTORY OF DATA COLLECTION

Since 1987, CDC's National Center for Chronic Disease Prevention and Health Promotion (NCCDPHP) has provided fiscal and technical assistance to every state department of education and 16 of the nation's largest local departments of education in order to support school health education programs targeting the prevention of HIV infection and other important health problems (9).

In 1988, CDC began developing the Youth Risk Behavior Surveillance System (YRBSS) to 1) focus the nation on specific behavior that causes the most important health problems among youths; 2) assess whether this behavior increases, decreases, or remains the same over time; and 3) provide comparable data among national, state, and local samples of youths.

After reviewing the leading causes of mortality and morbidity among youths and persons in all age-groups, we realized that nearly all contributing behaviors could be categorized in six areas: 1) behavior that results in unintentional and intentional injuries; 2) tobacco use; 3) use of alcohol and other drugs; 4) sexual behavior that contributes to unintended pregnancy and STDs, including HIV infection; 5) dietary behavior that results in disease; and 6) physical inactivity.

A panel of experts was established for each of the six areas and was asked to identify the highest priority risk behaviors in each category and to develop survey questions to measure this behavior. These panels consisted of scientific experts from relevant federal agencies, scientists from outside the federal government, representatives of state and local education agencies, survey research specialists from CDC's National Center for Health Statistics (NCHS), and staff from NCCDPHP. Because students would have a class period of about 45 minutes to complete the questionnaire covering all six categories of behavior, each panel was asked to identify only the highest priority behaviors and to suggest a limited number of questions to measure the prevalence of these behaviors.

The first version of the YRBSS questionnaire was completed in October 1989 and was reviewed at a national conference by representatives of each state department of education and 16 local departments of education. Survey research specialists from NCHS also provided comments and suggestions on that version of the questionnaire. Following this conference, the questionnaire was revised, and a second version was completed in November 1989. This questionnaire was used the following spring to generate data from national, state, and local samples of students in grades 9–12. This questionnaire also was sent to the Questionnaire Design Research Laboratory at NCHS for four waves of laboratory and field-testing with high school students. A review of student responses led to the development of recommendations to improve the wording of questions, set recall periods, and identify response categories. The field tests sought to identify survey conditions that could be expected to encourage students to be honest in answering survey questions.

In October 1990, the core questionnaire was completed. It reflected the national health objectives (4), a review of data collected during spring 1990, information from NCHS's laboratory and field tests, and input from the panel members and the representatives of each state and the 16 local departments of education. The core questionnaire is self-administered, contains 84 multiple-choice questions, and has about a grade-7 reading level. A standard computer scannable bubble sheet or questionnaire booklet can be used to record responses. Skip patterns are not included in the questionnaire to help ensure that students do not lose their place on the answer sheet when recording responses and to prevent students from looking at other youths' answer sheets or questionnaire booklets to detect a pattern of blank responses that might identify the risk behavior of those students.

CDC SURVEILLANCE ACTIVITIES

The YRBSS currently has three complementary components: national school-based surveys, state and local school-based surveys, and a national household-based survey. Each of these components provides unique information about different subpopulations of adolescents in the United States.

National School-Based Surveys

In spring 1990, CDC conducted the first national school-based Youth Risk Behavior Survey. Results from this survey were published in the *Morbidity and Mortality Weekly Report* in 1991 and 1992 *(10)*.

In spring 1991, CDC conducted the second national school-based Youth Risk Behavior Survey, using the core questionnaire that was revised and completed in October 1990. Results from this survey are described elsewhere *(10,11)*. The survey will be conducted biennially during odd-numbered years throughout the decade and will involve national probability samples of students in grades 9–12 from public and private schools.

State and Local School-Based Surveys

In 1990, CDC began offering each state and the 16 funded local departments of education the YRBSS questionnaire as well as fiscal and technical assistance to conduct the Youth Risk Behavior Survey. During 1990, 24 states and 8 cities conducted surveys, sometimes with the assistance of area departments of health. In 1991, 29 states and 10 cities conducted surveys. In 1993, 43 states and 13 cities conducted surveys. Results from the 1991 surveys are described elsewhere *(10)*. Each state and the 16 local departments of education will be able to conduct Youth Risk Behavior Surveys biennially throughout the decade.

Although use of the same questionnaire allows better comparability across sites, each department of education determines which questions will be asked. Questions may be added, deleted, or modified. Each survey year, however, more and more sites are using the questionnaire unchanged.

To help improve the quality of the surveys and increase the usefulness of the data, CDC provides several types of technical assistance to interested departments of education. For example, CDC has developed a *Handbook for Conducting Youth Risk Behavior Surveys (12)* to help state and local departments of education plan surveys; obtain clearance; select schools, classes, and students; contact or notify parents about the surveys; conduct surveys; prepare data for analysis; and report survey results. CDC has also developed *PCSample (13)*, personal computer-based software that helps program directors in departments of education draw probability samples of schools and students.

CDC offers data analysis services that include scanning answer sheets and cleaning, editing, weighting, and analyzing data. Standard procedures are used to help make results comparable across sites. CDC provides a detailed technical report to each site and can help departments of education interpret, apply, and disseminate results. The data generated from these surveys remain the property of the respective state or local department of education.

National Household-Based Survey

CDC included the Youth Risk Behavior Survey as a supplement in the 1992 National Health Interview Survey (NHIS). This supplemental survey was conducted among persons 12–21 years of age from a national probability sample of households. Data were obtained from youths attending school, youths who had dropped out of school, and college-age youths, including those who had not completed high school, those who had completed high school but were not attending college, and those attending college. School-age youths not attending school were oversampled.

Field staff administered the questionnaire using individual portable cassette players with earphones; respondents listened to the questions and marked their answers on a standardized answer sheet. This method helped to compensate for reading problems among respondents, helped to ensure confidentiality during household surveys, and allowed youths to avoid disclosing their responses to interviewers.

GENERAL FINDINGS

General results from the 1991 national Youth Risk Behavior Survey are described for each of the six categories (see the tables in reference 11 for detailed findings).

Unintentional and Intentional Injuries

Slightly more than one quarter (27.7%) of all students reported "always" using safety belts when riding in a car or truck driven by someone else. Among students who rode motorcycles, 39.2% "always" wore a motorcycle helmet. Among students who rode a bicycle, 1.1% "always" wore a bicycle helmet.

Among all students, 42.5% were in at least one physical fight during the 12 months preceding the survey. Male students (50.2%) were significantly more likely than female students (34.4%) to have been in a physical fight. Fighting decreased as the grade increased. An estimated 137 physical fights occurred per 100 students per year.

Among all students, 26.1% carried a weapon at least 1 day during the 30 days preceding the survey. Male students (40.6%) were significantly more likely than female students (10.9%) to have carried a weapon. Students in grade 12 (21.3%) were significantly less likely than those in grades 9 (27.5%) or 11 (29.0%) to have carried a weapon. An estimated 107 weapon-carrying incidents occurred per 100 students per month.

During the 12 months preceding the survey, 29.0% of students had thought seriously about attempting suicide; 8.6% had made a specific plan to attempt suicide; 7.3% had actually attempted suicide; and 1.7% had made a suicide attempt that resulted in an injury, poisoning, or overdose that required treatment by a physician or nurse. Female students were significantly more likely than male students to have thought about attempting suicide, to have made a specific plan to attempt suicide, to have actually attempted suicide, and to have made a suicide attempt requiring medical attention.

Tobacco Use

Among all students, 70.1% had ever tried cigarette smoking, 27.5% had smoked cigarettes on one or more of the 30 days preceding the survey (currently smoking), 12.7% had smoked cigarettes on 20 or more of the 30 days preceding the survey (frequent smoking), and 21.2% had ever smoked at least one cigarette every day for 30 days (regular smoking). Among all students, 10.5% had used smokeless tobacco (chewing tobacco or snuff) on one or more of the 30 days preceding the survey. Male students (19.2%) were significantly more likely than female students (1.3%) to use smokeless tobacco.

Alcohol and Other Drugs

Among all students, 81.6% had ever consumed alcohol during their lifetime, and 50.8% had consumed alcohol during the 30 days preceding the survey. Lifetime and current alcohol use increased significantly as the grade increased.

Among all students, 31.3% reported consuming five or more drinks of alcohol on at least one occasion during the 30 days preceding the survey (episodic heavy drinking). Episodic heavy drinking occurred significantly more often among male students (36.5%) than among female students (25.9%); it was also more common among students in grades 11 (36.3%) and 12 (39.3%) than among students in grade 9 (22.6%).

Among all students, 31.3% had ever used marijuana during their lifetime, 14.7% had used marijuana during the 30 days preceding the survey (current marijuana use), 5.9% had ever used cocaine during their lifetime, and 1.7% had used cocaine during the 30 days preceding the survey (current cocaine use). Lifetime and current marijuana use and lifetime cocaine use increased significantly as the grade increased.

Among all students, 2.7% had ever used steroids. Male students (4.1%) were significantly more likely than female students (1.2%) to use steroids.

Sexual Behavior

Among all students, 54.1% had ever had sexual intercourse, and 18.7% had had sexual intercourse with four or more sex partners during their lifetime. Among students who had had sexual intercourse, 69.3% had sexual intercourse during the 3 months preceding the survey (current sexual activity). Male students (23.4%) were significantly more likely than female students (13.8%) to have had sexual intercourse with four or more sex partners, whereas female students (75.3%) were significantly more likely than male students (64.1%) to be currently sexually active.

Among sexually active students, 81.8% used contraception (birth control pills, condoms, or withdrawal), and 46.2% used condoms during the last sexual intercourse. Contraceptive use increased significantly as the grade increased; 72.9% of students in grade 9, 81.8% of students in grade 10, 82.9% of students in grade 11, and 84.9% of students in grade 12 used contraceptives. Male students (54.6%) were significantly more likely than female students (38.0%) to have used condoms during the last sexual intercourse.

Dietary Behavior

Among all students, 12.9% consumed five or more servings of fruits and vegetables (fruit, fruit juice, green salads, and cooked vegetables) during the day preceding the survey. Male students (15.2%) were significantly more likely than female students (10.5%) to consume five or more servings per day of fruits and vegetables.

Among all students, 64.9% ate no more than two servings of foods typically high in fat content (hamburger, hot dogs, or sausage;

french fries or potato chips; and cookies, doughnuts, pie, or cake) during the day preceding the survey. Female students (72.9%) were significantly more likely than male students (57.2%) to eat no more than two servings per day of foods typically high in fat content.

Physical Activity

Among all students, 48.9% were enrolled in physical education (PE) class, and 41.6% attended PE class daily. Enrollment and daily attendance in PE class decreased significantly from grade 9 to grade 12. Among students enrolled in PE class, 49.4% exercised or played sports >30 minutes during an average PE class. Male students (56.5%) were significantly more likely than female students (40.7%) to exercise >30 minutes during an average PE class.

Among all students, 40.9% reported walking or bicycling for at least 30 minutes at a time during the day preceding the survey (moderate physical activity). Moderate physical activity decreased significantly from grade 9 (49.3%) to grade 12 (32.4%). Among all students, 43.0% performed stretching exercises (including toe touches, knee bending, or leg stretching) and 36.6% performed strengthening exercises (including push-ups, sit-ups, or weight lifting to tone or strengthen muscles) during 4 or more of the 7 days preceding the survey. Male students (43.9%) were significantly more likely than female students (28.9%) to perform strengthening exercises.

INTERPRETATION ISSUES

The YRBSS is an epidemiologic surveillance system that shares some of the strengths and limitations of other health-related surveys of youths:

- The surveillance system was designed to focus primarily on health risk behavior—rather than related knowledge, attitudes, or beliefs—for two reasons: behavior is the best predictor of related health outcomes, and so many knowledge, attitude, and belief variables have an unknown or tenuous association with related risk behavior. To improve the health status of youths and the adults that they will become, interventions must focus primarily on reducing risk behavior (14,15).

- By measuring six categories of priority health risk behavior, the questionnaire allows users to examine interrelationships among categories of risk behavior and reduces the burden on schools posed by multiple categorical surveys. Surveys that focus on one or two high-risk behaviors may provide more information about that behavior, but such surveys do not provide information for developing the more comprehensive interventions that might address simultaneously the multiple and interrelated risk behaviors exhibited by many youths (16,17).

- Collection of data from out-of-school adolescents is limited to the 1992 NHIS Youth Risk Behavior Supplement. In 1991, 98.8% of adolescents 14–15 years old, 93.3% of adolescents 16–17 years old, and 59.6% of adults 18–19 years old were enrolled in school (18). The 1992 supplement helps to determine the extent to which the risk behavior of out-of-school youths differ from the behavior of youths who remain in school.

- Some behavior, such as sexual intercourse and attempted suicide, may be controversial to measure. All behavior measured in the survey, however, is critical to the nation's health (4). We have no evidence that voluntarily responding to questions about any health risk behavior will encourage or discourage a respondent to practice that behavior. Schools that administer the survey may provide resource information, such as hot line numbers, to students who may have questions about any of the behavior measured in the questionnaire.

- YRBSS results are based on self-reported data that appear valid for estimating the prevalence of health risk behavior (19–21).

However, a respondent may underreport or overreport a behavior, depending in part on the perceived social stigma or support for that behavior and the perceived confidentiality of responses (19,22–25). Establishing criterion-related validity for responses to most of the questions on the questionnaire may be impractical, if not impossible. Survey administration procedures were developed carefully to protect confidentiality and, in the school-based surveys, to allow youths to respond anonymously. Data collected to date are similar to data from categorical school-based surveys and demonstrate subgroup trends consistent with data from other surveys (26–28).

- Information generated by the household-based NHIS Youth Risk Behavior Supplement may not be entirely comparable with information generated by the school-based Youth Risk Behavior Surveys. Previous research suggests that youths may be more likely to respond candidly to school-based surveys than to household-based surveys because they may consider school-based surveys a common school practice; they may be reassured by responding as a part of a large group; and they may have more confidence in the anonymity of school-based surveys.

- Although the YRBSS can provide information to help assess the effects of broad national, state, or local policies and programs, the system was not designed to evaluate the effectiveness of specific interventions, such as a teacher training program, school curriculum, or media campaign. Other instruments and protocols can measure more precisely the intended outcomes of such interventions.

EXAMPLES OF USING DATA

The YRBSS is the only ongoing surveillance system that provides national, state, and local information on such a broad range of health objectives. The YRBSS is being used to help monitor our progress in achieving the following objectives:

- Twenty-six of the national health objectives for the year 2000 *(4)*.

- Five student-related objectives in CDC's *Strategic Plan for Preventing Human Immunodeficiency Virus (HIV) Infection (29)*.

- Twenty-eight model standards presented in *Healthy Communities 2000 (30)*.

- Four primary goals in the American Cancer Society's comprehensive school health education initiative *(31,32)*.

- The National Education Goal 6 that states "by the year 2000, every school in America will be free of drugs and violence and will offer a disciplined environment conducive to learning" *(33,34)*. (At the request of the National Education Goals Panel, 10 questions were added to the national, state, and local YRBSS questionnaire in 1993 to provide even more information to measure Goal 6.)

The YRBSS also is being used increasingly to support state and local policies and programs that help to reduce health risk behavior among youths *(33,35–43)*. For example, Youth Risk Behavior Survey data have been used in the following ways:

- To inform the public of the need for effective health education programs.

- To provide state boards of education and state legislatures with information supporting comprehensive school health policies and programs.

- To support stricter enforcement of policies on minors' access to cigarette vending machines and alcohol.

- To update and improve teacher training and instructional materials.

- To target interventions to special populations that are at increased risk.

- To promote collaboration with institutions of higher education that are responsible for preparing teachers.

- To help health agencies and community organizations develop effective community-based programs to reduce health risk behavior.

FUTURE ISSUES

Data from the YRBSS will continue to be used to help measure progress, particularly among high school students, toward achieving 26 of the 111 national health objectives that focus on adolescents. The national data collected in 1991 suggest that, among high school students, few of these 26 national health objectives have been met. In the future, CDC plans to expand the surveillance system to include components that focus on college students at the national and state levels and middle school students at the state and local levels. In addition, we will continue our efforts to increase the quantity and quality of the state and local school-based surveys among high school students.

REFERENCES

1. NCHS. Advance report of final mortality statistics, 1989. Hyattsville, Maryland: US Department of Health and Human Services, Public Health Service, CDC, 1992. (Monthly vital statistics report; vol. 40, no. 8, suppl.)

2. Perrine M, Peck R, Fell J. Epidemiologic perspectives on drunk driving. In: Surgeon General's workshop on drunk driving: background papers. Rockville, Maryland: US Department of Health and Human Services, Public Health Service, Office of the Surgeon General, 1989.

3. Rice DP, Kelman S, Miller LS, Dunmeyer S. The economic costs of alcohol and drug abuse and mental illness: 1985. Washington, DC: US Department of Health and Human Services, Public Health Service, Alcohol, Drug Abuse, and Mental Health Administration, 1990; DHHS publication no. (ADM)90-1694.

4. Public Health Service. Healthy people 2000: national health promotion and disease prevention objectives—full report, with commentary. Washington, DC: US Department of Health and Human Services, Public Health Service, 1991; DHHS publication no. (PHS)91-50212.

5. Hoffereth SL. Teenage pregnancy and its resolution. In: Hoffereth SL, Hayes CD, eds. Risking the future: adolescent sexuality, pregnancy, and childbearing: working papers and statistical appendixes. Washington DC: National Academy Press, 1987: 78–92.

6. Center for Prevention Services. 1990 Division of STD/HIV Prevention annual report. Atlanta: US Department of Health and Human Services, Public Health Service, CDC, 1991.

7. National Center for Infectious Diseases. HIV/AIDS surveillance report. 1st quarter ed. Atlanta: US Department of Health and Human Services, Public Health Service, CDC, 1993. (US AIDS cases reported through March 1993; vol. 5, no. 1.)

8. CDC. AIDS and human immunodeficiency virus infection in the United States: 1988 update. MMWR 1989;38(suppl. no. S-4):1.

9. Moore JR, Daily L, Collins J, et al. Progress in efforts to prevent the spread of HIV infection among youth. Public Health Rep 1991;106:678–86.

10. National Center for Chronic Disease Prevention and Health Promotion. Chronic disease and health promotion: reprints from the MMWR: 1990–1991 Youth Risk Behavior Surveillance System. Atlanta: US Department of Health and Human Services, Public Health Service, CDC, 1993.

11. Kann L, Warren W, Collins J, Ross J, Collins B, Kolbe LJ. Results from the national school-based 1991 Youth Risk Behavior Survey and progress toward achieving related health objectives for the nation. Public Health Rep 1993;108(suppl. 1):47–67.

12. National Center for Chronic Disease Prevention and Health Promotion. Handbook for conducting Youth Risk Behavior Surveys. Atlanta: CDC, 1992.

13. National Center for Chronic Disease Prevention and Health Promotion. PCSample user's guide. Atlanta: CDC, 1992.

14. Kolbe LJ. Indicators for planning and monitoring school health programs. In: Kar SB, ed. Health promotion indicators and actions. New York: Springer Publishing Company, 1989:221–48.

15 Kolbe LJ. The application of health behavior research: health education and health promotion. In: Gochman DS, ed. Health behavior: emerging research perspectives. New York: Plenum Press, 1988:381–96.

16. Dryfoos JG. Adolescents at risk: prevalence and prevention. New York: Oxford University Press, 1990.

17. Jessor R, Jessor SL. Problem behavior and psychosocial development: a longitudinal study of youth. New York: Academic Press, 1977.

18. US Bureau of the Census. Statistical abstract of the United States: 1992. 112th ed. Washington, DC: US Government Printing Office, 1992.

19 Center for Chronic Disease Prevention and Health Promotion. Reducing the health consequences of smoking: 25 years of progress. A report of the Surgeon General. Washington, DC: US Department of Health and Human Services, Public Health Service, CDC 1989; DHHS publication no. (CDC)89-8411.

20. Harrell AV. Validation of self-report: the research record. In: Rouse BA, Kozel NJ, Richards LG, eds. Self-report methods of estimating drug use: meeting current challenges to validity. Washington, DC: US Government Printing Office, 1985:12–21; NIDA research monograph 57; DHHS publication no. (ADM)85-1402.

21. Bar-Or O. Fitness and activity assessment of children and adolescents. In: Drury TF, ed. Assessing physical fitness and physical activity in population-based surveys. Hyattsville, Maryland: US Department of Health and Human Services, Public Health Service, CDC, NCHS, 1989:213–28; DHHS publication no. (PHS)89-1253.

22. Johnston LD, O'Malley PM. Issues of validity and population coverage in student surveys of drug use. In: Rouse BA, Kozel NJ, Richards LG, eds. Self-report methods of estimating drug use: meeting current challenges to validity. Washington, DC: US Government Printing Office, 1985:31–54; NIDA research monograph 57; DHHS publication no. (ADM)85-1402.

23. Rootman I, Smart RG. A comparison of alcohol, tobacco and drug use as determined from household and school surveys. Drug Alcohol Depend 1985; 16:89–94.

24. Zanes A, Matsoukas E. Different settings, different results? A comparison of school and home responses. Public Opinion Q 1979;43:550–7.

25. Gfroerer J. Influence of privacy on self-reported drug use by youths. In: Rouse BA, Kozel NJ, Richards LG. Self-report methods of estimating drug use: meeting current challenges to validity. Washington DC: US Government Printing Office, 1985:22–30. NIDA research monograph 57; DHHS publication no. (ADM)85-1402.

26. American School Health Association, Association for the Advancement of Health Education, Society for Public Health Education. The national adolescent student health survey: a report on the health of America's youth. Oakland, California: Third Party Publishing Company, 1989.

27. Johnston LD, O'Malley PM, Bachman JG. Smoking, drinking, and illicit drug use among American secondary school students, college students, and young adults, 1975–1991. Vol. I. Rockville, Maryland: US Department of Health and Human Services, Public Health Service, National Institutes of Health, National Institute on Drug Abuse, 1992; NIH publication no. 93-3480.

28. CDC. Cigarette smoking among youth—United States, 1989. MMWR 1991;40:712–5.

29. CDC. Strategic plan for preventing human immunodeficiency virus (HIV) infection. Atlanta: US Department of Health and Human Services, Public Health Service, 1992.

30. American Public Health Association. Healthy communities 2000: model standards. Guidelines for community attainment of the year 2000 national health objectives. 3rd ed. Washington, DC: American Public Health Association, 1991.

31. CDC. Selected tobacco-use behaviors and dietary patterns among high school students—United States, 1991. MMWR 1992;41:417–21.

32. American Cancer Society. Cancer risk report: prevention and control. Atlanta: American Cancer Society, 1992.

33. CDC. Current tobacco, alcohol, marijuana, and cocaine use among high school students—United States, 1990. MMWR 1991;40:659–63.

34. National Education Goals Panel. Measuring progress toward the National Education Goals: potential indicators and measurement strategies—discussion document. Washington, DC: National Education Goals Panel, 1991.

35. Education Development Center. YRBSS: using adolescent risk behavior data. Network News: Comprehensive School Health Education 1991;2:7,9.

36. Nelson M. AIDS: an informational update and a look at AIDS infection during adolescence. Tennessee Teacher 1991:September;6–7,28–29.

37. Montana Office of Public Instruction, Montana Board of Crime Control. Montana Youth Risk Behavior Survey. Helena, Montana: Montana Office of Public Instruction and Montana Board of Crime, 1991.

38. Wyoming Department of Education. A healthy Wyoming: start with youth today. Results of the 1991 Wyoming Youth Risk Behavior and School Health Education Surveys. Cheyenne, Wyoming: Wyoming Department of Education, 1991.

39. Utah State Office of Education. Is this the place . . . for healthy kids? Results of the 1991 Utah Youth Risk Behavior and School Health Education Surveys. Salt Lake City, Utah: Utah State Office of Education, 1991.

40. Florida Department of Education. 1991 Florida Youth Risk Behavior Survey report. Tallahassee, Florida: Florida Department of Education, 1992.

41. Hawaii Department of Education. 1991 Hawaii Youth Risk Behavior Survey report. Honolulu, Hawaii: Department of Education, 1992.

42. New York State Education Department. New York State Youth Risk Behavior Survey: 1991 Findings. Albany, NY: New York State Education Department, 1992.

43. Felts WM, Chenier T, Barnes R. Drug use and suicide ideation and behavior among North Carolina public school students. Am J Public Health 1992; 82:870–2.

Pregnancy in Adolescents

Jacqueline B. Wilson, M.P.H.,[1] Stephanie J. Ventura, A.M.,[1]
Lisa M. Koonin, M.N., M.P.H.,[2] and Alison M. Spitz, M.S., M.P.H.[2]

PUBLIC HEALTH IMPORTANCE

In 1990, U.S. females aged 15–19 years had an estimated 1 million pregnancies and 521,826 births (1,2). More than 80% of these births were unintended—they occurred sooner than desired or were not wanted at any time (3). Surveillance data on adolescents' pregnancy, childbearing, and sexual behavior have been critical in assisting federal, state, and local agencies with program efforts to reduce pregnancy among teenagers. The monitoring of teenage pregnancy trends also provides a means for assessing the overall effects of intervention strategies to reduce unintended pregnancy among teens and for identifying subgroups of teens at special risk.

The adverse health and socioeconomic consequences of pregnancy and childbearing among teenagers are well recognized (4). Teenage mothers are more likely than older women to receive inadequate prenatal care and to experience inadequate weight gain during pregnancy, maternal anemia, and pregnancy-associated hypertension. Labor and delivery complications such as fetal distress are also reported more frequently for teenage mothers (5). Moreover, babies born to young mothers are at an increased risk of low birth weight, preterm birth, newborn anemia, respiratory distress syndrome, meconium aspiration, and assisted ventilation (1,4–7).

In addition to the substantial medical risks that pregnancy and childbearing pose to teenage mothers and their infants, other factors, such as socioeconomic status, also may play a major role in the high costs of pregnancy among teenagers (4). Adolescent mothers are more likely than older mothers to leave high school before graduation, to have decreased earning potential, and to live in poverty (4). Furthermore, early sexual activity can result in a higher risk for sexually transmitted diseases (STDs) (8), which can impair the future fertility and health of adolescents.

To gain some perspective on the public health importance of pregnancy among adolescents in the United States, we must evaluate the problem in a world context. In a 1985 study of pregnancy among teenagers in the United States and Western Europe, investigators found that although teenage fertility rates declined in both the United States and Western Europe in the early 1980s, the United States still had teenage pregnancy and birthrates considerably higher than rates in Canada, England, Wales, France, the Netherlands, and Sweden (9). Although U.S. rates of sexual activity were not dramatically different from rates in these countries, the effective use of contraceptives and access to contraceptive and abortion services differed considerably (9). More recent data show that U.S. teenage fertility rates continue to exceed European teenage fertility rates (10). For additional information about related topics and surveillance activities, see the Contraception, Sexually Transmitted Diseases, Human Immunodeficiency

---

[1] Division of Vital Statistics
National Center for Health Statistics
Centers for Disease Control and Prevention
Hyattsville, Maryland

[2] Division of Reproductive Health
National Center for Chronic Disease Prevention
    and Health Promotion
Centers for Disease Control and Prevention
Atlanta, Georgia

Virus, Unintended Pregnancy and Child-bearing, Legal Induced Abortion, Low Birth Weight and Intrauterine Growth Retardation, and Youth Risk Behavior chapters.

HISTORY OF DATA COLLECTION

The surveillance of pregnancy among adolescents requires the collection of data on live births, abortions, and sexual experience. Historically, these components have been collected by different organizations at different points in time. Since 1933, annual data on live births to teenage mothers and birthrates for teens have been available from CDC's National Center for Health Statistics.*

The national birth-registration area, established in 1915 with 10 states and the District of Columbia, contained all 48 states and the District of Columbia by 1933; data were added from Alaska in 1959 and from Hawaii in 1960.

Over the past three decades, CDC has established several surveillance systems for collecting information on adolescent pregnancy, child-bearing, abortion, and sexual experience. In the late 1960s, CDC established a mission of reducing unintended pregnancies among teens. In meeting that mission, CDC has assisted state and local family planning programs by providing them with analyses of state statistics on teenage pregnancy and evaluations of state and local programs. CDC has released national and state pregnancy and fertility data in a series of publications for federal, state, and local program planners and evaluators of family planning services (2,11–19).

In 1969, CDC began abortion surveillance activities to document the number and characteristics of women obtaining legal induced abor-

tions and in 1970 published CDC's first report on legal induced abortions. The term legal was used to contrast the reported abortions with the illegal or self-induced procedures that were frequent during that period. Since then, reports of annual abortion data have been published regularly. CDC and the Alan Guttmacher Institute, an independent nonprofit research organization, also report national abortion data (20–22). (For details about these collection and reporting activities, see the Legal Induced Abortion chapter.)

Data on the sexual behaviors of adolescents who have ever had sexual intercourse contribute to our understanding of adolescents at risk of becoming pregnant. The first surveys that measured sexual behavior among adolescent girls were the National Surveys of Young Women, conducted in 1971, 1976, and 1979 (23). These studies collected data on a variety of reproductive health issues, including sexual intercourse, contraceptive use, and pregnancy among females aged 15–19 years living in the United States.† Since 1982, the National Surveys of Family Growth (NSFGs) have collected data on these issues (as well as on fetal losses) from a sample of all U.S. females aged 15–44 years. The NSFG data have allowed us to calculate sexual experience and contraceptive use estimates for all adolescent girls and young women. In addition, CDC's school-based Youth Risk Behavior Surveys, first conducted in 1990, collect information from adolescents and young adults concerning their sexual behaviors and other risk factors for health (24). (For details about the NSFGs and the Youth Risk Behavior Surveys, see the Contraception and Youth Risk Behavior chapters.)

CDC SURVEILLANCE ACTIVITIES

Live Births

The birth data collected and reported by CDC are based on 100% of the birth certificates filed with state health departments. These data are

---

* CDC's National Center for Health Statistics (NCHS) and National Center for Chronic Disease Prevention and Health Promotion (NCCDPHP) are both involved in surveillance of pregnancy among adolescents. NCHS's pregnancy estimates are based on a composite of three outcomes of pregnancy—live births, induced abortions, and fetal losses. NCCDPHP estimates pregnancies as the sum of live births plus induced abortions (excluding spontaneous abortions or stillbirths); these estimates are based on the assumption that spontaneous abortions and stillbirths do not vary substantially for any group during the reporting period.

† The 1971 and 1976 surveys sampled women living in both metropolitan and nonmetropolitan areas; the 1979 survey included only women in metropolitan areas (23).

provided to CDC through the Vital Statistics Cooperative Program, which began in 1975 and has included all states since 1985. A birth certificate is filed for every birth occurring in the United States and includes maternal age, race, Hispanic origin, educational attainment, marital status, pregnancy history, and other basic sociodemographic and health information on infants and their mothers. The completeness of reporting is quite high for all of the information, although the accuracy of some variables has been questioned (see the Prenatal Care chapter). CDC periodically evaluates the quality and accuracy of the data (25).

Beginning in 1989, birth data by race have been tabulated primarily by race of the mother, as reported directly on the birth certificate. Before 1989, births were tabulated by race of the child, which was determined from the race of the parents as entered on the birth certificate. Details of current and former procedures concerning the tabulation of births by race are described elsewhere (1).

Abortions

CDC compiles annual tables of legal induced abortion data from 52 reporting areas: 50 states, New York City, and the District of Columbia (see the Legal Induced Abortion chapter). The total numbers of legal induced abortions are available from all reporting areas, most of which provide information on the characteristics of women obtaining abortions. Each year, for about 45 reporting areas, data are provided from central health agencies (i.e., state health departments and the health departments of New York City and the District of Columbia). For the remaining reporting areas, data are provided from hospitals and other medical facilities. No patient or physician identifiers are provided to CDC. Data are reported by the state in which the abortion occurred and are tabulated by the state of occurrence.

Population Estimates

Pregnancy and birthrates for 1990 and other census years are based on U.S. population

counts as of April 1 of each year. The 1990 census counts by race and age were modified to be consistent with the Office of Management and Budget's historical categories for birth data. The modification procedures are described in detail in a census bureau report (26). After each census, birthrates for the previous decade are revised on the basis of population counts for those years which have been revised to levels consistent with the latest census (27). Birth and fertility rates based on revised population counts for 1981–1989 have been published elsewhere (1,27).

GENERAL FINDINGS

National Data

Small declines in pregnancy and birthrates among teenagers during the early 1980s subsequently reversed, resulting in relatively little net change in these rates over the decade (1,2). Women who were teenagers in the late 1980s were born during the early 1970s, after the baby boom and during a period when birthrates dropped to historic low levels. The actual number of pregnancies among adolescent females declined about 14% between 1980 and 1988 (the most recent year for which national pregnancy data are available), as the number of teenage women fell. The total teenage pregnancy rate was about the same in 1980 and 1988 (110 per 1,000 females aged 15–19 years) and showed only slight changes in rates among ethnic groups. Although overall pregnancy rates changed little during the 1980s, distinctive differences were observed in the trends for live birth and abortion rates—the two principal components of the pregnancy rate (1,2,28–31).

Live Births

Despite the declining number of U.S. teenagers, the number of births among teens aged 15–19 years increased by 12% between 1986 and 1991 (the most recent year for which live birth data are available), to 519,577 (4). After declining 5% between 1980 and 1986, the birthrate for teenagers (the number of live births per 1,000 females aged 15–19 years) increased

20% between 1986 and 1990, to 59.9 births per 1,000 females aged 15–19 years, and increased an additional 4% in 1991, to 62.1 per 1,000. The birthrate for teens aged 15–17 years increased 27% between 1986 and 1991, to 38.7 per 1,000, and the rate for older teens aged 18–19 years increased to 94.4 per 1,000 *(32)*. The 27% rise in birthrates for teens aged 15–17 years translated into >40,000 additional births in 1991 than would have occurred had the 1991 rate equaled the 1986 rate.

Two factors, in particular, have contributed to the continued rise in birthrates among U.S. teenagers—the growing proportion of teenagers who are sexually experienced and the growing proportion of Hispanic teenage births:

- In 1990, 52% of teens aged 15–19 years were sexually experienced (had ever had sexual intercourse) (Figure 1), compared with 42% in 1982 *(29)*. The proportion of females aged 15–19 years who were sexually experienced increased between 1982 and 1990, with 42% of 15-year-old girls and 69% of 19-year-old women being sexually experienced in 1990. Although the pregnancy rate for sexually experienced teens actually declined during the 1980s, from 262 pregnancies per 1,000 females

in 1980 to 215 per 1,000 in 1988 *(2)*, a higher proportion of teens were sexually experienced, so the overall pregnancy rate stayed about the same.

- In 1991, 20% of teenage births were among Hispanics *(32)*. Hispanics, who are predominantly white (97%), have much higher fertility rates than non-Hispanic whites at all ages, but particularly at ages <20 years. For example, the birthrate for Hispanic teenagers 15–19 years of age was 106.7 per 1,000 in 1991, compared with 42.7 per 1,000 for non-Hispanic white teenagers *(32)*. Moreover, the Hispanic teenage population has increased considerably in recent years, while the non-Hispanic white teenage population has declined *(27)*. Thus, the rapid rise in birthrates for white teenagers since the mid-1980s results in part from the combined effects of the growing proportion of white teenagers who are Hispanic and the higher fertility rates in this population.

Legal Induced Abortions

The abortion rate for young women aged 15–19 years (the number of abortions per 1,000 teenagers) increased slightly from 42.7 per 1,000

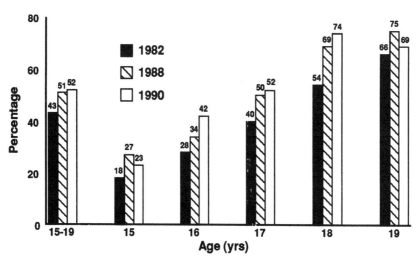

FIGURE 1. Percentage of females 15–19 years of age who have had sex — United States, 1982, 1988, and 1990

Source: National Surveys of Family Growth.

372

teenagers in 1980 to 44.0 per 1,000 in 1988 *(2)*. The teenage abortion ratio (the number of abortions per 1,000 live births among women 15–19 years of age) rose from 491 per 1,000 in 1974 to a peak of 727 per 1,000 in 1983 *(30)*, then declined to 515 per 1,000 by 1990 *(28)*. This decrease in the abortion ratio indicates that a greater proportion of teenage pregnancies are ending in live births. Although the abortion ratios for this age-group remain higher than those for older women, the proportion of all legal abortions obtained by teenagers has steadily decreased over time—from 31% of all legal induced abortions in 1974 to 21% in 1990 *(28,30)*

State Data

From 1980 to 1990, state pregnancy rates for U.S. teenagers aged 15–19 years have changed little. However, because declines in abortion rates were generally greater than declines in pregnancy rates, state birthrate trends between 1980 and 1990 were most likely to reflect increases *(17,19)*.

In 1990, pregnancy, live birth, and abortion rates for females 15–19 years old varied widely by state, race, and Hispanic origin (Table 1). For example, rates of pregnancy ranged from 56 pregnancies per 1,000 females to 111 per 1,000. Birthrates ranged from 33 births per 1,000 females to 81 per 1,000. Abortion rates varied even more, ranging from 6 abortions per 1,000 females to 49 per 1,000. In most states, rates of pregnancy and live births for blacks were higher than rates for whites and Hispanics (Table 1); these racial and ethnic differences are related to socioeconomic factors rather than to race per se *(19)*.

INTERPRETATION ISSUES

When evaluating pregnancy trends among adolescents, we must consider whether the pregnancy rates are based on the entire adolescent population or just sexually experienced adolescents. With the first method, the rate represents the number of pregnancies (or live births

or abortions) to females in a given age-group (e.g., aged 15–19 years) per 1,000 females in that group. With the second method, the rate represents the number of pregnancies (or live births or abortions) among women in a given age-group per 1,000 sexually experienced females in that group.

Monitoring pregnancy rates among sexually experienced teenagers provides a more accurate picture of trends in pregnancy rates because it describes the experience of the population actually at risk for becoming pregnant. In addition, this measure enhances the evaluation of the efficacy of family planning programs that target subgroups of teens at high risk for pregnancy.

The current CDC system for collecting and analyzing data on pregnancies among adolescents has some limitations. For example, the timeliness and availability of birth certificate data pose methodologic challenges. Birth certificate data have an important advantage in that virtually all births are registered in the United States. However, the availability and timeliness of birth certificate data for the country as a whole are directly affected by how quickly each state provides its data to CDC. Currently, detailed birth data for a given year are available about 18 months after the end of that year.

Another limitation is that the total number of legal abortions reported to CDC in a given year is lower than the number of abortions actually performed. The total number of abortions reported by CDC remains about 16%–18% lower than the number reported by the Alan Guttmacher Institute, which obtains information directly from abortion providers *(30)*.[§] Although 10 states do not collect data on the age of women obtaining abortions, CDC has developed procedures to calculate national estimates of pregnancy among teenagers rates *(2,17,19)*. In 1990, the abortion reports from states that lacked age information represented about 39% of the abortions reported to CDC.

There are also limitations in interpreting data on adolescent pregnancy, related, in part, to the

---

[§] The last year for which the Alan Guttmacher Institute reported abortion survey data was 1988.

TABLE 1. Pregnancy rates* and birthrates† for females 15–19 years old, by race and Hispanic origin§ — United States, 1990

	Pregnancy Rate				Birthrate			
	Total¶	White**	Black	Hispanic	Total	White	Black	Hispanic
Alabama	††	††	††	††	71.0	55.3	105.3	33.8
Alaska	††	††	††	††	65.3	53.8	§§	§§
Arizona	101.8	99.9	153.5	145.0	75.5	72.3	115.1	123.3
Arkansas	98.4	82.7	157.2	¶¶	80.1	66.2	131.9	§§
California	††	††	††	††	70.6	73.9	101.0	112.3
Colorado	82.3	¶¶	¶¶	¶¶	54.5	52.1	105.9	110.6
Connecticut	††	††	††	††	38.8	30.5	102.5	121.9
Delaware	††	††	††	††	54.5	37.4	120.4	§§
District of Columbia	255.2	††	††	††	93.1	11.8	121.4	88.7
Florida	††	††	††	††	69.1	52.9	135.0	60.2
Georgia	110.8	86.2	162.5	87.5	75.5	56.6	116.2	73.0
Hawaii	88.2	¶¶	¶¶	¶¶	61.2	42.0	§§	§§
Idaho	58.8	58.6	§§	126.0	50.6	50.3	§§	118.6
Illinois	††	††	††	††	62.9	44.3	144.2	94.8
Indiana	74.3	65.5	158.0	76.4	58.6	51.9	122.4	64.5
Iowa	††	††	††	††	40.5	38.5	119.1	79.9
Kansas	81.1	74.5	181.1	99.3	56.1	50.8	131.9	86.1
Kentucky	91.0	84.3	164.1	††	67.6	63.5	115.8	§§
Louisiana	92.1	68.7	128.8***	††	74.2	52.1	109.1	20.9
Maine	68.4	67.6	§§	††	43.0	42.7	§§	§§
Maryland	84.7	61.5	141.8	††	53.2	36.0	95.5	46.0
Massachusetts	71.1	††	††	††	35.1	30.9	89.5	121.1
Michigan	85.2	††	††	††	59.0	43.1	131.1	94.4
Minnesota	62.0	55.3	219.4	89.9	36.3	30.6	151.7	79.4
Mississippi	97.8	71.6	130.5	§§	81.0	55.5	112.7	§§
Missouri	82.6	64.8	197.5	57.0	62.8	50.3	143.9	46.4
Montana	81.7	¶¶	¶¶	¶¶	48.4	39.7	§§	§§
Nebraska	74.2	††	††	††	42.3	36.9	135.1	81.7
Nevada	107.5	105.8	156.8	112.8	73.3	68.9	129.3	107.5
New Hampshire	††	††	††	††	33.0	33.1	§§	†††
New Jersey	75.3	52.7	181.6	115.1	40.5	28.1	99.6	79.9
New Mexico	100.4	99.6	115.5	122.2	78.2	75.6	94.6	96.9
New York	92.9	76.3	166.4	136.8	43.6	36.7	75.6	81.6
North Carolina	106.4	86.3	157.3	§§	67.6	52.0	106.6	106.1
North Dakota	56.4	50.4	§§	§§	35.4	29.2	§§	§§
Ohio	74.5	60.5	170.1	83.2	57.9	47.7	129.4	73.9
Oklahoma	††	††	††	††	66.8	60.2	116.0	†††
Oregon	89.2	88.7	178.0	134.3	54.6	54.0	108.0	113.9
Pennsylvania	74.6	††	††	††	44.9	35.1	124.8	126.1
Rhode Island	87.7	80.4	198.9	134.9	43.9	38.7	114.3	129.8
South Carolina	95.0	76.6	127.0	84.5	71.3	54.3	101.1	66.8
South Dakota	56.9	46.0	§§	††	46.8	35.0	§§	§§
Tennessee	101.8	86.3	165.6	56.2	72.3	60.3	121.3	40.9
Texas	102.8	96.1	153.6	124.5	75.3	70.6	114.0	103.8

374

TABLE 1. Pregnancy rates* and birthrates† for females 15–19 years old, by race and Hispanic origin§ — United States, 1990 — continued

	Pregnancy Rate				Birthrate			
	Total¶	White**	Black	Hispanic	Total	White	Black	Hispanic
Utah	63.0	62.2	§§	128.7	48.5	47.8	§§	115.0
Vermont	72.1	72.7	§§	§§	34.0	34.3	§§	§§
Virginia	86.5	70.4	149.1	74.4	52.9	41.1	98.5	55.5
Washington	95.4	¶¶	¶¶	¶¶	53.1	52.2	94.3	113.4
West Virginia	67.4	66.4	103.9	§§	57.3	57.1	74.4	§§
Wisconsin	66.6	††	††	††	42.6	31.2	174.7	90.4
Wyoming	62.2	††	††	††	56.3	54.5	§§	94.2

* Pregnancy rate equals live births plus legal induced abortions per 1,000 females aged 15–19 years; fetal losses are excluded.
† Birthrate equals live births per 1,000 females aged 15–19 years.
§ Persons of Hispanic origin may be of any race.
¶ Includes all racial/ethnic groups.
** In the calculation of pregnancy rates, abortions by white race included women of Hispanic origin. Kentucky, Louisiana, Maine, Maryland, North Carolina, and South Dakota did not report abortion data by Hispanic origin.
†† Pregnancy rates for states with unknown abortion data could not be calculated.
§§ Pregnancy rates and birthrates were not calculated for states with ≤20 births among teenagers in 1990 or ≤1,000 females aged 15–19 years in the respective racial/ethnic group.
¶¶ Pregnancy rates were not calculated because ≥15% of abortions were of unknown race/ethnicity.
*** Includes black and other races.
††† New Hampshire and Oklahoma did not report Hispanic origin on the birth certificate.

lack of a coordinated national pregnancy surveillance system. The data used to monitor adolescent pregnancy are obtained by several data collection systems that have different methodologies. In addition, the frequency of data collection varies greatly among the systems; some systems collect data annually, whereas others collect data only periodically.

EXAMPLES OF USING DATA

By periodically evaluating pregnancy and birthrates, states can improve their policy and program planning for health services, prevention activities, and support programs for pregnant teenagers and teenage mothers. Many state and local health departments have used these data extensively:

- To evaluate program interventions for pregnancy among adolescents.

- To assist with targeting program efforts among subpopulations of teenagers at high risk of pregnancy.

- To increase awareness of adolescent pregnancy among parents, teachers, community leaders, and legislators.

FUTURE ISSUES

The year 2000 national health objectives, which have helped us to establish guidelines to monitor the nation's health, include several goals related to adolescent pregnancy. These include objectives to decrease adolescent and unintended pregnancies, delay the onset of sexual activity among adolescents, reduce the number of adolescents who have sex at young ages, and increase the proportion of sexually active adolescents who use contraceptives effectively *(33)*. Anticipated improvements in surveillance methodology, expansion of surveillance activities, and technological advances are likely to help us better measure our progress toward meeting these goals.

Improvements in Surveillance Methodology

A major improvement to vital statistics reporting is reflected in the 1989 revision of the U.S. Standard Certificate of Live Birth (Figure 2). It includes a number of new items on medical and lifestyle risk factors related to pregnancy and birth as well as items on obstetric procedures performed, method of delivery, abnormal conditions and congenital anomalies of the

FIGURE 2.

TYPE/PRINT IN PERMANENT BLACK INK FOR INSTRUCTIONS SEE HANDBOOK

U.S. STANDARD
CERTIFICATE OF LIVE BIRTH

LOCAL FILE NUMBER | BIRTH NUMBER

CHILD

1. CHILD'S NAME (First, Middle, Last)
2. DATE OF BIRTH (Month, Day, Year)
3. TIME OF BIRTH ___ M
4. SEX
5. CITY, TOWN, OR LOCATION OF BIRTH
6. COUNTY OF BIRTH
7. PLACE OF BIRTH: ☐ Hospital ☐ Freestanding Birthing Center ☐ Clinic/Doctor's Office ☐ Residence ☐ Other (Specify) _____
8. FACILITY NAME (If not institution, give street and number)

CERTIFIER/ATTENDANT

DEATH UNDER ONE YEAR OF AGE Enter State File Number of death certificate for this child

9. I certify that this child was born alive at the place and time and on the date stated. Signature ▶
10. DATE SIGNED (Month, Day, Year)
11. ATTENDANT'S NAME AND TITLE (If other than certifier) (Type/Print) Name _____ ☐ M.D. ☐ D.O. ☐ C.N.M. ☐ Other Midwife ☐ Other (Specify)
12. CERTIFIER'S NAME AND TITLE (Type/Print) Name _____ ☐ M.D. ☐ D.O. ☐ Hospital Admin. ☐ C.N.M. ☐ Other Midwife ☐ Other (Specify)
13. ATTENDANT'S MAILING ADDRESS (Street and Number or Rural Route Number, City or Town, State, Zip Code)
14. REGISTRAR'S SIGNATURE ▶
15. DATE FILED BY REGISTRAR (Month, Day, Year)

MOTHER

16a. MOTHER'S NAME (First, Middle, Last)
16b. MAIDEN SURNAME
17. DATE OF BIRTH (Month, Day, Year)
18. BIRTHPLACE (State or Foreign Country)
19a. RESIDENCE—STATE
19b. COUNTY
19c. CITY, TOWN, OR LOCATION
19d. STREET AND NUMBER
19e. INSIDE CITY LIMITS? (Yes or no)
20. MOTHER'S MAILING ADDRESS (If same as residence, enter Zip Code only)

FATHER

21. FATHER'S NAME (First, Middle, Last)
22. DATE OF BIRTH (Month, Day, Year)
23. BIRTHPLACE (State or Foreign Country)

INFORMANT

24. I certify that the personal information provided on this certificate is correct to the best of my knowledge and belief. Signature of Parent or Other Informant ▶

INFORMATION FOR MEDICAL AND HEALTH USE ONLY

MULTIPLE BIRTHS Enter State File Number for Mate(s) LIVE BIRTH(S)

FETAL DEATH(S)

MOTHER

25. OF HISPANIC ORIGIN? (Specify No or Yes—If yes, specify Cuban, Mexican, Puerto Rican, etc.)
26. RACE—American Indian, Black, White, etc. (Specify below)
27. EDUCATION (Specify only highest grade completed) Elementary/Secondary (0-12) | College (1-4 or 5+)

25a. ☐ No ☐ Yes Specify:
26a.
27a.

FATHER

25b. ☐ No ☐ Yes Specify:
26b.
27b.

28. PREGNANCY HISTORY (Complete each section)

LIVE BIRTHS (Do not include this child)

OTHER TERMINATIONS (Spontaneous and induced at any time after conception)

28a. Now Living Number _____ ☐ None
28b. Now Dead Number _____ ☐ None
28d. Number _____ ☐ None

28c. DATE OF LAST LIVE BIRTH (Month, Year)
28e. DATE OF LAST OTHER TERMINATION (Month, Year)

29. MOTHER MARRIED? (At birth, conception, or any time between) (Yes or no)
30. DATE LAST NORMAL MENSES BEGAN (Month, Day, Year)
31. MONTH OF PREGNANCY PRENATAL CARE BEGAN—First, Second, Third, etc. (Specify)
32. PRENATAL VISITS—Total Number (If none, so state)
33. BIRTH WEIGHT (Specify unit)
34. CLINICAL ESTIMATE OF GESTATION (Weeks)
35a. PLURALITY—Single, Twin, Triplet, etc. (Specify)
35b. IF NOT SINGLE BIRTH—Born First, Second, Third, etc. (Specify)

36. APGAR SCORE
36a. 1 Minute
36b. 5 Minutes

37a. MOTHER TRANSFERRED PRIOR TO DELIVERY? ☐ No ☐ Yes If Yes, enter name of facility transferred from:
37b. INFANT TRANSFERRED? ☐ No ☐ Yes If Yes, enter name of facility transferred to:

38a. MEDICAL RISK FACTORS FOR THIS PREGNANCY (Check all that apply)

Anemia (Hct. <30/Hgb. <10)	01 ☐
Cardiac disease	02 ☐
Acute or chronic lung disease	03 ☐
Diabetes	04 ☐
Genital herpes	05 ☐
Hydramnios/Oligohydramnios	06 ☐
Hemoglobinopathy	07 ☐
Hypertension, chronic	08 ☐
Hypertension, pregnancy-associated	09 ☐
Eclampsia	10 ☐
Incompetent cervix	11 ☐
Previous infant 4000+ grams	12 ☐
Previous preterm or small for gestational age infant	13 ☐
Renal disease	14 ☐
Rh sensitization	15 ☐
Uterine bleeding	16 ☐
None	00 ☐
Other	17 ☐
(Specify)	

38b. OTHER RISK FACTORS FOR THIS PREGNANCY (Complete all items)

Tobacco use during pregnancy ☐ Yes ☐ No
Average number cigarettes per day _____
Alcohol use during pregnancy ☐ Yes ☐ No
Average number drinks per week _____
Weight gained during pregnancy _____ lbs.

39. OBSTETRIC PROCEDURES (Check all that apply)

Amniocentesis	01 ☐
Electronic fetal monitoring	02 ☐
Induction of labor	03 ☐
Stimulation of labor	04 ☐
Tocolysis	05 ☐
Ultrasound	06 ☐
None	00 ☐
Other	07 ☐
(Specify)	

40. COMPLICATIONS OF LABOR AND/OR DELIVERY (Check all that apply)

Febrile (>100°F. or 38°C.)	01 ☐
Meconium, moderate/heavy	02 ☐
Premature rupture of membrane (>12 hours)	03 ☐
Abruptio placenta	04 ☐
Placenta previa	05 ☐
Other excessive bleeding	06 ☐
Seizures during labor	07 ☐
Precipitous labor (<3 hours)	08 ☐
Prolonged labor (>20 hours)	09 ☐
Dysfunctional labor	10 ☐
Breech/Malpresentation	11 ☐
Cephalopelvic disproportion	12 ☐
Cord prolapse	13 ☐
Anesthetic complications	14 ☐
Fetal distress	15 ☐
None	00 ☐
Other	16 ☐
(Specify)	

41. METHOD OF DELIVERY (Check all that apply)

Vaginal	01 ☐
Vaginal birth after previous C-section	02 ☐
Primary C-section	03 ☐
Repeat C-section	04 ☐
Forceps	05 ☐
Vacuum	06 ☐

42. ABNORMAL CONDITIONS OF THE NEWBORN (Check all that apply)

Anemia (Hct. <39/Hgb. <13)	01 ☐
Birth injury	02 ☐
Fetal alcohol syndrome	03 ☐
Hyaline membrane disease/RDS	04 ☐
Meconium aspiration syndrome	05 ☐
Assisted ventilation <30 min	06 ☐
Assisted ventilation ≥30 min	07 ☐
Seizures	08 ☐
None	00 ☐
Other	09 ☐
(Specify)	

43. CONGENITAL ANOMALIES OF CHILD (Check all that apply)

Anencephalus	01 ☐
Spina bifida/Meningocele	02 ☐
Hydrocephalus	03 ☐
Microcephalus	04 ☐
Other central nervous system anomalies (Specify)	05 ☐
Heart malformations	06 ☐
Other circulatory/respiratory anomalies (Specify)	07 ☐
Rectal atresia/stenosis	08 ☐
Tracheo esophageal fistula/Esophageal atresia	09 ☐
Omphalocele/Gastroschisis	10 ☐
Other gastrointestinal anomalies (Specify)	11 ☐
Malformed genitalia	12 ☐
Renal agenesis	13 ☐
Other urogenital anomalies (Specify)	14 ☐
Cleft lip/palate	15 ☐
Polydactyly/Syndactyly/Adactyly	16 ☐
Club foot	17 ☐
Diaphragmatic hernia	18 ☐
Other musculoskeletal/integumental anomalies (Specify)	19 ☐
Down's syndrome	20 ☐
Other chromosomal anomalies (Specify)	21 ☐
None	00 ☐
Other	22 ☐
(Specify)	

DEPARTMENT OF HEALTH AND HUMAN SERVICES PUBLIC HEALTH SERVICE NATIONAL CENTER FOR HEALTH STATISTICS – 1989 REVISION

PHS T-002 REV 1/89

infant, birth attendants, place of delivery, and Hispanic origin of the parents. This major enhancement of medical and health data on mothers and babies greatly expands the scope of information on pregnancy outcomes among both teenagers and adults in the United States *(34)*.

In addressing data needs for the year 2000 health objectives, the NSFG is improving the collection of data on a number of topics related to the risk of pregnancy among adolescents. New questions will collect information on the respondent's family background, such as the family members with whom the girl lived during childhood *(35)*. Data on the characteristics of the respondent's first sexual partner and the nature of that relationship may help us better understand adolescent sexuality and pregnancy; the 1994 NSFG includes questions related to this topic. Previous NSFGs have oversampled black women to permit better group-specific estimates on reproductive health concerns; the 1994 survey is oversampling Hispanic women as well.

Expansion of Surveillance Activities

In addition to releasing reports of state pregnancy and birthrates, CDC also plans to publish national 1980–1990 estimates of pregnancy rates for sexually experienced teens aged 15–19 years as well as national pregnancy and birth trends among girls <15 years of age.

Technologic Advances

The electronic collection and reporting of data will promote more timely collection and more rapid dissemination of surveillance data. A number of states have already started electronically transmitting birth certificate data to help speed up preparation of vital statistics data, which is especially important in monitoring trends in adolescent pregnancy.

Among the technologies that will improve survey research and data collection are computer-

assisted personal interviewing, computer-assisted telephone interviewing, and audio computer-assisted self-interviewing. All of these technologies will be used in the upcoming NSFGs this decade.

Trends in Reproductive Health

Changes in contraceptive technology—such as the use of longer-acting contraceptives (e.g., the Norplant® System and Depo-Provera®) and postcoital contraceptives—are likely to affect pregnancy rates among young women and may enable them to postpone childbirth until they are out of their teens. If additional contraceptive methods or nonsurgical methods of abortion become available in this country, they may also affect teenage pregnancy rates and may require alterations in pregnancy surveillance methodology *(36)*.

Given that adolescent girls are becoming sexually active at younger ages and that their use of barrier contraceptives is less effective than use among adult women, their risk of exposure to STDs is a valid concern *(8)*. Rates of STDs such as chlamydia and syphilis have been increasing among teenage girls. Several STDs have long-term effects on fertility, but whether this increasing rate of STD infection will alter the fertility rate of teens remains to be determined (see the Sexually Transmitted Diseases chapter). Reproductive health issues such as these will challenge adolescent pregnancy surveillance and reporting in the 1990s.

Teenage pregnancy remains a significant and complex public health concern. Timely surveillance of teenage pregnancy—at both the national and state levels—is crucial for monitoring pregnancy, birth, and abortion trends and for assessing the effects of efforts to reduce unintended pregnancy. By monitoring all of the components of teenage pregnancy, states can collect data that are critical to monitoring and evaluating family planning programs, identifying and assisting adolescents at high risk, and implementing additional activities to reduce teenage pregnancy.

377

REFERENCES

1. NCHS. Advance report of final natality statistics, 1990. Hyattsville, Maryland: US Department of Health and Human Services, Public Health Service, CDC, 1993. (Monthly vital statistics report; vol. 41, no. 9, suppl.)

2. Ventura SJ, Taffel SM, Mosher WD, Henshaw S. Trends in pregnancies and pregnancy rates, United States, 1980–88. Hyattsville, Maryland: US Department of Health and Human Services, Public Health Service, CDC, NCHS, 1992. (Monthly vital statistics report; vol. 41, no. 6, suppl.)

3. Piccinino LJ. Unintended pregnancy and childbearing in the United States: 1973–1990. Hyattsville, Maryland: US Department of Health and Human Services, Public Health Service, CDC, NCHS, 1994 (in press). (Advance data from vital and health statistics.)

4. Hofferth SL, Hayes CD, eds. Risking the future: adolescent sexuality, pregnancy, and childbearing. Washington, DC: National Academy Press, 1987.

5. NCHS. Advance report of maternal and infant health data from the 1990 birth certificate. Hyattsville, Maryland: US Department of Health and Human Services, Public Health Service, CDC, 1992. (Monthly vital statistics report; vol. 42 no. 2, suppl.)

6. NCHS. Vital statistics of the United States, 1988. Vol. I, natality. Hyattsville, Maryland: US Department of Health and Human Services, Public Health Service, CDC, 1990.

7. Taffel SM. Trends in low birth weight, United States, 1975–85. Hyattsville, Maryland: US Department of Health and Human Services, Public Health Service, CDC, NCHS, 1989. (Vital and health statistics; Series 21, no. 48.)

8. Kost K, Forrest JD. American women's sexual behavior and exposure to sexually transmitted diseases. Fam Plann Perspect 1992;24:244–54.

9. Jones EF, Forrest JD, Goldman N, et al. Teenage pregnancy in developed countries: determinants and policy implications. Fam Plann Perspect 1985;17: 53–63.

10. David HP. European perspectives. Presented at the CPR/NICHD Workshop on Negotiating the Paths to Parenthood, Bethesda, Maryland, February 8–9, 1993.

11. Ventura SJ, Taffel SM, Mosher WD. Estimates of pregnancies and pregnancy rates for the United States, 1976–81. Public Health Rep 1985;100:31–4.

12. Ventura SJ, Taffel SM, Mosher WD. Estimates of pregnancies and pregnancy rates for the United States, 1976-85. Am J Public Health 1988;78: 506–11.

13. CDC. Teenage pregnancy and fertility in the United States: 1970, 1974, 1980. Regional and state variations and unintended fertility. Atlanta: CDC, 1987.

14. Maciak BJ, Spitz AM, Strauss LT, Morris L, Warren CW, Marks JS. Pregnancy and birth rates among sexually experienced US teenagers—1974, 1980, and 1983. JAMA 1987;285:2069–71.

15. CDC. Teenage fertility in the United States. Atlanta: CDC, 1978.

16. CDC. Texas fertility: childbearing patterns and trends. Atlanta: CDC, 1980.

17. CDC. Teenage pregnancy and birth rates—United States, 1990. MMWR 1993;42:733-7.

18. Spitz AM, Strauss LT, Maciak BJ, Morris L. Teenage pregnancy and fertility in the United States, 1970, 1974, and 1980. MMWR 1987;36(No. 1SS): 1-10.

19. Spitz AM, Ventura SJ, Koonin L, et al. State teenage pregnancy and birth rates—United States, 1980 and 1990. MMWR 1993;42(No. SS-6): in press.

20. Kochanek KD. Induced terminations of pregnancy: reporting states, 1988. Hyattsville, Maryland: US Department of Health and Human Services, Public Health Service, CDC, NCHS, 1991; DHHS publication no.(PHS)91-1120. (Monthly vital statistics report; vol. 39, no. 12, suppl.)

21. Henshaw SK, Forrest JD, Van Vort J. Abortion services in the United States, 1987 and 1988. Fam Plann Perspect 1990;22:102–8.

22. Henshaw SK, Van Vort J, eds. Abortion factbook, 1992 edition: readings, trends, and state and local data to 1988. New York: Alan Guttmacher Institute, 1993.

23. Zelnik M, Kantner JF. Sexual activity, contraceptive use and pregnancy among metropolitan-area teenagers: 1971–1979. Fam Plann Perspect 1980; 12:230–1, 233–7.

24. Kolbe LJ. An epidemiological surveillance system to monitor the prevalence of youth behaviors that most affect health. Health Educ 1990;21:44–8.

25. Schoendorf KC, Parker JD, Batkhan LZ, Kiely JL. Comparability of the birth certificate and 1988 Maternal and Infant Health Survey. Hyattsville, Maryland: US Department of Health and Human Services, Public Health Service, CDC, NCHS, 1993. (Vital and health statistics; series 2, no. 116.)

26. US Bureau of the Census. Age, sex, race, and Hispanic origin information from the 1990 census: a comparison of results with results where age and race have been modified. Washington, DC: US Department of Commerce, 1991.

27. US Bureau of the Census. U.S. population estimates, by age, sex, race, and Hispanic origin: 1980 to 1991. Washington, DC: US Department of Commerce, Economics and Statistics Administration, US Bureau of the Census, 1992. (Current population reports; series P25, no. 1095.

28. Koonin L, Smith JC, Ramick M. Abortion surveillance—United States, 1990. MMWR 1993;42(No. SS-6) (in press).

29. Forrest JD, Singh S. The sexual and reproductive behavior of American women, 1982–1988. Fam Plann Perspect 1990;22:206-14.

30. CDC. Abortion surveillance: United States, 1974. Atlanta: CDC, 1976.

31. Atrash HK, Lawson HW, Smith JC. Legal abortion in the US: trends and mortality. Contemp Obstet Gynecol 1990;35:58–69.

32. NCHS. Advance report of final natality statistics, 1991. Hyattsville, Maryland: US Department of Health and Human Services, Public Health Service, CDC, 1993. (Monthly vital statistics report; vol. 42, no. 3, suppl.)

33. Public Health Service. Healthy people 2000: national health promotion and disease prevention objectives. Washington, DC: US Department of Health and Human Services, Public Health Service, 1990; DHHS Publication No.(PHS)91-50212.

34. Taffel SM, Ventura SJ, Gay GA. Revised US Certificate of Birth: new opportunities for research on birth outcome. BIRTH 1989;16:188–93.

35. Young EW, Jensen LC, Olsen JA, Cundick BP. The effects of family structure on the sexual behavior of adolescents. Adolescence 1991;26:977–86.

36. Klitsch M. RU486: the science and the politics. New York: Alan Guttmacher Institute, 1989.

Unintentional Injuries and Violence

Suzanne M. Smith, M.D., M.P.H.,[1] Joseph E. Sniezek, M.D., M.P.H.,[2]
Arlene I. Greenspan, P.T., M.P.H., Dr.P.H.,[2]
Julie C. Russell, Ph.D.,[1] David Thurman, M.D., M.P.H.,[2]
Christine M. Branche-Dorsey, Ph.D., M.S.P.H.,[1]
and Juan G. Rodriguez, M.D., M.P.H.[1,3]

PUBLIC HEALTH IMPORTANCE

Whereas injuries are the leading cause of death for all Americans <45 years of age, the overall injury rate is highest among older adolescents and young adults (1).[*] Among children and adolescents, injuries have different patterns in different age-groups, largely as a result of varying developmental levels and the activities that these levels influence. Adolescents engage in activities that reflect the turbulence of the transition from childhood to adulthood. Compared with younger children, adolescents are more frequently exposed to certain risk factors, such as motor vehicles and firearms, yet they may not have developed the skills, experience, or judgment to reduce their injury risks. Early experiences with alcohol and other drugs may further increase their risk for injury.

Injury-Related Mortality

Unintentional injuries are the leading cause of death among young persons 10–14, 15–19, and 20–24 years of age (Table 1). Fifty-six percent of injury deaths before 20 years of age occur among adolescents, even though they account for only 26% of the pediatric (under 20 years of age) population (1). The overall rate of fatal injuries among adolescents increases dramatically with age. The injury fatality rate is almost five times greater among adolescents 15–19 years of age than it is among those aged 10–14 years; the injury fatality rate then increases about 20% for persons 20–24 years of age. Injuries account for more than three fourths of all deaths

among adolescents 15–19 years of age. Older adolescents and young adults are at a particularly increased risk of death from motor vehicle crashes, suicides, and homicides. Of all motor vehicle crash deaths that occur before the age of 20 years, 75% occur among adolescents 15–19 years of age, compared with 87% of suicides and 62% of homicides occurring before the age of 20 years (1).

Injury-Related Morbidity

Nonfatal injury data are not available nationally. Estimates based on certain hospital-based studies demonstrate injury hospitalization rates to be six to nine times higher for adolescents than for younger children (2). Adolescents 15–19 years of age account for more than three fourths of nonfatal injuries and direct care costs among persons <20 years of age.

Rates of severe disabling conditions such as traumatic head and spinal cord injuries increase

[1] Division of Unintentional Injury Prevention
National Center for Injury Prevention and Control
Centers for Disease Control and Prevention
Atlanta, Georgia

[2] Division of Acute Care, Rehabilitation Research,
and Disability Prevention
National Center for Injury Prevention and Control
Centers for Disease Control and Prevention
Atlanta, Georgia

[3] Deceased

Acknowledgments

For their contributions to this chapter, we thank David Lawrence, R.N., M.P.H., Louisiana Department of Health and Hospitals; and Marcella Hammett, M.P.H., Kenneth E. Powell, M.D., M.P.H., and Joseph L. Annest, Ph.D., National Center for Injury Prevention and Control, Centers for Disease Control and Prevention.

[*] In this chapter, we focus on older children, adolescents, and young adults in three age-groups: 10–14, 15–19, and 20–24 years.

TABLE 1. Ten leading causes of death,* by age-group — United States, 1990

Rank	Age-groups (years)		
	10–14	15–19	20–24
1	Unintentional injuries 1,897	Unintentional injuries 7,561	Unintentional injuries 8,680
2	Malignant neoplasms 525	Homicide 3,042	Homicide 4,312
3	Homicide 356	Suicide 1,979	Suicide 2,890
4	Suicide 258	Malignant neoplasms 759	Malignant neoplasms 1,060
5	Heart disease 184	Heart disease 344	Heart disease 573
6	Congenital anomalies 182	Congenital anomalies 224	Human immunodeficiency virus 493
7	Bronchitis, emphysema, and asthma 81	Pneumonia and influenza 85	Congenital anomalies 267
8	Pneumonia and influenza 58	Bronchitis, emphysema, and asthma 82	Cerebrovascular disease 160
9	Benign neoplasms 47	Cerebrovascular disease 74	Pneumonia and influenza 146
10	Cerebrovascular disease 40	Human immunodeficiency virus 48	Bronchitis, emphysema, and asthma 96

* Cause and number of deaths are represented in each cell.

Source: NCHS mortality tapes.

dramatically among adolescents compared with younger children. Preliminary data reported to CDC from four states indicate that in 1990–1991, the rate of spinal cord injury (per 1 million population) was 5.3 for children <5 years of age, 9.8 for children 5–14 years of age, and 71.1 for adolescents 15–19 years of age *(Sniezek JE, unpublished data, 1993)*. This increase in traumatic spinal cord injuries was particularly dramatic for males.

Cross-National Comparisons

Adolescent rates of death from natural causes are similar in the United States, France, Netherlands, England, Wales, Sweden, Canada, Japan, and Australia (3). However, adolescent rates of death from injuries and violence are significantly higher in the United States than in these other countries. For example, suicide and homicide rates among youths aged 15–19 years are higher in the United States than in most other industrialized countries. Excess homicide among adolescents is particularly striking. In 1985, 1,579 homicides among adolescents aged 15–19 years were reported in the United States, compared with 159 homicides among adolescents in the same age-group in the Federal Republic of Germany, France, England, Wales, Sweden, Canada, and Japan combined—even though the combined population of these countries is 1.4 times that of the United States (3).

HISTORY OF DATA COLLECTION

The history of injury surveillance systems and data gathering is similar for all childhood and adolescent age-groups. For a summary of this historical perspective, see the Injury and Child Abuse chapter.

CDC SURVEILLANCE ACTIVITIES

CDC's injury surveillance activities are described in detail in the Injury and Child Abuse chapter. Details about the Youth Risk Behavioral Surveillance System can be found in the Youth Risk Behavior chapter.

GENERAL FINDINGS

Unintentional Injuries

The magnitude of unintentional injuries dwarfs all other causes of death among adolescents. Unintentional injuries alone account for more fatalities among youths aged 10–19 years than the next nine leading causes of death combined (Table 1).

For adolescents and young adults, motor vehicle crashes are the leading cause of injury fatalities, accounting for >40% of injury deaths among those 10–24 years of age (Table 2). For young adolescents 10–14 years of age, motor vehicle-related fatalities occur principally among vehicle passengers (42%) and pedestrians (22%). Bicycle-related fatalities among young adolescents (149 in 1990) often involve motor vehicles. From 1979 through 1988, motor vehicle-related death rates for youths aged 10–24 years declined 15.5%, with the greatest decreases occurring among those aged 15–19 years (16.6%) and 20–24 years (15.0%) (4).

Alcohol use increases the risk for a motor vehicle crash for all drivers, but for young drivers the risk begins to increase at very low blood alcohol concentrations (5). Data from the Fatal Accident Reporting System of the National Highway Traffic Safety Administration show that the proportion of alcohol-related traffic fatalities among young persons 15–24 years old decreased from 1982 to 1989. Reductions in the proportion of these deaths were greater for persons aged 15–17 years (31%) and 18–20 years (22%) than for those aged 21–24 years (7%) and ≥25 years (11%) (5).

Data from the 1990 Youth Risk Behavior Survey demonstrated that we could expect even greater reductions in motor vehicle-related fatalities if more adolescents adopted known preventive measures (6). In the survey, less than one fourth (24.3%) of students in grades 9–12 reported "always" using safety belts when riding in a car or truck driven by someone else; 13.4% reported "never" using safety belts. Other students reported that they did not use safety belts regularly. Observational studies from 1989 in 19 cities indicate that adolescents have the lowest safety-belt use of any age-group (28.9%), even in locations with mandatory safety-belt laws (7).* Among students who rode motorcycles, 59.8% wore motorcycle helmets "always" or "most of the time." Only 2.3% of bicycle riders wore helmets "always" or "most of the time."

---

* Observers categorized subjects into age-groups (<1, 1–4, 5–12, 13–18, and >18 years) to the best of their ability by observation alone.

TABLE 2. Leading causes of injury-related deaths among youths aged 10–24 years, by age and sex — United States, 1990

| | Numbers (and rates)* of injuries | | | | | | | | |
| | 10–14 years | | | 15–19 years | | | 20–24 years | | |
	Males	Females	Total	Males	Females	Total	Males	Females	Total
All injury causes	1,736 (19.87)	792 (9.52)	2,528 (14.82)	9,884 (107.75)	2,823 (32.42)	12,707 (71.06)	13,217 (135.66)	2,850 (30.35)	16,067 (83.98)
Motor vehicle crash	665 (7.61)	424 (5.10)	1,089 (6.38)	4,172 (45.48)	1,746 (20.05)	5,918 (33.10)	5,189 (53.26)	1,500 (15.98)	6,689 (34.96)
Drivers	50 (0.57)	21 (0.25)	71 (0.42)	1,636 (17.84)	593 (6.81)	2,229 (12.47)	2,228 (22.87)	663 (7.06)	2,891 (15.11)
Passengers	208 (2.38)	254 (3.05)	462 (2.71)	1,116 (12.17)	674 (7.74)	1,790 (10.01)	935 (9.60)	431 (4.59)	1,366 (7.14)
Pedestrians	162 (1.85)	78 (0.94)	240 (1.41)	244 (2.66)	95 (1.09)	339 (1.90)	402 (4.13)	104 (1.11)	506 (2.64)
Motorcyclists	27 (0.31)	1 (0.01)	28 (0.16)	297 (3.24)	6 (0.07)	303 (1.69)	569 (5.84)	8 (0.09)	577 (3.02)
Bicyclists	131 (1.50)	18 (0.22)	149 (0.87)	113 (1.23)	11 (0.13)	124 (0.69)	58 (0.60)	7 (0.07)	65 (0.34)
Firearms	441 (5.05)	119 (1.43)	560 (3.28)	3,678 (40.10)	495 (5.68)	4,173 (23.34)	4,781 (49.07)	588 (6.26)	5,369 (28.06)
Homicide	229 (2.62)	127 (1.53)	356 (2.09)	2,571 (28.03)	471 (5.41)	3,042 (17.01)	3,651 (37.47)	661 (7.04)	4,312 (22.54)
Suicide	191 (2.19)	67 (0.81)	258 (1.51)	1,656 (18.05)	323 (3.71)	1,979 (11.07)	2,504 (25.70)	386 (4.11)	2,890 (15.11)
Drowning	207 (2.37)	53 (0.64)	260 (1.52)	439 (4.79)	39 (0.45)	478 (2.67)	393 (4.03)	37 (0.39)	430 (2.25)
Fire/burns	66 (0.76)	41 (0.49)	107 (0.63)	114 (1.24)	51 (0.59)	165 (0.92)	231 (2.37)	51 (0.54)	282 (1.47)
Poisoning	23 (0.26)	9 (0.11)	32 (0.19)	144 (1.57)	47 (0.54)	191 (1.07)	259 (2.66)	69 (0.73)	328 (1.71)
Falls	17 (0.19)	7 (0.08)	24 (0.14)	105 (1.14)	18 (0.21)	123 (0.69)	156 (1.60)	13 (0.14)	169 (0.88)

* Rates per 100,000 population; categories may not be mutually exclusive.

Sources: NCHS mortality tapes and US Bureau of the Census decennial census data for 1990.

Young persons also are overrepresented among firearm-related injuries nationwide. In 1990, firearms use was second only to motor vehicle crashes as a specific cause of death among adolescents (Table 2). From 1985 to 1990, adolescent rates of death caused by firearms use increased 18% for youths 10–14 years old and 77% for those 16–19 years old *(8)*. Of all unintentional firearm-related deaths, 30% occurred among youths aged 10–19 years *(9)*. Firearm-related death rates among young male adolescents are up to 10 times higher than for females of the same race *(8)*. Overall, adolescents living in nonmetropolitan regions were more than twice as likely to die from an unintentional gunshot wound as those living in metropolitan areas *(9)*. Specific behavioral characteristics associated with adolescence—such as impulsivity, feelings of invincibility, and curiosity about firearms—combined with easy access to firearms place adolescents at a particularly high risk for firearm-related injuries *(10)*.

Drowning rates increase among children aged 1–3 years, and a secondary rise in rates occurs among adolescents aged 15–19 years, but only among boys. Unlike drownings among toddlers and young children that are most likely to occur in swimming pools, drownings among adolescent boys occur in a wide variety of locations: rivers, lakes, canals, and oceans *(11)*. Even in states with substantial coastlines, the vast majority of adolescent drownings occur in fresh water *(11)*. Drowning rates for adolescent blacks are twice those for adolescent whites and may be related to blacks' exposure to more dangerous, unsupervised open bodies of water and lack of access to swimming skills programs, although these hypotheses are largely unexplored. Boating incidents play a larger role in drownings among adolescents when compared with younger children, and alcohol use is believed to be a major contributing factor in 40%–50% of drownings among adolescent boys (11).

Sports are the leading cause of injuries requiring medical treatment among youths aged 12–17 years (12). Each year, one child in 27 sustains a sports injury severe enough to result in hospital treatment. Almost two thirds of all sports injuries result from team contact sports such as football, basketball, or soccer. During the 6 academic years from fall 1982 to spring 1988, an average of 49 catastrophic injuries (death or severe functional disability) were reported annually among high school participants, and an average of 13 such injuries were reported annually among college participants (12). Most sports-related deaths among adolescents were not caused by trauma, but, rather, were caused by cardiac failure or heat exhaustion.

Injuries Caused by Violence

Homicide follows only unintentional injuries as a cause of death among persons 15–24 years of age (Table 1). Among black males and females aged 10–24 years, homicide ranks first as a cause of death for reasons that are not yet clear but are being explored (13). In 1990, 31% of all homicides occurred among young persons aged 10–24 years; >95% of these persons were 15 years of age or older. Unlike adolescent unintentional injury and overall fatality rates, which have been declining in recent years, adolescent homicide rates have increased. From 1984 to 1990, homicide rates increased 40.3% for youths aged 10–14 years, 72% for those aged 15–19 years, and 28.2% for those aged 20–24 years. In 1990, most adolescent homicides were related to firearms—82% among persons 15–19 years of age and 76% among persons 20-24 years of age (8). Homicide rates for black males have increased sharply. In each youth age-sex category, firearm-related homicide rates were higher for blacks than for youths of other races: eleven times higher for males aged 15–24 years, eight times higher for females

aged 10–14 years, and five times higher for males aged 10–14 years and females aged 15–24 years.

Suicide is the third leading cause of adolescent deaths, with rates increasing most profoundly among younger adolescents. From 1979 to 1988, suicide rates for young adolescents 10–14 years of age increased >75% (4). At the same time, suicide rates for youths aged 15–19 years increased 34.5%, whereas suicide rates for persons 20–24 years of age showed a slight decline (8.5%). In 1990, male:female rate ratios for adolescent suicide were 2.7 for youths aged 10–14 years, 4.9 for those aged 15–19 years, and 6.3 for those aged 20–24 years. Most suicides were related to firearms (8). Firearm-related suicide rates, unlike firearm-related homicide rates, were higher for white males than for black males aged 15–24 years, although the race differences were considerably smaller than for firearm homicides.

INTERPRETATION ISSUES

Among all age groups, adolescents and young adults are at the highest risk for traumatic head and spinal cord injuries. Despite the severe consequences of central nervous system injuries, no surveillance systems adequately monitor their effects in the United States. Many states maintain specialized registries of persons sustaining these injuries (14). Although these are potentially valuable sources of injury surveillance data, the key purpose of these systems is to identify the affected persons to allow the delivery of services. Moreover, registries may not provide ongoing population-based incidence and etiology information that is useful for public health programs. Registry data may only reflect those persons seeking treatment at a particular hospital or group of hospitals. The data characterize only a limited segment of all affected persons and do not include information on persons who receive treatment elsewhere. In addition, the data may not be comparable across states. Other states are developing population-based surveillance systems to address these issues. The following example illustrates the need for population-based surveillance systems.

During a 6-week period in 1988, eight patients with cervical spinal cord injuries received treatment at two spinal cord injury centers in Milwaukee, Wisconsin (15). During similar periods the centers reported five spinal cord injuries in 1986 and three in 1987. Seven of the injuries in 1988 occurred in natural bodies of water, and some investigators hypothesized that the increased frequency was a result of diving into bodies of water with reduced levels caused by a drought. Because no statewide data were available for Wisconsin before 1988, investigators were unable to make comparisons to previous years. After conducting a case-control study to assess this hypothesis, they concluded that the increase in reported water-related spinal cord injuries at the two centers was a reporting artifact caused by a change in referral patterns for the treatment of spinal cord injury (16). The presence of a population-based spinal cord injury surveillance system would have allowed comparisons to previous years, thus facilitating the detection of clusters of such injuries.

EXAMPLES OF USING DATA

Football-Related Spinal Cord Injuries in Louisiana

Louisiana law requires the reporting of all spinal cord injuries to the Office of Public Health of the Louisiana Department of Health and Hospitals. Four high school football players sustained cervical spinal cord injuries during the 1989 high school football season (17). All injuries resulted in quadriplegia; in three of the injuries, no motor or sensory function was preserved below the zone of injury. The injuries occurred when players were tackling or blocking with the head as a point of contact. Their heads were not, however, in the typical head-down or spearing position typically associated with spinal cord injury.

On the basis of Louisiana's experience from 1978 through 1988, one spinal cord injury would be expected during a period of <4 years. Reasons for the occurrence of the four spinal cord injuries during the 1989 high school football season in Louisiana are not known. In response to these injuries, the state produced and

distributed an instructional video, targeted to high school coaches and trainers, explaining safe tackling techniques. Other suggestions for prevention included 1) enforcing existing tackling rules; 2) educating officials, coaches, and players about the mechanisms of injury; 3) requiring proper conditioning exercises to strengthen players' necks; 4) requiring medical examinations of players before participating in football and before resuming participation after injury; and 5) increasing awareness among school administrators and coaches about the proper handling of any injured player during practice or competition.

Traumatic Head Injuries in Utah

Traumatic head injury is a reportable condition in Utah. Cases are ascertained through a statewide injury reporting system maintained by the Utah Department of Health's Bureau of Epidemiology. The system identifies cases from discharge data from all of the state's acute care hospitals and death certificates.

In 1990–1991, overall rates of traumatic head injury (fatal and nonfatal) were higher for adolescents aged 15–19 years than for persons aged 20–24 years (209.4 per 100,000 vs. 119.6). Among persons aged 15–19 years, rates for males were almost twice those for females (276.9 vs. 141.0). Among persons 20–24 years old, rates for males were almost three times those for females (181.6 vs. 59.5). Major causes of traumatic head injury were motor vehicle crashes and firearms use. The state is using these data to develop interventions based on the leading causes of traumatic head injury. The surveillance system will be useful for evaluating the effectiveness of these intervention programs.

FUTURE ISSUES

Over the coming decade, the major challenges in injury surveillance will be diverse, ranging from the modification of mechanisms used to collect data on nonfatal injuries to the development of new systems for the surveillance of childhood injuries. For details about these future challenges and the national year 2000 health objectives see the Injury and Child Abuse chapter. Of particular relevance to the prevention of adolescent injuries will be the surveillance of firearm-related injuries and traumatic head and spinal cord injuries.

Firearm-Related Injuries

As is true for other nonfatal injuries, national data are not available to adequately depict the incidence and distribution of nonfatal firearm-related injuries. Consequently, the Firearm Injury Surveillance Study is being conducted to determine the usefulness of the National Electronic Injury Surveillance System (NEISS) to obtain national estimates of the incidence, cost, and disability associated with nonfatal firearm-related injuries treated in hospital emergency departments. The U.S. Consumer Product Safety Commission (CPSC) operates NEISS and uses the data to track product-related injuries. Although the CPSC has regulatory authority for other consumer products but does not regulate firearms, it collects data on firearm injuries for CDC through an interagency agreement.

In June 1992, the CPSC began collecting data for the Firearm Injury Surveillance Study, ascertaining information on nonfatal firearm injuries in all 91 NEISS hospital emergency departments; the commission continued data collection through September 1993. The 91 NEISS hospitals represent a national probability sample drawn from approximately 6,100 U.S. hospitals that have emergency departments and are located in metropolitan, smaller urban, suburban, and rural areas.

The NEISS provides useful information on the incidence of nonfatal firearm injuries, characteristics of the persons injured, as well as morbidity and circumstances about the injury event, such as the intent of injury, the type of firearms used to inflict injuries, and victim-perpetrator relationships. Preliminary results based on NEISS data obtained in 1992 suggest that approximately 102,000 nonfatal gunshot wounds occur annually in the United States. About 25,000 of these gunshot wounds involve persons 19 years

of age and younger; this is about five times the number of fatalities that occurred in this age-group during 1990. The data also indicate that at least 35% of these children and adolescents were shot by a handgun and that at least 40% were the result of assaults.

The magnitude and severity of these nonfatal firearm injuries emphasize the need for effective prevention strategies. Of the 102,000 persons receiving gunshot wounds in 1992, 64% were transported to the emergency department by emergency medical services, and 58% were severe enough to require hospitalization. Of those hospitalized, at least 17% had primary injuries to the head and neck region. The morbidity and disability associated with these severe nonfatal injuries—especially among children and adolescents—have a tremendous effect on society in terms of human suffering, medical-care costs, and loss of productivity.

Traumatic Head and Spinal Cord Injuries

Because of the devastating effects of injuries to the central nervous system, a number of states are developing registries or surveillance systems to provide services and plan prevention programs. CDC currently receives spinal cord injury data from five states—Arkansas, Colorado, Louisiana, Mississippi, and Utah. Some states use the traditional reportable disease model, whereas others use hospital discharge data and abstract medical records to obtain more complete information. Although the purposes and methods of data collection may differ across jurisdictions, a standardized approach (i.e., case definitions and minimum data sets) would allow data comparisons among states and facilitate national surveillance.

To meet these needs, CDC's National Center for Injury Prevention and Control has worked with government agencies, professional organizations, and consumer groups to develop standard guidelines—including case definitions and a minimum data set—for the surveillance of traumatic head and spinal cord injuries. These guidelines, which are based on the CDC

National Electronic Telecommunications Surveillance System format, are being field-tested and should be finalized in 1994.

REFERENCES

1. Guyer B, Ellers B. Childhood injuries in the United States: mortality, morbidity, and cost. Am J Dis Child 1990;144:649–52.

2. Rodriguez JG, Brown ST. Childhood injuries in the United States. Am J Dis Child 1990;144:627–46.

3. Public Health Service. Childhood injuries in the United States. Atlanta: US Department of Health and Human Services, Public Health Service, Centers for Disease Control, 1990.

4. CDC. Mortality trends and leading causes of death among adolescents and young adults—United States, 1979–1988. MMWR 1993;42:459–62.

5. CDC. Alcohol-related traffic fatalities among youth and young adults—United States, 1982–1989. MMWR 1991;40:178–82.

6. CDC. Safety-belt and helmet use among high school students—United States, 1990. MMWR 1992;41:111–4.

7. National Highway Traffic Safety Administration. Restraint use in 19 US cities: 1989 annual report. Washington, DC: US Department of Transportation, National Highway Traffic Safety Administration; DOT publication no. HS-807-595.

8. Fingerhut LA. Firearm mortality among children, youth, and young adults 1–34 years of age, trends and current status: United States, 1985–1990. Hyattsville, Maryland: US Department of Health and Human Services, Public Health Service, CDC, NCHS, 1993. (Advance data from vital and health statistics; no. 231.)

9. CDC. Unintentional firearm-related fatalities among children and teenagers—United States, 1982–1988. MMWR 1992;41:442–5,451.

10. Committee on Adolescence, American Academy of Pediatrics. Firearms and adolescents. AAP News 1992;(January):20–1.

11. Wintemute GJ. Childhood drowning and near-drowning in the United States. Am J Dis Child 1990;144:663–9.

12. Baker SP, O'Neill B, Ginsburg MJ, Li G. The injury fact book. 2nd ed. New York: Oxford University Press, 1992.

13. Hammett M, Powell KE, O'Carroll PW, Clanton ST. Homicide surveillance—United States, 1979–1988. MMWR 1992;41(No. SS-3):1–33.

14. Harrison CL, Dijkers M. Spinal cord injury surveillance in the United States: an overview. Paraplegia 1991;29:233–46.

15. CDC. Diving-associated spinal cord injuries during drought conditions—Wisconsin, 1988. MMWR 1988;37:453–4.

16. Branche CM, Sniezek JE, Sattin RW, Mirkin IR. Water recreation-related spinal injuries: risk factors in natural bodies of water. Accid Anal & Prev 1991;23(1):13–7.

17. CDC. Football-related spinal cord injuries among high school players—Louisiana, 1989. MMWR 1990;39:586–7.

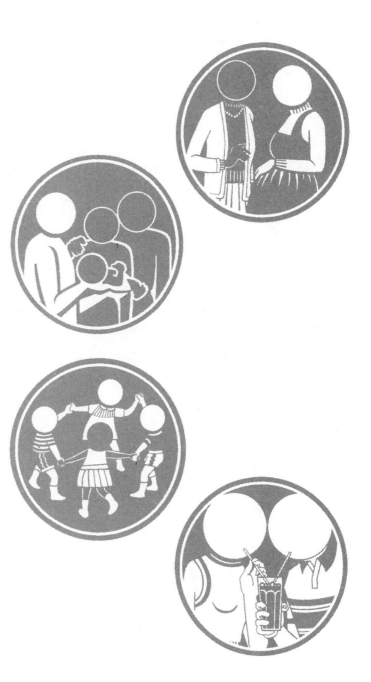

Appendix A
Contact Persons for CDC Surveillance and Data Programs in Women and Children's Health (1994)

Abortion Surveillance
Lisa M. Koonin, M.N., M.P.H.
Division of Reproductive Health
National Center for Chronic Disease Prevention
and Health Promotion
(404)488-5188

Adolescent Pregnancy
Alison M. Spitz, M.S., M.P.H.
Division of Reproductive Health
National Center for Chronic Disease Prevention
and Health Promotion
(404)488-5258

AIDS and National Surveys
Ronald W. Wilson, M.A.
Office of Analysis, Epidemiology and Health
Promotion
National Center for Health Statistics
(301)436-7032

AIDS Case Reporting
Patricia L. Fleming, Ph.D.
Division of HIV/AIDS
National Center for Infectious Diseases
(404)639-2050

Birth Defects Monitoring Program
M. Louise Martin, D.V.M.
Division of Birth Defects and Developmental
Disabilities
National Center for Environmental Health
(404)488-7176

Cesarean Section Statistics
Selma M. Taffel, B.B.A.
Division of Vital Statistics
National Center for Health Statistics
(301)436-8954

Environmental and Occupational Exposures
Diane K. Wagener, Ph.D.
Office of Analysis, Epidemiology and Health
Promotion
National Center for Health Statistics
(301)436-7032

Fetal Alcohol Syndrome
R. Louise Floyd, R.N., D.S.N.
Division of Birth Defects and Developmental
Disabilities
National Center for Environmental Health
(404)488-7370

M. Louise Martin, D.V.M.
Division of Birth Defects and Developmental
Disabilities
National Center for Environmental Health
(404)488-7176

Gonococcal Isolate Surveillance Project
Allyn K. Nakashima, M.D.
Division of Sexually Transmitted Diseases
and HIV Prevention
National Center for Prevention Services
(404)639-8356

Healthy People 2000 Objectives
Mary Anne Freedman, M.A.
Division of Health Promotion
National Center for Health Statistics
(301)436-3548

State and Local Support
Kenneth G. Keppel, Ph.D.
Division of Health Promotion
National Center for Health Statistics
(301)436-3548

Data Monitoring and Analysis
Richard J. Klein, M.P.H.
Division of Health Promotion
National Center for Health Statistics
(301)436-3548

HIV Reporting
Patricia A. Sweeney, M.P.H.
Division of HIV/AIDS
National Center for Infectious Diseases
(404)639-2050

HIV Seroprevalence Surveillance
Lyle R. Petersen, M.D., M.P.H.
Division of HIV/AIDS
National Center for Infectious Diseases
(404)639-2090

Infant Mortality
Marion F. MacDorman, Ph.D.
Division of Vital Statistics
National Center for Health Statistics
(301)436-8884

Diane L. Rowley, M.D., M.P.H.
Division of Reproductive Health
National Center for Chronic Disease Prevention
and Health Promotion
(404)488-5149

Invasive Bacterial Diseases Reporting
Katherine A. Deaver-Robinson, M.P.H.
Division of Bacterial and Mycotic Diseases
National Center for Infectious Diseases
(404)639-2215

Low Birth Weight
John L. Kiely, Ph.D.
Division of Health and Utilization Analysis
National Center for Health Statistics
(301)436-3650

Kate M. Brett, Ph.D.
Division of Epidemiology
National Center for Health Statistics
(301)436-5975

Diane L. Rowley, M.D., M.P.H.
Division of Reproductive Health
National Center for Chronic Disease Prevention
and Health Promotion
(404)488-5149

Metropolitan Atlanta Congenital Defects Program
M. Louise Martin, D.V.M.
Division of Birth Defects and Developmental
Disabilities
National Center for Environmental Health
(404)488-7176

Metropolitan Atlanta Developmental Disabilities Surveillance Program
Coleen A. Boyle, Ph.D.
Division of Birth Defects and Developmental
Disabilities
National Center for Environmental Health
(404)488-7365

Minority Health Statistics
Patricia M. Golden, B.A., M.P.H.
Office of Analysis, Epidemiology and Health
  Promotion
National Center for Health Statistics
(301)436-7032

National Bacterial Meningitis Reporting System
Jay D. Wenger, M.D.
Division of Bacterial and Mycotic Diseases
National Center for Infectious Diseases
(404)639-2215

National Childhood Lead Poisoning Prevention Program
Carol A. Pertowski, M.D.
Division of Environmental Hazards and
  Health Effects
National Center for Environmental Health
(404)488-7330

National Electronic Injury Surveillance System
J. Lee Annest, Ph.D.
Office of Statistics, Programming, and Graphics
National Center for Injury Prevention and
  Control
(404)488-4656

National Electronic Telecommunication System for Surveillance
Donna F. Stroup, Ph.D., M.Sc.
Division of Surveillance and Epidemiology
Epidemiology Program Office
(404)639-0080

National Health and Nutrition Examination Surveys
Susan S. Eslami, Ph.D.
Division of Health Examination Statistics
National Center for Health Statistics
(301)436-7075

NHANES I Epidemiologic Follow-up Study
  Christine S. Cox, M.A.
  Division of Epidemiology
  National Center for Health Statistics
  (301)436-5975

National Health Interview Survey
Gerry E. Hendershot, Ph.D.
Division of Health Interview Statistics
National Center for Health Statistics
(301)436-7085

National Hospital Discharge Survey
Maria F. Owings, Ph.D.
Division of Health Care Statistics
National Center for Health Statistics
(301)436-7125

National Maternal and Infant Health Survey
James A. Weed, Ph.D.
Division of Vital Statistics
National Center for Health Statistics
(301)436-8951

Analytic Issues
  Kenneth C. Schoendorf, M.D., M.P.H.
  Division of Health and Utilization Analysis
  National Center for Health Statistics
  (301)436-3650

Longitudinal Follow-up
  Michael D. Kogan, Ph.D., M.A.
  Division of Vital Statistics
  National Center for Health Statistics
  (301)436-7464

National Notifiable Diseases Surveillance System
Donna F. Stroup, Ph.D., M.Sc.
Division of Surveillance and Epidemiology
Epidemiology Program Office
(404)639-0080

National Survey of Family Growth
Adolescent Pregnancy
  Jacqueline B. Wilson, M.P.H.
  Division of Vital Statistics
  National Center for Health Statistics
  (301)436-8731

Contraception
  Linda S. Peterson, M.A.
  Division of Vital Statistics
  National Center for Health Statistics
  (301)436-8731

Infertility
  Anjani Chandra, Ph.D.
  Division of Vital Statistics
  National Center for Health Statistics
  (301)436-8731

Unintended Pregnancy
  Linda J. Piccinino, M.P.S.
  Division of Vital Statistics
  National Center for Health Statistics
  (301)436-8731

Obstetric Service Areas
Diane M. Makuc, Dr.P.H.
Division of Health and Utilization Analysis
National Center for Health Statistics
(301)436-7035

Pediatric Nutrition Surveillance System
Ibrahim Parvanta, M.S.
Division of Nutrition
National Center for Chronic Disease Prevention
  and Health Promotion
(404)488-4867

Paralytic Poliomyelitis Surveillance System
Hector Izurieta, M.D.
National Immunization Program
(404)639-8255

Pregnancy Nutrition Surveillance System
Linda D. Clark, M.P.H., R.D.
Division of Nutrition
National Center for Chronic Disease Prevention
  and Health Promotion
(404)488-4867

Pregnancy Risk Assessment Monitoring System
Eileen P. Gunter, R.N., M.P.H.
Division of Reproductive Health
National Center for Chronic Disease Prevention
  and Health Promotion
(404)488-5227

Pregnancy Morbidity and Mortality
Hani K. Atrash, M.D., M.P.H.
Division of Reproductive Health
National Center for Chronic Disease Prevention
  and Health Promotion
(404)488-5186

Pregnancy Morbidity and Mortality — continued
Cynthia J. Berg, M.D.
Division of Reproductive Health
National Center for Chronic Disease Prevention
  and Health Promotion
(404)488-5146

Lisa M. Koonin, R.N., M.P.H.
Division of Reproductive Health
National Center for Chronic Disease Prevention
  and Health Promotion
(404)488-5188

Prenatal Care
John L. Kiely, Ph.D.
Division of Health and Utilization Analysis
National Center for Health Statistics
(301)436-3650

Preterm Birth
Cheryl A. Blackmore, Ph.D., M.P.H., M.S.N.
Division of Reproductive Health
National Center for Chronic Disease Prevention
  and Health Promotion
(404)488-5141

Diane L. Rowley, M.D., M.P.H.
Division of Reproductive Health
National Center for Chronic Disease Prevention
  and Health Promotion
(404)488-5149

John L. Kiely, Ph.D.
Division of Health and Utilization Analysis
National Center for Health Statistics
(301)436-3650

Sexually Transmitted Diseases Surveillance
Allyn K. Nakashima, M.D.
Division of Sexually Transmitted Diseases
  and HIV Prevention
National Center for Prevention Services
(404)639-8356

Vaccination Coverage Surveillance
Elizabeth R. Zell, M.Stat.
National Immunization Program
(404)639-8235

Vaccine-Preventable Diseases
Diphtheria
  Iain R. Hardy, M.D.
  National Immunization Program
  (404)639-8255

Haemophilus influenzae Type B
  Jay D. Wenger, M.D.
  Division of Bacterial and Mycotic Diseases
  National Center for Infectious Diseases
  (404)639-2215

Hepatitis B
  Patrick J. Coleman, Ph.D.
  Division of Viral and Rickettsial Diseases
  National Center for Infectious Diseases
  (404)639-3048

Measles
  William L. Atkinson, M.D.
  National Immunization Program
  (404)639-8230

Mumps
  Sandra J. Holmes, Ph.D.
  National Immunization Program
  (404)639-8247

Pertussis
  Iain R. Hardy, M.D.
  National Immunization Program
  (404)639-8255

Rubella and Congenital Rubella Syndrome
  Sandra J. Holmes, Ph.D.
  National Immunization Program
  (404)639-8247

Tetanus
  Hector Izurieta, M.D.
  National Immunization Program
  (404)639-8255

Vital Statistics
Birth Certificates
  Robert L. Heuser, M.A.
  Division of Vital Statistics
  National Center for Health Statistics
  (301)436-8954

Death Certificates
  Harry M. Rosenberg, Ph.D.
  Division of Vital Statistics
  National Center for Health Statistics
  (301)436-8884

Deaths in Childhood and Adolescence
  Lois A. Fingerhut, M.A.
  Office of Analysis, Epidemiology and
    Health Promotion
  National Center for Health Statistics
  (301)436-7026

Fetal Death Reports
  Donna L. Hoyert, Ph.D.
  Division of Vital Statistics
  National Center for Health Statistics
  (301)436-8884

Injury Deaths
  Lois A. Fingerhut, M.A.
  Office of Analysis, Epidemiology and
    Health Promotion
  National Center for Health Statistics
  (301)436-7026

Linked Birth-Death Files
  Marian F. MacDorman, Ph.D.
  Division of Vital Statistics
  National Center for Health Statistics
  (301)436-8884

Women's Health
Julie Dawson Weeks, M.A.
Division of Epidemiology
National Center for Health Statistics
(301)436-5979

Youth Risk Behavior Surveillance System
Laura Kann, Ph.D.
Division of Adolescent and School Health
National Center for Chronic Disease Prevention
  and Health Promotion
(404)488-5330

Appendix B
CDC Surveillance Programs

Public Health Topics	Abortion Surveillance	AIDS Case Reporting	Birth Certificate	BDMP	Death Certificate	Fetal Death Reports	GISP	HIV Reporting	HIV Seroprevalence Surveillance	Invasive Bacterial Disease Reporting	Lead Poisoning	Linked Birth/ Infant Death File	MACDP
Abortion	X												
Adolescent Pregnancy	X		X			X						X	
Adolescent Injury					X								
Birth Defects			X	X									X
Childhood Infections										X			
Childhood Injury and Abuse					X							X	
Contraception													
Developmental Disabilities													
Fetal Alcohol Syndrome			X	X								X	X
Fetal Death						X							
HIV Infection (Women and Children)		X						X	X				
Infant Mortality					X							X	
Infertility													
Lead Poisoning											X		
Low Birth Weight			X									X	
Pediatric Nutrition													
Periconceptional Behaviors (Women)			X			X							
Pregnancy Morbidity			X			X							
Pregnancy Mortality					X								
Pregnancy Nutrition													
Prenatal Care			X			X						X	
Preterm Birth			X									X	
Sexually Transmitted Diseases							X						
Unintended Pregnancy or Birth	X												
Vaccination Coverage (Children)													
Vaccine- Preventable Diseases													
Youth Risk Behavior													

See Glossary for definition of abbreviations.

MADDSP	NBMRS	NEISS	NETSS	NHANES	NHDS	NIHS	NMIHS	NNDSS	NSFG	PedNSS	PNSS	PRAMS	Pregnancy Mortality Surveillance	STD Surveillance	YRBSS
									X						
							X		X						
		X			X	X									
							X								
	X		X			X	X								
		X			X	X	X								
									X						
X						X	X								
					X										
							X								
							X								
									X						
			X		X	X									
						X	X		X	X	X				
			X				X			X					
							X				X	X			
					X		X				X	X			
					X								X		
							X				X				
						X	X		X		X	X			
							X					X			
														X	
							X		X			X			
					X										
								X							
					X				X		X	X			X

Appendix C
Organizational Location of Authors and
Contact Persons Included in Monograph

CENTERS FOR DISEASE CONTROL AND PREVENTION
OFFICE OF THE DIRECTOR

Epidemiology Program Office

National Immunization Program

National Center for Chronic Disease Prevention and Health Promotion

      Division of Adolescent and School Health

      Division of Nutrition

      Division of Reproductive Health

National Center for Environmental Health

      Division of Birth Defects and Developmental Disabilities

      Division of Environmental Hazards and Health Effects

National Center for Health Statistics

      Office of Analysis, Epidemiology and Health Promotion

          Division of Epidemiology

          Division of Health and Utilization Analysis

          Division of Health Promotion

      Office of Vital and Health Statistics Systems

          Division of Health Examination Statistics

          Division of Health Interview Statistics

          Division of Vital Statistics

National Center for Infectious Diseases

      Division of Bacterial and Mycotic Diseases

      Division of HIV/AIDS

      Division of Viral and Rickettsial Diseases

      Hospital Infections Program

National Center for Injury Prevention and Control

      Division of Acute Care, Rehabilitation Research, and Disability Prevention

      Division of Unintentional Injury Prevention

      Office of Statistics, Programming, and Graphics

National Center for Prevention Services

      Division of Sexually Transmitted Diseases and HIV Prevention

This list includes the organizational location of authors and contact persons listed in this monograph. It does not include all programs of the Centers for Disease Control and Prevention.

Appendix D
Glossary

ACOG. American College of Obstetricians and Gynecologists.

AGI. Alan Guttmacher Institute.

AIDS. Acquired immunodeficiency syndrome.

antepartum fetal death. Fetal death occurring before the initiation of labor.

Audio-CASI. Audio computer-assisted self-interviewing.

birth cohort prevalence rate. In developmental disabilities surveillance, the prevalence of a specific disorder in a geographic area, among children of a specific age who were born in that geographic area, within a specified time interval.

birth defect. A structural abnormality present at birth.

birth weight-specific mortality. The number of infant deaths that occurred among live births in a specific birth weight category in a calendar year, divided by the total number of live births that occurred in that category in that year, multiplied by 1,000.

BDMP. Birth Defects Monitoring Program.

BMI. Body mass index, expressed as kilograms of body mass per height in meters squared ($kg1m^2$).

CAPI. Computer-assisted personal interviewing.

case ascertainment. Identification of cases of an exposure or health outcome in public health surveillance, usually according to a specific case definition.

CATI. Computer-assisted telephone interviewing.

cause-of-death. As defined by the World Health Organization, the underlying cause of death, indicated on the death certificate, and defined as a) the disease or injury which initiated the train of morbid events leading directly to death, or b) the circumstances of the accident or violence which produced the fatal injury.

CI. Confidence interval; a range of values for a variable of interest, constructed so that this range has a specified probability of including the true value of the variable (1).

CNS. Central nervous system.

cohort infant mortality rate. The number of infant deaths that occurred among live births in a calendar year, divided by the total number of live births that year, multiplied by 1,000.

contraceptive failure rate. The average probability of having an unintended pregnancy in a year of using a specific contraceptive method.

coverage survey. In population vaccination assessment, a survey using population-based sampling techniques to identify vaccination coverage in a specific target population.

CSTE. Council of State and Territorial Epidemiologists.

current mortality sample. A 10% systematic sample of death certificates filed in state vital records offices and coded by the National Center for Health Statistics.

developmental disability. One of a group of heterogeneous conditions that 1) are attributable to mental and/or physical impairments, 2) are manifested before the person reaches 22 years of age, 3) are likely to continue indefinitely, 4) result in substantial functional limitations in three or more areas of self-care, and 5) reflect the need for specialized services.

DTP. Diphtheria-tetanus-pertussis vaccine.

E-codes. The current standard of coding external causes of injury for nonfatal cases, from the ICD-9-CM Supplemental Classification of External Causes of Injury and Poisoning.

EPSDT. Early and Periodic Screening, Diagnosis, and Treatment.

FAE. Fetal alcohol effects.

FAS. Fetal alcohol syndrome.

fetal death. As defined by the World Health Organization; "death prior to the complete expulsion or extraction from its mother of a product of conception, irrespective of the duration of pregnancy. The death is indicated by the fact that after such separation, the fetus does not breathe or show any other evidence of life such as beating of the heart, pulsation of the umbilical cord, or definite movement of voluntary muscles." This definition includes stillbirths, spontaneous abortions, and miscarriages as fetal deaths.

fetal mortality rate. The number of fetal deaths divided by the sum of the number of live births plus the number of fetal deaths in a specified time period, multiplied by 1,000.

fetal mortality ratio. The ratio of the number of fetal deaths to live births in a specified period, multiplied by 1,000.

final data. Complete data from vital records (such as birth and death certificates and fetal death reports) that have been reviewed by the National Center for Health Statistics for validity and consistency; available about 2 years after the close of a data year.

gestational weight gain. Maternal weight gain during pregnancy.

GISP. Gonococcal Isolate Surveillance Project.

Healthy People 2000. An extensive description of health goals for the U.S. population in the year 2000, identified by the Public Health Service.

height-for-age. Pediatric measurement of a child's height at a specified age, allows for the comparison of a child's height to the reference population of the same age and sex.

HIV. Human immunodeficiency virus.

ICD-9. International Statistical Classification of Diseases, Injuries, and Causes of Death, 9th revision (published by the World Health Organization). This classification system is used primarily for mortality coding.

ICD-9-CM. International Classification of Diseases, 9th revision, Clinical Modification (published by the Health Care Financing Administration, U.S. Public Health Service). This classification system is used primarily for morbidity coding.

impaired fecundity. In the National Survey of Family Growth, the status of a woman who is either part of an infertile couple or who reports that it is physically difficult or impossible to conceive or deliver a baby or who has been told by a physician that pregnancy would pose a danger to her or the baby.

incidence. The number of new events occurring during a specified period (1).

infant mortality. The death of a live-born infant before its first birthday.

infertile. The status of a married couple who is not surgically sterilized, has not used contraception, and has not become pregnant for at least 12 months.

intentional injury. An injury arising from purposeful action, such as interpersonal or self-directed violence.

intrapartum fetal death. Fetal death occurring after the initiation of labor and before delivery.

IUD. Intrauterine device.

IUGR. Intrauterine growth retardation: in epidemiologic surveillance, IUGR is most commonly defined as intrauterine fetal growth below the 10th percentile for gestational age, or gestational age of ≥37 weeks and birth weight of <2,500 g.

Kessner index. A classification of prenatal care developed by the Institute of Medicine in 1973 that adjusts the timing and quantity of prenatal care for the length of gestation to determine levels of adequate, inadequate, and intermediate prenatal care. David Kessner was the first author of the Institute of Medicine report.

LBW. Low birth weight; birth weight <2,500 g.

lead poisoning case. In CDC surveillance, a lead poisoning case is defined in children by a venous sample containing 10 micrograms or more per deciliter of serum lead or two capillary samples taken within 12 weeks of each other, both containing this level.

legal induced abortion. An abortion conducted by a licensed health provider under conditions consistent with the legal requirements of the state.

LMP. Last menstrual period.

MACDP. Metropolitan Atlanta Congenital Defects Program.

MADDSP. Metropolitan Atlanta Developmental Disabilities Surveillance Program.

mistimed pregnancy. According to questions included in the National Survey of Family Growth, a pregnancy that was intended but occurred sooner than the mother would have liked.

MLBW. Moderately low birth weight; birth weight ≥1,500 grams and <2,500 g.

MMWR. Morbidity and Mortality Weekly Report.

NAS. National Academy of Science.

NBMRS. National Bacterial Meningitis Reporting System.

NEISS. National Electronic Injury Surveillance System.

neonatal death. Death of a live-born infant from birth to <28 days of life.

net pregnancy weight gain. Total weight gain of the mother during pregnancy after the birth weight of the infant is subtracted.

NETSS. National Electronic Telecommunications System for Surveillance.

NHANES (I, II, III). National Health and Nutrition Examination Surveys.

NHDS. National Hospital Discharge Survey.

NHIS. National Health Interview Survey.

NLSY. National Longitudinal Survey of Youth.

NMIHS. National Maternal and Infant Health Survey.

NNDSS. National Notifiable Diseases Surveillance System.

NNS. National Natality Survey.

NSFG. National Survey of Family Growth.

NTD. Neural tube defect.

nulligravida. A woman who has never been pregnant.

OCs.   Oral contraceptives.

PedNSS.   Pediatric Nutrition Surveillance System.

periconceptional.   Occurring around the time of conception.

period infant mortality rates.   The number of infant deaths occurring in a calendar year per the number of live births occurring during the same period, multiplied by 1,000.

PID.   Pelvic inflammatory disease.

PNSS.   Pregnancy Nutrition Surveillance System.

point prevalence rate.   In developmental disabilities surveillance, the prevalence of a specific disorder among all children of a specific age in a geographic area, regardless of where the children were born.

postneonatal death.   Death of a live-born infant after 28 days of life and before its first birthday.

PRAMS.   Pregnancy Risk Assessment Monitoring System.

pregnancy-associated mortality.   The death of a woman from any cause while pregnant or within one calendar year of termination of pregnancy, regardless of the duration and site of pregnancy.

pregnancy mortality rate.   The number of pregnancy-related deaths per 100,000 pregnancies.

pregnancy mortality ratio.   The number of pregnancy-related deaths per 100,000 live births.

pregnancy-related mortality.   A pregnancy-associated death resulting from 1) complications of the pregnancy itself; 2) the chain of events initiated by the pregnancy that led to death; or 3) aggravation of an unrelated condition by the physiologic or pharmacologic effects of the pregnancy that subsequently caused death.

preterm delivery.   Termination of pregnancy before the 37th completed week of gestation.

prevalence.   The number of cases of a condition in a specified population at a designated time (1).

primary infertility.   The status of an infertile couple who has not previously conceived.

provisional data.   Limited, early data from filed death certificates; provisional data on infant mortality are provided by the National Center for Health Statistics 3-4 months after the death certificates are filed in the states and include estimates of the number of infant deaths and selected causes of death.

rate ratio.   The ratio of two rates, expressed in epidemiology as the ratio of the rate of a health outcome in an exposed population to the rate in the unexposed population (1).

RDS.   Respiratory distress syndrome.

registry.   A system of ongoing registration of cases of a specific disease or health-relevant condition in a defined population (1).

relative risk.   The ratio of the risk of disease in the exposed population to the risk in an unexposed population (see rate ratio).

RR.   Relative risk or relative ratio.

secondary infertility.   The status of an infertile couple who has had one or more previous conceptions.

seroprevalence.   The prevalence of HIV in anonymous surveys of blood serum from selected populations such as child-bearing women, patients of sentinel hospitals, and clients of clinics treating sexually transmitted diseases, tuberculosis, and substance abuse.

SES.   Socioeconomic status.

SIDS.   Sudden infant death syndrome.

spontaneous abortion.   Spontaneous death prior to the complete expulsion or extraction from its mother of a product of conception. In some surveillance systems, this term indicates such deaths at gestational age less than 20 weeks.

STD.   Sexually transmitted diseases.

STELLAR.   System for Tracking Elevated Lead Levels and Remediation (a software program).

stillbirth.   Death prior to the complete expulsion or extraction from its mother of a product of conception. In some surveillance systems, this term indicates such deaths at gestational age of 20 weeks or more.

teratogen.   An exposure that causes birth defects.

TSS.   Toxic shock syndrome.

unintentional injury.   Injury arising from unintentional events.

unintended pregnancy.   According to questions included in the National Survey of Family Growth, a pregnancy identified as either unwanted or mistimed.

unwanted pregnancy.   According to questions included in the National Survey of Family Growth, a pregnancy occurring when the mother reported that she did not want a child at the time of conception or any time in the future.

VBAC.   Vaginal birth after cesarean section.

VLBW.   Very low birth weight; birth weight <1,500 g.

weight-for-height.   Pediatric measurement of weight for height, adjusts a child's weight relative to his or her height and thus is a measurement of body mass.

WHO.   World Health Organization.

WIC.   Special Supplemental Food Program for Women, Infants, and Children.

YRBSS.   Youth Risk Behavior Surveillance System.

References

1.   Last JM. A dictionary of epidemiology. 2nd edition. New York: Oxford University Press, 1988.

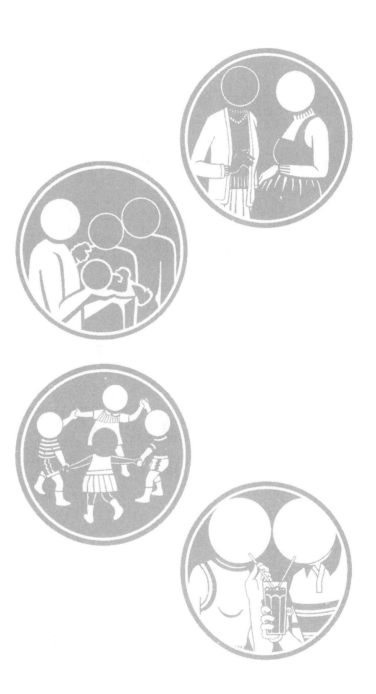

Index

G

H

I

S

sentinel surveillance   5, 16, 18, 47

seroprevalence   16, 18, 50, 53, 55, 58, 60

services, health

    adolescent   355

    child   293

    developmental disability   341

    family planning   iii, 25, 26, 29, 32, 33, 73, 83

    infant   9, 246

    infertility   63, 66, 69

    maternal   189, 246

    tracking use of   14

screening   53

sexually transmitted diseases (see also names of specific diseases)   iii, 7, 11, 16, 29, 39–61, 64, 359, 369, 377

    incidence   39, 359

    racial and ethnic differences   11, 359

    surveillance   11, 16, 359

SIDS   238, 271

smoking

    among adolescents   vi, 359, 362

    and low birth weight   93, 96, 105, 113, 185, 191, 196, 197

    association with infertility   67, 68, 70

    during pregnancy   vi, 76, 93–96, 105, 113, 185, 191, 196, 197

Social Security   10

socioeconomic status   v, 9, 11, 14, 25, 35, 67, 77, 87, 105, 108, 119, 191, 231, 321, 369

South Carolina   89, 94, 107, 161, 220, 251, 258–260

South Dakota   87, 89, 220, 298

Special Supplemental Food Program for Women, Infants, and Children (WIC)   15, 16, 121, 122, 126, 127, 162, 237, 252, 315, 323

spina bifida   211, 217

state health departments   15, 130

state-specific surveillance   15, 130

sterilization   29, 32, 69

stillbirth   39, 79, 141, 164

sudden infant death syndrome (SIDS)   238, 271

suicide   359, 362, 381, 382, 385

surveillance, public health (see also names of specific surveillance programs)   iii, vi, 7, 12, 14, 15, 18, 29, 47, 142, 217–229, 267, 355

    CDC's definition of   12

    convenience sample   7, 29

    disease-reporting   7, 16, 29

    feasibility issues related to   7, 29

    history of   29

    measurement issues related to   29

    race and ethnicity reporting   14, 29, 97, 243

    registries   16, 29, 293, 297, 298

    sentinel   16, 18, 47, 278

survey (see also names of specific surveys)

    coverage   17, 292

    cross-sectional   17, 93

    hospital discharge-based   5, 14, 16, 17, 131, 132, 203, 267, 305

    limitations   17

    mail   132

    methods   18

    population-based   5, 15, 16, 18

    response rates   18

    school-based   18, 361

syphilis

    congenital   39, 40, 43, 46

    primary   39, 42

    secondary   39, 42

System for Tracking Elevated Lead Levels and Remediation (STELLAR)   314

T

teen pregnancy   v, 5, 12, 26, 83, 108, 359, 369–379

Tennessee   15, 90, 115, 181, 192, 220

Ten-State Nutrition Survey   11, 322

tetanus   11, 282, 285, 286

Texas   35, 87, 90, 96, 220

time trends in health outcomes   163

toxic shock syndrome (TSS)   272

U

unintended pregnancy   iii, v, vi, 5, 11, 25, 73–83, 369

unintentional injury

    among children   299–310

    among adolescents   362, 381–388

United States Immunization Survey   291

U.S. Virgin Islands   179

Utah   35, 90, 220, 386

V

vaccination
coverage among children   iii, v, 7, 9, 11, 12, 14, 267, 271, 278, 281, 291–298
surveillance   267, 292–294, 296

Vaccine Assistance Act   11

vaccine-preventable diseases (see also names of specific diseases)   iii, 267, 281–291
surveillance   282–285, 287–288

varicella   282, 283

Vermont   90, 220

very low birth weight (VLBW)   119, 185, 188, 254

violence
toward adolescents   v, 11, 381–388
toward children   11, 299–310

Virginia   90, 220

vision impairment   335, 337, 340

vital statistics
analysis   15
collection   15, 25, 141
systems   5, 93, 151, 164, 232, 233

W

Washington   90, 94, 107, 131, 220, 348

weight-for-height   325, 327

weight gain during pregnancy   93–95, 119, 121, 194, 195, 369

well-baby programs   9

West Virginia   90, 94, 97, 100, 102, 107, 220, 223, 260

WIC   15, 16, 121, 122, 126, 127, 162, 237, 252, 315, 323

Wisconsin   46, 90, 220, 386

World Health Organization (WHO)   15, 64, 130, 142, 163, 179, 185, 233

Wyoming   87, 90, 220

Y

year 2000 objectives   3, 12, 27, 36, 64, 103, 119, 141, 198, 199, 225, 246, 288, 291, 298, 318, 321, 322, 331, 341, 344, 349, 357, 365, 375

youth risk behavior   5, 16, 35, 359–367, 370

Youth Risk Behavior Surveillance System (YRBSS)   5, 16, 35, 359–364, 370